Oncological Medicine: Beyond the Basics

Oncological Medicine: Beyond the Basics

Editor: Maria Walters

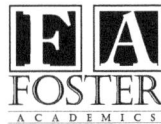

FA

FOSTER
ACADEMICS

www.fosteracademics.com

www.fosteracademics.com

FA
FOSTER
ACADEMICS

Cataloging-in-Publication Data

Oncological medicine : beyond the basics / edited by Maria Walters.
    p. cm.
Includes bibliographical references and index.
ISBN 978-1-63242-736-6
1. Oncology. 2. Cancer. 3. Cancer--Treatment. 4. Tumors. I. Walters, Maria.
RC256 .O53 2019
616.994--dc23

Foster Academics,
118-35 Queens Blvd., Suite 400,
Forest Hills, NY 11375, USA

ISBN 978-1-63242-736-6 (Hardback)

Contents

Preface

This book has been an outcome of determined endeavour from a group of educationists in the field. The primary objective was to involve a broad spectrum of professionals from diverse cultural background involved in the field for developing new researches. The book not only targets students but also scholars pursuing higher research for further enhancement of the theoretical and practical applications of the subject.

Oncology is a branch of medicine that is concerned with the diagnosis, treatment and prevention of cancer. An important domain within oncology is medical oncology, which is a modality of cancer treatment that involves hormonal therapy, targeted therapy, chemotherapy and immunotherapy. Chemotherapy uses drugs to kill cancer cells by stopping or slowing down their growth. It can however harm healthy cells of the body thereby resulting in many side-effects. It can be of two types- neoadjuvant and adjuvant chemotherapies. Immunotherapy is a unique technique in cancer care that activates the immune cells of the body to fight against cancer cells. This is done using vaccines, drug therapy and dendritic cell therapy. Targeted therapy targets specific genes and proteins associated with cancer growth, while hormone therapy slows down the growth of the cancer by reducing or blocking the hormones essential to its growth. This book explores all the important aspects of oncological medicine in the present day scenario. Different approaches, evaluations, methodologies and advanced studies on oncological medicine have been included herein. The extensive content of this book provides the readers with a thorough understanding of the recent advances in this domain.

It was an honour to edit such a profound book and also a challenging task to compile and examine all the relevant data for accuracy and originality. I wish to acknowledge the efforts of the contributors for submitting such brilliant and diverse chapters in the field and for endlessly working for the completion of the book. Last, but not the least; I thank my family for being a constant source of support in all my research endeavours.

Editor

Metastasis of Gastric Signet-Ring Cell Carcinoma to the Urinary Bladder: A Case Report and Review of the Literature

Kerem Okutur,[1] **Orhan Onder Eren,**[2] **and Gokhan Demir**[1]

[1]*Department of Medical Oncology, Acibadem University School of Medicine, Buyukdere Cad, No. 40, Sariyer, 34453 Istanbul, Turkey*
[2]*Department of Medical Oncology, Yeditepe University School of Medicine, Devlet Yolu, Ankara Caddesi, No. 102-104, Kozyatagi, 34652 Istanbul, Turkey*

Correspondence should be addressed to Kerem Okutur; keremokutur@gmail.com

Academic Editor: Jose I. Mayordomo

Although signet-ring cell (SRC) adenocarcinoma is commonly seen in the stomach, it is a very rarely seen histologic entity in the bladder. It is difficult to distinguish primary SRC adenocarcinoma of the bladder from bladder metastasis of SRC carcinoma of the stomach only based on histological findings. In such cases, clinical findings and immunohistochemical studies may be helpful. We present here a 48-year-old male patient presenting with hematuria and abdominal pain. Computerised tomography of the patient revealed a gastric mass, peritoneal involvement, and thickening of the bladder wall, and histopathological analysis revealed SRC adenocarcinoma in both of the endoscopic biopsies taken from the stomach and bladder. Immunohistochemical analyses confirmed the diagnosis of SRC adenocarcinoma of the bladder secondary to gastric cancer.

1. Introduction

Ninety-five percent of primary bladder tumors have transitional cell carcinoma histology. Adenocarcinomas of the bladder constitute only 1% of all bladder tumors and usually emerge as a result of metastatic involvement of the bladder. Metastatic bladder tumors are responsible for less than 2% of all bladder tumors and originate most commonly from melanoma, breast cancer, and gastric cancer. Curative surgery is the gold standard in the treatment of primary bladder adenocarcinomas; on the other hand, secondary bladder adenocarcinomas have no chance of cure and chemotherapy or radiotherapy is administered for palliative purposes [1].

Signet-ring cell (SRC) carcinoma is a subtype of mucin producing adenocarcinomas. Ninety percent of SRC tumors arise from stomach, colon, and breast. SRC form is associated with aggressive clinical course and early metastatic disease particularly in tumors of gastrointestinal origin [2, 3]. In bladder tumors, SRC histologic type is very rare. When SRC carcinoma histology is encountered in the bladder of a patient, primary SRC carcinoma of the bladder and bladder metastasis of a malignancy of gastrointestinal system origin

are primarily included in the differential diagnosis [4]. It is important to distinguish these two conditions because their treatment and prognosis are different. It is however difficult to differentiate between primary and secondary SRC carcinomas of the bladder both clinically and histologically.

We present here a case presenting with urinary system symptoms and found to have bladder metastasis secondary to SRC of the stomach.

2. Case Report

48-year-old male patient presented to the urology clinic with complaints of gross hematuria and abdominal pain of duration of a few weeks. In addition, he also described loss of appetite, weight loss, and fatigue. His ECOG performance status was 1. Physical examination revealed mild abdominal distention and tenderness in the hypogastric region with deep palpation; there was no defence or rebound. Laboratory workup was as follows: hemoglobin 10.5 g/dL, creatinine 1.0 mg/dL, carcinoma antigen (CA) 19.9 168 mg/dL, and carcinoembryonic antigen (CEA) 9.2 mg/dL. Abdominal tomography revealed a malignant tumoral mass in gastric corpus,

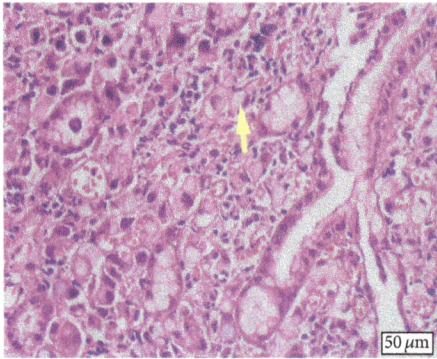

FIGURE 1: Primary signet-ring cell (arrow) carcinoma of the stomach (H&E, ×20).

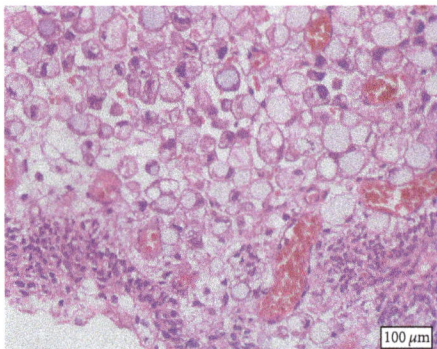

FIGURE 2: Signet-ring cell carcinoma infiltrating bladder subepithelium (H&E, ×20).

peritoneal involvement and ascites, multiple abdominal lymphadenopathies, bilateral grade 1 hydronephrosis, and diffuse thickening of the bladder wall. Endoscopy of the upper gastrointestinal system revealed an infiltrating mass of malignant appearance in the gastric corpus. Pathologic examination of endoscopic biopsy material taken from the mass was consistent with SRC carcinoma (Figure 1). In immunohistochemical analyses, cell blocks obtained from mass biopsy and ascites fluid stained positive for CEA and cytokeratin 7 (CK7) and negative for cytokeratin 20 (CK20); in addition, there was focal staining with mucicarmine (MUC). All these findings were suggestive of a gastric primary carcinoma. Papillary-nodular lesions diffusely covering the bladder wall were noted in cystoscopy. Transurethral biopsy was consistent with glandular differentiation and intact urothelial epithelium with SRC carcinoma infiltrating the subepithelium (Figure 2). In immunohistochemical analyses, CEA and CK7 were positive and CK20 was negative, similar to the biopsy taken from the stomach. The patient was started on systemic chemotherapy consisting of docetaxel, cisplatin, and 5-fluorouracil (modified DCF) with the diagnosis of metastatic gastric cancer. A partial response was noted in the radiologic imaging performed after the second cycle. The patient whose hydronephrosis regressed and hematuria did not recur is in the seventh month of his diagnosis and his clinical status is stable.

3. Discussion

Most of the information about metastatic tumors of the bladder is derived from autopsy series. When the primary tumor is prostate, colon, rectum, or cervix, bladder is involved with direct extension; on the other hand, in melanomas and breast and gastric cancers, bladder metastases occur as a result of lymphatic/hematogenous spread or peritoneal dissemination [5]. In a series of 282 patients including secondary tumors of the bladder, the tumors most commonly causing bladder involvement with direct extension were colon (21%), prostate (19%), rectum (12%), and cervix (11%) [6]. However, when tumors involving the bladder with metastatic spread are investigated, gastric cancer is the leading cause (4.3%) followed by melanoma (3.9%), lung (2.8%), and breast (2.5%) cancer. In this series, SRC histology is present in only 3 of 12 reported cases of gastric cancer. In our case, the presence of ascites of malignant nature and intra-abdominal metastatic lymph nodes suggests that bladder metastasis may have developed as a result of lymphatic/hematogenous and/or peritoneal dissemination. While the usual metastatic pattern of gastric cancer generally occurs in the form of lymph nodes and peritoneal and liver metastases, gastric cancers with SRC histology have been reported to exhibit a different pattern of metastasis. Peritoneal metastases are more commonly seen in SRC gastric cancers; in addition, pulmonary involvement via lymphatic route, ovarian metastases, and atypical metastases are more common [7].

Including our case, there are 16 cases in the English literature reporting bladder metastasis secondary to gastric cancer [8–19] (Table 1). The majority of the cases are above 50 years of age. Synchronous bladder metastasis was noted during the diagnosis of primary gastric tumor in only 5 cases, and, in the remaining 11 cases, bladder metastasis was noted at a time frame later (median 24 months later, range 7–120 months) than the diagnosis of gastric cancer. While there was isolated bladder metastasis in nine cases, metastatic disease was present at the time of diagnosis in the other 7 cases. Ten of sixteen cases have SRC adenocarcinoma. Metastatic disease was present at the time of diagnosis in 6 of these 10 cases and peritoneal involvement was detected in six cases; however, metastatic disease was encountered at the time of diagnosis in only 1 of 6 cases without SRC histology. This is consistent with the aggressive clinical course of SRC gastric cancers.

In bladder metastases, urinary system findings are present at the time of diagnosis in approximately 20% of the cases [11]. In cases where the tumor is a focal protuberant lesion, macroscopic hematuria is a common sign and this facilitates the diagnosis; on the other hand, symptoms may be more subtle and diagnosis may be more difficult in cases where the bladder wall is diffusely involved. In these cases, irritative symptoms and hydronephrosis are predominant [15]. Hematuria appears to be the most common presenting symptom in cases with bladder metastasis due to gastric cancer reported in the literature. Hydronephrosis was noted in seven cases at the time of presentation and the tumor in the bladder is characterized with diffuse wall thickening in 5 of these 7 cases. Our case presented with macroscopic hematuria and papillary-nodular metastatic lesions diffusely involving

TABLE 1: Cases of bladder metastasis secondary to gastric cancer in the literature.

Author/year	Number of patients	Age	Gender	Histology/IHC	Interval between primary gastric tumor and bladder metastasis	Distant metastatic sites at the time of diagnosis	Macroscopic features of bladder metastasis	Urinary symptoms	Presence of hydronephrosis	Treatment of bladder metastasis	Prognosis
Saba et al. [8] (1997)	1	52	M	SRCC/no	7 years	Peritoneum, pleura, lymph nodes	Protuberant mass	Hematuria	No	No treatment	Died
Ota et al. [9] (1999)	1	57	F	Adenoca/no	2 years	No distant metastasis	Diffuse wall thickening	Incontinence	Yes	Chemotherapy	Alive after 12-month follow-up
Kim et al. [10] (2001)	3	60	M	Adenoca/no	1 year	No distant metastasis	Protuberant mass	Dysuria, sense of residual urine	NR	NR	NR
		57	F	SRCC/no	15 months	No distant metastasis	Diffuse wall thickening	Dysuria, frequency	NR	NR	NR
		42	M	SRCC/no	2 years	No distant metastasis	Diffuse wall thickening	Dysuria	NR	Total cystectomy	NR
Antunes et al. [11] (2004)	1	63	F	SRCC/no	21 months	Peritoneum	Diffuse wall thickening	Dysuria, lumbar pain	Yes	No treatment	Alive after 8-month follow-up
Matsuhashi et al. [12] (2005)	1	90	F	Adenoca/no	Synchronous metastasis	No distant metastasis	Protuberant mass (in a bladder diverticulum)	Hematuria	No	No treatment	Died 3 months after the diagnosis
Farhat et al. [13] (2007)	1	58	M	Adenoca/no	15 months	No distant metastasis	Protuberant mass	Hematuria	No	TUR	NR
Lim et al. [14] (2011)	1	51	M	Adenoca/no	2 years	Peritoneum, bone	Protuberant mass	Hematuria	Yes	Partial cystectomy	Died 7 months after the surgery
Sharma et al. [15] (2011)	1	30	M	SRCC/no	2 years	No distant metastasis	Protuberant mass	Hematuria	No	TUR, chemotherapy	Alive after 5 months after the chemotherapy
Neves et al. [16] (2011)	2	62	F	SRCC/yes	Synchronous metastasis	Peritoneum, ovary (Krukenberg)	Diffuse wall thickening	Dysuria, infrequency, lumbar pain	Yes	No treatment	Died
		41	M	SRCC/no	Synchronous metastasis	No distant metastasis	Protuberant mass	Hematuria	No	Partial cystectomy	Died
András et al. [17] (2013)	1	59	M	Adenoca/yes	10 years	No distant metastasis	Protuberant mass	Hypogastric pain	No	TUR, chemotherapy	NR

TABLE 1: Continued.

Author/year	Number of patients	Age	Gender	Histology/IHC	Interval between primary gastric tumor and bladder metastasis	Distant metastatic sites at the time of diagnosis	Macroscopic features of bladder metastasis	Urinary symptoms	Presence of hydronephrosis	Treatment of bladder metastasis	Prognosis
Vigliar et al. [18] (2013)	1	38	M	SRCC/yes	7 months	Peritoneum, pleura, lymph nodes	Protuberant mass	Hematuria	Yes	No treatment	Died 2 months after the diagnosis
Kalra et al. [19] (2015)	1	60	M	SRCC/yes	Synchronous metastasis	Peritoneum	Diffuse wall thickening	LUTS	Yes	Chemotherapy	Alive (follow-up NR)
Present case	1	48	M	SRCC/yes	Synchronous metastasis	Peritoneum, lymph nodes	Diffuse wall thickening	Hematuria	Yes	Chemotherapy	Alive 5 months after the diagnosis

M, male; F, female; IHC, immunohistochemical studies; SRCC, signet-ring cell carcinoma; Adenoca, adenocarcinoma; LUTS, lower urinary tract symptoms; TUR, transurethral resection; NR, not reported.

the bladder wall were noted in cystoscopy. In addition, there was hydronephrosis associated with wall thickening due to the diffuse involvement of the bladder. Double J stent was not found to be necessary because hydronephrosis was still at an early stage and renal functions and urinary output were normal. Imaging performed after systemic chemotherapy revealed that hydronephrosis disappeared and thickening of the bladder wall regressed.

Histologically, bladder adenocarcinomas represent less than 2% of primary bladder tumors and 54% of secondary tumors [17]. Primary SRC bladder adenocarcinomas are much more rare and account for 0.24% of all bladder malignancies [18, 19]. SRC histology is more common in gastrointestinal system tumors and particularly in gastric cancer and is seen in 3.4% to 39% of the patients [20]. As is true for gastrointestinal tumors, SRC histology is also associated with "unfavorable outcomes" in primary bladder adenocarcinomas [21]. However, long-term survival is possible with radical cystectomy in primary SRC bladder cancers [1]. Since the treatment approaches are very different, it is important to distinguish between primary and secondary bladder adenocarcinoma. Mostofi et al. have reported that polypoid formation or presence of Brunn's nests in the tumor and glandular or mucous metaplasia in the adjacent mucosa and presence of epithelial cell foci such as squamous or transitional cells should suggest primary origin [22]. Still, despite all these clues, it may not be possible to histologically differentiate between primary and secondary adenocarcinomas of the bladder. Immunohistochemical studies may be helpful at this stage. CK7 is positive in 82% and CK20 in 73% of primary bladder tumors, whereas 29% of the cases are CK7 negative and CK20 positive [23]. In addition to immunohistochemical CK7 and CK20 positivity, negative caudal-type homeobox 2 (CDX2) which is frequently expressed in tumors of gastrointestinal origin suggests primary bladder tumor. CK7 negativity, CK20 positivity, and CDX-2 positivity are a frequently seen pattern in gastrointestinal cancers and particularly in colorectal cancer. In gastric cancer, CK7 is usually positive and CK20 is negative. Positive expression rates of CK7 and CK20 in intestinal type of primary gastric cancer are 63% and 32%, respectively, whereas these rates are 75% and 42% in diffuse SRC type [24]. MUC is positive at a high rate in mucin producing tumors and particularly in gastrointestinal malignancies [25]. With their introduction into frequent use, immunohistochemical studies have been used for confirming the diagnosis in nearly all the patients with bladder metastases due to gastric cancer reported in the literature since 2011. Our case also had typical SRC adenocarcinoma histology in both the stomach and bladder tumors. On the other hand, the tumor in the bladder had typical glandular differentiation and urothelial epithelium was intact. While the tumor in the stomach stained positively with CK7, CEA, and MUC, there was no staining with CK20; immunohistochemical staining pattern of the biopsy taken from the bladder was the same as that taken from the stomach and this staining pattern was consistent with primary gastric adenocarcinoma.

Prognosis is poor in bladder metastases of gastric origin. In localized primary SRC carcinoma of the bladder, long-term disease-free survival is possible with radical surgery and adjuvant therapy [1]. However it is not possible to obtain cure with surgery in bladder metastases because of the aggressive biology of SRC gastric cancer and rapid metastatic burden. Chemotherapy and radiotherapy can slow progression of the disease in some cases and control hematuria and irritative symptoms.

In conclusion, bladder metastasis originating from SRC gastric carcinoma is a rarely seen clinical condition with poor prognosis. Bladder metastasis is frequent particularly in cases with gastric cancer presenting with thickening of bladder wall or a mass accompanying peritoneal involvement. Immunohistochemical studies should be used in cases where it is difficult to clinically and histologically distinguish it from primary SRC adenocarcinoma of the bladder because treatment approaches are different.

References

[1] J. Michels, S. Barbour, D. Cavers, and K. N. Chi, "Metastatic signet-ring cell cancer of the bladder responding to chemotherapy with capecitabine: case report and review of literature," *Journal of the Canadian Urological Association*, vol. 4, no. 2, pp. E55–E57, 2010.

[2] G. Piessen, M. Messager, E. Leteurtre, T. Jean-Pierre, and C. Mariette, "Signet ring cell histology is an independent predictor of poor prognosis in gastric adenocarcinoma regardless of tumoral clinical presentation," *Annals of Surgery*, vol. 250, no. 6, pp. 878–887, 2009.

[3] W. Song, S.-J. Wu, Y.-L. He et al., "Clinicopathologic features and survival of patients with colorectal mucinous, signet-ring cell or non-mucinous adenocarcinoma: experience at an institution in southern China," *Chinese Medical Journal*, vol. 122, no. 13, pp. 1486–1491, 2009.

[4] J. Singh, V. Zherebitskiy, D. Grynspan, and P. M. Czaykowski, "Metastatic signet ring cell adenocarcinoma of the bladder: responsive to treatment?" *Journal of the Canadian Urological Association*, vol. 6, no. 1, pp. E15–E19, 2012.

[5] F. F. Leddy, N. E. Peterson, and T. C. Ning, "Urogenital linitis plastica metastatic from stomach," *Urology*, vol. 39, no. 5, pp. 464–467, 1992.

[6] A. W. Bates and S. I. Baithun, "Secondary neoplasms of the bladder are histological mimics of nontransitional cell primary tumours: clinicopathological and histological features of 282 cases," *Histopathology*, vol. 36, no. 1, pp. 32–40, 2000.

[7] I. Duarte and O. Llanos, "Patterns of metastases in intestinal and diffuse types of carcinoma of the stomach," *Human Pathology*, vol. 12, no. 3, pp. 237–242, 1981.

[8] N. F. Saba, D. M. Hoenig, and S. I. Cohen, "Metastatic signet-ring cell adenocarcinoma to the urinary bladder," *Acta Oncologica*, vol. 36, no. 2, pp. 219–220, 1997.

[9] T. Ota, M. Shinohara, K. Kinoshita, T. Sakoma, M. Kitamura, and Y. Maeda, "Two cases of metastatic bladder cancers showing diffuse thickening of the bladder wall," *Japanese Journal of Clinical Oncology*, vol. 29, no. 6, pp. 314–316, 1999.

[10] H.-C. Kim, S. H. Kim, S.-I. Hwang, H. J. Lee, and J. K. Han, "Isolated bladder metastases from stomach cancer: CT

demonstration," *Abdominal Imaging*, vol. 26, no. 3, pp. 333–335, 2001.

[11] A. A. Antunes, T. M. Siqueira Jr., and E. Falcão, "Vesical metastasis of gastric adenocarcinoma," *International Braz J Urol*, vol. 30, no. 5, pp. 403–405, 2004.

[12] N. Matsuhashi, K. Yamaguchi, T. Tamura, K. Shimokawa, Y. Sugiyama, and Y. Adachi, "Adenocarcinoma in bladder diverticulum, metastatic from gastric cancer," *World Journal of Surgical Oncology*, vol. 3, article 55, 2005.

[13] M. H. Farhat, G. Moumneh, R. Jalloul, and Y. El Hout, "Secondary adenocarcinoma of the urinary bladder from a primary gastric cancer," *Journal Medical Libanais*, vol. 55, no. 3, pp. 162–164, 2007.

[14] E.-K. Lim, V. C.-H. Lin, C.-T. Shu, T.-J. Yu, and K. Lu, "Gastric cancer with bladder metastasis: case report and literature review," *Urological Science*, vol. 22, no. 2, pp. 80–82, 2011.

[15] P. K. Sharma, M. K. Vijay, R. K. Das, and U. Chatterjee, "Secondary signet-ring cell adenocarcinoma of urinary bladder from a gastric primary," *Urology Annals*, vol. 3, no. 2, pp. 97–99, 2011.

[16] T. R. Neves, A. Covita, M. Soares et al., "Bladder metastasis of gastric adenocarcinoma. Report of 2 cases and bibliographic review," *Archivos Espanoles de Urologia*, vol. 64, no. 6, pp. 544–550, 2011.

[17] C. András, L. Tóth, J. Pósán et al., "Occurrence of bladder metastasis 10 years after surgical removal of a primary gastric cancer: a case report and review of the literature," *Journal of Medical Case Reports*, vol. 7, article 204, 2013.

[18] E. Vigliar, G. Marino, E. Matano, C. Imbimbo, D. C. Rossella, and L. Insabato, "Signet-ring-cell carcinoma of stomach metastatic to the bladder: a case report with cytological and histological correlation and literature review," *International Journal of Surgical Pathology*, vol. 21, no. 1, pp. 72–75, 2013.

[19] S. Kalra, R. Manikandan, L. N. Dorairajan, and B. Badhe, "Synchronously detected secondary signet ring cell urinary bladder malignancy from the stomach masquerading as genitourinary tuberculosis," *BMJ Case Reports*, vol. 2015, Article ID 206120, 2015.

[20] K.-J. Kwon, K.-N. Shim, E.-M. Song et al., "Clinicopathological characteristics and prognosis of signet ring cell carcinoma of the stomach," *Gastric Cancer*, vol. 17, no. 1, pp. 43–53, 2014.

[21] L. A. Busto Martín, M. Janeiro Pais, J. González Dacal, V. Chantada Abal, and L. Busto Castañón, "Signet-ring cell adenocarcinoma of the bladder: case series between 1990–2009," *Archivos Espanoles de Urologia*, vol. 63, no. 2, pp. 150–153, 2010.

[22] F. K. Mostofi, R. V. Thomson, and A. L. Dean Jr., "Mucous adenocarcinoma of the urinary bladder," *Cancer*, vol. 8, no. 4, pp. 741–758, 1955.

[23] M. L. Marques, G. S. D'Alessandro, D. C. Chade, V. P. Lanzoni, S. Saiovici, and C. J. R. de Almeida, "Primary mucinous adenocarcinoma of the bladder with signet-ring cells: case report," *Sao Paulo Medical Journal*, vol. 125, no. 5, pp. 297–299, 2007.

[24] H. H. Wong and P. Chu, "Immunohistochemical features of the gastrointestinal tract tumors," *Journal of Gastrointestinal Oncology*, vol. 3, no. 3, pp. 262–284, 2012.

[25] T. Terada, "An immunohistochemical study of primary signet-ring cell carcinoma of the stomach and colorectum: II. Expression of MUC1, MUC2, MUC5AC, and MUC6 in normal mucosa and in 42 cases," *International Journal of Clinical and Experimental Pathology*, vol. 6, no. 4, pp. 613–621, 2013.

2

Oxaliplatin-Induced Pulmonary Toxicity in Gastrointestinal Malignancies: Two Case Reports and Review of the Literature

Mor Moskovitz, Mira Wollner, and Nissim Haim

Division of Oncology, Rambam Health Care Campus, 3109601 Haifa, Israel

Correspondence should be addressed to Mor Moskovitz; m_moskovitz@rambam.health.gov.il

Academic Editor: David Lindquist

Oxaliplatin is a common chemotherapy drug, used mainly for colon and gastric cancer. Most common side effects are peripheral sensory neuropathy, hematological toxicity, and allergic reactions. A less common side effect is pulmonary toxicity, characterized mainly by interstitial pneumonitis. The incidence of this side effect is unknown, but the toxicity can be fatal. Twenty-six cases of pulmonary toxicity have been described in the literature, seven in the setting of adjuvant treatment. We describe two fatal cases of pulmonary injury related to oxaliplatin and a review of the literature.

1. Introduction

Oxaliplatin is a common chemotherapy drug of the platinum salts class and is used for the treatment of colon cancer and other gastrointestinal malignancies, usually in combination with 5-fluorouracil [1, 2]. The main dose-limiting toxicities of oxaliplatin are peripheral sensory neuropathy and hematological toxicity [3]. A less common side effect is pulmonary toxicity, characterized mainly by interstitial pneumonitis. The incidence of this side effect is unknown, as well as the risk factors, but the pulmonary toxicity can be fatal. Hereby we present two fatal cases of pulmonary injury related to oxaliplatin and a review of the literature.

2. Case 1

A 65-year-old female, never smoker, with a history of hypertension, was diagnosed with colon cancer metastatic to the liver in June 2007. The patient commenced chemotherapy treatment according to the FOLFIRI protocol (bevacizumab/5-fluorouracil/irinotecan). From July 2007 to July 2009, she received 19 cycles of therapy with good response. Then she underwent liver metastasectomy and, in October 2009, she started chemotherapy according to the FOLFOX protocol (bevacizumab/5-fluorouracil/oxaliplatin) [1, 2]. No treatment related side effects were noted and the patient was in very good performance status (WHO 1) until the 6th cycle

of chemotherapy. On day 15 of the 6th cycle, she developed dyspnea and fever immediately after the treatment with oxaliplatin. She was treated with intravenous corticosteroids and promethazine with symptomatic improvement of the dyspnea. The following day her dyspnea worsened, with several episodes of near-syncope. Her saturation without oxygen was measured as low as 73%, and blood pressure was as low as 100/50 mm/Hg, but no tachycardia was observed. On physical examination, the patient was dyspneic, rales were heard on auscultation to the lungs, and mild pitting edema was noticed on the lower limbs. Initial blood tests revealed respiratory alkalosis, moderate acute-on-chronic renal failure, and hyponatremia of 122 mEq/L. Troponin and brain natriuretic peptide levels, as well as echocardiography, did not show cardiac failure or ischemia. Chest X-ray showed no pulmonary congestion (following treatment with loop diuretics) or infection. Chest CT scan showed diffused bilateral ground glass infiltrates and no pulmonary emboli (Figure 1). After ruling out cardiac and thromboembolic etiology of the dyspnea, diagnostic bronchoscopy was performed. Bronchoalveolar lavage analysis, along with blood cultures, revealed no sign of bacterial, viral, or *Pneumocystis carinii* infection, and no eosinophilia. *Candida* infection was present in fungal cultures. Pulmonary biopsy showed organizing diffuse alveolar damage. A diagnosis of interstitial pneumonitis was concluded, most probably drug-induced.

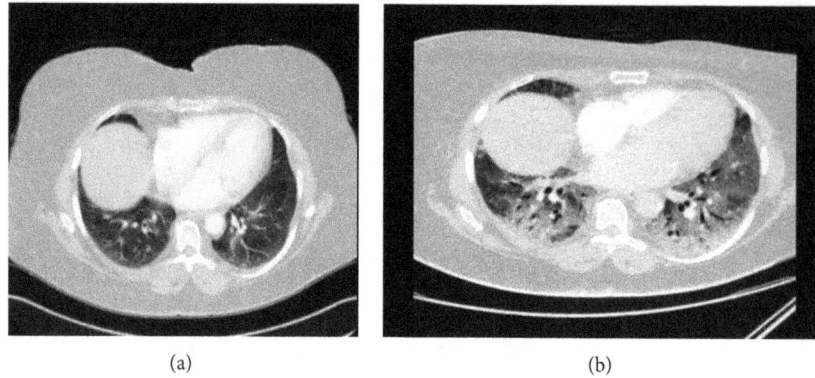

(a)   (b)

FIGURE 1: (a) Chest CT scan of patient 1, three months prior to symptoms of pneumonitis. (b) Chest CT scan of patient 1, at the beginning of respiratory symptoms: diffuse interstitial infiltrates and ground glass opacities shown in both lung fields.

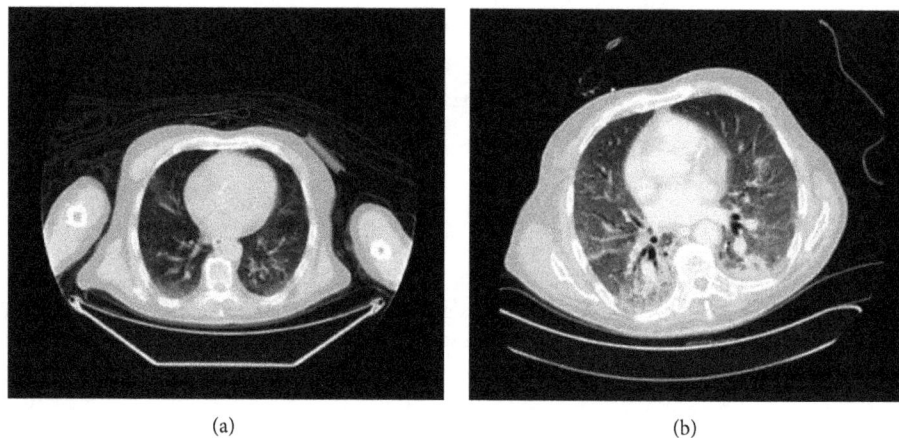

(a)   (b)

FIGURE 2: (a) Chest CT scan of patient 2, three months prior to development of respiratory symptoms. (b) Chest CT scan of patient 2, at the beginning of respiratory symptoms: diffuse interstitial infiltrates shown in both lungs.

The patient was treated with high-dose corticosteroids and wide ranging antibiotics, until the diagnosis of bacterial infection was ruled out, antifungal drugs, and loop diuretics. She received respiratory support with oxygen and continuous positive airway pressure. The patient's respiratory failure did not improve with treatment and she died 15 days following initial presentation.

3. Case 2

An 80-year-old male, never smoker, with a history of hypertension was diagnosed in September 2005 with adenocarcinoma of the rectum, stage IIIB. He received standard neoadjuvant treatment of a combination of radiation therapy and 5-fluorouracil and then underwent total mesorectal excision. In July 2006, the patient had local recurrence of the rectal cancer confirmed by rectoscopy, and biopsy from the rectum and inguinal lymph node revealed well-differentiated adenocarcinoma of the rectum, with bilateral inguinal lymph node involvement, a nonresectable disease. CT scan of the chest, abdomen, and pelvis was normal

except for the rectal mass and enlarged inguinal lymph nodes. The patient started treatment with chemotherapy for metastatic disease, the FOLFIRI protocol (bevacizumab/5-fluorouracil/irinotecan) for two cycles. Due to the severe side effects of diarrhea, the treatment was changed to FOL-FOX protocol (bevacizumab/5-fluorouracil/oxaliplatin). The patient was treated with this protocol for nine months with no side effects reported. Following the 17th treatment cycle, he was hospitalized due to fever, cough, and dyspnea. Physical examination revealed mild dyspnea, and blood tests showed mild respiratory acidosis and acute-on-chronic renal failure. Chest X-ray showed diffuse bilateral interstitial infiltrates. CT scan showed a picture consistent with diffuse alveolar damage without pulmonary fibrosis, with a differential diagnosis of atypical infection or drug-induced pneumonitis (Figure 2). These findings did not appear on the previous CT scan taken three months earlier. Blood and urine cultures were negative. Bronchoscopy including bronchoalveolar lavage was performed. Bronchoalveolar lavage analysis as well as blood cultures revealed no sign of bacterial, viral, or *Pneumocystis carinii*, *Legionella*, and *Aspergillus* infection and no eosinophilia. *Candida* infection was present on lavage analysis. There was no sign of malignancy on bronchial cytology. The patient was treated with wide spectrum empiric antibiotics, glucocorticosteroids, and oxygen, with continuous clinical deterioration and respiratory failure. He died 27 days following his initial presentation.

4. Discussion

Oxaliplatin (third generation platin, like trans-L-1,2 diaminocyclohexane, Eloxatin) was first introduced in the year 2000 as part of the treatment in metastatic colorectal carcinoma and demonstrated efficacy both in the metastatic and adjuvant settings [1, 2]. Oxaliplatin demonstrated efficacy in other gastrointestinal malignancies as well, such as gastric and pancreatic cancer. Most common side effects reported in Phase 3 randomized controlled trials were peripheral sensory neuropathy, hematological toxicity, and allergic reactions, including acute laryngeal spasm, mostly at the beginning of therapy, gastrointestinal toxicity, increase in transaminase and alkaline phosphatase levels, and fatigue [3]. Pulmonary fibrosis and grade IV pulmonary toxicity were reported in less than 1% of patients treated in trials that included oxaliplatin, and one patient died of eosinophilic pneumonia [3]. The oxaliplatin prescribing information indicates discontinuation of the drug in any case of unexplained respiratory symptoms, such as nonproductive cough, dyspnea, crackles, or radiological pulmonary infiltrates, until further pulmonary investigation excludes interstitial lung disease or pulmonary fibrosis. Data collected in Phase 4 trials revealed more cases with pulmonary interstitial lung disease. Twenty-six cases of oxaliplatin-related pulmonary toxicity have been described in the English literature [4–21] and are presented in Table 1. Sixteen of these cases (61.5%) were fatal. The real incidence is probably higher and, very likely, only selected cases were described in the literature. Most patients were males (20/26, 77%), were older than 60 years (24/26, 92.3%), with a diagnosis of metastatic colorectal carcinoma (16/26, 61.5%), and were treated with oxaliplatin for less than six months (20/26, 76%). As shown in Table 1, seven of these 26 (27%) patients had previous lung disease, two (8%) were smokers, and 4 (15%) were hypertensive. In the current report, both our patients were hypertensive but none had previous lung disease or smoking history. It was suggested that previous lung disease can be a risk factor for oxaliplatin-induced pulmonary toxicity [15]. However, due to the small number of reported patients, it is difficult to draw firm conclusions regarding such correlation. Of the 26 patients described above, 10 received oxaliplatin as part of adjuvant therapy, and seven died as a result of pulmonary toxicity.

Drug-induced pneumonitis is a diagnosis of exclusion. All the patients described above, including the two patients in this report, underwent extensive workup to exclude the more common causes for pneumonitis: infections, pulmonary emboli, pulmonary bleeding, lymphangitic carcinomatosis, and heart failure. All underwent CT scan and most, including

the first patient in this report, underwent bronchoscopy with a lung biopsy that confirmed the less common diagnosis of drug-induced interstitial pneumonitis. Fifteen of the 26 patients were treated according to the FOLFOX protocol (oxaliplatin/5-fluorouracil/leucovorin), and five of the 26 patients were treated with the FOLFOX protocol with the addition of bevacizumab, a vascular endothelial growth factor inhibitor monoclonal antibody. Few incidents of acute lung fibrosis have been reported in patients treated with 5-FU and cisplatin, although 5-fluorouracil is a widely used agent. In two cases of interstitial lung disease that improved with therapy, 5-fluorouracil was reintroduced without additional pulmonary toxicity. This implies that the most likely agent to cause the pulmonary toxicity is oxaliplatin [5, 14].

The mechanism for this pulmonary injury is not yet determined. One study that examined liver specimens of patients with colorectal carcinoma who underwent neoadjuvant chemotherapy and metastasectomy of liver lesions suggested that oxaliplatin may cause sinusoidal injury complicated by fibrosis and veno-occlusive lesions [22]. This injury may be related to oxidative damage and glutathione depletion caused by oxaliplatin. It is possible that this kind of damage may be the pathological base of the pulmonary injury of oxaliplatin.

Some chemotherapy agents are known to cause pulmonary toxicity (bleomycin, busulfan) and have well-established guidelines for follow-up and treatment of this side effect of the drug [23]. There are few case reports on the pulmonary toxicity of oxaliplatin, but this side effect is less recognized. In addition, oxaliplatin is usually given in a multidrug regimen, usually 5-fluorouracil, leucovorin, bevacizumab, or cetuximab; thus the offending agent is not clear. Since this drug is widely administered as the treatment for metastatic colorectal cancer, as well as adjuvant therapy for stage 3 resectable disease and other malignancies, it is important to be aware of this rare but potentially fatal side effect of the drug. It is important to take action for early detection and treatment of this complication.

Our recommendations to reduce the risk of death from pulmonary toxicity of oxaliplatin are as follows:

(1) awareness of the potential of pulmonary toxicity of oxaliplatin, which is probably underestimated;

(2) discontinuation of the drug in any case of respiratory symptoms associated with radiology findings consistent with interstitial lung injury and considering early treatment with corticosteroids.

In summary, treatment with oxaliplatin for early or metastatic colorectal carcinoma can cause pulmonary toxicity, often fatal, as a rare side effect of the drug. Of the 26 cases reported in the English literature, most patients were males, were older than 60 years, had metastatic disease, and had no previous lung disease. Sixteen patients died of pulmonary toxicity related to oxaliplatin, 10 in the course of adjuvant therapy for resected colon cancer.

TABLE 1: Reported cases of pulmonary toxicity related to oxaliplatin*.

References number	Patient age/gender	Aim of treatment*	Cumulative dose of oxaliplatin (mg/m^2)	Number of cycles	Regimen**	Previous lung disease	Outcome
[4]	60/M	Metastatic disease	910	7	FOLFOX	None	Resolved
[5]	60/F	Metastatic disease	NA	NA	FOLFOX	None	Resolved
[6]	68/F	Adjuvant	510	6	FOLFOX/single agent oxaliplatin	None	Death
[7]	64/M	Metastatic disease (gastric ca)	200	2	FOLFOX	None	Resolved
	75/M	Metastatic disease (gastric ca)	100	1	FOLFOX	None	Resolved
[8]	74/M	Adjuvant	510	6	FOLFOX	None	Death
[9]	67/M	Metastatic disease (HCC)	1100	11	FOLFOX	Pulmonary artery stenosis, lung metastases	Resolved
[10]	62/M	Adjuvant	595	7	FOLFOX	None	Death
	77/M	Metastatic disease	595	7	FOLFOX	None	Resolved
[11]	30/F	Adjuvant	510	6	FOLFOX	None	Resolved
[12]	66/M	Metastatic disease	1020	12	FOLFOX	None	Death
[13]	73/F	Metastatic disease	340	4	FOLFOX	Lung metastases	Death
	71/M	Adjuvant	340	4	FOLFOX	Wegener's granulomatosis, mild COPD	Death
[14]	82/M	Metastatic disease	850	10	FOLFOX	None	Resolved
[15]	71/M	Adjuvant	510	6	FOLFOX	Mild interstitial lung disease	Death
	77/F	Adjuvant	1020	12	FOLFOX	Asymptomatic ground glass opacities at right lung base	Resolved
	69/M	Adjuvant	NA	6	FOLFOX	Asymptomatic subpleural infiltrate	Resolved partially
[16]	76/M	Metastatic disease	260	2	XELOX	None	Death
[17]	47/M	Metastatic disease	NA	NA	XELOX + bevacizumab	Lung metastases	Resolved
[18]	55/M	Metastatic disease	1105	13	FOLFOX	None	Death
	73/M	Adjuvant	765	9	FOLFOX	Emphysematous lungs	Death
[19]	69/F	Metastatic disease	595	7	FOLFOX + cetuximab	Malignant pleural effusion	Death
[20]	73/F	Metastatic disease	1785	11	FOLFOX + bevacizumab	Smoking, suspected lung metastases	Death
	75/M	Metastatic disease (gastric ca)	765	9	FOLFOX	Lung metastases	Death
	64/M	Adjuvant	1020	12	FOLFOX	Smoking	Death
[21]	57/M	Metastatic disease	765	9	NA	None	Resolved
Current paper	65/F	Metastatic disease	1020	12	FOLFOX + bevacizumab	None	Death
	80/M	Advanced locoregional disease	1445	17	FOLFOX + bevacizumab	None	Death

Note. *If not stated otherwise, the patient was treated for colon cancer.
**FOLFOX-oxaliplatin/5-fluorouracil/leucovorin, XELOX-oxaliplatin/capecitabine.
ca: cancer.

References

[1] A. De Gramont, A. Figer, M. Seymour et al., "Leucovorin and fluorouracil with or without oxaliplatin as first-line treatment in advanced colorectal cancer," *Journal of Clinical Oncology*, vol. 18, no. 16, pp. 2938–2947, 2000.

[2] T. André, C. Boni, L. Mounedji-Boudiaf et al., "Oxaliplatin, fluorouracil, and leucovorin as adjuvant treatment for colon cancer," *The New England Journal of Medicine*, vol. 350, no. 23, pp. 2343–2351, 2004.

[3] R. K. Ramanathan, J. W. Clark, N. E. Kemeny et al., "Safety and toxicity analysis of Oxaliplatin combined with fluorouracil or as a single agent in patients with previously treated advanced colorectal cancer," *Journal of Clinical Oncology*, vol. 21, no. 15, pp. 2904–2911, 2003.

[4] R. Trisolini, L. Lazzari Agli, D. Tassinari et al., "Acute lung injury associated with 5-fluorouracil and oxaliplatinum combined chemotherapy," *European Respiratory Journal*, vol. 18, no. 1, pp. 243–245, 2001.

[5] F. Gagnadoux, C. Roiron, E. Carrie, L. Monnier-Cholley, and B. Lebeau, "Eosinophilic lung disease under chemotherapy with oxaliplatin for colorectal cancer," *American Journal of Clinical Oncology*, vol. 25, no. 4, pp. 388–390, 2002.

[6] X. H. Yagüe, E. Soy, B. Q. Merino, J. Puig, M. B. Fabregat, and R. Colomer, "Interstitial pneumonitis after oxaliplatin treatment in colorectal cancer.," *Clinical & Translational Oncology*, vol. 7, no. 11, pp. 515–517, 2005.

[7] K. H. Jung, S. Y. Kil, I. K. Choi et al., "Interstitial lung diseases in patients treated with oxaliplatin, 5-fluorouracil and leucovorin (FOLFOX)," *International Journal of Tuberculosis and Lung Disease*, vol. 10, no. 10, pp. 1181–1182, 2006.

[8] L. M. Pasetto and S. Monfardini, "Is acute dyspnea related to oxaliplatin administration?" *World Journal of Gastroenterology*, vol. 12, no. 36, pp. 5907–5908, 2006.

[9] A. Ruiz-Casado, M. D. García, and M. A. Racionero, "Pulmonary toxicity of 5-fluoracil and oxaliplatin," *Clinical and Translational Oncology*, vol. 8, no. 8, p. 624, 2006.

[10] C. Pena Álvarez, H. J. Suh Oh, A. Sáenz de Miera Rodríguez et al., "Interstitial lung disease associated with oxaliplatin: description of two cases," *Clinical and Translational Oncology*, vol. 11, no. 5, pp. 332–333, 2009.

[11] M. Garrido, A. O'Brien, S. González, J. M. Clavero, and E. Orellana, "Cryptogenic organizing pneumonitis during oxaliplatin chemotherapy for colorectal cancer: case report," *Chest*, vol. 132, no. 6, pp. 1997–1999, 2007.

[12] P. Mundt, H.-C. Mochmann, H. Ebhardt, M. Zeitz, R. Duchmann, and M. Pauschinger, "Pulmonary fibrosis after chemotherapy with oxaliplatin and 5-fluorouracil for colorectal cancer," *Oncology*, vol. 73, no. 3-4, pp. 270–272, 2008.

[13] S. A. Lobera, N. S. Mariñelarena, I. E. Echeberría et al., "Fatal pneumonitis induced by oxaliplatin," *Clinical and Translational Oncology*, vol. 10, no. 11, pp. 764–767, 2008.

[14] K. Muneoka, Y. Shirai, M. Sasaki, T. Wakai, J. Sakata, and K. Hatakeyama, "Interstitial pneumonia arising in a patient treated with oxaliplatin, 5-fluorouracil, and, leucovorin (FOLFOX)," *International Journal of Clinical Oncology*, vol. 14, no. 5, pp. 457–459, 2009.

[15] B. E. Wilcox, J. H. Ryu, and S. Kalra, "Exacerbation of pre-existing interstitial lung disease after oxaliplatin therapy: a report of three cases," *Respiratory Medicine*, vol. 102, no. 2, pp. 273–279, 2008.

[16] A. Shah, Z. F. Udwadia, and S. Almel, "Oxaliplatin-induced lung fibrosis," *Indian Journal of Medical and Paediatric Oncology*, vol. 30, no. 3, pp. 116–118, 2009.

[17] M. H. Fekrazad, S. Eberhardt, D. Jones, and F.-C. Lee, "Development of bronchiolitis obliterans organizing pneumonia with platinum-based chemotherapy for metastatic rectal cancer," *Clinical Colorectal Cancer*, vol. 9, no. 3, pp. 177–178, 2010.

[18] C.-G. Ryu, E.-J. Jung, G. Kim, S. R. Kim, and D.-Y. Hwang, "Oxaliplatin-induced pulmonary fibrosis: two case reports," *Journal of the Korean Society of Coloproctology*, vol. 27, no. 5, pp. 266–269, 2011.

[19] J.-I. Lai, W.-S. Wang, Y.-C. Lai, P.-C. Lin, and S.-C. Chang, "Acute interstitial pneumonitis in a patient receiving a FOLFOX-4 regimen plus cetuximab treated with pulse therapy," *International Journal of Clinical Pharmacology and Therapeutics*, vol. 48, no. 7, pp. 425–428, 2010.

[20] L. B. Pontes, D. P. D. Armentano, A. Soares, and R. C. Gansl, "Fatal pneumonitis induced by oxaliplatin: description of three cases," *Case Reports in Oncology*, vol. 5, no. 1, pp. 104–109, 2012.

[21] E. J. Lee, S. Y. Lee, K. H. In, C. H. Kim, and S. Park, "Organizing pneumonia associated with oxaliplatin-combined chemotherapy: a case report," *Medical Principles and Practice*, vol. 21, no. 1, pp. 89–92, 2012.

[22] L. Rubbia-Brandt, V. Audard, P. Sartoretti et al., "Severe hepatic sinusoidal obstruction associated with oxaliplatin-based chemotherapy in patients with metastatic colorectal cancer," *Annals of Oncology*, vol. 15, no. 3, pp. 460–466, 2004.

[23] M. Meadors, J. Floyd, and M. C. Perry, "Pulmonary toxicity of chemotherapy," *Seminars in Oncology*, vol. 33, no. 1, pp. 98–105, 2006.

3

A Case Report of Long-Term Survival following Hepatic Arterial Infusion of *L*-Folinic Acid Modulated 5-Fluorouracil Combined with Intravenous Irinotecan and Cetuximab Followed by Hepatectomy in a Patient with Initially Unresectable Colorectal Liver Metastases

Kobe Van Bael,[1] Yanina Jansen,[2] Teofila Seremet,[2] Benedikt Engels,[3] Georges Delvaux,[1] and Bart Neyns[2]

[1] *Department of Surgery, Laarbeeklaan 101, 1090 Brussels, Belgium*
[2] *Department of Medical Oncology, Laarbeeklaan 101, 1090 Brussels, Belgium*
[3] *Department of Radiotherapy, Laarbeeklaan 101, 1090 Brussels, Belgium*

Correspondence should be addressed to Kobe Van Bael; kobe.van.bael@gmail.com and Bart Neyns; bart.neyns@uzbrussel.be

Academic Editor: Raffaele Palmirotta

A 43-year-old women admitted to our hospital for weight loss, anorexia, and abdominal pain was diagnosed with sigmoid neoplasm and multiple bilobar liver metastases. This patient received six cycles of systemic FOLFOX prior to a laparoscopically assisted anterior resection of the rectosigmoid for a poorly differentiated invasive adenocarcinoma T2N2M1, K-RAS negative (wild type). Hepatic arterial infusion (HAI) of *L*-folinic acid modulated 5-fluorouracil (LV/5-FU) with intravenous (iv) irinotecan (FOLFIRI) and cetuximab as adjuvant therapy resulted in a complete metabolic response (CR) with CEA normalization. A right hepatectomy extended to segment IV was performed resulting in (FDG-)PET negative remission for 7 months. Solitary intrahepatic recurrence was effectively managed by local radiofrequent ablation following 6c FOLFIRI plus cetuximab iv. Multiple lung lesions and recurrence of pulmonary and local lymph node metastases were successfully treated with fractionated stereotactic radiotherapy (50 Gy) and iv LV/5-FU/oxaliplatin (FOLFOX) plus cetuximab finally switched to panitumumab with CR as a result. At present the patient is in persistent complete remission of her stage IV colorectal cancer, more than 5 years after initial diagnosis of the advanced disease. Multidisciplinary treatment with HAI of chemotherapy (LV/5-FU + CPT-11) plus EGFR-inhibitor can achieve CR of complex unresectable LM and can even result in hepatectomy with possible long-term survival.

1. Introduction

The 5-year survival rate of patients with advanced colorectal cancer (CRC) that has metastasized to the liver is determined by the possibility of resection of the primary tumor and liver metastases (LM). Up to 50% of patients with CRC develop LM synchronously or metachronously during the course of their disease. In a majority of stage IV CRC patients, the LM determines the life expectancy [1].

Complete resection of colorectal hepatic metastases, when possible (10–20% of patients presenting with LM), is a standard of care as it can offer the only potential for cure and improve the long-term survival. Reported 5-year survival rates after hepatectomy for CRC-LM are in the order of 27 to 40% [2]. Protoadjuvant treatment with the FOLFOX4 chemotherapy regimen improves the disease-free survival (PFS) rate in patients who are eligible for upfront hepatectomy. There was no difference in the overall survival (OS) in the patients with perioperative chemotherapy compared with the surgery-only group with resectable CRC-LM [3]. A major challenge represents the group of patients with liver-confined metastases that are unresectable at first diagnosis. Despite the improvement in systemic treatment for metastasized CRC, the 5-year survival rates for these patients are below 10%

[4, 5]. Patients who cannot undergo upfront resection of their LM may become eligible for resection following systemic treatment with cytotoxic chemotherapy and biological agents targeting the epidermal growth factor receptor (EGFR; cetuximab or panitumumab) or vascular growth factor (VEGF; bevacizumab or aflibercept) (bio)chemotherapy. Over the past few years the so-called downstaging of CRC-LM has been an intense focus of clinical research. Series reported in the literature have suggested that the outcome of patients who become amenable for hepatectomy following response to systemic (bio)chemotherapy is at the level of patients who can undergo upfront hepatectomy resulting in sparking enthusiasm for this sequential therapy approach. However, controversy exists regarding the optimal (bio)chemotherapy regimen to be used and the duration of treatment. In particular the concern for chemotherapy mediated toxicity to the liver compromising the residual functional liver capacity following hepatectomy has been raised [6].

Contemporary neoadjuvant systemic (bio)chemotherapy allows for resection of initially unresectable CRC-LM in about 5–22% of patients. Despite a high rate of recurrence, 5- and 10-year overall survival are, respectively, 33% and 23% with a wide use of repeat hepatectomies and extrahepatic resections (median survival of 39 months) [7]. This strategy has become incorporated in the treatment of CRC with LM, although randomized studies that demonstrate the superiority of this approach are lacking.

With the increasing number of patients with LM receiving surgery, another question concerning the discrepancy between a complete radiologic response and a complete pathologic clearance of cancer comes up. In up to 83% of cases, patients with a complete radiologic response are not found to be in a complete pathologic response following chemotherapy for CRC-LM [8]. This makes the timing for hepatic resection a controversial issue with a high risk of missing "dormant" LM that will progress after the discontinuing the chemotherapy. An Expert Consensus Statement recommends that hepatic metastases should be resected directly when they become resectable [9].

Hepatic arterial chemotherapy infusion (HAI) using fluoropyrimidines (5-fluorouracil or FUDR) has been widely explored for the treatment of CRC-LM. HAI offers the advantage of achieving a high concentration of cytotoxic agents within the CRC-LM, thus providing higher intraliver response rates of up to 83% [10]. A 2-year survival benefit in patients with unresectable metastasis of 48% versus 37% for HAI over systemic chemotherapy was reported [11]. Because of the added complexity and lack of survival advantage in other randomized trials HAI was not adapted as a standard of care. More recently phase I/II studies have demonstrated the feasibility of combining HAI of 5-FU with systemic administration of irinotecan or oxaliplatin and the EGFR targeted monoclonal antibodies cetuximab or panitumumab in patients with RASwt CRC [12, 13]. Our group reported a promising activity with such an approach. A partial response was documented in 62% with median time to progression of 8.7 months. We though also need to note the association of specific toxicity [14].

We here report on a case where HAI of 5-FU-based chemotherapy could downstage the initially unresectable CRC-LM and rendered the patient amenable for hepatectomy achieving an overall survival of more than 5 years.

2. Case Presentation

A 43-year-old woman without any prior disease history was admitted to our institution in March 2008 because of a short-lived history of weight loss, anorexia, nausea, and epigastric pain for only a few weeks. Physical examination revealed a hepatomegaly measuring 7 cm under the right costal border. The patient has no familial history of cancer or polyps. Laboratory data showed a strongly elevated carcinoembryonic antigen (CEA) of 1987 μg/L (normal range 0–3.0 μg/L) and disturbed liver tests (LDH 6017 U/L; AST 245 U/L; ALT 135 U/L; ALP 719 U/L; GGT 712 U/L; bilirubin 1.43). Further investigation by Computed Tomography (CT) presumed a tumor of the sigmoid which was confirmed at colonoscopy (at 15 cm of the anal marge, biopsy indicating a poorly differentiated invasive adenocarcinoma). CT examination also visualized voluminous diffuse liver metastases in both left and right lobes with almost complete involvement of segments 4a, 8, and 7 and smaller lesions in segment 2 with a big spur of the left lobe up to the spleen. No extrahepatic metastases were diagnosed (Figure 1).

Because of the involvement of both liver lobes, the patient was ineligible for hepatectomy and six cycles of systemic chemotherapy according to the FOLFOX regimen (LV modulated 5-fluorouracil + oxaliplatin) were administered.

Following an initially rapid decline of the elevated CEA and LDH during FOLFOX therapy, values stabilized. A partial tumor response was obtained but FDG-PET indicated a persistent metabolic activity in the liver. Furthermore, a grade 3 sensorial polyneuropathy became treatment limiting with respect to the oxaliplatin containing chemotherapy regimen. In June 2008, following multidisciplinary consultation, resecting the primary tumor (laparoscopy assisted anterior resection of the rectosigmoid) and inserting an arterial catheter in the gastroduodenal artery (including cholecystectomy) were decided [15]. Pathological staging indicated a poorly differentiated invasive adenocarcinoma stage pT2N2M1, K-RAS wild type.

Intra-arterial treatment was initiated in July 2008 based on the FOLFIRI scheme (LV modulated 5-FU (2400 mg/m^2 over 48 hours) by hepatic arterial infusion (HAI) + irinotecan (180 mg/m^2 ~300 mg over 90 minutes) by intravenous (iv) infusion biweekly). Cetuximab (400 mg/m^2 over 2 hours once weekly, iv) was added to the treatment regimen.

After three cycles of therapy the patient experienced multiple episodes of palpitations complicated by a few short-lived syncopes. A 48-hour in-hospital Holter-ECG monitoring during treatment of 5-FU by HAI revealed repetitive episodes of sustained and nonsustained monomorphic ventricular tachycardia (frequency of 220–230 beats per minute) at the fourth cycle. An urgent electrophysiologic exploration was done and the focus of the idiopathic right ventricular outflow tract tachycardia was successfully ablated. After five cycles of 5-FU by HAI, treatment administration had to be

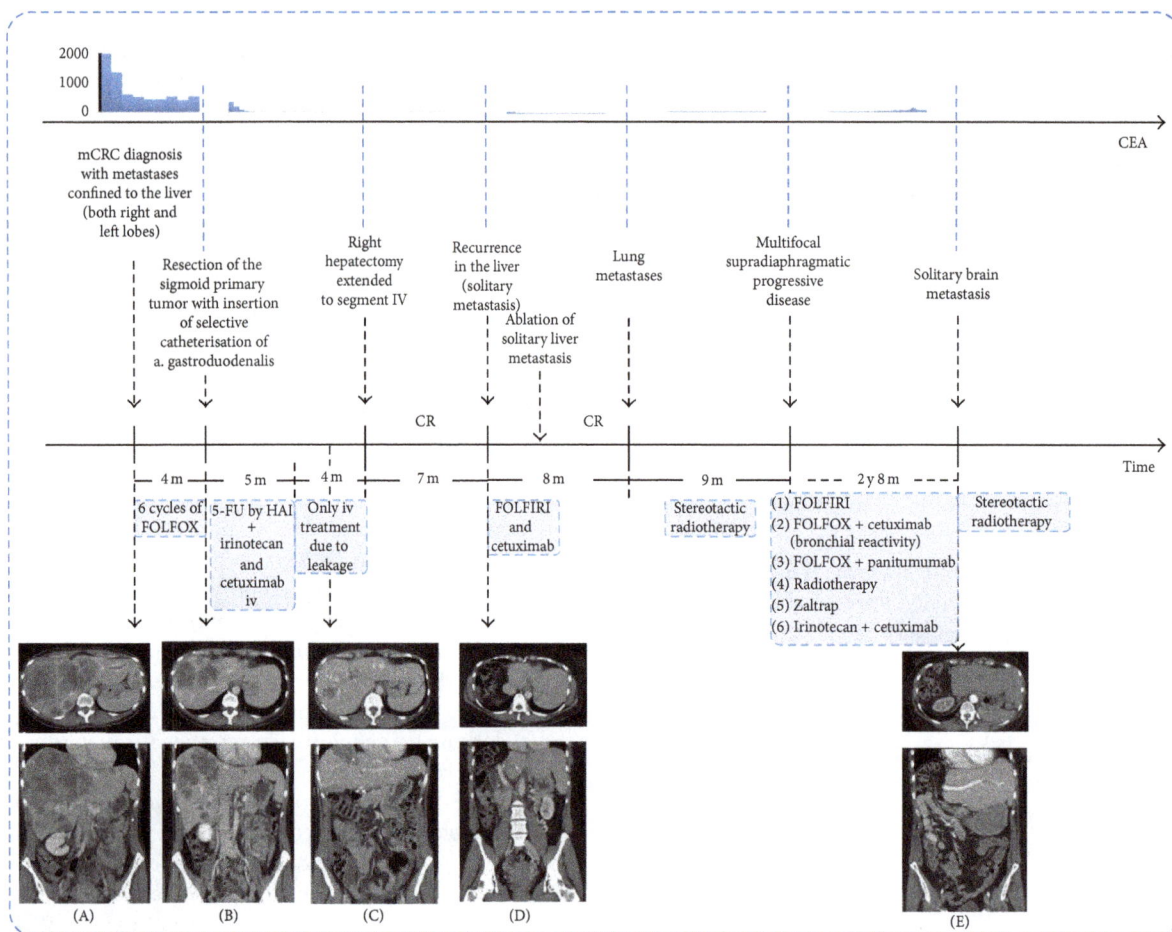

FIGURE 1

switched back to iv-administration because of a leak at the catheter tip (diagnosed after the occurrence of abdominal pain associated with administration of chemotherapy by HAI). At this moment, 4 months after surgery and start of HAI, a partial response according to RECIST was obtained with further regression of remnant LM that were no longer characterized by increased fluoro-18-deoxyglucose (FDG) uptake on PET image (providing evidence of a complete metabolic response). In addition, sustained CEA normalization was documented on repeated measurements. Systemic chemotherapy was continued for another 6 months. In April 2009 after a persistent favorable clinical, biological, and radiological evolution, a right hepatectomy extended to segment IV was performed. The postoperative period was complicated with a small bile leak that was effectively managed by ERCP with mini sphincterotomy and intrahepatic placement of a short prosthesis. Otherwise, postoperative recovery was uneventful without hepatic failure. Anatomopathological examination of the liver showed mainly scar tissue after chemotherapy with rare nests of tumoral cells. A complete metabolic response and CEA remission were maintained in the absence of further therapy until November 2009. Recurrence of a solitary liver metastasis was suggested by an

elevation in the CEA and confirmed by FDG-PET. The combination of FOLFIRI plus cetuximab was restarted for six cycles after which a stable disease was documented and a successful radiofrequent ablation was performed in February 2010, obtaining a complete response according to RECIST until June 2010 when FDG-PET revealed extrahepatic progression in the lungs (four lung lesions).

In the following years the patient developed additional lung metastasis treated with the combination of systemic chemotherapy and fractionated radiotherapy. A PET-CT in December 2013 showed solitary brain metastases, confirmed on MRI. We treated this patient with stereotactic radiotherapy. The patient was alive and received further systemic therapy at the latest follow-up in November 2014. No recurrence in the liver was documented.

3. Discussion

The therapeutic objectives in patients with CRC and upfront unresectable liver-confined metastases have shifted from palliation to maximization of the chance of resection (including also local ablative therapies such as RFA or cryoablation) by applying preoperative systemic (bio)chemotherapy to downsize the LM. In the case described here with initially unresectable voluminous LM, sequential, multimodal treatment including HAI of chemotherapy achieved over-6-year survival. Remarkably, after more than 5 years, the liver remains disease-free. The role of HAI in the treatment of metastatic CRC remains controversial [16]. A recent phase I study of Kemeny et al. demonstrated the conversion to resectability in 47% (even 57% in chemotherapy-naïve patients) with HAI of FUDR in combination with systemic treatment of oxaliplatin and irinotecan [17, 18]. In a previous manuscript, we also described a patient treated in a phase 1 study who experienced an unexpected durable remission after combined-modality treatment involving HAI for synchronous inoperable LM and a solitary lung metastasis of a rectal adenocarcinoma [19].

The reason for the switch from cetuximab to panitumumab was dual. The patient developed a progressive bronchial hyperreactivity. Incidence of hypersensitivity in panitumumab is lower because of its fully humanized nature of the IgG backbone [20]. Whether or not this adjustment results in higher efficacy cannot be confirmed. But it is now safe to say that panitumumab and cetuximab are equally effective and interchangeable in clinical practice, either as monotherapy or in combination with cytotoxic chemotherapy. A switch in idiotype can potentially generate a renewed activity from an anti-EGFR mAb, but this is not supported by scientific evidence.

Today, costs in public health care are of great concern. General cost of overall treatment is beyond the scope of this case report but the increment in survival with good quality of life obviously justifies the financial burden. As a matter of fact, this treatment allowed the patient to remain economically active.

With this technique and contemporarily available efficient biochemotherapy in combination with a dedicated oncosurgical approach, more patients are likely to be able to benefit from extended survival that did not seem achievable at initial diagnosis. A multidisciplinary approach is necessary to obtain such results.

References

[1] E. van Cutsem, C.-H. Köhne, I. Láng et al., "Cetuximab plus irinotecan, fluorouracil, and leucovorin as first-line treatment for metastatic colorectal cancer: updated analysis of overall survival according to tumor KRAS and BRAF mutation status," *Journal of Clinical Oncology*, vol. 29, no. 15, pp. 2011–2019, 2011.

[2] J. S. Tomlinson, W. R. Jarnagin, R. P. DeMatteo et al., "Actual 10-year survival after resection of colorectal liver metastases defines cure," *Journal of Clinical Oncology*, vol. 25, no. 29, pp. 4575–4580, 2007.

[3] B. Nordlinger, H. Sorbye, B. Glimelius et al., "Perioperative FOLFOX4 chemotherapy and surgery versus surgery alone for resectable liver metastases from colorectal cancer (EORTC 40983): long-term results of a randomised, controlled, phase 3 trial," *The Lancet Oncology*, vol. 14, no. 12, pp. 1208–1215, 2013.

[4] E. K. Abdalla, J.-N. Vauthey, L. M. Ellis et al., "Recurrence and outcomes following hepatic resection, radiofrequency ablation, and combined resection/ablation for colorectal liver metastases," *Annals of Surgery*, vol. 239, no. 6, pp. 818–827, 2004.

[5] R. M. Goldberg, "Therapy for metastatic colorectal cancer," *Oncologist*, vol. 11, no. 9, pp. 981–987, 2006.

[6] J.-N. Vauthey, T. M. Pawlik, D. Ribero et al., "Chemotherapy regimen predicts steatohepatitis and an increase in 90-day mortality after surgery for hepatic colorectal metastases," *Journal of Clinical Oncology*, vol. 24, no. 13, pp. 2065–2072, 2006.

[7] R. Adam, V. Delvart, G. Pascal et al., "Rescue surgery for unresectable colorectal liver metastases downstaged by chemotherapy: a model to predict long-term survival," *Annals of Surgery*, vol. 240, no. 4, pp. 644–658, 2004.

[8] S. Benoist, A. Brouquet, C. Penna et al., "Complete response of colorectal liver metastases after chemotherapy: does it mean cure?" *Journal of Clinical Oncology*, vol. 24, no. 24, pp. 3939–3945, 2006.

[9] E. K. Abdalla, R. Adam, A. J. Bilchik, D. Jaeck, J.-N. Vauthey, and D. Mahvi, "Improving resectability of hepatic colorectal metastases: expert consensus statement," *Annals of Surgical Oncology*, vol. 13, no. 10, pp. 1271–1280, 2006.

[10] F. D. Barber, G. Mavligit, and R. Kurzrock, "Hepatic arterial infusion chemotherapy for metastatic colorectal cancer: a concise overview," *Cancer Treatment Reviews*, vol. 30, no. 5, pp. 425–436, 2004.

[11] A. P. Venook, "Induction therapy in patients with metastatic colorectal cancer," *Seminars in Oncology*, vol. 30, no. 4, pp. 25–29, 2003.

[12] L. B. Saltz, S. Clarke, E. Díaz-Rubio et al., "Bevacizumab in combination with oxaliplatin-based chemotherapy as first-line therapy in metastatic colorectal cancer: a randomized phase III study," *Journal of Clinical Oncology*, vol. 26, no. 12, pp. 2013–2019, 2008.

[13] H. Hurwitz, L. Fehrenbacher, W. Novotny et al., "Bevacizumab plus irinotecan, fluorouracil, and leucovorin for metastatic colorectal cancer," *The New England Journal of Medicine*, vol. 350, no. 23, pp. 2335–2342, 2004.

[14] B. Neyns, M. Aerts, Y. Van Nieuwenhove et al., "Cetuximab with hepatic arterial infusion of chemotherapy for the treatment of colorectal cancer liver metastases," *Anticancer Research*, vol. 28, no. 4, pp. 2459–2467, 2008.

[15] Y. Van Nieuwenhove, M. Aerts, B. Neyns, and G. Delvaux, "Techniques for the placement of hepatic artery catheters for regional chemotherapy in unresectable liver metastases," *European Journal of Surgical Oncology*, vol. 33, no. 3, pp. 336–340, 2007.

[16] D. J. Gallagher, M. Capanu, G. Raggio, and N. Kemeny, "Hepatic arterial infusion plus systemic irinotecan in patients with unresectable hepatic metastases from colorectal cancer previously treated with systemic oxaliplatin: a retrospective analysis," *Annals of Oncology*, vol. 18, no. 12, pp. 1995–1999, 2007.

[17] N. E. Kemeny, F. D. Huitzil Melendez, M. Capanu et al., "Conversion to resectability using hepatic artery infusion plus systemic chemotherapy for the treatment of unresectable liver metastases from colorectal carcinoma," *Journal of Clinical Oncology*, vol. 27, no. 21, pp. 3465–3471, 2009.

[18] J. B. Ammori, N. E. Kemeny, Y. Fong et al., "Conversion to complete resection and/or ablation using hepatic artery infusional chemotherapy in patients with unresectable liver metastases from colorectal cancer: a decade of experience at a single institution," *Annals of Surgical Oncology*, vol. 20, no. 9, pp. 2901–2907, 2013.

[19] K. van Bael, M. Aerts, M. de Ridder, J. de Gréve, G. Delvaux, and B. Neyns, "Durable remission of inoperable liver metastasis from rectal cancer after hepatic arterial infusion of oxaliplatin and 5-fluorouracil in combination with intravenous cetuximab," *Current Oncology*, vol. 18, no. 5, pp. E256–E259, 2011.

[20] R. Kim, "Cetuximab and panitumumab: are they interchangeable?" *The Lancet Oncology*, vol. 10, no. 12, pp. 1140–1141, 2009.

4

A Rare Case of Undifferentiated Carcinoma of the Colon with Rhabdoid Features: A Case Report and Review of the Literature

E. Moussaly and J. P. Atallah

Staten Island University Hospital, 475 Seaview Avenue, Staten Island, NY 10305, USA

Correspondence should be addressed to J. P. Atallah; jeanpaul_atalla@yahoo.com

Academic Editor: Jorg Kleeff

Malignant rhabdoid tumors were originally described in children. Subsequently, the same histological pattern was described in adults. Malignant rhabdoid tumors are aggressive neoplasms that have been reported in multiple organs. To our best knowledge, only 16 previous cases of rhabdoid tumor in the colon have been described in the literature. We present the case of an 87-year-old lady who was diagnosed with a rhabdoid tumor of the colon that relapsed rapidly after surgical resection. The literature concerning this unusual neoplasm was subsequently reviewed with comparison of all known cases in the literature.

1. Introduction

In 1978, Beckwith and Palmer first described Wilms' tumors with "rhabdomyosarcomatoid" features in children. This pattern was characterized by diffuse sheets of polygonal cells with acidophilic cytoplasm and rounded vesicular nuclei [1]. Subsequently, this pattern was described in adults and in multiple extrarenal locations such as the gastrointestinal tract, urinary tract, skin, and central nervous system and termed malignant rhabdoid tumors (MRT) [2, 3]. These malignant rhabdoid tumors can be pure or mixed with other malignancies. The existence of MRT as a distinct oncological entity is still under debate [4, 5]. MRT are invariably associated with unfavorable prognosis [2, 3]. The first case of MRT in the colon was described in 1994 by Yang et al. [6]. Since this publication, 15 cases of malignant colon cancer with rhabdoid features have been published in the literature to our knowledge [5–19]. We present the case of an 87-year-old female who was complaining of abdominal pain and was found to have undifferentiated carcinoma of the transverse colon with rhabdoid features.

2. Case Presentation

The patient was an 87-year-old Caucasian female of Russian descent who presented to our hospital with a two-day history of generalized weakness, profuse nonbilious nonbloody vomiting, and decreased oral intake. The patient complained of diffuse abdominal pain but had no change in bowel movement. The patient had been suffering from decreased appetite for weeks. The patient's past medical and surgical history are noncontributory because the patient had not seen a physician nor taken a medication in many years. In the emergency department, vital signs showed blood pressure of 88/54, pulse rate of 115 bpm, a respiratory rate of 20, and a temperature of 98.8 F. Physical examinations showed a frail looking lady with pale conjunctiva and skin, lungs were clear to auscultation bilaterally, and heart auscultation did not elicit any murmur rubs or gallop. Abdominal examination elicited a right upper quadrant mass on deep palpation without associated tenderness or distention and with positive bowel sounds in all quadrants. The rest of the physical exam was unremarkable. A stool guaiac test performed at bedside was negative. On further interrogation of the family, we were informed that the patient was a nonsmoker and occasional alcohol user and had no known drug allergies. The patient had no family history of malignancy.

The patient was urgently stabilized in the emergency department with intravenous fluids, transfusion therapy, and antibiotics and was admitted to the intensive care unit for monitoring.

Blood tests on admission were as shown in Table 1.

TABLE 1

Sodium	130 mmol/L
Chloride	90 mmol/L
Potassium	3.8 mmol/L
Bicarbonate	20 mmol/L
Creatinine	1.83 mg/dL
BUN	51 mg/dL
Lactic acid	1.5 mmol/L
Glucose	175 mg/dL
Magnesium	2.9 mg/dL
ALT	45 IU/L
AST	20 IU/L
Alkaline phosphatase	95 IU/L
Total bilirubin	0.7 mg/dL
Albumin	2.8 g/dL
Lipase	14 U/L
WBC	14.54 TH/mm3
Hb	6.3 g/dL
MCV	75.3 MCM3
RDW	14.2%
Platelets	576 TH/mm3
Segmented neutrophils	74%
Lymphocytes	1%
Band neutrophils	19%
CEA	4.3

An emergent CT scan of the abdomen and pelvis done without contrast showed a large concentric and enveloping 12.1 × 9.3 × 8.4 cm mass along the hepatic flexure of the transverse colon with associated mass-effect and obstruction along a portion of the distal jejunum and innumerable splenic hypodensities. A chest radiograph done on admission did not show any suspicious nodules. A colonoscopy showed a friable, infiltrative, and ulcerated tumor which occupied 100% of the circumference of the transverse colon and caused a severe 80% obstruction of the lumen. Biopsies were taken. Additional findings included diverticulosis in the sigmoid and descending colon and incidental polyps which were removed. The patient underwent right hemicolectomy, partial omentectomy, small bowel resection with primary anastomosis, and a twelve-lymph node resection. The post-operative course was unremarkable. Macroscopically, the mass was a 12 × 9 × 9 cm necrotic tumor. Pathological findings showed a high grade malignant neoplasm, in favor of undifferentiated carcinoma with rhabdoid features involving ulcerated mucosal and submucosal fragments with extensive necrosis. The tumor was positive for calretinin, pancytokeratin, vimentin, CAM 5.2, and neuron specific enolase which are in favor of the aforementioned diagnosis. The tumor was focally positive for epithelial membrane antigen. One of twelve lymph nodes that were found in the resected specimen was positive for micrometastasis. The tumor extended to the free serosal surface of the right colon and a loop of small bowel with extensive vascular involvement and no perineural involvement. Surgical margins were negative microscopically.

The final pathologic stage was pT4B, pN1 (mic), and pMx with microsatellite instability. The initial staging was stage IIIC without ruling out metastasis since the splenic masses were never evaluated with pathology. Upon follow-up with the oncologist and further discussion of the case with the family, a trial of capecitabine was suggested. The family opted not to undergo any treatment but decided to follow with the oncologist closely and manage symptoms.

Upon follow-up with the oncologist one month after the initial assessment, a repeat CT of the abdomen showed development of moderate amount of intra-abdominal pelvic ascites and interval development of 6.1 × 3.1 cm heterogenous mass in the right abdominal wall consistent with tumor recurrence associated with new mesenteric, gastrohepatic ligament and retropritoneal adenoapthies. Multiple low-density splenic lesions stable in appearance from the previous study were identified. A repeat CT of the chest showed a 1.2 cm solid nodule in the left lung apex. Physical exam in the clinic elicited effectively a 5 cm nontender palpable mass at the surgical scar. Repeat CEA was 11. The patient passed away two months later from complications of her disease.

3. Discussion

Colon carcinoma with rhabdoid features is an uncommon pathological entity. It is almost always associated with unfavorable prognosis. The existence of this tumor as an independent pathological entity is still under debate since it is considered by some experts to be merely a phenotypical variation of the tumor [4]. Malignant rhabdoid tumors have been described in a variety of organs. They share common histology and immunophenotype and can be mixed with different types of neoplasms (carcinomas, melanomas, and sarcomas). These tumors are described as "composite" when the rhabdoid phenotype is mixed with another type of identifiable neoplasm and termed "pure" when the rhabdoid features are the only identifiable phenotype. Histologically, the rhabdoid phenotype is characterized by the presence of pleomorphic cells with large, eccentric nuclei, prominent nucleoli, abundant and eosinophilic cytoplasm, paranuclear inclusions of intermediate filaments, and abundant mitotic figures [7]. Cytokeratin and vimentin are frequently found on immunochemistry [8].

Table 2 shows the clinical characteristics of all the cases of poorly differentiated carcinoma of the colon with rhabdoid features that we found in the literature [5–19]. This entity seems to be a disease of the elderly with a mean age of 70 years at presentation. It is equally distributed between both sexes with 9 males and 8 females. Almost all patients presented with abdominal symptoms including abdominal pain, abdominal mass, and gastrointestinal bleed. This is quite an unusual presentation of colon cancer that tends to have more occult presentation and could be a reflection of the aggressive nature of this type of tumor. In fact, the average size at presentation, which we calculated based on the tumor's longest diameter, was 8.8 cm. The largest tumor is 12 cm and the smallest one is 3 cm. These tumors were distributed equally along the colon. Tumors were described from the cecum all the way to the

TABLE 2: Clinical characteristics of all cases of poorly differentiated carcinoma of the colon with rhabdoid features described in the literature, to our knowledge. Age is in years. Size means the largest diameter of the tumor in centimeters. *DNS: did not specify.* [5–19].

	Age	Sex	Size	Location	Presentation	Metastasis	Type	Survival
Baba et al.	45	F	—	—	Abdominal pain	—	—	6 weeks
Romera Barba et al.	77	M	DNS	Descending colon	Abdominal pain	No	Pure	2 months
Lee et al. case 1	62	M	4.5	Sigmoid colon	Occult blood in stool	No	Composite	36 months still alive
Lee et al. case 2	83	M	6.5	Rectum	Rectal mass	Yes	Composite	one month
Remo et al.	73	F	10	Right colon	Rectal bleed	No	Composite	6 months
Pancione et al.	71	F	10	Right colon	Abdominal pain	Yes	Pure	8 months
Nakamura et al.	76	M	14	Cecum	Abdominal pain	Yes	Pure	3 months
Marcus et al.	84	F	7	Transverse colon	Abdominal mass	No	Composite	12 months still alive
Yang et al.	75	M	15	Transverse colon	DNS	No	Pure	2 weeks
Agaimy et al.	79	M	9	Cecum	—	No	Composite	6 months
Mastoraki et al.	62	F	10	Descending colon	Abdominal pain	Yes	Pure	4 months
Lee et al.	63	M	3	Right colon	Weakness	Yes	Pure	DNS
Chetty and Bhathal	72	F	6	Cecum	Abdominal mass	Yes	Composite	DNS
Kono et al.	66	M	13	Cecum	Abdominal mass	No	Composite	6 weeks
Oh et al.	69	F	3.5	Sigmoid colon	Blood in stools	No	Composite	6 months
Macák and Kodet	50	M	—	Rectum	—	—	Composite	—
Our case	87	F	12	Transverse colon	Abdominal mass	No	Composite	2 months

rectum. Six of the patients had identifiable metastasis on presentation. Twelve patients had at least one positive lymph node invasion, 2 were negative, and 3 were not specified. These facts also reflect the aggressive nature of this particular phenotype. Nine patients had composite rhabdoid tumors of the colon, 6 had pure rhabdoid tumors, and one case was not specified. The overall survival from this tumor even after surgical intervention seems to be unfavorable with a large majority of the patients surviving for less than six months even after surgery. Only three patients were documented to have received chemotherapy. One patient received 12 cycles of FOLFOX and was still alive at the time the paper was written surviving 36 months [8]. Another received a trial of capecitabine and oxaliplatin with a survival of 6 months [9]. The third patient received a trial of bevacizumab and cetuximab and had an 8-month survival [10]. The uncommon occurrence of malignant extrarenal rhabdoid tumors (MERT) has made it complicated to establish adequate survival-improving protocols. Horazdovsky et al. concluded in their meta-analysis that surgery and actinomycin might improve survival in MERT [20].

Imaging does not seem to be particularly helpful in diagnosing tumors with rhabdoid features since it does not present any specific radiological findings [21]. The rhabdoid phenotype is characterized in pathology by the presence of pleomorphic cells with large eccentric nuclei, prominent nucleoli, a large eosinophilic cytoplasm, and intermediate filament inclusions. Cytokeratin and vimentin are found regularly on immunochemistry, although in variable degrees [22]. Other markers described in the rhabdoid phenotype are epithelial membrane antigen, CAM5.2, CD99, synaptophysin, and neuron specific enolase. Some tumors express the p53 gene mutation and others show microsatellite instability [8]. Since a wide variety of tumors may exhibit

rhabdoid features, the WHO recommends, in its classification of soft tumors, that the rhabdoid phenotype be reflected in the final pathological diagnosis, either as composite extrarenal rhabdoid tumor (if the tumor appears to be a mix of rhabdoid and non-rhabdoid elements) or as a modifier (if the rhabdoid phenotype is more diffuse in the tumor) [23].

In 1998, Versteege et al. described *SMARCB1* biallelic inactivation in rhabdoid tumors [24, 25]. *SMARCB1* (also known as BAF47) is a core subunit of the SWI/SNF chromatin remodeling complex which regulates chromatin structure and thus plays an important role in gene expression [26]. The inactivation of other SWI/SNF subunits such as the BRM gene has also been implicated in rhabdoid tumor oncogenesis [25]. The SWI/SNF chromatin remodeling complex has been hypothesized to play a key role in the formation of a variety of neoplasms [27]. Even though rhabdoid tumors are aggressive tumors, they present a simple genetic configuration with lack of chromosomal instability and a mutation rate among the lowest in all sequenced cancer genomes with loss of *SMARCB1* as the only consistently recurrent event [28, 29]. Up to one-third of patients with rhabdoid tumors have been found to have a genetic predisposition to these tumors secondary to a germline *SMARCB1* alteration [30]. Germline *SMARCB1* mutations strongly predispose to rhabdoid tumors [31] and subsequent somatic loss of the other allele can lead to cancer formation. *SMARCB1* biallelic loss is now used in diagnosing these tumors by detecting loss of protein expression in the nucleus by immunostaining [32]. Thus atypical teratoid/rhabdoid tumors (central nervous system rhabdoid tumors) and renal and extrarenal rhabdoid tumors seem to be genetically related and *SMARCB1* loss detection can thus play an integral part in differentiating rhabdoid tumors from other tumors with similar histologic features [33]. This low mutation rate could imply that even limited genetic disturbances can drive cancer formation. This argument is also supported by the fact that other cancers also have low mutation rates such as retinoblastoma, neuroblastoma, and AML [34]. The oncogenic properties of *SMARCB1* loss seem to be related to its effect on p16 INK4a and cyclin D1 which play a significant role in the cell cycle and on RhoA signaling which enhances cell migration [33]. Understanding the epigenetic consequences of *SMARCB1* loss might provide insight to oncogenesis and may help in developing therapies for a multitude of SWI/SNF mutant neoplasms [34]. *SMARCB1* losses have also been described in other tumors such as renal medullary carcinoma, epithelioid sarcomas, and nerve sheath neoplasms [33].

4. Conclusion

Tumors with rhabdoid features have been described in multiple organs. The rhabdoid feature seems to be associated with poor prognosis. We present the case of an 87-year-old female who was found to have an undifferentiated carcinoma of the colon with rhabdoid features. To our best knowledge, this case is the seventeenth case of a tumor with rhabdoid phenotype to be described in the colon.

References

[1] J. B. Beckwith and N. F. Palmer, "Histopathology and prognosis of Wilms tumor: results from the first national Wilms' tumor study," *Cancer*, vol. 41, no. 5, pp. 1937–1948, 1978.

[2] D. M. Parham, D. A. Weeks, and J. B. Beckwith, "The clinicopathologic spectrum of putative extrarenal rhabdoid tumors: an analysis of 42 cases studied with immunohistochemistry or electron microscopy," *The American Journal of Surgical Pathology*, vol. 18, no. 10, pp. 1010–1029, 1994.

[3] M. R. Wick, J. H. Ritter, and L. P. Dehner, "Malignant rhabdoid tumors: a clinicopathologic review and conceptual discussion," *Seminars in Diagnostic Pathology*, vol. 12, no. 3, pp. 233–248, 1995.

[4] D. A. Weeks, J. B. Beckwith, and G. W. Mierau, "Rhabdoid tumor: an entity or a phenotype?" *Archives of Pathology and Laboratory Medicine*, vol. 113, no. 2, pp. 113–114, 1989.

[5] R. Chetty and P. S. Bhathal, "Caecal adenocarcinoma with rhabdoid phenotype: an immunohistochemical and ultrastructural analysis," *Virchows Archiv—A Pathological Anatomy and Histopathology*, vol. 422, no. 2, pp. 179–182, 1993.

[6] A. H. Yang, W. Y. K. Chen, and H. Chiang, "Malignant rhabdoid tumour of colon," *Histopathology*, vol. 24, no. 1, pp. 89–91, 1994.

[7] E. Romera Barba, A. S'anchez P'erez, C. Duque P'erez, J. A. Garc'ia Marcilla, and J. L. V'azquez Rojas, "Malignant rhabdoid tumor of the colon: a case report," *Cirugia Espanola*, vol. 92, no. 9, pp. 638–640, 2014.

[8] S. H. Lee, H. Seol, W. Y. Kim et al., "Rhabdoid colorectal carcinomas: reports of two cases," *Korean Journal of Pathology*, vol. 47, no. 4, pp. 372–377, 2013.

[9] A. Remo, C. Zanella, E. Molinari et al., "Rhabdoid carcinoma of the colon: a distinct entity with a very aggressive behavior: a case report associated with a polyposis coli and review of the literature," *International Journal of Surgical Pathology*, vol. 20, no. 2, pp. 185–190, 2012.

[10] M. Pancione, A. Di Blasi, L. Sabatino et al., "A novel case of rhabdoid colon carcinoma associated with a positive CpG island methylator phenotype and BRAF mutation," *Human Pathology*, vol. 42, no. 7, pp. 1047–1052, 2011.

[11] Y. Baba, T. Uchiyama, K. Hamada et al., "A case report of undifferentiated carcinoma of the sigmoid colon with rhabdoid features," *Nihon Shokakibyo Gakkai Zasshi*, vol. 111, no. 7, pp. 1384–1390, 2014.

[12] I. Nakamura, K. Nakano, K. Nakayama et al., "Malignant rhabdoid tumor of the colon: report of a case," *Surgery Today*, vol. 29, no. 10, pp. 1083–1087, 1999.

[13] V. A. Marcus, J. Viloria, D. Owen, and M.-S. Tsao, "Malignant rhabdoid tumor of the colon. Report of a case with molecular analysis," *Diseases of the Colon & Rectum*, vol. 39, no. 11, pp. 1322–1326, 1996.

[14] A. Agaimy, T. T. Rau, A. Hartmann, and R. Stoehr, "SMARCB1 (INI1)-negative rhabdoid carcinomas of the gastrointestinal tract: clinicopathologic and molecular study of a highly aggressive variant with literature review," *American Journal of Surgical Pathology*, vol. 38, no. 7, pp. 910–920, 2014.

[15] A. Mastoraki, O. Kotsilianou, I. S. Papanikolaou, P. G. Foukas, G. Sakorafas, and M. Safioleas, "Malignant rhabdoid tumor of the large intestine," *International Journal of Colorectal Disease*, vol. 24, no. 11, pp. 1357–1358, 2009.

[16] S. J. Lee, T. H. Kim, D. H. Ko et al., "Undifferentiated adenocarcinoma of the colon with rhabdoid features," *Korean Journal of Gastrointestinal Endoscopy*, vol. 40, no. 1, pp. 49–53, 2010.

[17] T. Kono, Y. Imai, J. Imura et al., "Cecal adenocarcinoma with prominent rhabdoid feature: report of a case with immunohistochemical, ultrastructural, and molecular analyses," *International Journal of Surgical Pathology*, vol. 15, no. 4, pp. 414–420, 2007.

[18] H.-K. Oh, C.-H. Cho, and Y.-S. Kum, "Adenocarcinoma of the sigmoid colon with prominent rhabdoid features—a case report," *Korean Journal of Pathology*, vol. 42, no. 1, pp. 63–65, 2008.

[19] J. Mac'ak and R. Kodet, "Rectal adenocarcinoma with rhabdoid phenotype," *Pathologica*, vol. 87, no. 6, pp. 696–699, 1995.

[20] R. Horazdovsky, J. C. Manivel, and E. Y. Cheng, "Surgery and actinomycin improve survival in malignant rhabdoid tumor," *Sarcoma*, vol. 2013, Article ID 315170, 8 pages, 2013.

[21] D. J. Roebuck, "The role of imaging in renal and extra-renal rhabdoid tumours," *Australasian Radiology*, vol. 40, no. 3, pp. 310–318, 1996.

[22] C. Voglino, M. Scheiterle, G. Di Mare et al., "Malignant rhabdoid tumor of the small intestine in adults: a brief review of the literature and report of a case," *Surgery Today*, 2014.

[23] C. Fletcher, K. Unni, and F. Mertens, *Pathology and Genetics of Tumours of Soft Tissue and Bone*, IARC Press, Lyon, France, 2002.

[24] I. Versteege, N. S'evenet, J. Lange et al., "Truncating mutations of hSNF5/INI1 in aggressive paediatric cancer," *Nature*, vol. 394, no. 6689, pp. 203–206, 1998.

[25] B. Kahali, J. Yu, B. Stefanie et al., "The silencing of the SWI/SNF subunit and anticancer gene BRM in Rhabdoid tumors," *Oncotarget*, vol. 5, no. 10, pp. 3316–3332, 2014.

[26] M. L. Phelan, S. Sif, G. J. Narlikar, and R. E. Kingston, "Reconstitution of a core chromatin remodeling complex from SWI/SNF subunits," *Molecular Cell*, vol. 3, no. 2, pp. 247–253, 1999.

[27] B. G. Wilson and C. W. M. Roberts, "SWI/SNF nucleosome remodellers and cancer," *Nature Reviews Cancer*, vol. 11, no. 7, pp. 481–492, 2011.

[28] R. S. Lee, C. Stewart, S. L. Carter et al., "A remarkably simple genome underlies highly malignant pediatric rhabdoid cancers," *The Journal of Clinical Investigation*, vol. 122, no. 8, pp. 2983–2988, 2012.

[29] E. M. Jackson, A. J. Sievert, X. Gai et al., "Genomic analysis using high-density single nucleotide polymorphism-based oligonucleotide arrays and multiplex ligation-dependent probe amplification provides a comprehensive analysis of INI1/SMARCB1 in malignant rhabdoid tumors," *Clinical Cancer Research*, vol. 15, no. 6, pp. 1923–1930, 2009.

[30] K. W. Eaton, L. S. Tooke, L. M. Wainwright, A. R. Judkins, and J. A. Biegel, *Spectrum of SMARCB1/INI1 mutations in familial and sporadic rhabdoid tumors [Ph.D. thesis]*, 2011.

[31] N. S'evenet, E. Sheridan, D. Amram, P. Schneider, R. Handgretinger, and O. Delattre, "Constitutional mutations of the hSNF5/INI1 gene predispose to a variety of cancers," *The American Journal of Human Genetics*, vol. 65, no. 5, pp. 1342–1348, 1999.

[32] J. A. Biegel, G. Kalpana, E. S. Knudsen et al., "The role of INI1 and the SWI/SNF complex in the development of rhabdoid tumors: meeting summary from the workshop on childhood atypical teratoid/rhabdoid tumors," *Cancer Research*, vol. 62, no. 1, pp. 323–328, 2002.

[33] C. W. M. Roberts and J. A. Biegel, "The role of SMARCB1/INI1 in development of rhabdoid tumor," *Cancer Biology & Therapy*, vol. 8, no. 5, pp. 412–416, 2009.

[34] R. S. Lee and C. W. M. Roberts, "Rhabdoid tumors: an initial clue to the role of chromatin remodeling in cancer," *Brain Pathology*, vol. 23, no. 2, pp. 200–205, 2013.

5

Primary Mesenteric Undifferentiated Pleomorphic Sarcoma Masquerading as a Colon Carcinoma: A Case Report and Review of the Literature

Robert Diaz-Beveridge,[1] Marcos Melian,[1] Carlos Zac,[2] Edwin Navarro,[1] Dilara Akhoundova,[1] Melitina Chrivella,[2] and Jorge Aparicio[1]

[1]Medical Oncology Department, University Hospital La Fe, Avinguda de Fernando Abril Martorell, No. 106, 46026 Valencia, Spain
[2]Pathology Department, University Hospital La Fe, Avinguda de Fernando Abril Martorell, No. 106, 46026 Valencia, Spain

Correspondence should be addressed to Robert Diaz-Beveridge; diaz‑rob@gva.es

Academic Editor: Francesca Micci

Undifferentiated pleomorphic sarcoma (UPS) is the most common sarcoma that appears in older patients, usually in the extremities and the retroperitoneum. Other locations are rare. By definition, in UPS, although the malignant cells tend to appear fibroblastic or myofibroblastic, they should not show differentiation towards a more specific line of differentiation. In this sense, we report the case of an 80-year-old patient with an initial clinical diagnosis of a locally advanced colonic neoplasm that was later confirmed as a primary mesenteric UPS. Primary mesenteric UPS are extremely rare with less than 20 cases reported. We also review the pathologic and radiologic diagnostic criteria and the natural history of these tumours.

1. Introduction

Undifferentiated pleomorphic sarcoma (UPS), previously known as malignant fibrous histiocytoma, is the most common sarcoma appearing in late adult life. By definition, although the malignant cells tend to appear fibroblastic or myofibroblastic, they should not show differentiation towards a more specific line of differentiation. In this sense, as the pathological and molecular diagnostic techniques have improved in the last few years, in many cases previously classified as malignant fibrous histiocytoma, a more specific diagnosis can be confidently made. In those remaining true cases of UPS, the most frequent localization is the extremities, followed by the retroperitoneum. On the other hand, visceral and intra-abdominal primary involvement is rare. We report the case of an elderly gentleman with the diagnosis of a primary mesenteric UPS, an extremely rare site of involvement by this tumour. We also review the pathologic and radiologic diagnostic criteria and the natural history of these tumours.

2. Case Report

A 75-year-old male was referred to our hospital in May 2010 with a two-month history of diffuse abdominal pain and intermittent rectal bleeding. He also reported low-grade fever in the evenings. No weight loss or other symptoms were noted. His previous medical history was unremarkable except for hypertension and type 2 diabetes. On physical examination, the patient had a good general status and was not septic. A painful, poorly defined, and nontender mass was noted in the right hypochondrium; there were no signs of peritoneal irritation. Blood counts, renal and hepatic biochemistry tests, LDH levels, and tumour markers values were all within the normal range. Only the fibrinogen level and the C-reactive protein were elevated (841 mg/dL and 209.1 mg/L, resp.).

A full-body CT scan revealed a heterogeneous, well-circumscribed mass in the right abdominal loin that seemed to originate from the hepatic flexure colon and descended towards the anterosuperior iliac spine (Figure 1). The mass

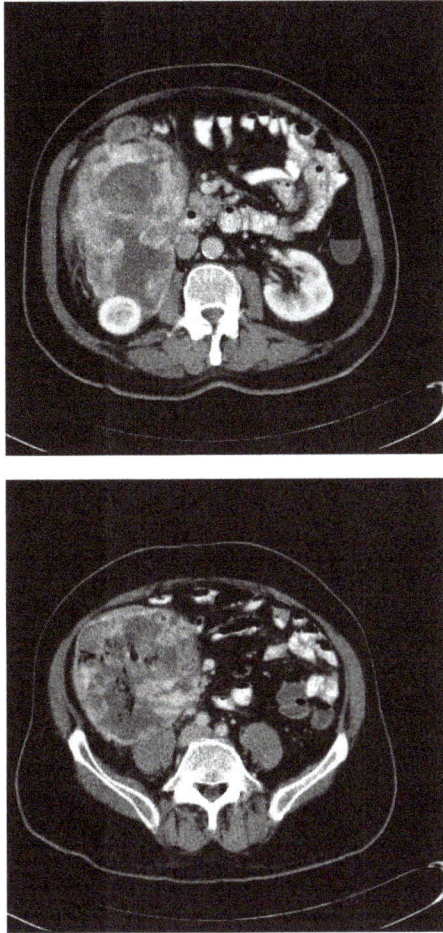

FIGURE 1: A CT scan shows a heterogeneous, well-circumscribed mass in the right abdominal loin that seems to originate from the hepatic flexure colon and descends towards the anterosuperior iliac spine. Note the presence of air bubbles due to the colonic invasion.

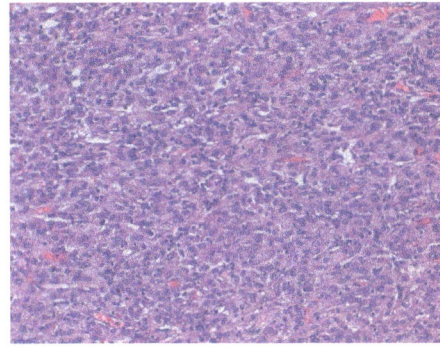

FIGURE 2: H&E stain (100 hpf). A poorly differentiated mesenchymal tumour, with ample zones of necrosis and with an extensive mononuclear inflammatory component. The malignant cells form different morphological patterns, from highly cellular epithelioid areas to pleomorphic-storiform areas. The malignant cells are large, with highly atypical nuclei.

displaced the right kidney and appeared to infiltrate the anterior renal capsule. There were air bubbles in the interior of the tumour. There were no other imaging abnormalities. The colonoscopy revealed in the transverse colon, near the hepatic flexure, both an extrinsic compression of the colonic lumen and more proximally an intraluminal tumour that occupied the whole of the circumference and did not allow the further passage of the colonoscope. Biopsies of the mass, however, revealed only necrosis but no malignant cells.

An exploratory laparotomy was performed in May 2010. A right colonic mass was seen that occupied the whole right abdominal flank and infiltrated the distal ileum. There was a small quantity of ascitic fluid. The right kidney was not infiltrated. An extended right hemicolectomy with a distal ileal resection was performed. The postoperative course was uneventful and the patient was quickly discharged.

The pathologic analysis showed a poorly delimitated 14 × 13 cm tumoural mass, covered by the colonic mesentery. The lesion was lobulated and heterogeneous, with intertwined gelatinous and solid zones. Cavitated and necrotic areas in the interior and in the outer surface of the tumour were readily

seen. The tumour was extrinsic to the colon and originated from the mesentery. However, when the intestinal lumen was inspected, fungating masses were seen in the right colon and in the caecum, secondary to the mesenteric tumour. The surgical margins were free.

The microscopic study revealed a poorly differentiated mesenchymal tumour, with ample zones of necrosis and with an extensive mononuclear inflammatory component. Some zones were abscessified. The malignant cells formed different morphological patterns, from highly cellular epithelioid areas to pleomorphic-storiform areas (Figure 2). Although some mucin could be seen, no typical lipoblasts were evident. The malignant cells were large, with highly atypical nuclei and microvacuolated cytoplasm. The immunohistochemical studies performed only showed a high positivity to vimentin and focal positivity to CD68 (Figure 3). Epithelial (cytokeratin and epithelial membrane antigen (EMA)), melanoma (S100 and HMB45), lymphoid (CD34), and neurogenic and myogenic markers (myogenin, actin, and desmin) expression were all negative. The study of both synovial sarcoma and Ewing sarcoma-specific translocations was negative. The final diagnosis was a primary mesenteric undifferentiated pleomorphic sarcoma with inflammation associated with a secondary obstructive endophytic colonic mass.

The patient began follow-up in our outpatient clinic. No adjuvant treatment was given. Unfortunately, an unresectable local and peritoneal recurrence was diagnosed in August 2010. Palliative chemotherapy was begun with pegylated doxorubicin, with little effect, and the patient died in October, 2010, six months after the original diagnosis.

3. Discussion

The mesentery is a frequent avenue of spread for malignant neoplasms through the peritoneal cavity and between the peritoneal spaces and the retroperitoneum. On the other hand, primary tumours arising from the mesentery are rare. Most of these are mesenchymal in origin, and the majority are histologically benign [1]. The most frequent

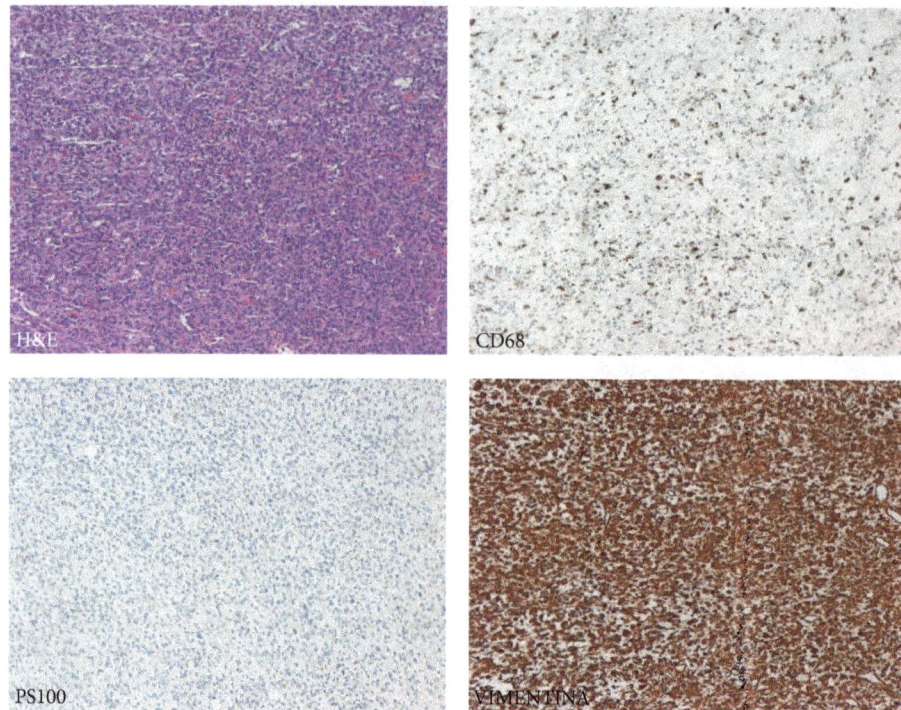

FIGURE 3: Immunohistochemical analysis: The malignant cells show strong positivity to vimentin and focal patchy positivity to CD68, a nonspecific marker of fibrohistiocytic differentiation. S100 expression was negative.

primary mesenteric neoplasms are desmoid tumours, usually in patients with familial adenomatous polyposis (Gardner syndrome), occurring in 9 to 18% of patients [1]. Other primary mesenteric tumours are very uncommon and include lipomas, schwannomas, smooth muscle tumours (both gastrointestinal stromal tumours and leiomyomas), and other sarcomas, both low and high grade [1, 2].

In our case, we report a primary mesenteric undifferentiated high-grade pleomorphic sarcoma (UPS). UPS, previously known as a malignant fibrous histiocytoma, is defined as a high-grade pleomorphic neoplasm with no identifiable lines of differentiation using currently available diagnostic techniques [3] and accounts for up to 20% of all soft-tissue sarcomas, although, with better diagnostic techniques, this frequency is expected to fall in the future. Although the cells of origin are currently unknown, gene expression profiling and functional analysis suggest that mesenchymal stem cells may be the precursors of UPS [4]. It usually appears in the deep soft tissues of older patients, with a special predilection for the extremities, followed by the trunk and in the subcutaneous tissues [5]. Men are more affected than women. Abdominal presentations are less common and usually affect retroperitoneal structures. Less than 20 cases of primary mesenteric UPS, as was our case, have been described in the medical literature [1, 2, 6–12].

In our patient, the clinical presentation was a locally advanced primary colonic tumour, due to the presence of fungating tumours in the colonic lumen secondary to the primary tumour invasion, a rare occurrence. The CT appearance was similar to that in other published cases and showed a well-circumscribed soft-tissue mass, with hypodense areas

due to necrosis and cystic degeneration [10, 11]. However, we did not observe eccentrically located lumpy and ring calcifications due to osteoid and chondroid metaplasia, a finding found in other cases of abdominal UPS [10, 11]. There were air bubbles in the tumour due to the colonic invasion, which confounded the radiological diagnosis.

Histologically, tumours are composed of a haphazard, storiform, or fascicular arrangement of highly pleomorphic and spindle-shaped cells with numerous typical or atypical mitosis; areas with necrosis and hemorrhage are frequent. In our case, the stroma had an important inflammatory component and the final diagnosis is UPS with prominent inflammation [3, 5, 13, 14]. As defined, there is neither reproducible immunophenotype nor any pattern of protein expression that would allow a more specific subclassification. Usually, as was our case, only vimentin is convincingly positive [13]. We observed focal positivity for CD68, a marker of fibrohistiocytic differentiation, although its specificity is poor. Karyotypes are usually highly complex and nonspecific [3]. As such, it is a diagnosis of exclusion and should be used only when all efforts to identify a specific line of differentiation have failed and when pleomorphic variants of other tumours such as poorly differentiated carcinoma, melanoma, or lymphoma have been excluded. In our case, after extensive sampling and the use of immunohistochemistry, all nonsarcoma markers were negative and we did not identify foci with neurogenic or myogenic features (leiomyosarcoma-rhabdomyosarcoma or malignant peripheral nerve sheath tumours), lipoblasts (pleomorphic liposarcoma), contiguous foci of well-differentiated liposarcoma (dedifferentiated liposarcoma), or areas with myxoid stroma and curvilineal vessels (myxofibrosarcoma).

Although numbers are limited, most reports suggest that intra-abdominal UPS is a rare but aggressive tumour, the prognosis of which is poorer than that seen in tumours in the extremities, due presumably to late detection [6–10]. Tumour size is the major prognostic factor alongside high grade [3, 4]. Wide surgical resection with free margins is the primary therapeutic modality of choice [4, 15]. The use of adjuvant radiotherapy is controversial in the abdominal cavity, compared to limb presentations, and is not routinely used, although neoadjuvant radiotherapy may be considered in locally advanced retroperitoneal tumours in order to achieve a radical resection [15].

Adjuvant chemotherapy with the combination of anthracyclines-ifosfamide is also controversial and was not offered in our patient's case due to his advanced age. Unfortunately, although the tumour was completely resected with clear margins, our patient developed local and systemic recurrence with rapid progression after one month of surgery, with little effect of the palliative chemotherapy given. He died six months after the original diagnosis, highlighting the extremely aggressive nature of the tumour.

References

[1] S. Sheth, K. M. Horton, M. R. Garland, and E. K. Fishman, "Mesenteric neoplasms: CT appearances of primary and secondary tumors and differential diagnosis," *Radiographics*, vol. 23, no. 2, pp. 457–473, 2003.

[2] J. S. Liles, C.-W. D. Tzeng, J. J. Short, P. Kulesza, and M. J. Heslin, "Retroperitoneal and intra-abdominal sarcoma," *Current Problems in Surgery*, vol. 46, no. 6, pp. 445–503, 2009.

[3] "Undifferentiated/unclassified sarcomas," in *WHO Classification of Tumours of Soft Tissue and Bones*, C. D. M. Fletcher, J. A. Bridge, P. C. W. Hogendoorn, and F. Mertens, Eds., IARC, Lyon, France, 2013.

[4] G. K. Zagars, J. R. Mullen, and A. Pollack, "Malignant fibrous histiocytoma: outcome and prognostic factors following conservation surgery and radiotherapy," *International Journal of Radiation Oncology Biology Physics*, vol. 34, no. 5, pp. 983–994, 1996.

[5] M. T. Henderson and S. T. Hollmig, "Malignant fibrous histiocytoma: changing perceptions and management challenges," *Journal of the American Academy of Dermatology*, vol. 67, no. 6, pp. 1335–1341, 2012.

[6] K. S. Atmatzidis, T. E. Pavlidis, I. N. Galanis, B. T. Papaziogas, and T. B. Papaziogas, "Malignant fibrous histiocytoma of the abdominal cavity: report of a case," *Surgery Today*, vol. 33, no. 10, pp. 794–796, 2003.

[7] A. Agaimy, A. Gaumann, J. Schroeder et al., "Primary and metastatic high-grade pleomorphic sarcoma/malignant fibrous histiocytoma of the gastrointestinal tract: an approach to the differential diagnosis in a series of five cases with emphasis on myofibroblastic differentiation," *Virchows Archiv*, vol. 451, no. 5, pp. 949–957, 2007.

[8] J. H. Kweon, C. S. Choi, C. J. Im, G. S. Seo, and S. C. Choi, "Malignant fibrous histiocytoma arising from the omentum presenting as hemoperitoneum," *Gut and Liver*, vol. 4, no. 2, pp. 241–244, 2010.

[9] N. S. Salemis, S. Gourgiotis, E. Tsiambas, N. Panagiotopoulos, A. Karameris, and E. Tsohataridis, "Primary intra-abdominal malignant fibrous histiocytoma: a highly aggressive tumor," *Journal of Gastrointestinal Cancer*, vol. 41, no. 4, pp. 238–242, 2010.

[10] B. Karki, Y. K. Xu, Y. K. Wu, and W. W. Zhang, "Primary malignant fibrous histiocytoma of the abdominal cavity: CT findings and pathological correlation," *World Journal of Radiology*, vol. 4, no. 4, pp. 151–158, 2012.

[11] S.-F. Ko, Y.-L. Wan, T.-Y. Lee, S.-H. Ng, J.-W. Lin, and W.-J. Chen, "CT Features of calcifications in abdominal malignant fibrous histiocytoma," *Clinical Imaging*, vol. 22, no. 6, pp. 408–413, 1998.

[12] S. M. Goldman, D. S. Hartman, and S. W. Weiss, "The varied radiographic manifestations of retroperitoneal malignant fibrous histiocytoma revealed through 27 cases," *Journal of Urology*, vol. 135, no. 1, pp. 33–38, 1986.

[13] J. R. Goldblum, "An approach to pleomorphic sarcomas: can we subclassify, and does it matter?" *Modern Pathology*, vol. 27, no. 1, pp. S39–S46, 2014.

[14] I. Matushansky, E. Charytonowicz, J. Mills, S. Siddiqi, T. Hricik, and C. Cordon-Cardo, "MFH classification: differentiating undifferentiated pleomorphic sarcoma in the 21st century," *Expert Review of Anticancer Therapy*, vol. 9, no. 8, pp. 1135–1144, 2009.

[15] A. F. Nascimento and C. P. Raut, "Diagnosis and management of pleomorphic sarcomas (so-called 'MFH') in adults," *Journal of Surgical Oncology*, vol. 97, no. 4, pp. 330–339, 2008.

6

Dysphagia and Neck Swelling in a Case of Undiagnosed Lhermitte-Duclos Disease and Cowden Syndrome

Zishuo Ian Hu,[1] Lev Bangiyev,[2] Roberta J. Seidman,[3] and Jules A. Cohen[4]

[1]Department of Medicine, Mount Sinai St. Luke's Roosevelt Hospital Center, New York, NY 10019, USA
[2]Department of Radiology, Stony Brook University Medical Center, Stony Brook, NY 11794, USA
[3]Department of Pathology, Stony Brook University Medical Center, Stony Brook, NY 11794, USA
[4]Division of Hematology/Oncology, Department of Medicine, Stony Brook University Medical Center, Stony Brook, NY 11794, USA

Correspondence should be addressed to Zishuo Ian Hu; ian.hu6@gmail.com

Academic Editor: Raffaele Palmirotta

We report a case of a 37-year-old woman presenting with dysphagia and thyroid masses who was subsequently diagnosed with Lhermitte-Duclos disease (LDD) based on MRI scan and histopathology. Additional imaging subsequently revealed the presence of thyroid nodules and bilateral breast cancers. Genetic testing later confirmed the diagnosis of Cowden syndrome. This case illustrates the importance of the overlap between LDD, Cowden syndrome, thyroid disease, and breast cancer.

1. Introduction

Somatic mutations in the phosphate and tensin homologue deleted on chromosome 10 (*PTEN*) gene have been implicated in a number of human cancers, including those of the breast, endometrium, skin, and prostate [1, 2]. PTEN predominantly functions as a tumor suppressor through its role in the phosphatidylinositol 3-kinase (PI3K) pathway [3]. By regulating PI3K signaling, PTEN inhibits the recruitment of Akt, influencing cell survival, growth, and proliferation.

Germline mutations in PTEN manifest as PTEN hamartoma tumor syndromes (PHTS), a spectrum of syndromes which includes Cowden syndrome, Bannayan-Riley-Ruvalcaba syndrome, Proteus syndrome, and Proteus-like Syndrome [4]. Cowden syndrome is an autosomal dominant syndrome characterized by multiorgan hamartomas affecting all three germ layers. Adult dysplastic gangliocytoma of the cerebellum, or Lhermitte-Duclos disease (LDD), is considered a major criterion for diagnosis of Cowden syndrome. Here, we report a case of LDD in a patient with Cowden syndrome.

2. Case Report

A 37-year-old East Asian woman presented with 3 days of dysphagia and 2 months of bilateral neck swelling. She denied any nausea, vomiting, headache, or gait disturbances.

The patient's family history was unknown as she was adopted. The patient's medical history was significant for bipolar disorder. On physical exam, patient was alert and oriented and cranial nerves were found to be intact. Palpable, nontender masses in the anterior neck were appreciated on head and neck examination. A mobile, nontender, 1 cm lump was also present on the left breast.

CT, MRI, and fine needle aspiration of the thyroid masses revealed bilateral nonmalignant nodules measuring 1.9 cm and 1.7 cm on the right side and 2.2 cm and 2.3 cm on the left (Figure 1). The nodules abutted the esophagus bilaterally.

MRI of the head revealed mild hydrocephalus and a right 3.8 cm cerebellar mass with a "tiger-stripe" appearance consistent with LDD (Figure 2). Total resection of the lesion was performed and histopathologic evaluation confirmed the diagnosis (Figure 3).

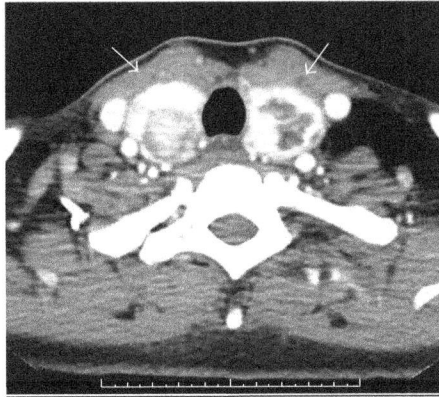

FIGURE 1: Axial postcontrast CT image through the thyroid gland demonstrates enlarged thyroid lobes that contain heterogeneously enhancing nodules bilaterally.

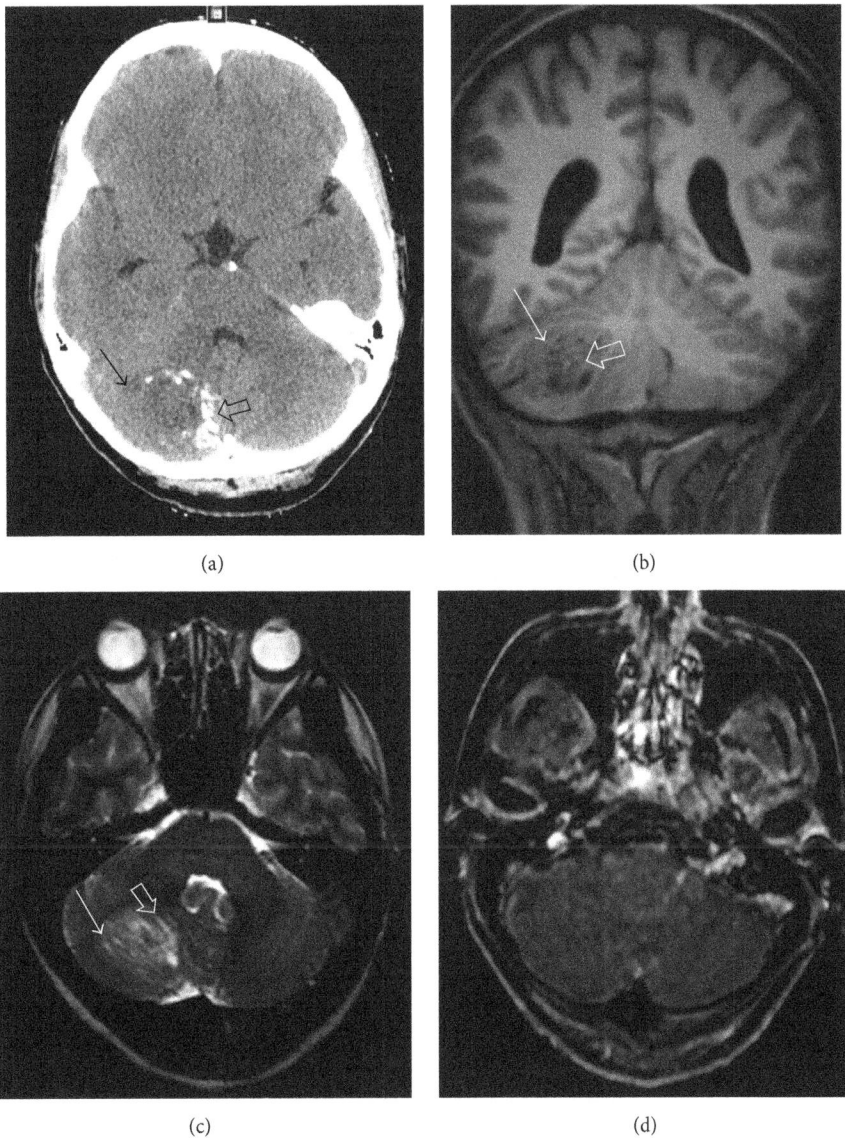

(a)

(b)

(c)

(d)

FIGURE 2: Noncontrast head CT (a) demonstrates a slightly hypodense (solid arrow) mass with calcifications (open arrow) centered in the right cerebellum. MRI of the brain demonstrates the typical striated-appearing right cerebellar mass with alternating isointense (solid arrow) and hypointense (open arrow) striations on coronal precontrast T_1 weighted image (b) and isointense (solid arrow) and hyperintense (open arrow) signal on axial T_2 weighted image (c). There is no appreciable enhancement of the mass on postcontrast axial T_1 weighted image (d).

(a) (b) (c)

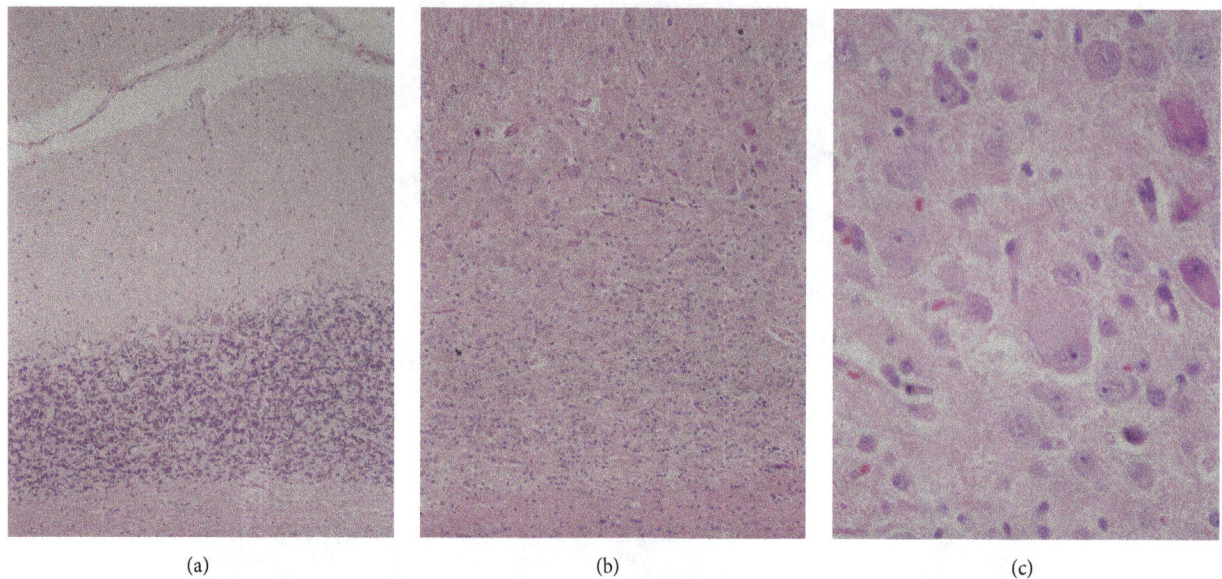

FIGURE 3: The surgical resection specimen includes a region of almost normal cerebellar parenchyma (a), with a normal granule cell layer that consists of fairly densely packed small neurons that are seen as blue nuclei separated by synaptic zones that are pink. The normal single layer of large Purkinje cells is located at the interface with the low cellularity molecular layer, here minimally more cellular than usual. Compare this with the images of the lesion (b and c). (b) The cerebellar granule cell layer in this region of the lesion is dysmorphic. Granule cells are scant and dispersed among ganglionic cells of varying sizes that expand this layer. (c) Detail of a region featured in upper right quadrant of panel (b) highlights the variable size of the abnormal ganglionic neurons characterized by relatively abundant cytoplasm and large nuclei with prominent nucleoli, some with abnormal irregularly shaped nuclei, that replace and expand the granule cell layer (hematoxylin and eosin paraffin sections; original magnifications: (a) 100x, (b) 200x, and (c) 400x).

Mammogram, MRI, and core biopsy of the breasts were also performed, which showed bilateral invasive ductal carcinoma. The patient subsequently underwent bilateral mastectomy. Histology revealed a 0.8 cm invasive ductal carcinoma of the right breast (T1bN0), estrogen positive, progesterone positive, and HER2 negative, and a 1.5 cm invasive ductal carcinoma of the left breast (T1cN0), estrogen positive, progesterone positive, and HER2 negative. Her Oncotype DX breast cancer recurrence score was 24 for her left breast carcinoma, corresponding with a 15% risk of distant recurrence over 10 years. She was given 4 doses of Taxotere and Cytoxan. The patient declined tamoxifen therapy.

Genetic testing results confirmed the presence of the R335X (c.1003C>T) mutation in the PTEN gene and the patient was diagnosed with Cowden syndrome. The patient also chose to undergo risk-reducing thyroidectomy and hysterectomy with bilateral salpingectomy.

3. Discussion

Lhermitte and Duclos originally reported LDD in a 36-year-old man suffering from occipital headaches and diminished hearing on the left side in 1920 [5]. LDD is a hamartomatous overgrowth of the cerebellum that causes a mass effect in the posterior fossa. Patients typically present with headache, nausea, vomiting, and papilledema [6].

MRI of LDD lesions typically shows a striated appearance with hyperintense/hypointense signal on T_1/T_2 images [7].

Pathologically, LDD is noted for its dysplastic expansion of ganglion cells, leading to replacement of the internal granule cell layer in the cerebellum. Large neuronal cells with vesicular nuclei and prominent nucleoli are usually seen.

Lloyd and Dennis named Cowden syndrome after its first reported patient, Rachel Cowden, in 1963 [8]. About 87% of Cowden syndrome patients have a germline mutation either in the PTEN gene or in its promoter region [9–11]. Individuals with Cowden syndrome are at an increased risk of developing thyroid, breast, and endometrial malignancies [11, 12]. Cowden syndrome patients have a 10% lifetime risk of developing thyroid cancer [13]. Female patients have a 25% to 50% lifetime risk of developing breast cancer and an estimated lifetime risk of 5 to 10% of developing endometrial cancer [14–16]. Estimated lifetime risk for any cancer in PTEN patients has been reported as high as 89% [17].

Due to the high risk of malignancy in Cowden syndrome, the National Comprehensive Cancer Network (NCCN) recommends regular monthly breast self-exams beginning at age 18, semiannual clinical breast exams starting at age 25 or 5 to 10 years earlier than the earliest known breast cancer in the family, and annual mammograms and breast MRI screening starting at age 30–35 years or 5 to 10 years earlier than the earliest known breast cancer in the family for female patients. For women treated for breast cancer, mammography and breast MRI should be done on remaining breast tissue [18]. Annual thyroid ultrasounds should be started at time of diagnosis. Annual random endometrial biopsies or ultrasound starting at age 30–35 years are recommended for women with Cowden syndrome. In addition, colonoscopy is recommended starting at age 35 at 5-year intervals, or more often frequently when patients are symptomatic or polyps are present. Renal ultrasound can be given every one or two years after the age of 40.

A 2007 literature review found 53 reported cases of LDD associated with Cowden syndrome [19]. Derrey et al. reported a mean age of 36.7 years at the diagnosis of LDD in Cowden syndrome patients [20]. Our patient was 37 years old on presentation and found to have LDD, thyroid nodules, and bilateral breast cancers. The delay in diagnosis for our patient was likely due to underrecognition of Cowden syndrome in the clinical setting. The incidence of Cowden syndrome has been reported to be 1 in 200,000 and likely to be underestimated due to its variable expression.

Symptomatic LDD patients are recommended to have surgical resection. Thyroid cancer has the earlier onset and second greatest cumulative lifetime risks compared with other Cowden syndrome-associated malignancies [21]. For selecting patients with Cowden syndrome, including patients with developmental disorders, patients difficult to monitor routinely, and patients who have nodules and are aware of the risks and benefits of the procedure, prophylactic total thyroidectomy may be considered. Prophylactic hysterectomy should be discussed with the patient on a case-to-case basis.

References

[1] J. Li, C. Yen, D. Liaw et al., "PTEN, a putative protein tyrosine phosphatase gene mutated in human brain, breast, and prostate cancer," *Science*, vol. 275, no. 5308, pp. 1943–1947, 1997.

[2] I. U. Ali, L. M. Schriml, and M. Dean, "Mutational spectra of PTEN/MMAC1 gene: a tumor suppressor with lipid phosphatase activity," *Journal of the National Cancer Institute*, vol. 91, no. 22, pp. 1922–1932, 1999.

[3] T. Maehama and J. E. Dixon, "The tumor suppressor, PTEN/MMAC1, dephosphorylates the lipid second messenger, phosphatidylinositol 3,4,5-trisphosphate," *The Journal of Biological Chemistry*, vol. 273, no. 22, pp. 13375–13378, 1998.

[4] G. M. Blumenthal and P. A. Dennis, "PTEN hamartoma tumor syndromes," *European Journal of Human Genetics*, vol. 16, no. 11, pp. 1289–1300, 2008.

[5] J. Lhermitte and P. Duclos, "Sur un ganglioneurome diffus du cortex du cervelet," *Bulletin de l'Association Française pour l'Étude du Cancer*, vol. 9, pp. 99–107, 1920.

[6] D. A. Nowak and H. A. Trost, "Lhermitte-Duclos disease (dysplastic cerebellar gangliocytoma): a malformation, hamartoma or neoplasm?" *Acta Neurologica Scandinavica*, vol. 105, no. 3, pp. 137–145, 2002.

[7] K. Kulkantrakorn, E. E. Awwad, B. Levy et al., "MRI in lhermitte-duclos disease," *Neurology*, vol. 48, no. 3, pp. 725–731, 1997.

[8] K. M. Lloyd II and M. Dennis, "Cowden's disease. A possible new symptom complex with multiple system involvement," *Annals of Internal Medicine*, vol. 58, pp. 136–142, 1963.

[9] D. J. Marsh, V. Coulon, K. L. Lunetta et al., "Mutation spectrum and genotype-phenotype analyses in Cowden disease and Bannayan-Zonana syndrome, two hamartoma syndromes with germline PTEN mutation," *Human Molecular Genetics*, vol. 7, no. 3, pp. 507–515, 1998.

[10] X.-P. Zhou, K. A. Waite, R. Pilarski et al., "Germline PTEN promoter mutations and deletions in Cowden/Bannayan-Riley-Ruvalcaba syndrome result in aberrant PTEN protein and dysregulation of the phosphoinositol-3-kinase/Akt pathway," *The American Journal of Human Genetics*, vol. 73, no. 2, pp. 404–411, 2003.

[11] D. Liaw, D. J. Marsh, J. Li et al., "Germline mutations of the PTEN gene in Cowden disease, an inherited breast and thyroid cancer syndrome," *Nature Genetics*, vol. 16, no. 1, pp. 64–67, 1997.

[12] J. I. Risinger, A. K. Hayes, A. Berchuck, and J. C. Barrett, "PTEN/MMAC1 mutations in endometrial cancers," *Cancer Research*, vol. 57, no. 21, pp. 4736–4738, 1997.

[13] C. Eng, "PTEN: one gene, many syndromes," *Human Mutation*, vol. 22, no. 3, pp. 183–198, 2003.

[14] T. M. Starink, J. P. van der Veen, F. Arwert et al., "The Cowden syndrome: a clinical and genetic study in 21 patients," *Clinical Genetics*, vol. 29, no. 3, pp. 222–233, 1986.

[15] M. H. Brownstein, M. Wolf, and J. B. Bikowski, "Cowden's disease: a cutaneous marker of breast cancer," *Cancer*, vol. 41, no. 6, pp. 2393–2398, 1978.

[16] R. Pilarski and C. Eng, "Will the real Cowden syndrome please stand up (again)? Expanding mutational and clinical spectra of the PTEN hamartoma tumour syndrome," *Journal of Medical Genetics*, vol. 41, no. 5, pp. 323–326, 2004.

[17] D. L. Riegert-Johnson, F. C. Gleeson, M. Roberts et al., "Cancer and Lhermitte-Duclos disease are common in Cowden syndrome patients," *Hereditary Cancer in Clinical Practice*, vol. 8, no. 1, article 6, 2010.

[18] National Comprehensive Cancer Network, *Genetic/Familial High-Risk Assessment: Breast and Ovarian. Clinical Practice Guidelines in Oncology*, National Comprehensive Cancer Network, Fort Washington, Pa, USA, 2015.

[19] T.-C. Tan and L.-C. Ho, "Lhermitte-Duclos disease associated with Cowden syndrome," *Journal of Clinical Neuroscience*, vol. 14, no. 8, pp. 801–805, 2007.

[20] S. Derrey, F. Proust, B. Debono et al., "Association between Cowden syndrome and Lhermitte-Duclos disease: report of two cases and review of the literature," *Surgical Neurology*, vol. 61, no. 5, pp. 447–454, 2004.

[21] M. Milas, J. Mester, R. Metzger et al., "Should patients with Cowden syndrome undergo prophylactic thyroidectomy?" *Surgery*, vol. 152, no. 6, pp. 1201–1210, 2012.

7

Left Vocal Cord Paralysis Detected by PET/CT in a Case of Lung Cancer

Ali Ozan Oner,[1] **Adil Boz,**[2] **Evrim Surer Budak,**[3] **and Gulnihal Hale Kaplan Kurt**[4]

[1]*Nuclear Medicine Department, School of Medicine, Afyon Kocatepe University, 03200 Afyon, Turkey*
[2]*Nuclear Medicine Department, School of Medicine, Akdeniz University, 07070 Antalya, Turkey*
[3]*Nuclear Medicine Department, Antalya Training and Research Hospital, Antalya, Turkey*
[4]*Nuclear Medicine Department, Isparta State Hospital, Isparta, Turkey*

Correspondence should be addressed to Adil Boz; boz@akdeniz.edu.tr

Academic Editor: Jose I. Mayordomo

We report a patient with lung cancer. The first PET/CT imaging revealed hypermetabolic mass in the left aortopulmonary region and hypermetabolic nodule in the anterior segment of the upper lobe of the left lung. After completing chemotherapy and radiotherapy against the primary mass in the left lung, the patient underwent a second PET/CT examination for evaluation of treatment response. This test demonstrated, compared with the first PET/CT, an increase in the size and metabolic activity of the primary mass in the left lung in addition to multiple, pathologic-sized, hypermetabolic metastatic lymph nodes as well as multiple metastatic sclerotic areas in bones. These findings were interpreted as progressive disease. In addition, an asymmetrical FDG uptake was noticed at the level of right vocal cord. During follow-up, a laryngoscopy was performed, which demonstrated left vocal cord paralysis with no apparent mass. Thus, we attributed the paralytic appearance of the left vocal cord to infiltration of the left recurrent laryngeal nerve by the primary mass located in the apical region of the left lung. In conclusion, the knowledge of this pitfall is important to avoid false-positive PET results.

1. Introduction

Vocal cord paralysis occurs due to pathologies of the nerves that innervate vocal cords. The nerves that make vocal cords vibrate consist of neurons originating from the region of nucleus ambiguus in the brainstem. The nerve arising from the nucleus is called the "vagus nerve," which is the thickest nerve in the human body and extends to thoracic and abdominal cavities [1]. The nerve gives off 2 thin branches for larynx at the base of the skull. The first one is called the "superior laryngeal nerve" and the second one is called the "recurrent laryngeal nerve (RLN)." The latter conveys orders to both opening and closure muscles. The problems in that nerve cause paralysis of both opening and closure muscles, leading to loss of their basic functions. Hence, respiratory difficulty and hoarseness and aspiration problems due to failure of closure arise. Problems of superior laryngeal nerve, on the other hand, become manifest, with a monotonous, thin voice as well as difficulty in tone control and singing songs.

Causes of Vocal Cord Paralysis:

  (i) Idiopathic diseases.

 (ii) Viral neuritis.

(iii) Masses, tumors compressing vocal nerves in brain, base of the skull, neck, thyroid region, and thoracic cavity.

(iv) Surgical interventions (especially thyroid surgery).

 (v) Being secondary to intubation in certain surgical operations [1].

^{18}F-fluorodeoxyglucose positron emission tomography/computed tomography (^{18}FDG-PET/CT) scans are utilized for identification of stage cancers clinically but the causes of false-positive and false-negative results must be identified to evaluate the results of the test. As a result of the increased glucose consumption, FDG accumulates in benign and malignant conditions. The degree of muscle work is

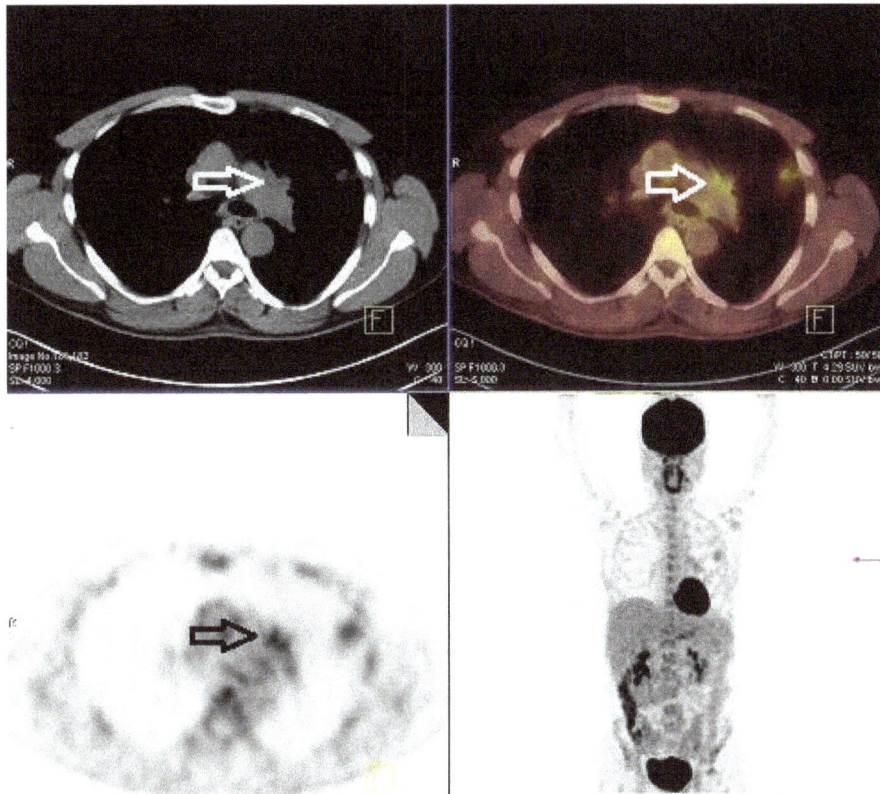

FIGURE 1: First PET/CT: axial CT, pet, fused PET/CT, and coronal MIP images revealed a hypermetabolic mass (arrows) in the left aortopulmonary region and hypermetabolic nodule in the anterior segment of the upper lobe of the left lung.

directly commensurate with the amount of glucose being dealt with [2].

The lack of FDG activity in the paralyzed cord and compensatory activation of the nonparalyzed vocal cord causes asymmetric FDG uptake seen in vocal cord paralysis. In vocal cord paralysis, workload of the nonparalyzed cord increases and so glucose consumption increases which is seen as a focal hotspot on FDG PET images [3].

We report a case of lung cancer in a patient with a false-positive PET scan in the larynx due to increased workload of the right vocal cord as it compensates for the paralyzed left vocal cord.

2. Case History

A 46-year-old man presented to Faculty of Medicine, Akdeniz University, with dyspnea, cough, and sputum. He was diagnosed with small cell lung cancer as a result of examination of a left lung biopsy. The first PET/CT imaging dating revealed hypermetabolic mass in the left aortopulmonary region and hypermetabolic nodule in the anterior segment of the upper lobe of the left lung (Figure 1).

After completing chemotherapy and radiotherapy against the primary mass in the left lung, the patient underwent a second PET/CT examination for evaluation of treatment response. It revealed, compared with the first PET/CT, an increase in the size and metabolic activity of the primary mass

in the left lung, multiple, pathologic-sized, hypermetabolic metastatic lymph nodes (Figure 2), and multiple metastatic sclerotic areas in bones, consistent with progression of disease.

In addition, an asymmetrical FDG uptake was noticed at the level of right vocal cord (Figure 3). During follow-up, the patient was sent for laryngoscopy, which demonstrated left vocal cord paralysis with no apparent mass. Thus, we considered that the paralytic appearance of the left vocal cord may have been due to infiltration of the left recurrent laryngeal nerve by the primary mass observed in the apical region of the left lung. The asymmetrical FDG uptake in the right vocal cord was attributed to overactivity of right vocal cord muscles to compensate left vocal cord paralysis.

3. Discussion

In the course of PET/CT scans, the patient must rest in silence, without any movement during the uptake period of FDG. After injection of isotope, if the patient coughs, talks, or chews, we can see a normal glucose uptake by larynx, tongue, and pharyngeal musculature. Generally this uptake is symmetric and can be intense, moderate, or mild [4].

The suspicion of a primary neoplastic or inflammatory cord pathology should be always enhanced by asymmetric increased FDG uptake. In identifying primary and recurrent laryngeal cancer, FDG PET has been found to be useful [5, 6].

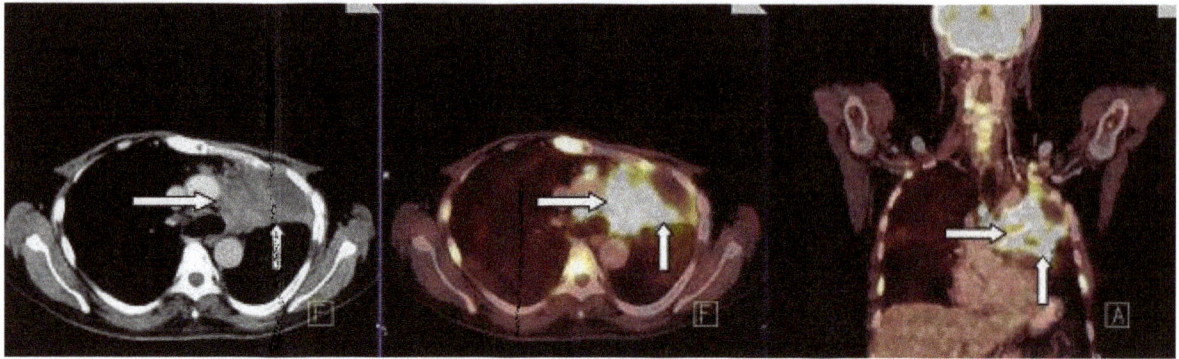

FIGURE 2: Second PET/CT: axial CT, axial PET/CT, and coronal PET/CT images revealed an increase in the size and metabolic activity of the primary mass in the left lung and mediastinal lymph nodes (arrows) when we compared with first PET/CT images.

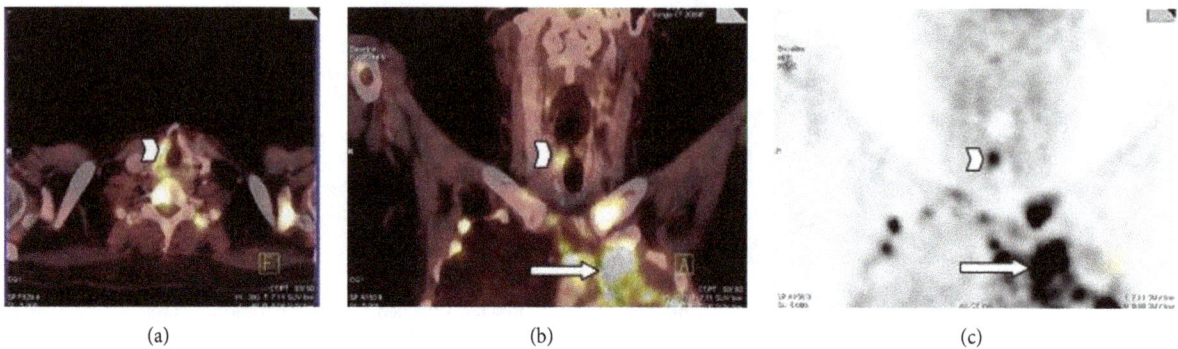

(a)   (b)   (c)

FIGURE 3: Second PET/CT: (a) transverse, (b) coronal PET/CT fusion, and (c) coronal PET images show intense FDG uptake in the left lung tumor (arrow) and in the right vocal cord (arrowhead).

Asymmetric increased uptake can be observed due to impaired movement or paralysis of the contralateral vocal cord [7–11]. When there is incidental detection of asymmetric vocal cord activity, the clinical history often helps us. An evolution of prior surgery, hoarseness, or intervention in the thyroid, larynx, neck, or mediastinum are marks to indicate injury of one of the recurrent laryngeal nerves. Laryngoscopic examination will help us to see impaired movement or paralysis of the contralateral vocal cord and, at the same time, we can also see if there is a primary pathology in the ipsilateral cord [3].

Symmetric vocal cord uptake is the possibility of physiologic, either in patients with normal resting cords or in patients vocalizing at or soon after FDG injection. If there is asymmetric FDG uptake in vocal cord activity in an oncology patient, we should suspect for RLN palsy. Pathologies being found throughout the course of the recurrent laryngeal nerves, such as enlarged lymph nodes or masses in the root of the neck or the mediastinum, can infiltrate the nerves which trigger vocal cord paralysis.

Vocal cord paralysis is more common due to left recurrent laryngeal nerve infiltration than right recurrent laryngeal nerve infiltration. This is because the left recurrent laryngeal nerve has a longer anatomical pathway and passes through the aortopulmonary window. Kamel et al., in a study on 184 patients with lung cancer, reported 6 cases of vocal cord paralysis, all of which were due to infiltration of left recurrent laryngeal nerve [11].

However, there are also cases of vocal cord paralysis due to right recurrent laryngeal nerve paralysis in the literature. Purandare et al. reported a hypermetabolic metastatic lymph node of pathologic size at level 4 in neck in a patient with esophagus cancer. They reported that that lymph node infiltrated and paralyzed right recurrent laryngeal nerve and led to asymmetrical FDG uptake [3].

Minamimoto et al., in a study in 59 patients with vocal cord paralysis, observed that the asymmetrical FDG uptake was on the ipsilateral side with the lesion when the primary lesion was in laryngeal region whereas on the contralateral side with the lesion when the lesion infiltrated recurrent laryngeal nerve. Both conditions in that study were characterized by a significant difference in maximum standardized uptake values (SUVmax) of FDG uptake in vocal cords [12].

4. Conclusion

In this case, PET/CT images demonstrated that the focal FDG uptake was localized in the right vocal cord muscles. This focal FDG uptake was a result of increased workload of vocal cord muscles caused by contralateral RLN palsy due to direct nerve invasion by lung cancer of the left lung apices. The knowledge of this pitfall is important to avoid false-positive PET results.

References

[1] M. Komissarova, K. K. Wong, M. Piert, S. K. Mukherji, and L. M. Fig, "Spectrum of18F-FDG PET/CT findings in oncology-related recurrent laryngeal nerve palsy," *American Journal of Roentgenology*, vol. 192, no. 1, pp. 288–294, 2009.

[2] T. Fujimoto, M. Itoh, M. Tashiro, K. Yamaguchi, K. Kubota, and H. Ohmori, "Glucose uptake by individual skeletal muscles during running using whole-body positron emission tomography," *European Journal of Applied Physiology*, vol. 83, no. 4-5, pp. 297–302, 2000.

[3] N. C. Purandare, V. Rangarajan, and S. Shah, "Case report: right vocal cord paralysis detected by PET/CT in a case of esophageal cancer," *Indian Journal of Radiology and Imaging*, vol. 17, no. 3, pp. 166–168, 2007.

[4] L. Kostakoglu, J. C. H. Wong, S. F. Barrington, B. F. Cronin, A. M. Dynes, and M. N. Maisey, "Speech-related visualization of laryngeal muscles with fluorine-18-FDG," *Journal of Nuclear Medicine*, vol. 37, no. 11, pp. 1771–1773, 1996.

[5] V. J. Lowe, H. Kim, J. H. Boyd, J. F. Elsenbeis, F. R. Dunphy, and J. W. Fletcher, "Primary and recurrent early stage laryngeal cancer: preliminary results of 2-[fluorine 18]fluoro-2-deoxy-D-glucose pet imaging," *Radiology*, vol. 212, no. 3, pp. 799–802, 1999.

[6] M. T. Truong, J. J. Erasmus, H. A. Macapinlac, and D. A. Podoloff, "Teflon injection for vocal cord paralysis: false-positive finding on FDG PET-CT in a patient with non-small cell lung cancer," *American Journal of Roentgenology*, vol. 182, no. 6, pp. 1587–1589, 2004.

[7] M. T. Heller, C. C. Meltzer, M. B. Fukui et al., "Superphysiologic FDG uptake in the non-paralyzed vocal cord. Resolution of a false-positive PET result with combined PET-CT imaging," *Clinical Positron Imaging*, vol. 3, no. 5, pp. 207–211, 2000.

[8] I. Igerc, G. Kumnig, M. Heinisch et al., "Vocal cord muscle activity as a drawback to FDG-PET in the followup of differentiated thyroid cancer," *Thyroid*, vol. 12, no. 1, pp. 87–89, 2002.

[9] B. B. Chin, P. Patel, and D. Hammoud, "Combined positron emission tomography-computed tomography improves specificity for thyroid carcinoma by identifying vocal cord activity after laryngeal nerve paralysis," *Thyroid*, vol. 13, no. 12, pp. 1183–1184, 2003.

[10] M. Lee, D. L. Lilien, M. R. Ramaswamy, and C.-A. O. Nathan, "Unilateral vocal cord paralysis causes contralateral false-positive positron emission tomography scans of the larynx," *Annals of Otology, Rhinology and Laryngology*, vol. 114, no. 3, pp. 202–206, 2005.

[11] E. M. Kamel, G. W. Goerres, C. Burger, G. K. Von Schulthess, and H. C. Steinert, "Recurrent laryngeal nerve palsy in patients with lung cancer: detection with PET-CT image fusion—report of six cases," *Radiology*, vol. 224, no. 1, pp. 153–156, 2002.

[12] R. Minamimoto, K. Kubota, M. Morooka et al., "Reevaluation of FDG-PET/CT in patients with hoarseness caused by vocal cord palsy," *Annals of Nuclear Medicine*, vol. 26, no. 5, pp. 405–411, 2012.

8

Rhabdomyolysis due to Trimethoprim-Sulfamethoxazole Administration following a Hematopoietic Stem Cell Transplant

Alexander Augustyn,[1,2] Mona Lisa Alattar,[2,3] and Harris Naina[2,3]

[1]Hamon Center for Therapeutic Oncology Research, University of Texas Southwestern Medical Center, Dallas, TX 75390, USA
[2]Simmons Comprehensive Cancer Center, University of Texas Southwestern Medical Center, Dallas, TX 75390, USA
[3]Department of Hematology and Oncology, University of Texas Southwestern Medical Center, Dallas, TX 75390, USA

Correspondence should be addressed to Harris Naina; harrisvk2002@yahoo.com

Academic Editor: Marcel W. Bekkenk

Rhabdomyolysis, a syndrome of muscle necrosis, is a life-threatening event. Here we describe the case of a patient with chronic myeloid leukemia who underwent a haploidentical stem cell transplant and subsequently developed rhabdomyolysis after beginning trimethoprim-sulfamethoxazole (TMP/SMX) prophylaxis therapy. Rechallenge with TMP/SMX resulted in a repeat episode of rhabdomyolysis and confirmed the association. Withdrawal of TMP/SMX led to sustained normalization of creatine kinase levels in the patient. A high index of suspicion is necessary to identify TMP/SMX as the cause of rhabdomyolysis in immunocompromised patients.

1. Introduction

Rhabdomyolysis is a potentially life-threatening syndrome of muscle necrosis characterized by the release of intracellular muscle contents into the systemic circulation and can result in significant muscle pain, electrolyte imbalance, acute renal failure, and even death [1, 2]. Many medications, including salicylates, statins, neuroleptics, and fibrates, are associated with rhabdomyolysis although few reports indicate trimethoprim-sulfamethoxazole (TMP/SMX), a commonly used antibiotic, as the culprit [2–8]. Here we describe the case of a patient with blast phase chronic myeloid leukemia and subsequent haploidentical stem cell transplant maintained on dasatinib who developed rhabdomyolysis when concurrent TMP/SMX prophylaxis was initiated.

The classic triad of rhabdomyolysis includes muscle pain, weakness, and dark urine although the presentation can vary from asymptomatic elevations of muscle enzymes to severe muscle pain with acute kidney failure [1, 2]. In addition to characteristic symptoms, about half of patients also present with myoglobinuria, while more severe cases can present with electrolyte imbalances such as hyperkalemia, acute renal failure, and/or swelling of the extremities [9, 10]. The trademark

laboratory diagnosis is an elevation of creatine phosphokinase (CK) to levels 5 times the normal limit, with a range of approximately 1,000 to 100,000 international units per liter (IU) [11].

The association of TMP/SMX with rhabdomyolysis is rare, and most cases have been reported in patients with human immunodeficiency virus (HIV) who receive TMP/SMX as prophylaxis against *Toxoplasma gondii* and prophylaxis or treatment for *Pneumocystis jirovecii* pneumonia (PJP) [3, 4, 6, 7]. TMP/SMX was also reported as the cause of rhabdomyolysis in one patient with CML who subsequently underwent an unrelated donor allogeneic stem cell transplant, developed PJP, and was treated with high-dose TMP/SMX although without concurrent tyrosine kinase inhibitor (TKI) therapy [5]. A diagnosis of rhabdomyolysis was made after the patient developed lactic acidosis, acute renal failure, and hypotension with dramatic elevation of CK levels. Discontinuation of TMP/SMX led to CK normalization within five days [5]. Here, we report the case of a patient with CML and haploidentical stem cell transplant who developed rhabdomyolysis while receiving TMP/SMX for PJP prophylaxis. Discontinuation of all medications resulted in CK normalization while the rechallenge with TMP/SMX caused repeated elevation of CK levels, supporting the diagnosis.

2. Case Presentation

A 28-year-old male with a past medical history significant only for benign hypertension presented at our institution for swelling of the left mandible in 2011. Routine blood work revealed a white blood cell count (WBC) of 298,000 with 2% blasts. Peripheral blood polymerase chain reaction (PCR) was positive for the t(9; 22) BCR-ABL translocation. The patient was started on imatinib after bone marrow biopsy confirmed the diagnosis of chronic myeloid leukemia, chronic phase (CML-CP). He initially achieved a complete hematologic response but six months later was found to have a WBC of 59,000 with 37% blasts and an elevated lactate dehydrogenase. Bone marrow biopsy revealed a mixed phenotype acute leukemia (B-cell/myeloid) most consistent with CML in blast phase. Due to progression on imatinib, he was treated with the R-hyper-CVAD regimen plus dasatinib while awaiting bone marrow transplantation.

Two years later, in January 2013, our patient received a haploidentical transplant and his course was free from graft versus host disease and major infections. He achieved major molecular response and was maintained on dasatinib. Six months after transplantation, his cytopenias resolved, immunosuppressive agents were tapered completely, and he was started on TMP/SMX and valacyclovir prophylaxis. Of note, the patient did not use any herbal remedies.

In September of 2013, the dasatinib dose was increased from 75 mg daily to 100 mg after tacrolimus was discontinued and he received five vaccinations (influenza, TDaP, HepB, Hib, and IPV). Four days later, our patient presented at his usual follow-up clinic visit with complaints of dark urine despite adequate water intake with no diarrhea or other symptoms. He did not report any abnormal exercise routines. Initial laboratory evaluation revealed LDH 3172 international units/L (IU/L), AST 1532 IU/L, and ALT 321 IU/L. The patient's baseline AST and ALT were 22 IU/L and 21 IU/L, respectively, measured three months prior to admission. Immediately, all medications including dasatinib, TMP/SMX, amlodipine, valacyclovir, and pantoprazole were discontinued. CK was found to be markedly elevated at 132,400 IU/L. Fluids were administered and his CK dropped to 76,600 IU/L overnight; he was discharged one day later with CK at 43,700 IU/L along with instructions to avoid strenuous exercise and be followed up closely in the clinic. 11 days later, his CK levels normalized at 502 IU/L and the decision was made to restart dasatinib at 100 mg per day. No other medications were restarted. Four days later, his CK was measured at 301 IU/L, and PJP prophylaxis with TMP/SMX was restarted. One week later, the patient presented for a scheduled laboratory workup and was found to have a CK of 34,300 IU/L but was otherwise asymptomatic, with clear yellow urine.

The patient was admitted and TMP/SMX and dasatinib were once again held, fluids were administered, and his CK levels decreased to 8,300 IU/L when he was discharged two days later. Due to the temporal association of CK elevation

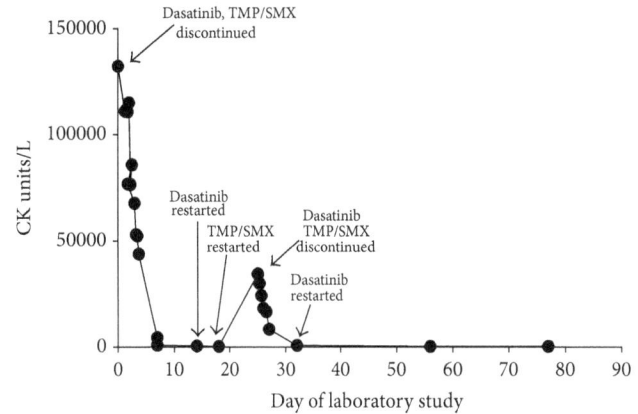

FIGURE 1: Plot of creatine kinase levels versus day of laboratory study. Relationship of creatine kinase levels to medication administration or cessation is indicated by arrows.

following rechallenge with TMP/SMX, the decision was made to not provide prophylaxis for PJP. The patient was continued on valacyclovir and dasatinib. Since TMP/SMX was completely stopped, his CK levels have remained normal (Figure 1). Complete medication dosing and CK, LDH, AST, and ALT levels for both inpatient hospitalizations are provided in Table 1.

3. Discussion

In a study involving 475 patients with rhabdomyolysis, exogenous toxins including medically administered drugs, alcohol, and illicit substances were determined to be the cause in 46% of cases [11]. Prior cases of TMP/SMX-induced rhabdomyolysis have occurred in patients with HIV receiving prophylaxis or treatment for toxoplasmosis or PJP [3, 4, 6, 7]. One prior report detailed rhabdomyolysis in a patient with AML who underwent allogeneic stem cell transplant and developed PJP, necessitating treatment with TMP/SMX [5]. In our patient, before the discovery of TMP/SMX as the likely causative agent of rhabdomyolysis, we considered other etiologies, such as dasatinib, vaccination, or extreme exercise. Dasatinib use has been associated with rare occurrences of rhabdomyolysis (<1% of patients), according to the official drug data sheet, although no case reports currently detail such an association [12]. Vaccines for influenza and TDaP have also been temporally associated with the development of rhabdomyolysis in isolated case reports [13–15]. Based on the Naranjo probability scale of adverse drug reactions, TMP/SMX was the likely causative agent of rhabdomyolysis in our patient with a score of 6 (probable adverse drug reaction) [16]. This was confirmed by rechallenge with TMP/SMX, which resulted in elevation of CK to over 30,000 IU/L.

Several reports implicated imatinib as the cause of rhabdomyolysis. These patients were treated with imatinib for CML and aggressive fibromatosis [17–19]. In each case, withdrawal of imatinib or transition from imatinib to the second-generation tyrosine kinase inhibitor dasatinib resulted in

TABLE 1: Complete medication and dosing history with relevant laboratory values for our patient during first inpatient admission for rhabdomyolysis (September 9, 2013), discharge (September 12, 2013), and outpatient clinic follow-up visit (September 27, 2013). The same information is also presented for the second inpatient admission for rhabdomyolysis (October 3, 2013), discharge (October 6, 2013), and outpatient clinic follow-up visit (October 14, 2013).

	September 9	September 12	September 27	October 3	October 6	October 14
Medications						
Dasatinib	100 mg daily	—	100 mg daily	100 mg daily	100 mg daily	100 mg daily
TMP/SMX	160/800 MWF	—	160/800 MWF	160/800 MWF	—	—
Valacyclovir	500 mg daily	—	—	—	—	500 mg daily
Amlodipine	5 mg daily	—	5 mg daily	5 mg daily	5 mg daily	5 mg daily
Pantoprazole	40 mg daily	—	40 mg daily	40 mg daily	40 mg daily	40 mg daily
Lab values (IU/L)						
CK	132,400	43,700	301	34,308	8,329	285
LDH	3,172	—	203	647	—	210
AST	1,532	978	26	535	198	26
ALT	321	351	28	230	149	37

resolution of rhabdomyolysis. Gordon et al. also identified a high number of CK abnormalities in patients treated with imatinib for CML or gastrointestinal stromal tumors, suggesting that this drug is associated with rare development of severe rhabdomyolysis [19]. However, to date, no report has directly linked dasatinib to rhabdomyolysis, and this remains true in the case of our patient whose CK levels have remained within normal limits on dasatinib maintenance therapy.

Drug-drug interactions such as those identified between cytochrome P450 isoform 3A4 inhibitors and HMG-CoA reductase inhibitors (statins) are known to cause rhabdomyolysis. For example, cotreatment with simvastatin and fluconazole, a known CYP isoenzyme 3A4 (CYP3A4) inhibitor, can cause rhabdomyolysis in patients likely due to elevated plasma levels of simvastatin [20]. Dasatinib is metabolized primarily by CYP3A4 and is a known time-dependent inhibitor of CYP3A4 [12, 21, 22]. TMP/SMX is a potent inhibitor of CYP2C8 and CYP2C9 and also inhibits CYP3A4 at higher concentrations [23]. However, the steady state plasma concentrations of both TMP (approximately 6 μM) and SMX (approximately 270 μM) are below that required to appreciably inhibit CYP3A4 in human cells (over 250 μM for TMP, over 500 μM for SMX, resp.), suggesting that a drug-drug interaction elevating levels of TMP/SMX and/or dasatinib leading to rhabdomyolysis is unlikely [23, 24]. Of course, wide variability exists in cytochrome P450 enzymatic capacity among humans, so this possibility cannot be completely excluded at the present time [25]. The occurrence of drug-drug interactions increases as the number of medications increases and factors such as gastrointestinal absorption, drug distribution, and drug metabolism can enhance this effect [26]. Further study is needed to determine if a drug-drug interaction occurs between dasatinib and TMP/SMX, especially since both drugs are known to modulate CYP family members *in vitro*. If such an interaction is found to occur, pentamidine may be the preferred mode of PJP prophylaxis instead of TMP/SMX in the setting of concurrent TKI usage.

Authors' Contribution

Alexander Augustyn, Mona Lisa Alattar, and Harris Naina analyzed data, obtained funding, and wrote the paper.

Acknowledgments

Alexander Augustyn is supported by the UTSW Medical Scientist Training Program and the Ruth L. Kirschstein National Research Service Award for Individual Predoctoral MD/PhD Fellows (1F30CA168264).

References

[1] F. Y. Khan, "Rhabdomyolysis: a review of the literature," *Netherlands Journal of Medicine*, vol. 67, no. 9, pp. 272–283, 2009.

[2] R. Zutt, A. J. van der Kooi, G. E. Linthorst, R. J. A. Wanders, and M. de Visser, "Rhabdomyolysis: review of the literature," *Neuromuscular Disorders*, vol. 24, no. 8, pp. 651–659, 2014.

[3] S. Walker, J. Norwood, C. Thornton, and D. Schaberg, "Trimethoprim-sulfamethoxazole associated rhabdomyolysis in a patient with AIDS: case report and review of the literature," *The American Journal of the Medical Sciences*, vol. 331, no. 6, pp. 339–341, 2006.

[4] S. J. Singer, J. A. Racoosin, and R. Viraraghavan, "Rhabdomyolysis in human immunodeficiency virus—positive patients taking trimethoprim-sulfamethoxazole," *Clinical Infectious Diseases*, vol. 26, no. 1, pp. 233–234, 1998.

[5] P. J. Kiel, N. Dickmeyer, and J. E. Schwartz, "Trimethoprim-sulfamethoxazole-induced rhabdomyolysis in an allogeneic stem cell transplant patient," *Transplant Infectious Disease*, vol. 12, no. 5, pp. 451–454, 2010.

[6] S. P. Jen and R. Sharma, "Trimethoprim-sulphamethoxazole-associated rhabdomyolysis in an HIV-infected patient," *International Journal of STD and AIDS*, vol. 22, no. 7, pp. 411–412, 2011.

[7] H. J. Anders, J. R. Bogner, and F. D. Goebel, "Mild rhabdomyolysis after high-dose trimethoprim-sulfamethoxazole in a patient with HIV infection," *European Journal of Medical Research*, vol. 2, no. 5, pp. 198–200, 1997.

[8] B. Ainapurapu and U. B. Kanakadandi, "Trimethoprim-sulfamethoxazole induced rhabdomyolysis," *American Journal of Therapeutics*, vol. 21, no. 3, pp. e78–e79, 2014.

[9] J. P. Knochel, "Rhabdomyolysis and myoglobinuria," *Annual Review of Medicine*, vol. 33, pp. 435–443, 1982.

[10] G. D. Giannoglou, Y. S. Chatzizisis, and G. Misirli, "The syndrome of rhabdomyolysis: pathophysiology and diagnosis," *European Journal of Internal Medicine*, vol. 18, no. 2, pp. 90–100, 2007.

[11] G. Melli, V. Chaudhry, and D. R. Cornblath, "Rhabdomyolysis: an evaluation of 475 hospitalized patients," *Medicine*, vol. 84, no. 6, pp. 377–385, 2005.

[12] Y. Fujii, M. Amano, and T. Seriu, "Pharmacological properties and clinical efficacy of dasatinib hydrate (Sprycel), an anticancer drug for chronic myelogenous leukemia and Philadelphia chromosome-positive acute lymphoblastic leukemia," *Nihon Yakurigaku Zasshi*, vol. 134, no. 3, pp. 159–167, 2009.

[13] K. S. Raman, T. Chandrasekar, R. S. Reeve, M. E. Roberts, and P. A. Kalra, "Influenza vaccine-induced rhabdomyolysis leading to acute renal transplant dysfunction," *Nephrology Dialysis Transplantation*, vol. 21, no. 2, pp. 530–531, 2006.

[14] H. Kulkarni, N. Lenzo, and A. McLean-Tooke, "Causality of rhabdomyolysis and combined tetanus, diphtheria and acellular pertussis (Tdap) vaccine administration," *Journal of Clinical Pharmacology*, vol. 53, no. 10, pp. 1099–1102, 2013.

[15] R. B. Callado, T. G. Ponte Carneiro, C. C. Da Cunha Parahyba, N. De Alcantara Lima, G. B. Da Silva Junior, and E. De Francesco Daher, "Rhabdomyolysis secondary to influenza A H1N1 vaccine resulting in acute kidney injury," *Travel Medicine and Infectious Disease*, vol. 11, no. 2, pp. 130–133, 2013.

[16] C. A. Naranjo, U. Busto, and E. M. Sellers, "A method for estimating the probability of adverse drug reactions," *Clinical Pharmacology and Therapeutics*, vol. 30, no. 2, pp. 239–245, 1981.

[17] N. Penel, J.-Y. Blay, and A. Adenis, "Imatinib as a possible cause of severe rhabdomyolysis," *The New England Journal of Medicine*, vol. 358, no. 25, pp. 2746–2747, 2008.

[18] U. Y. Malkan, G. Gunes, S. Etgul, T. Aslan, S. Balaban, and I. C. Haznedaroglu, "Management of de novo CML and imatinib-induced acute rhabdomyolysis with the second-generation TKI, dasatinib," *Annals of Pharmacotherapy*, vol. 49, no. 6, pp. 740–742, 2015.

[19] J. K. Gordon, S. K. Magid, R. G. Maki, M. Fleisher, and E. Berman, "Elevations of creatine kinase in patients treated with imatinib mesylate (Gleevec)," *Leukemia Research*, vol. 34, no. 6, pp. 827–829, 2010.

[20] A. Shaukat, M. Benekli, G. D. Vladutiu, J. L. Slack, M. Wetzler, and M. R. Baer, "Simvastatin-fluconazole causing rhabdomyolysis," *Annals of Pharmacotherapy*, vol. 37, no. 7-8, pp. 1032–1035, 2003.

[21] A. M. Filppula, P. J. Neuvonen, and J. T. Backman, "In vitro assessment of time-dependent inhibitory effects on CYP2C8 and CYP3A activity by fourteen protein kinase inhibitors," *Drug Metabolism and Disposition*, vol. 42, no. 7, pp. 1202–1209, 2014.

[22] J. R. Kenny, S. Mukadam, C. Zhang et al., "Drug-drug interaction potential of marketed oncology drugs: in vitro assessment of time-dependent cytochrome P450 inhibition, reactive metabolite formation and drug-drug interaction prediction," *Pharmaceutical Research*, vol. 29, no. 7, pp. 1960–1976, 2012.

[23] X. Wen, J.-S. Wang, J. T. Backman, J. Laitila, and P. J. Neuvonen, "Trimethoprim and sulfamethoxazole are selective inhibitors of CYP2C8 and CYP2C9, respectively," *Drug Metabolism and Disposition*, vol. 30, no. 6, pp. 631–635, 2002.

[24] R. B. Patel and P. G. Welling, "Clinical pharmacokinetics of co-trimoxazole (trimethoprim-sulphamethoxazole)," *Clinical Pharmacokinetics*, vol. 5, no. 5, pp. 405–423, 1980.

[25] U. M. Zanger and M. Schwab, "Cytochrome P450 enzymes in drug metabolism: regulation of gene expression, enzyme activities, and impact of genetic variation," *Pharmacology and Therapeutics*, vol. 138, no. 1, pp. 103–141, 2013.

[26] C. Palleria, A. Di Paolo, C. Giofrè et al., "Pharmacokinetic drug-drug interaction and their implication in clinical management," *Journal of Research in Medical Sciences*, vol. 18, no. 7, pp. 601–610, 2013.

9

Cutaneous Angiosarcoma of the Foot: A Case Report and Review of the Literature

Sharang Tenjarla,[1] Lucy Ashley Sheils,[2] Theresa M. Kwiatkowski,[1] and Sheema Chawla[1]

[1]*Department of Radiation Oncology, Rochester General Hospital, 1425 Portland Avenue, Rochester, NY 14621, USA*
[2]*Department of Pathology, Rochester General Hospital, 1425 Portland Avenue, Rochester, NY 14621, USA*

Correspondence should be addressed to Sheema Chawla; sheemachawla@gmail.com

Academic Editor: Ossama W. Tawfik

Primary Angiosarcoma of the skin of the foot is very rare. Angiosarcoma is typically treated with resection and wide-field postoperative radiation therapy. Chemotherapy and radiation therapy have also been used. Regardless of the treatment, the risk of local and distant relapse remains high for this disease. We present a case of an elderly patient who developed cutaneous angiosarcoma of the foot. It posed as a diagnostic dilemma at presentation. Chronic lymphedema was a possible predisposing factor. Given his age, preexisting renal dysfunction, refusal of surgery, and preference not to receive chemotherapy, the patient was ultimately treated with definitive radiotherapy. We present this case because of its rare site, unique presentation and delay in diagnosis of the condition, and attainment of an excellent response to radiation at the time of follow-up. We also review the current literature on this topic.

1. Introduction

Angiosarcoma is a rare, malignant neoplasm comprising 1–3% of adult soft tissue sarcomas [1–4]. This is typically a tumor of older individuals with a median age of 70–75 years and a male predominance, having a predilection for the scalp and central area of the face. Cutaneous angiosarcoma is clinically aggressive. The reported 5-year survival rate ranges from 12 to 24% [1, 5]. The neoplasm tends to invade tissue more widely than is clinically apparent and is thus prone to incomplete excision. Majority of patients present with locally advanced disease, regional lymph node involvement, or distant metastases at the time of initial diagnosis, all of which are associated with a poor prognosis [4]. The present study describes a case of cutaneous angiosarcoma of the foot in the setting of chronic lymphedema which was treated with definitive radiation alone. The patient was informed that data from the case would be submitted for publication and he provided the required consent.

2. Case Presentation

A 90-year-old Caucasian gentleman with a past medical history of prostatectomy 20 years ago for prostate cancer, chronic venous insufficiency, and lymphedema since a few years presented to the dermatology office with a nonhealing wound in the left medial foot since a few months. He was initially diagnosed with a fungal infection and was given a 4-week course of antifungal agent and wound dressings, not yielding any response to treatment. Bacterial cultures performed a month later showed mixed infection with aerobic and anaerobic flora. He was then given a course of oral and topical antibiotics for 4 weeks, bearing a minimal response to treatment. In the last 2 months before presentation to the clinic, the lesion progressed. On examination, the epicenter of the lesion was located in the medial aspect of the foot. There were two major areas of ulceration in medial foot measuring approximately 5 × 5 cm that emanated a serosanguinous discharge (Figure 1), with blistering satellite lesions in the medial

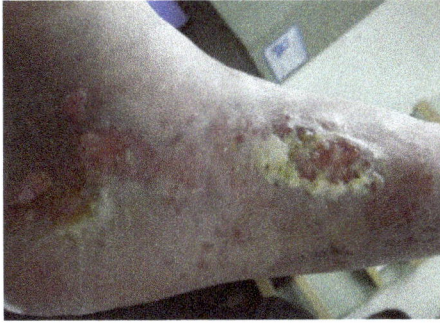

FIGURE 1: Pretreatment: 5 × 5 cm ulcer on the medial left foot emanating a serosanginous discharge and similar ulcer present posteriorly along with blistering satellite lesions on the plantar surface of the foot.

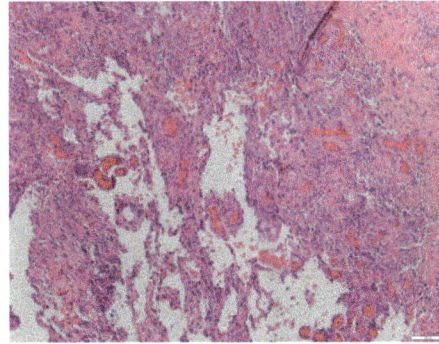

FIGURE 2: Low power view showing extensive spindle cell proliferation involving dermis, subcutis, and deeper fibroadipose tissue.

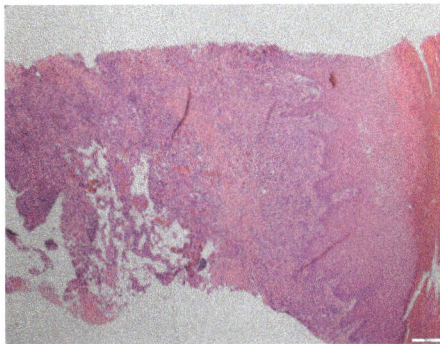

FIGURE 3: High power view showing multiple vascular sinuses lined by tufts of neoplastic endothelial cells.

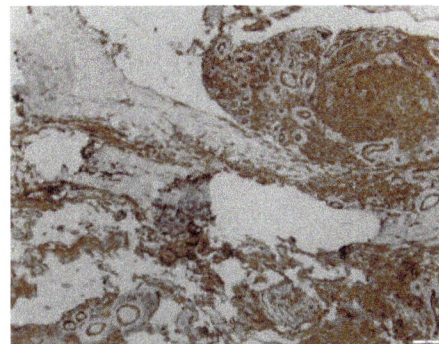

FIGURE 4: Positivity for vascular marker CD-31.

and lateral aspect of the foot. Smaller lesions were also present on the plantar surface of foot. There was nonpitting edema in both extremities. Marked restriction in the movement of the left ankle was noted.

Subsequently, a punch biopsy of the one of the ulcers revealed cutaneous angiosarcoma, moderate to high grade in differentiation. Microscopically, there was extensive spindle cell proliferation involving dermis, subcutis, and deeper fibroadipose tissue (Figure 2). There were multiple vascular sinuses lined by tufts of neoplastic endothelial cells (Figure 3). Immunohistochemical stains revealed negative staining for cytokeratin while vascular markers CD31 (Figure 4), CD34, and D2-40 were strongly positive. No necrosis was identified in the specimen. Mitotic rate was 0 to 9 mitoses per 10 high power fields. Lymphovascular invasion was indeterminate.

The patient was referred to the radiation oncology center with the above clinical and pathological data. MRI of the left foot with contrast revealed diffuse soft tissue T1 hypointense (Figure 5) and T2 hyperintense signal within both medial and lateral subcutaneous tissues. This was more prominent in the fat anterior to the Achilles tendon. There was no evidence of invasion in the tendon or the bone. Flourodeoxyglucose (FDG) PET and CT scan revealed heterogeneous uptake in the medial and lateral foot with a more focal uptake in the medial foot, anterior to the Achilles tendon (Figure 6). Two subcentimeter lymph nodes, one in the popliteal region

and the other in left groin, showed minimum FDG labelling and were thought to be reactive in nature. No abnormal uptake was seen throughout the body to suggest distant metastases.

Given the diffuse dermal involvement of the foot, the patient was not considered a candidate for upfront surgery. He declined surgical evaluation after preoperative radiation. He was not considered a candidate for chemotherapy because of comorbid conditions, poor renal functions, old age, and reluctance to pursue systemic therapy. He was planned for radiation therapy to both medial and lateral aspects of the foot in addition to the plantar surface using a custom immobilization device. This was done with a combination of photons of 6 MV and electrons of 9 Mev energy to achieve a homogenous dose distribution. A custom bolus was used to build up the radiation dose to the surface. The dose prescribed was 50.4 Gy in 1.8 Gy per fraction to the medial and lateral aspect in 5.5 weeks. The plantar surface of the foot was irradiated to a dose of 30.6 Gy at 1.8 Gy per fraction in 3.5 weeks. He was assessed clinically each week.

At the end of the course of radiation, there was anticipated radiation related moist desquamation of the radiated skin which was managed by the wound care center. There was good subjective and objective response to radiation with decline in discharge and excellent diminishment of cutaneous ulceration one month after radiation. At the end of two-month follow-up there was almost complete response

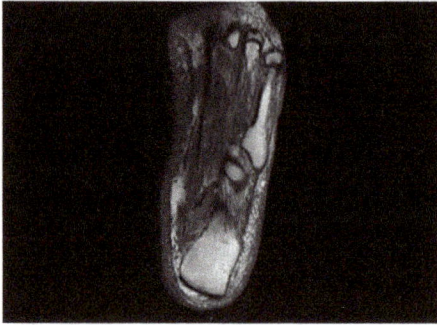

FIGURE 5: MRI of the left foot with contrast showing diffuse soft tissue T1 hypointense signal within both medial and lateral subcutaneous tissues, which is more prominent in the fat anterior to the Achilles tendon.

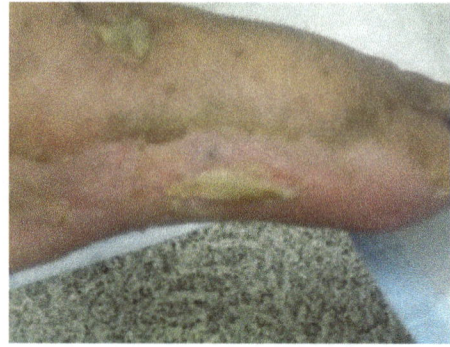

FIGURE 7: Two months postradiation: marked diminishment of cutaneous ulceration with decline in discharge and drying of satellite nodules.

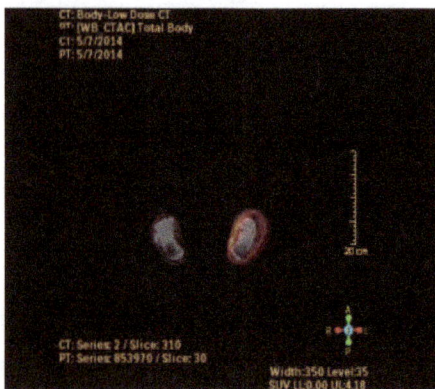

FIGURE 6: FDG-PET and CT scan showing heterogeneous uptake in the medial and lateral foot with a more focal uptake in the medial foot, anterior to the Achilles tendon.

and drying of the cutaneous ulceration and satellite nodules in his foot (Figure 7).

3. Discussion

Angiosarcoma is a rare and aggressive malignant tumor of vascular endothelial origin. Among all cases of angiosarcoma, one-third occur in the skin, one-fourth in soft tissue, and the remainder in other sites [6]. Radiation therapy, especially for breast cancer, is a predisposing factor. Vascular insufficiency and chronic lymphedema are other predisposing factors in addition to trauma and sun exposure [7]. In many cases, however, the exact cause is unknown [8]. In our case, advanced and chronic venous insufficiency leading to vascular stasis and lymphedema was perhaps the predisposing factor.

As regards clinical appearance, the appearance of cutaneous angiosarcoma can be variable [4] and it can manifest as bruise-like lesions [8], raised purplish-red papules [9], and rosacea-like lesions [10]. Due to the variability in the appearance of cutaneous angiosarcoma, the correct diagnosis can often be delayed. Differential diagnoses include, but are not limited to, eczema [4], Kaposi sarcoma [11], scarring alopecia [12], sebaceous cysts [13], and amelanotic melanoma

[14]. Our case is unique that it presented with cutaneous ulceration.

Majority of the patients are noted to be elderly males [15, 16] with Caucasians or fairer skinned people being more commonly affected than darker or black race [17, 18]. More than 90% of the cutaneous lesions are located in the head and neck region. Other non-cutaneous regions are breast and liver. It arises infrequently in the lower extremity [7]. Our case presented in the skin of foot which is very rare although angiosarcoma arising in bones of the foot or femoral artery have been described in the literature [19, 20].

The most common histological patterns include atypical and pleomorphic (rounded, polygonal, or fusiform) endothelial cells exhibiting a diffuse epithelioid or spindle cell proliferation [4, 9, 13, 15]. Immunohistochemical markers include Von Willebrand factor, CD34, CD31, Ulex europaeus agglutinin 1, vascular endothelial growth factor (VEGF), and factor VIII antigen [4, 8]. Our case showed spindle cell proliferation with interspersed vascular sinuses and positivity for CD31 and CD34.

Histological grade [1, 21] and tumor size are important prognostic factors with tumors > 10 cm portending a poor prognosis and tumors < 5 cm correlated with better outcomes [13, 22–24]. High mitotic counts are associated with worse outcomes [25]. In a case series, lymphocytic infiltrate was associated with a good prognosis [26]. Age, sex, and clinical appearance have no prognostic significance [5, 7]. Presence of metastasis, local recurrence, and positive surgical margins correlate with poor outcome [15]. Multifocal disease and depth of invasion (>3 mm) are other poor prognostic features [27]. Local recurrences have been observed in 35% to 86% of cases [16, 28]. Prognosis of angiosarcoma is poor with a reported 5-year survival rate ranging from 12 to 24% [5, 15, 21]. In a series of 48 patients with cutaneous angiosarcoma, 45 patients (94%) had disease recurrences [16]. In the same series, 37 of those patients had distant metastases to the lungs and a median survival time of 4 months. Lung metastases as a common site of spread have also been reported in other series [29, 30]. Other rare reported sites of spread were cardiac and/or vascular metastases [2, 15]. Mendenhall et al. reported a 5-year locoregional control of 40 to 50%, 5-year distant metastasis-free survival of 20 to 40%, and 5-year overall survival of 10 to 30% [31].

Treatment of cutaneous angiosarcoma is based on retrospective data because of the rarity of this disease. Complete resection of the disease is recommended whenever possible, since this disease has a high propensity to recur locally. Surgical excision may not be a feasible option since resectable cutaneous angiosarcoma lesions constitute only a fraction of all cases [4]. Recent studies of primary tumors have reported success with a combined-modality approach of surgical resection followed by postoperative radiation therapy [1, 4, 23, 32]. A retrospective study reported on survival outcomes of 48 patients who were treated for angiosarcoma of face and scalp with either a single modality or a combination of surgery, radiotherapy, chemotherapy, and immunotherapy [16]. The median follow-up for all 48 patients was 13.7 months. Patients who underwent both surgery and radiotherapy (2-year overall survival: 45.8%) had a significantly more favorable overall survival ($P < 0.0001$) compared with patients treated with either surgery or radiotherapy (2-year overall survival: 11.1%) alone and patients who received no surgery or radiotherapy (2-year overall survival: 0%).

Although the combined modality therapy is associated with a better outcome, patients are still at risk for the development of distant metastases [24]. Radiotherapy is a reasonable approach in unresectable or metastatic cases. Care must be taken to achieve full dose to the lesion and to use wide margins due to the diffuse nature of the tumor [33, 34]. It appears to improve local control and possibly overall survival based on the retrospective series in the literature [4, 16, 28, 35], however radiation employed as a single modality of treatment rarely results in complete remission [36, 37]. Radiation doses of > 50 Gy are usually recommended [4] but because of the poor tolerance of hands and feet to radiation [38, 39] we kept our radiation dose to about 50 Gy. Data on the role of chemotherapy in the definitive treatment of cutaneous angiosarcoma is limited and varied. Doxorubicin and Taxanes have been used for treatment in unresectable and metastatic setting [3, 4, 40].

Promising results with bevacizumab [41], sunitinib [42], and sorafenib [43] have also been reported, and their efficacy may be linked to VEGF production in most cases of angiosarcoma. Although single agent therapy with these agents is tolerable, toxicity is significant and patients with advanced age and comorbidities may not qualify for therapy [4]. Photodynamic therapy has been tried by Thong et al. for primary cutaneous angiosarcoma and tumor eradication was achieved with spontaneous remission of neighboring and distant untreated lesions [44].

Since surgery for diffuse involvement of the foot would have resulted in significant morbidity and poor functional outcome, our patient was not considered a candidate for surgery. He refused surgical evaluation after radiation. Systemic therapy and radiotherapy were the next available options. However, he did not want to consider chemotherapy and in any event it he was not a good candidate for aggressive therapy. Therefore, the patient underwent successful treatment with radiotherapy alone as a single modality.

4. Conclusion

A rare case of cutaneous angiosarcoma of the foot has been described in this case report. This case portrayed a clinical picture of a nonhealing ulcer with superadded infection. Physicians should be aware of this diagnosis while managing nonhealing skin lesions in patients with chronic lymphedema and vascular insufficiency. A delay in the diagnosis of angiosarcoma could culminate in significant treatment challenges. Radiotherapy alone may be an effective treatment in a select group of patients with cutaneous angiosarcoma of the foot in cases where surgery is not feasible. An excellent subjective and objective response to radiation was achieved in our case.

References

[1] R. J. Mark, J. C. Poen, L. M. Tran, Y. S. Fu, and G. F. Juillard, "Angiosarcoma: a report of 67 patients and a review of the literature," *Cancer*, vol. 77, no. 11, pp. 2400–2406, 1996.

[2] S. W. Weiss, J. R. Goldblum, and A. L. Folpe, *Enzinger and Weiss's Soft Tissue Tumors*, Mosby, St. Louis, Mo, USA, 2007.

[3] N. Penel, A. Lansiaux, and A. Adenis, "Angiosarcomas and taxanes," *Current Treatment Options in Oncology*, vol. 8, no. 6, pp. 428–434, 2007.

[4] N. Q. Trinh, I. Rashed, K. A. Hutchens, A. Go, E. Meilan, and R. Tung, "Unusual clinical presentation of cutaneous angiosarcoma masquerading as eczema: a case report and review of the literature," *Case Reports in Dermatological Medicine*, vol. 2013, Article ID 906426, 5 pages, 2013.

[5] C. A. Holden, M. F. Spittle, and E. W. Jones, "Angiosarcoma of the face and scalp, prognosis and treatment," *Cancer*, vol. 59, no. 5, pp. 1046–1057, 1987.

[6] K. Nagao, K. Suzuki, T. Yasuda et al., "Cutaneous angiosarcoma of the buttock complicated by severe thrombocytopenia: a case report," *Molecular Clinical Oncology*, vol. 1, no. 5, pp. 903–907, 2013.

[7] K. Wolf and J. Pasquino, "Cutaneous angiosarcoma. A literature review and case report," *Journal of the American Podiatric Medical Association*, vol. 80, no. 9, pp. 501–504, 1990.

[8] A. Selim, A. Khachemoune, and N. A. Lockshin, "Angiosarcoma: A case report and review of the literature," *Cutis*, vol. 76, no. 5, pp. 313–317, 2005.

[9] R. J. Young, N. J. Brown, M. W. Reed, D. Hughes, and P. J. Woll, "Angiosarcoma," *The Lancet Oncology*, vol. 11, no. 10, pp. 983–991, 2010.

[10] T. Mentzel, H. Kutzner, and U. Wollina, "Cutaneous angiosarcoma of the face: clinicopathologic and immunohistochemical study of a case resembling rosacea clinically," *Journal of the American Academy of Dermatology*, vol. 38, no. 5, pp. 837–840, 1998.

[11] J. M. Shehan and I. Ahmed, "Angiosarcoma arising in a lymphedematous abdominal pannus with histologic features reminiscent of Kaposi's sarcoma: report of a case and review of the literature," *International Journal of Dermatology*, vol. 45, no. 5, pp. 499–503, 2006.

[12] T. E. Knight, H. M. Robinson Jr., and B. Sina, "Angiosarcoma (angioendothelioma) of the scalp. An unusual case of scarring alopecia," *Archives of Dermatology*, vol. 116, no. 6, pp. 683–686, 1980.

[13] Z. Pan, D. Albertson, A. Bhuller, B. Wang, J. M. Shehan, and D. P. Sarma, "Angiosarcoma of the scalp mimicking a sebaceous cyst," *Dermatology Online Journal*, vol. 14, no. 6, article 13, 2008.

[14] W. McCarthy and G. Pack, "Malignant blood vessel tumor," *Surgery Gynecology Obstetrics*, vol. 91, no. 4, pp. 465–482, 1950.

[15] M. B. Morgan, M. Swann, S. Somach, W. Eng, and B. Smoller, "Cutaneous angiosarcoma: a case series with prognostic correlation," *Journal of the American Academy of Dermatology*, vol. 50, no. 6, pp. 867–874, 2004.

[16] K. Ogawa, K. Takahashi, Y. Asato et al., "Treatment and prognosis of angiosarcoma of the scalp and face: A retrospective analysis of 48 patients," *The British Journal of Radiology*, vol. 85, no. 1019, pp. e1127–e1133, 2012.

[17] A. N. Freedman, "Angiosarcoma of the scalp: case report and literature review," *Canadian Journal of Surgery*, vol. 30, no. 3, pp. 197–198, 1987.

[18] C. Girard, W. C. Johnson, and J. H. Graham, "Cutaneous angiosarcoma," *Cancer*, vol. 26, no. 4, pp. 868–883, 1970.

[19] G. Balaji, J. S. V. Arockiaraj, A. C. Roy, and B. Deepak, "Primary epithelioid angiosarcoma of the calcaneum: a diagnostic dilemma," *Journal of Foot and Ankle Surgery*, vol. 53, no. 2, pp. 239–242, 2014.

[20] S. Y. Choi, S. K. Min, K. I. Kim, and H. Y. Kim, "Intimal angiosarcoma presenting with common femoral artery aneurysm," *Journal of Vascular Surgery*, vol. 56, no. 3, pp. 819–821, 2012.

[21] H. F. Köhler, R. I. Neves, E. R. Brechtbühl, N. V. M. Granja, M. K. Ikeda, and L. P. Kowalski, "Cutaneous angiosarcoma of the head and neck: report of 23 cases from a single institution," *Otolaryngology—Head and Neck Surgery*, vol. 139, no. 4, pp. 519–524, 2008.

[22] A. Kacker, C. R. Antonescu, and A. R. Shaha, "Multifocal angiosarcoma of the scalp: a case report and review of the literature," *Ear, Nose & Throat Journal*, vol. 78, no. 4, pp. 302–305, 1999.

[23] W. M. Lydiatt, A. R. Shaha, and J. P. Shah, "Angiosarcoma of the head and neck," *The American Journal of Surgery*, vol. 168, no. 5, pp. 451–454, 1994.

[24] B. A. Guadagnolo, G. K. Zagars, D. Araujo, V. Ravi, T. D. Shellenberger, and E. M. Sturgis, "Outcomes after definitive treatment for cutaneous angiosarcoma of the face and scalp," *Head and Neck*, vol. 33, no. 5, pp. 661–667, 2011.

[25] N. Naka, M. Ohsawa, Y. Tomita et al., "Prognostic factors in angiosarcoma: a multivariate analysis of 55 cases," *Journal of Surgical Oncology*, vol. 61, no. 3, pp. 170–176, 1998.

[26] J. C. Maddox and H. L. Evans, "Angiosarcoma of skin and soft tissue: a study of forty-four cases," *Cancer*, vol. 48, no. 8, pp. 1907–1921, 1981.

[27] V. Kharkar, P. Jadhav, V. Thakkar, S. Mahajan, and U. Khopkar, "Primary cutaneous angiosarcoma of the nose," *Indian Journal of Dermatology, Venereology and Leprology*, vol. 78, no. 4, pp. 496–497, 2012.

[28] T. M. Pawlik, A. F. Paulino, C. J. McGinn et al., "Cutaneous angiosarcoma of the scalp: a multidisciplinary approach," *Cancer*, vol. 98, no. 8, pp. 1716–1726, 2003.

[29] M. Kitagawa, I. Tanaka, T. Takemura, O. Matsubara, and T. Kasuga, "Angiosarcoma of the scalp: report of two cases with fatal pulmonary complications and a review of Japanese autopsy registry data," *Virchows Archiv A*, vol. 412, no. 1, pp. 83–87, 1987.

[30] M. Nomura, Y. Nakaya, K. Saito et al., "Hemopneumothorax secondary to multiple cavitary metastasis in angiosarcoma of the scalp," *Respiration*, vol. 61, no. 2, pp. 109–112, 1994.

[31] W. M. Mendenhall, C. M. Mendenhall, J. W. Werning, J. D. Reith, and N. P. Mendenhall, "Cutaneous angiosarcoma," *The American Journal of Clinical Oncology: Cancer Clinical Trials*, vol. 29, no. 5, pp. 524–528, 2006.

[32] J. R. Ward, S. J. Feigenberg, N. P. Mendenhall, R. B. Marcus Jr., and W. M. Mendenhall, "Radiation therapy for angiosarcoma," *Head and Neck*, vol. 25, no. 10, pp. 873–878, 2003.

[33] W. H. Morrison, R. M. Byers, A. S. Garden, H. L. Evans, K. K. Ang, and L. J. Peters, "Cutaneous angiosarcoma of the head and neck. Atherapeutic dilemma," *Cancer*, vol. 76, no. 2, pp. 319–327, 1995.

[34] J. Glickstein, M. E. Sebelik, and Q. Lu, "Cutaneous angiosarcoma of the head and neck: a case presentation and review of the literature," *Ear, Nose & Throat Journal*, vol. 85, no. 10, pp. 672–674, 2006.

[35] J. Romanyshyn, S. Wolden, N. Caria et al., "Radiation therapy in the treatment of angiosarcoma of the head and neck," *International Journal of Radiation Oncology, Biology, Physics*, vol. 78, no. 3, pp. S483–S483, 2010.

[36] S. Gkalpakiotis, P. Arenberger, O. Vohradnikova, and M. Arenbergerova, "Successful radiotherapy of facial angiosarcoma," *International Journal of Dermatology*, vol. 47, no. 11, pp. 1190–1192, 2008.

[37] V. B. Patel and T. W. Speer, "Successful treatment of an angiosarcoma of the nose with radiation therapy," *Case Reports in Oncology*, vol. 5, no. 3, pp. 570–575, 2012.

[38] J. C. Owens, M. H. Shiu, R. Smith, and S. I. Hajdu, "Soft tissue sarcomas of the hand and foot," *Cancer*, vol. 55, no. 9, pp. 2010–2018, 1985.

[39] M. A. Simon and W. F. Enneking, "The management of soft tissue sarcomas of the extremities," *Journal of Bone and Joint Surgery A*, vol. 58, no. 3, pp. 317–327, 1976.

[40] N. Penel, B. N. Bui, J.-O. Bay et al., "Phase II trial of weekly paclitaxel for unresectable angiosarcoma: the ANGIOTAX study," *Journal of Clinical Oncology*, vol. 26, no. 32, pp. 5269–5274, 2008.

[41] M. Agulnik, S. Okuno, M. Von Mehren et al., "An open-label multicenter phase II study of bevacizumab for the treatment of angiosarcoma," *Journal of Clinical Oncology*, vol. 27, supplement 15, Article ID 10522, 2009.

[42] S. George, P. Merriam, R. G. Maki et al., "Multicenter phase II trial of sunitinib in the treatment of nongastrointestinal stromal tumor sarcomas," *Journal of Clinical Oncology*, vol. 27, no. 19, pp. 3154–3160, 2009.

[43] R. G. Maki, D. R. D'Adamo, M. L. Keohan et al., "Phase II study of sorafenib in patients with metastatic or recurrent sarcomas," *Journal of Clinical Oncology*, vol. 27, no. 19, pp. 3133–3140, 2009.

[44] P. S.-P. Thong, K.-W. Ong, N. S.-G. Goh et al., "Photodynamic-therapy-activated immune response against distant untreated tumours in recurrent angiosarcoma," *The Lancet Oncology*, vol. 8, no. 10, pp. 950–952, 2007.

10

An Unusual Case of Invasive Kaposi's Sarcoma with Primary Effusion Lymphoma in an HIV Positive Patient: Case Report and Literature Review

Alexandra Millet,[1] Sanmeet Singh,[1] Genelle Gittens-Backus,[1] Kim Ann Dang,[1] and Babak Shokrani[2]

[1]Howard University College of Medicine, Washington, DC 20059, USA
[2]Department of Pathology, Howard University Hospital, Washington, DC 20060, USA

Correspondence should be addressed to Babak Shokrani; b_shokrani@howard.edu

Academic Editor: Francesco A. Mauri

We report a case of AIDS-related Kaposi's sarcoma (KS) with Primary Effusion Lymphoma (PEL) in a 28-year-old, African American male. Kaposi's sarcoma is an AIDS defining disease and typically will disseminate early in the course of the disease affecting the skin, mucous membranes, gastrointestinal tract, lymph nodes, and lungs. This case reports an unusual presentation of the disease along with primary effusion lymphoma. Although the most common organ systems affected by KS are the respiratory and the gastrointestinal systems, the lungs of this patient did not show any evidence of KS. Additionally, the patient demonstrates the rarely seen liver and unique pancreatic involvement by KS along with unusual synchronous bilateral pleural and peritoneal cavity involvement by PEL, adding to the distinct pattern of invasive AIDS-related Kaposi's sarcoma.

1. Introduction

Kaposi's sarcoma is a tumor caused by Human Herpesvirus-8 (HHV-8), also known as Kaposi's sarcoma associated herpesvirus (KSHV) [1]. It was originally described in the 1980s by Moritz Kaposi, a Hungarian dermatologist, and has widely become known as one of the AIDS defining diseases [2]. KS is a malignancy of lymphatic endothelial cells that is often highly aggressive in people with HIV and severe immunodeficiency.

Infection of an HIV patient by HHV-8 also provides the setting for the development of another AIDS-related disease, Primary Effusion Lymphoma (PEL). PEL accounts for less than 1–4 percent of all AIDS-related lymphomas. While the disease may occur independently, the overwhelming majority of cases occur in HIV-infected patients. Patients with PEL are often coinfected with HHV-8 and many with Epstein-Barr Virus (EBV) infection as well [3]. The mechanism of the proliferation of the disease with HHV-8 is uncertain.

We report a case of a noncompliant AIDS patient who died from pneumonia and was later found to have an unusual presentation of AIDS-related Kaposi's sarcoma with primary effusion lymphoma.

2. Case Presentation

A 28-year-old African American male with a past medical history of HIV/AIDS, *Pneumocystis jiroveci* pneumonia, and latent syphilis presented with shortness of breath, cough, and fever associated with chest pain for the past two weeks. He also complained of nausea, vomiting, and abdominal pain with generalized body swelling. He was noncompliant with his antiretroviral medications and was lost to follow-up with the Center for Infectious Disease Management and Research Clinic.

Upon physical examination, the patient was cachectic in appearance with notable dyspnea. Auscultation of the lungs revealed increased breathing effort with bilateral scattered

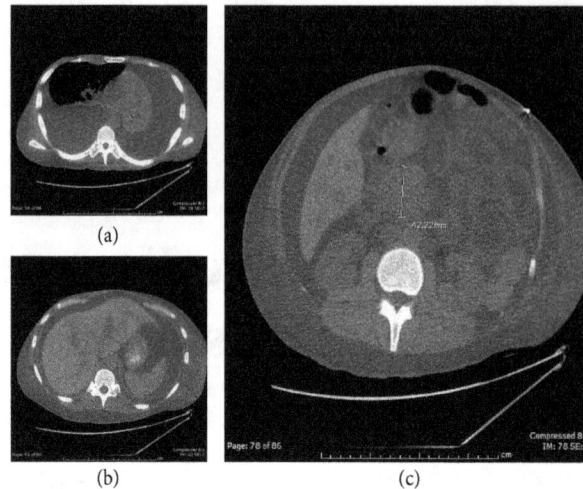

FIGURE 1: CT scans of the chest and abdomen show large bilateral pleural effusions (a) and severe ascites (b). There is a 4.2 cm mass in the head of the pancreas (c).

crepitation. Extremities showed bilateral pedal edema (1+). All other findings were within normal limits.

During the course of the hospital stay, the patient was treated and monitored for pneumocystis pneumonia. He was started on IV antibiotics Bactrim, Zithromax, and Rocephin. He had a CD4 count of $3/\mu L$ with a viral load of 73,965 copies. The infectious disease team was consulted and prophylaxis for MAC (*Mycobacterium avium* complex) was recommended. He was also found to have oral candidiasis which was subsequently treated with oral antifungal medication.

An EGD was performed showing esophageal ulceration and gastroduodenitis. The esophageal biopsy confirmed HSV esophagitis. CT of the chest revealed bilateral pleural effusions, severe ascites, and an enlarged head of the pancreas (Figure 1). Thoracentesis and ascitic taps yielded creamy fluid. Further cytologic evaluation of the pleural and ascitic fluid revealed scattered large atypical lymphoid cells expressing HHV-8, CD30, CD79A, MUM-1, CD56, and CD138 (Figure 2). Atypical cells showed positive staining for Epstein-Barr Virus (EBV) by in situ hybridization. The flow cytometry study on the pleural effusion sample also revealed a monoclonal B-cell population consisting of larger lymphocytes expressing CD45, HLA-DR, CD38, and both surface and cytoplasmic lambda light chain. These findings confirmed the diagnosis of Primary Effusion Lymphoma (PEL).

Subsequent bone marrow biopsy did not show bone marrow involvement. Bilateral chest pigtail tubes were inserted in response to rapidly accumulating pleural effusions.

His septic workup produced a blood culture positive for *Proteus mirabilis*. The patient continued to complain of shortness of breath and later became tachycardic and tachypneic. Following the diagnosis of PEL, Hematology Oncology team was consulted which recommended the chemotherapy with CHOP (cyclophosphamide, doxorubicin, vincristine, and prednisolone) regimen; however, the treatment could not be started since the patient's condition was deteriorated and

he developed septic shock associated with severe hypoxemia and hypotension. His respiratory status declined and he was intubated. Later, he was found pulseless with dilated pupils. Cardiopulmonary resuscitation (CPR) efforts were unsuccessful and he was pronounced dead 51 days after admission.

The major autopsy finding in our patient is one of invasive Kaposi's sarcomas involving the feet, the liver, the head of the pancreas, and the gastrointestinal system. Although the lungs are commonly involved in AIDS-associated invasive Kaposi's sarcoma, this patient's lungs did not show any indications of involvement of the disease. Of note, presentation of the disease extending to the liver is rarely reported, and an extensive literature review produced only a few cases of pancreatic involvement.

On gross examination of the patient, coalescing hyperpigmented skin changes on the feet and soles extending to the ankles were noted bilaterally. Tumorous growths were evident in the hepatobiliary system, pancreas, and gastrointestinal tract. The liver showed a well-demarcated perivascular infiltration marked by reddish-brown tumorous tissue (Figure 3). The head of the pancreas showed a 4×5 cm reddish-brown infiltrating lesion (Figure 3). The small and large intestine, along with stomach, showed widely separated, well-circumscribed, and circumferential areas of raised hemorrhagic mucosa (Figure 4). The small bowel mesentery was thickened.

In addition, a bilateral serosanguineous pleural effusion and ascitic fluid were present.

Histologically spindle cell proliferation consistent with Kaposi's sarcoma was found in a number of systems. Representative sections from the skin, vertebral bones, small intestine, stomach, colon, mesentery, liver, and the head of pancreas showed areas of interlacing bundles of spindle cells and slit-like vessels along with extravasated RBCs consistent with Kaposi's sarcoma. CD34 and HHV-8 immunostains provided a positive result confirming the diagnosis (Figure 3).

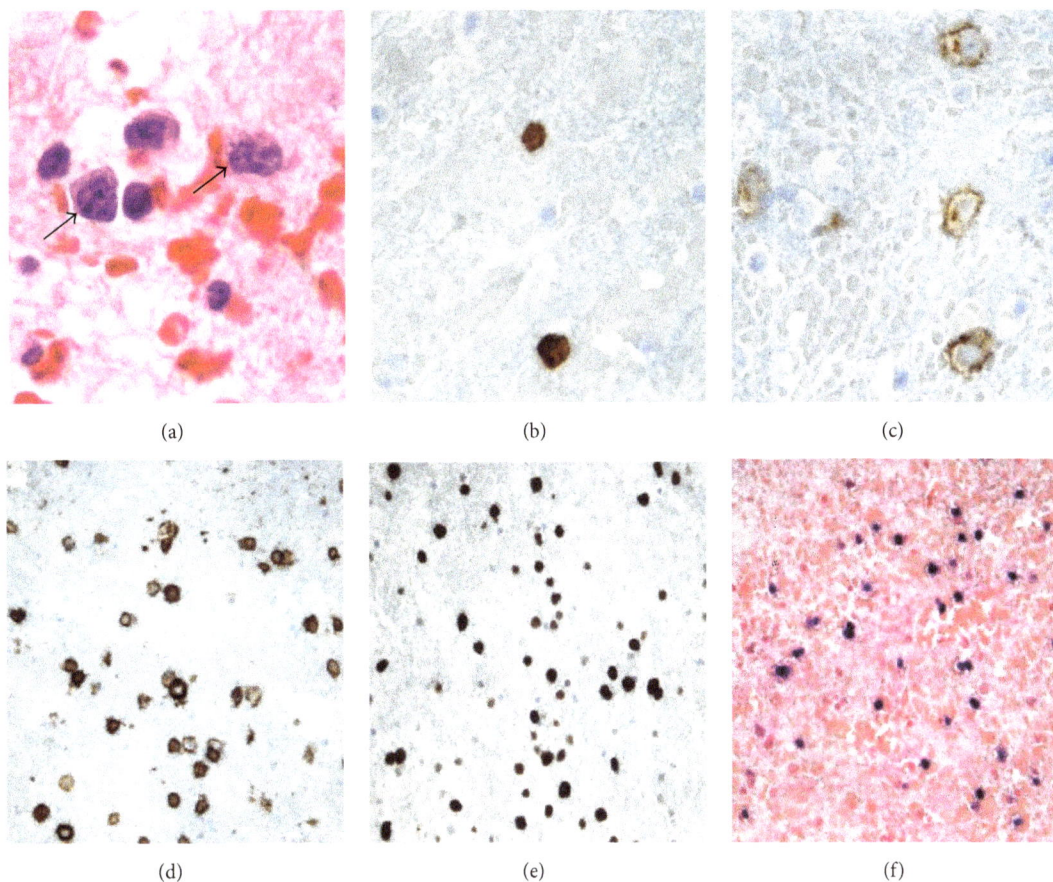

Figure 2: Cytologic evaluation of the pleural fluid shows large atypical lymphoid cells (arrows) ((a) H&E, ×100) expressing HHV8, CD30, and CD138 ((b), (c), and (d), resp.). The atypical cells show high proliferation index highlighted by Ki-67 immunostain (e) and positive staining for Epstein-Barr Virus (EBV) by in situ hybridization (f).

3. Discussion

Kaposi's sarcoma is the fourth most common malignancy associated with a viral infection [4].

There are four different types of Kaposi's sarcoma: classic, endemic, posttransplant, and lastly the AIDS-associated or epidemic. AIDS-associated or epidemic KS is the most common cause of tumor development in HIV infected individuals [5]. The manifestations of KS have changed considerably with the advent of highly active antiretroviral therapy (HAART). As a result of HAART, a smaller proportion of KS patients appear to present with visceral disease [6]. In particular, gastrointestinal tract and pulmonary involvement are less frequent among KS-HAART patients [6].

KS is a multifocal tumor that manifests most frequently in mucocutaneous sites, typically the skin of the lower extremities, face, trunk, genitalia, and oropharyngeal mucosa. KS also commonly involves lymph nodes and visceral organs, most notably the respiratory and gastrointestinal tracts [7]. Unusual presentations of KS reported in relation to the gastrointestinal tract involvement include primary KS of the pancreas [7].

Kaposi's sarcoma can be located in the gastrointestinal tract and cause identical symptoms to carcinoma of the same site. Kaposi's sarcoma of the pancreas mimics pancreatic cancer in an HIV-infected patient. Diagnosis can be made by identification of HHV-8 in pancreatic juice or bile, and a successful clinical outcome is possible with intensive antiviral and cytostatic treatment [8].

Our case is unique since the widespread visceral involvement by KS was not diagnosed until postmortem, and multiorgan involvement with symptoms related to each organ was interpreted separately and treated symptomatically.

Additionally the patient presented with an unusual involvement of the pancreas by KS that manifested as a pancreatic head mass, suggesting primary carcinoma of the head of the pancreas.

Primary Effusion Lymphoma (PEL) is a Human Herpesvirus-8 (HHV-8) associated lymphoma localized in body cavities and usually presenting as serous lymphomatous effusions without detectable tumor masses. It typically affects immunocompromised patients and usually involves only one body site, the most common being the pleural cavity; however, involvement of two body cavity sites has

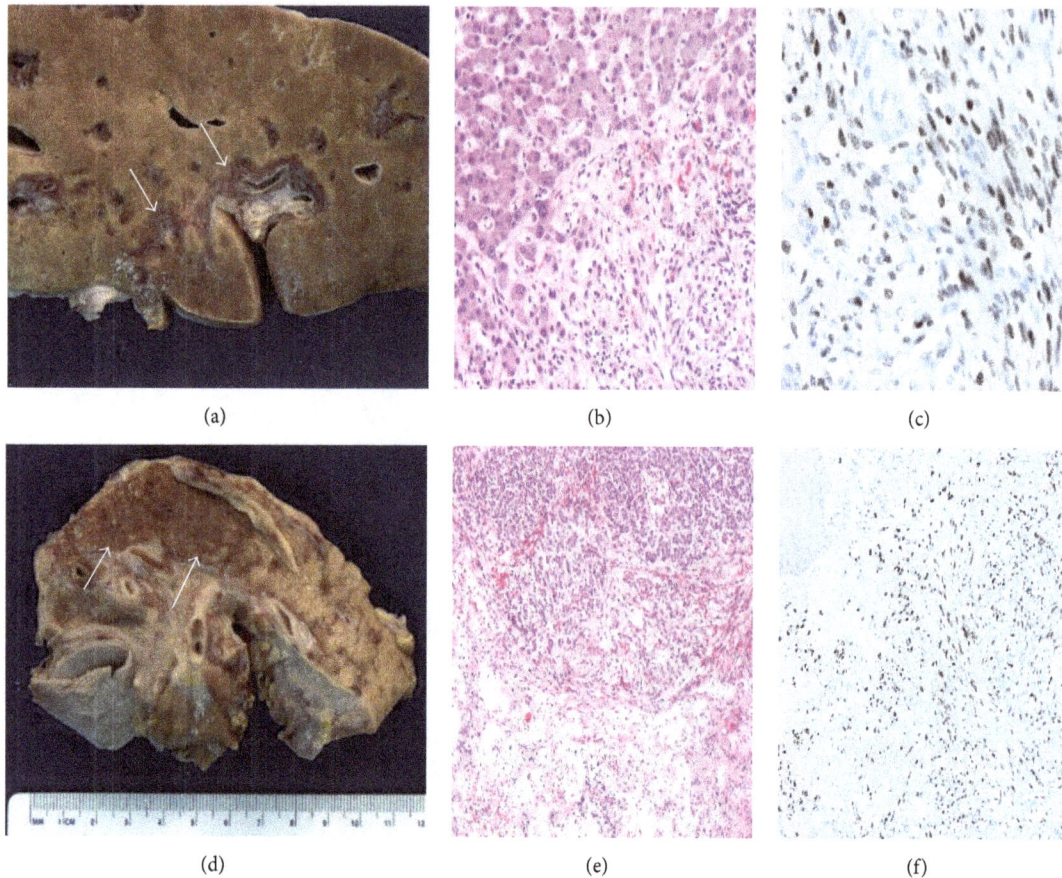

FIGURE 3: The cut surface of liver shows a well-demarcated perivascular infiltration marked by reddish-brown tumorous tissue (arrows) (a). The head of the pancreas shows a reddish-brown infiltrating lesion (arrows) (d). Representative microscopic sections show spindle cells proliferation involving hepatic lobules ((b) H&E, ×20) and pancreatic acini ((e) H&E, ×10) with positive staining for HHV-8 antibody consistent with Kaposi's sarcoma ((c), (f)).

been reported in some series [9, 10]. Herein we describe a case of PEL affecting three body cavity sites in an immunocompromised patient.

The majority of PEL cases arise in young or middle-aged homosexual or bisexual males with HIV infection and severe immunodeficiency [11, 12]. The neoplastic cells are positive for HHV-8 in all cases and most cases are coinfected with EBV [13–15]. Patients typically present with effusions in the absence of lymphadenopathy or organomegaly. Morphologically the neoplastic cells exhibit a range of appearance, from large immunoblastic or plasmablastic cells with markedly atypical features including large pleomorphic nuclei which may be lobated, one or more prominent nucleoli, and abundant amphophilic cytoplasm [11, 13].

Body cavity fluid is analyzed cytologically and by flow cytometry for the presence of clonal large neoplastic cells. To be given a diagnosis of PEL, an infection with HHV-8 must be present. A latency-associated nuclear antigen-1 (LANA-1) assay detects any evidence of HHV-8 in tissue samples. Complete blood counts and positron emission tomography/computed tomography (PET/CT) scans should also be performed to determine the extent of the disease [16].

Brimo et al. described a case of PEL in a 69-year-old HIV-negative man, who presented with peritoneal cavity involvement that progressed to involve the pleural and pericardial cavities despite being treated with chemotherapy and valganciclovir. The patient died 5 months following the initial diagnosis [17]. In contrast to our patient, this case was initially a peritoneal cavity disease that progressed to involve the pleural and pericardial spaces despite appropriate treatment.

Our case is unusual in its primary manifestation as synchronous involvement of bilateral pleural cavities and peritoneal space by PEL.

Learning Points

(1) In the presence of Kaposi's sarcoma in an HIV patient, the possibility of other HHV-8 related tumors such as Primary Effusion Lymphoma (PEL) should be considered.

(2) In our case, the patient had rare pancreatic and liver involvement of invasive Kaposi's sarcoma, as well as multiple cavitary involvement of PEL suggesting advanced disease.

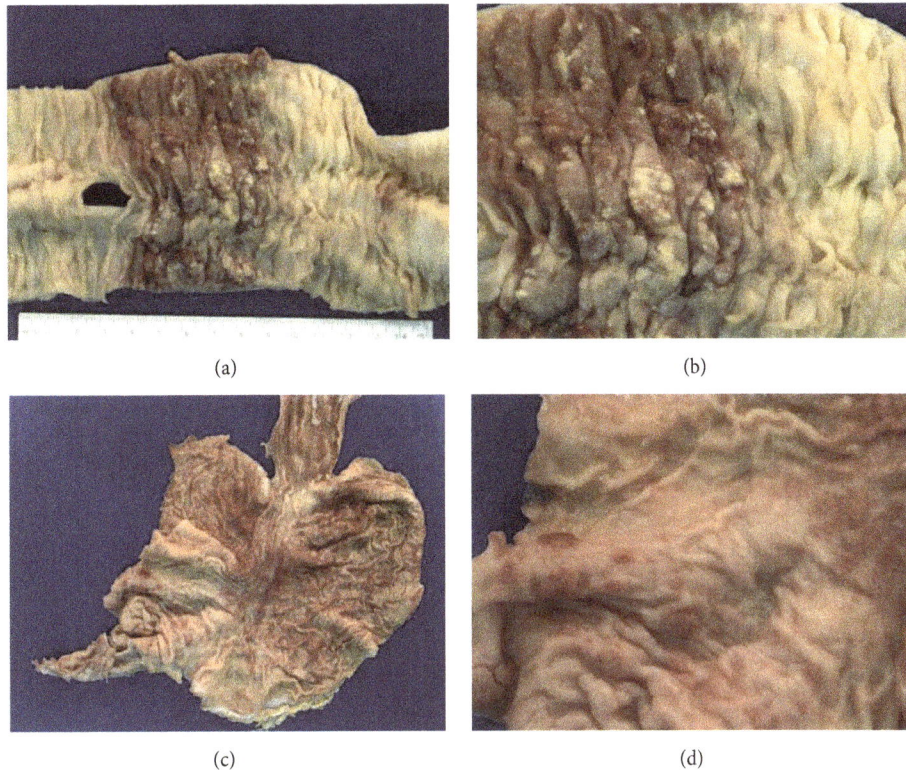

FIGURE 4: Kaposi's sarcoma with well-circumscribed areas of raised hemorrhagic mucosa in large intestine ((a), (b)) and stomach ((c), (d)).

References

[1] Y. Chang, E. Cesarman, M. S. Pessin et al., "Identification of herpesvirus-like DNA sequences in AIDS-associated Kaposi's sarcoma," *Science*, vol. 266, no. 5192, pp. 1865–1869, 1994.

[2] M. Kaposi, "Idiopathisches multiples Pigmentsarkom der Haut," *Archiv für Dermatologie und Syphilis*, vol. 4, no. 2, pp. 265–273, 1872.

[3] M. P. Menon, S. Pittaluga, and E. S. Jaffe, "The histological and biological spectrum of diffuse large B-cell lymphoma in the World Health Organization classification," *Cancer Journal*, vol. 18, no. 5, pp. 411–420, 2012.

[4] E. Cesarman, Y. Chang, P. S. Moore, J. W. Said, and D. M. Knowles, "Kaposi's sarcoma-associated herpesvirus-like DNA sequences in AIDS-related body-cavity-based lymphomas," *The New England Journal of Medicine*, vol. 332, no. 18, pp. 1186–1191, 1995.

[5] R. J. Sullivan, L. Pantanowitz, C. Casper, J. Stebbing, and B. J. Dezube, "Epidemiology, pathophysiology, and treatment of Kaposi sarcoma-associated herpesvirus disease: kaposi sarcoma, primary effusion lymphoma, and multicentric Castleman disease," *Clinical Infectious Diseases*, vol. 47, no. 9, pp. 1209–1215, 2008.

[6] G. Nasti, F. Martellotta, M. Berretta et al., "Impact of highly active antiretroviral therapy on the presenting features and outcome of patients with acquired immunodeficiency syndrome-related kaposi sarcoma," *Cancer*, vol. 98, no. 11, pp. 2440–2446, 2003.

[7] L. Pantanowitz and B. J. Dezube, "Kaposi sarcoma in unusual locations," *BMC Cancer*, vol. 8, article 190, 2008.

[8] M. Menges and H. W. Pees, "Kaposi's sarcoma of the pancreas mimicking pancreatic cancer in an HIV- infected patient: clinical diagnosis by detection of HHV 8 in bile and complete remission following antiviral and cytostatic therapy with paclitaxel," *International Journal of Pancreatology*, vol. 26, no. 3, pp. 193–199, 1999.

[9] J. Said, "Primary effusion lymphoma," in *WHO Classification of Tumours of Haematopoietic and Lymphoid Tissues*, S. H. Swerdlow, E. Campo, N. L. Harris et al., Eds., IARC, Lyon, France, 2008.

[10] F. Brimo, R. P. Michel, K. Khetani, and M. Auger, "Primary effusion lymphoma: a series of 4 cases and review of the literature with emphasis on cytomorphologic and immunocytochemical differential diagnosis," *Cancer Cytopathology*, vol. 111, no. 4, pp. 224–233, 2007.

[11] R. G. Nador, E. Cesarman, A. Chadburn et al., "Primary effusion lymphoma: a distinct clinicopathologic entity associated with the Kaposi's sarcoma-associated herpes virus," *Blood*, vol. 88, no. 2, pp. 645–656, 1996.

[12] J. W. Said, K. Chien, S. Takeuchi et al., "Kaposi's sarcoma-associated herpesvirus (KSHV or HHV8) in primary effusion lymphoma: ultrastructural demonstration of herpesvirus in lymphoma cells," *Blood*, vol. 87, no. 12, pp. 4937–4943, 1996.

[13] M. Q. Ansari, D. B. Dawson, R. Nador et al., "Primary body cavity-based AIDS-related lymphomas," *American Journal of Clinical Pathology*, vol. 105, no. 2, pp. 221–229, 1996.

[14] L. Arvanitakis, E. A. Mesri, R. G. Nador et al., "Establishment and characterization of a primary effusion (body cavity-based) lymphoma cell line (BC-3) harboring Kaposi's sarcoma-associated herpesvirus (KSHV/HHV-8) in the absence of Epstein-Barr virus," *Blood*, vol. 88, no. 7, pp. 2648–2654, 1996.

[15] M. G. Horenstein, R. G. Nador, A. Chadburn et al., "Epstein-Barr virus latent gene expression in primary effusion lymphomas containing Kaposi's sarcoma-associated herpesvirus/ human herpesvirus-8," *Blood*, vol. 90, no. 3, pp. 1186–1189, 1997.

[16] Y.-B. Chen, A. Rahemtullah, and E. Hochberg, "Primary effusion lymphoma," *The Oncologist*, vol. 12, no. 5, pp. 569–576, 2007.

[17] F. Brimo, G. Popradi, R. P. Michel, and M. Auger, "Primary effusion lymphoma involving three body cavities," *CytoJournal*, vol. 6, article 21, 2009.

11

Is It Safe to Restart Antivascular Endothelial Growth Factor Therapy in Patients with Renal Cell Carcinoma after Cardiac Ischemia?

Bo Zhao,[1] Laura S. Wood,[1] Karen James,[2] and Brian I. Rini[1]

[1]Department of Hematology and Oncology, Cleveland Clinic, 9500 Euclid Avenue R35, Cleveland, OH 44195, USA
[2]Department of Cardiovascular Medicine, Cleveland Clinic, 9500 Euclid Avenue J3-4, Cleveland, OH 44195, USA

Correspondence should be addressed to Bo Zhao; bozhaohp@gmail.com

Academic Editor: Raffaele Palmirotta

Agents targeting vascular endothelial growth factor (VEGF) represent active drugs in treating patients with advanced renal cell carcinoma (RCC). Studies have shown that sunitinib and axitinib can be associated with cardiac toxicity. Whether these agents should be restarted in patients who experience cardiac ischemia remains uncertain. Here, we present three patients with metastatic RCC who restarted sunitinib or axitinib after intervention of active ischemic cardiac disease without causing subsequent relevant cardiac events. This experience suggests that these agents can be continued after management of cardiac ischemia.

1. Introduction

The development of therapeutic agents targeting vascular endothelial growth factor (VEGF) represents a major advancement in treating patients with advanced renal cell carcinoma (RCC). The beneficial effects of these agents are balanced against acute and chronic toxicities, including cardiac toxicity. Bevacizumab, a recombinant humanized monoclonal antibody that targets VEGF, has been reported to be associated with an increased risk of cardiac events [1, 2]. The rate of cardiac ischemia/infarction was 1% (5/366) in a phase III study in patients receiving bevacizumab plus interferon alfa versus 0% in patients receiving interferon alfa alone, and the rate of left ventricular dysfunction was <1% (2/366) in patient receiving bevacizumab plus interferon alfa versus 0% in patients receiving interferon alone [1]. In a meta-analysis conducted in 4,617 patients with colorectal cancer, liver cancer, and RCC treated with bevacizumab-based therapy from 7 randomized controlled trials, ischemic heart disease was 1.7% (41/2417) in patients receiving bevacizumab versus 0.6% (13/2200) in patients receiving control therapies, with a calculated relative risk of 2.49 (95% CI 1.37–4.52) [2]. Tyrosine kinase inhibitors (TKIs) such as sunitinib, axitinib, and sorafenib target the VEGF receptor. Cardiac ischemia in

patients with RCC was not specifically reported from phase III studies for sunitinib or sorafenib [3–5]. In an observational study, 33.8% (25/74) patients receiving sunitinib or sorafenib experienced a cardiovascular event, including 7 patients who required coronary angiography [6]. In a recent analysis of pooled data from clinical trials in 672 patients with metastatic RCC and 1,304 patients with advanced solid tumors, 33 patients (1.7%) developed myocardial infarction (MI) on axitinib [7]. However, whether TKIs should be restarted in patients who receive successful intervention for cardiac ischemia remains uncertain, as such patients on clinical trials would have discontinued therapy. Here, we present three patients with metastatic RCC who safely restarted anti-VEGF TKIs after intervention of active ischemic cardiac disease.

2. Case Presentation

2.1. Case 1. A 55-year-old man was diagnosed with recurrent RCC in mediastinal lymph nodes one year after right partial nephrectomy for a Fuhrman grade 3, clear cell tumor. He was started on sunitinib 50 mg once daily, in cycles of 4 weeks on and two weeks off schedule on the phase III clinical trial of sunitinib versus interferon-alfa as a first-line systemic therapy for patients with metastatic RCC.

The dose was reduced to 37.5 mg after 11 cycles due to multiple recurrent grade 2 toxicities including fatigue, hand-foot syndrome, arthralgias, and myalgias. He had no known underlying coronary artery disease (CAD) at enrollment, and risk factors for CAD included a 25 pack-year smoking history, family history of premature CAD (brother < 55 years), and baseline hypertension of 140/85 mm Hg on moexipril 15 mg once daily. He developed grade 2 hypertension on sunitinib, which improved to 130/70 mm Hg after adding 25 mg of hydrochlorothiazide once daily. His creatinine was 1.3 mg/dL upon initiation of sunitinib with a calculated GFR of 61 mL/min/1.73 m^2, which remained relatively stable throughout his disease course. Five years later, he was noted to have developed coronary artery atherosclerotic calcifications on computed tomography scans. There were no symptoms to suggest angina at that time, and a stress test showed no evidence of ischemia. However, 14 months later, he developed acute onset chest pain and was found to have ST elevation indicative of myocardial infarction (MI) in the inferior wall. An emergent cardiac catheterization revealed 100% stenosis in right coronary artery (RCA) and 80% stenosis in left anterior descending artery (LAD). He received staged percutaneous coronary intervention (PCI) with two bare metal stents placement in the RCA and an everolimus-eluting stent in the LAD 10 days later. Sunitinib was restarted at the same dose after a holiday of ninety days when scans showed disease progression. An echocardiogram one day after the MI showed left ventricular ejection fraction (LVEF) of 50–55%, with hypokinesis of the posteriolateral and septal myocardium; a repeat echocardiogram 2 weeks before restarting sunitinib showed stable findings. He remained on sunitinib for another two years until disease progression, when he was switched to axitinib. The patient has been on axitinib for 2 years, currently on 8 mg twice daily. No further cardiac ischemia or other cardiac events have occurred.

2.2. Case 2.

A 52-year-old man was diagnosed with biopsy-proven, recurrent RCC in left adrenal gland one year after radical left nephrectomy. The primary tumor was Fuhrman grade 4, clear cell histology. He was started on axitinib through a randomized, double-blind, phase II study of axitinib with or without dose titration in patients with metastatic renal cell carcinoma. He had no known CAD at baseline, and risk factors for CAD included mixed type hyperlipidemia (normal cholesterol level on diet control) and a long-standing hypertension diagnosed at the age of 25. His blood pressure readings at baseline were 130/70 mm Hg on candesartan-hydrochlorothiazide 32 mg/25 mg. His creatinine was 1.2 mg/dL upon initiation of axitinib, and calculated GFR was 61 mL/min/1.73 m^2, which remained relatively stable throughout his disease course. He then developed grade 3 hypertension on axitinib, which improved to 120/70 mm Hg after adding once daily 5 mg amlodipine. He achieved an objective complete response per RECIST criteria v1.0 six months after the initiation of axitinib. Three years and 9 months later, he developed exertional chest pain. Axitinib was held, and two days later he underwent a cardiac catheterization evaluation, which revealed 99% stenosis of ostial/proximal LAD, 70% stenosis of proximal left circumflex

artery (LCx), and 90% stenosis in mid and distal RCA. EKG was sinus rhythm without evidence of ischemia, and LVEF was 60% on echocardiogram. He received successful staged PCI with placement of drug eluting stents (DES) in LAD and left circumflex artery (LCx), followed by mid and distal RCA with two more DES 4 days later. Axitinib was restarted 3 days after the second PCI at the same dose and schedule. Repeat lipid panel showed elevated cholesterol level of 345 mg/dL and triglyceride level of 362 mg/dL, ezetimibe-simvastatin 10–20 mg was added, and cholesterol and triglyceride levels were then normalized. The patient has remained on axitinib for one and half years since his cardiac ischemia with continued complete response. No subsequent cardiac ischemia or other cardiac events have been reported. A repeat echocardiogram one year later showed LVEF of 56 ± 5% with normal systolic function.

2.3. Case 3.

A 63-year-old man presented with low back pain and was found to have a vertebral soft tissue mass in the second lumbar vertebra (L2), a right kidney 7 cm contrast-enhancing tumor, multiple subcentimeter lung lesions, and bilateral adrenal nodules. Needle biopsy of the kidney tumor was consistent with RCC. He underwent palliative radiotherapy to the L2 vertebral lesion and debulking right nephrectomy, with pathology showing Fuhrman grade 3, clear cell RCC. He was started on front line axitinib through a randomized, double-blind phase II study of axitinib with or without dose titration in patients with metastatic renal cell carcinoma. At that time, he did not have symptoms to suggest active CAD, and risk factors for CAD included mixed type hyperlipidemia (normal cholesterol level on simvastatin 20 mg), a former 15 pack-year smoking history (quitted 30 years earlier), and hypertension. His blood pressure readings at baseline were 119/71 mm Hg on metoprolol tartrate 50 mg and hydrochlorothiazide 25 mg. His creatinine level was 1.68 mg/dL with a calculated GFR of 41 mL/min/1.73 m^2, which remained relatively stable throughout his disease course. Amlodipine 10 mg was added for grade 3 hypertension that developed on axitinib, and his blood pressure improved to 120/70 mm Hg. Two years and 5 months later, he experienced worsening recurrent chest pain 3 days after holding axitinib for grade 2 anorexia. EKG showed borderline T wave inversion in the anterior leads, and cardiac enzymes were within normal limits. A thallium stress test showed mild reversible changes involving the inferior wall. Further cardiac catheterization showed stenosis involving multiple vessels, including 95% of ostial RCA, 90% of mid and inferior segment of the posterolateral branch, 50% of distal left main, 50–60% of proximal and mid LAD, 90% of distal LAD, and 80% mid circumflex, and diffuse stenosis in distal LAD and mid circumflex. His calculated LVEF was 80% on stress test, and left ventricular systolic function was normally evaluated by ventriculogram. He was evaluated by cardiovascular surgery and deemed not a candidate for surgical intervention. Subsequently, he underwent staged PCI: stage I intervention with 4 DES was placed in ostial RCA, superior branch posterior left ventricular branch, inferior portion posterior left ventricular branch, and posterior descending artery. Stage II intervention with 2 DES was placed in mid-LAD and the circumflex

TABLE 1: Summary of ischemic events and interventions on anti-VEGF TKIs.

Case	1	2	3
Age at diagnosis (years)	54	51	63
TKI during cardiac event	Sunitinib	Axitinib	Axitinib
Ischemic event	MI	Angina	Angina
Intervention	Stent ×3	Stent ×4	Stent ×6
Known underlying CAD	No	No	No
Days on TKI before the event	2256	1384	885
Duration of break during cardiac event (days)	77	9	28
Days on the same TKI after the event	721	450	1080
LVEF after the event (%)	55	60	55
CHF at any time	No	No	No
Subsequent ischemia	No	No	Yes

VEGF: vascular endothelial growth factor; TKI: tyrosine kinase inhibitor; MI: myocardial infarction; CAD: coronary cardiac disease; CABG: coronary artery bypass graft; LVEF: left ventricular ejection fraction; CHF: congestive heart failure.

10 days later. Axitinib was held until 12 days after the stage II PCI. Metoprolol tartrate 50 mg and fenofibrate micronized 48 mg were added; his hypertriglyceridemia was improved from 408 mg/dL to 241 mg/dL. However, he subsequently experienced two more episodes of angina 6 months and 1 year and 10 months after the first angina and received 1 DES for a proximal 95%–99% LAD stenosis and 1 DES for a mid-LAD 95% stenosis, respectively. Axitinib was interrupted for 12 days and 24 days for these events, respectively. Both repeated echocardiograms after these two PCI interventions showed normal sized right and left ventricles with normal systolic function. He had disease progression after the third episode of angina, and the dose of axitinib was increased to 5 mg twice daily from 3 mg twice daily, which resulted in regression of his RCC. He is currently on axitinib 5 mg for an additional year without recurrent cardiac events. Table 1 summarizes the major clinical features of the three cases.

3. Discussion

The role of angiogenesis in ischemic heart disease has been controversial. While therapeutic angiogenesis has been thought to promote revascularization in ischemic cardiovascular disease, data from clinical trials have been inconclusive so far [8]. In the NORTHERN Trial, 93 patients with refractory Canadian Cardiovascular Society class 3 or 4 anginal symptoms were randomized to receive VEGF plasmid DNA or placebo (buffered saline) delivered via the endocardial route using an electroanatomical guidance catheter. There was no difference between the VEGF-treated and the placebo groups with respect to the change in myocardial perfusion, or improvements in exercise treadmill time and anginal symptoms [8]. On the other hand, studies suggest that neovascularization contributes to the growth of atherosclerotic lesions and is a key factor in plaque destabilization leading to rupture, which may cause acute coronary syndromes [9].

Although ischemic cardiac disease appears to be increased in patient receiving anti-VEGF TKIs [1–3], our patients did not experience ischemic cardiac events for at least two years after starting sunitinib or axitinib. Moreover, no patients experienced recurrent ischemia immediately after restarting these agents. This is consistent with the observation from another study, in which all 7 patients who experienced cardiac ischemia on sunitinib or sorafenib resumed the same TKI after medical intervention without causing subsequent clinically relevant cardiac events [6]. Another concern is that anti-VEGF TKIs may affect ventricular systolic function, as a normal angiogenic response has been proposed to be necessary to maintain an adequate response of cardiomyocytes to pressure load [10]. In fact, a decline in ejection fraction was reported in 10% patients receiving sunitinib in a randomized phase III study, as opposed to 3% in patients receiving interferon alfa [3]. No decreased ejection fraction was reported in the pooled analysis of axitinib [7]. For our patients, none of them had clinical evidence of congestive heart failure, with documented preserved and stable LVEF after resuming the same TKIs. Taken together, our experience suggests that after effective intervention of coronary artery stenosis, sunitinib or axitinib can be safely restarted without causing decline of ventricular systolic function or subsequent increased risk of recurrent cardiac ischemia. The suitability and timing of the resumption of treatment should be evaluated case by case, based on the clinical conditions of the individual patient.

References

[1] B. I. Rini, S. Halabi, J. E. Rosenberg et al., "Phase III trial of bevacizumab plus interferon alfa versus interferon alfa monotherapy in patients with metastatic renal cell carcinoma: final results of CALGB 90206," *Journal of Clinical Oncology*, vol. 28, no. 13, pp. 2137–2143, 2010.

[2] X.-L. Chen, Y.-H. Lei, C.-F. Liu et al., "Angiogenesis inhibitor bevacizumab increases the risk of ischemic heart disease associated with chemotherapy: a meta-analysis," *PLoS ONE*, vol. 8, no. 6, Article ID e66721, 2013.

[3] R. J. Motzer, T. E. Hutson, P. Tomczak et al., "Sunitinib versus interferon alfa in metastatic renal-cell carcinoma," *The New England Journal of Medicine*, vol. 356, no. 2, pp. 115–124, 2007.

[4] R. J. Motzer, T. E. Hutson, D. Cella et al., "Pazopanib versus sunitinib in metastatic renal-cell carcinoma," *The New England Journal of Medicine*, vol. 369, no. 8, pp. 722–731, 2013.

[5] B. Escudier, T. Eisen, W. M. Stadler et al., "Sorafenib in advanced clear-cell renal-cell carcinoma," *The New England Journal of Medicine*, vol. 356, no. 2, pp. 125–134, 2007.

[6] M. Schmidinger, C. C. Zielinski, U. M. Vogl et al., "Cardiac toxicity of sunitinib and sorafenib in patients with metastatic renal cell carcinoma," *Journal of Clinical Oncology*, vol. 26, no. 32, pp. 5204–5212, 2008.

[7] B. I. Rini, B. Escudier, S. Hariharan et al., "Long-term safety with axitinib in previously treated patients with metastatic renal cell carcinoma," *Clinical Genitourinary Cancer*, 2015.

[8] D. J. Stewart, M. J. B. Kutryk, D. Fitchett et al., "VEGF gene therapy fails to improve perfusion of ischemic myocardium in patients with advanced coronary disease: results of the NORTHERN trial," *Molecular Therapy*, vol. 17, no. 6, pp. 1109–1115, 2009.

[9] R. Khurana, M. Simons, J. F. Martin, and I. C. Zachary, "Role of angiogenesis in cardiovascular disease: a critical appraisal," *Circulation*, vol. 112, no. 12, pp. 1813–1824, 2005.

[10] I. Shiojima, K. Sato, Y. Izumiya et al., "Disruption of coordinated cardiac hypertrophy and angiogenesis contributes to the transition to heart failure," *Journal of Clinical Investigation*, vol. 115, no. 8, pp. 2108–2118, 2005.

12

Combination Trimodality Therapy Using Vismodegib for Basal Cell Carcinoma of the Face

Alec M. Block,[1] Fiori Alite,[1] Aidnag Z. Diaz,[2] Richard W. Borrowdale,[3]
Joseph I. Clark,[4] and Mehee Choi[1]

[1]Department of Radiation Oncology, Stritch School of Medicine, Loyola University Medical Center, 2160 S. First Avenue,
 Maywood, IL 60153, USA
[2]Department of Radiation Oncology, Rush University Medical Center, 500 S. Paulina Street, Ground Floor, Chicago, IL 60612, USA
[3]Department of Otolaryngology Head and Neck Surgery, Stritch School of Medicine, Loyola University Medical Center,
 2160 S. First Avenue, Maywood, IL 60153, USA
[4]Department of Medicine, Division of Hematology/Oncology, Stritch School of Medicine, Loyola University Medical Center,
 2160 S. First Avenue, Maywood, IL 60153, USA

Correspondence should be addressed to Mehee Choi; mehee.choi@gmail.com

Academic Editor: Marcel W. Bekkenk

Background. For large basal cell carcinomas (BCCs) of the head and neck, definitive surgery often requires extensive resection and reconstruction that may result in prolonged recovery and limited cosmesis. Vismodegib, a small-molecule inhibitor of the hedgehog pathway, is approved for advanced and metastatic BCCs. We present a case of advanced BCC treated with combination of vismodegib, radiotherapy, and local excision resulting in excellent response and cosmesis. *Case Presentation.* A 64-year-old gentleman presented with a 5-year history of a 7 cm enlarging right cheek mass, with extensive vascularization, central ulceration, and skin, soft tissue, and buccal mucosa involvement. Biopsy revealed BCC, nodular type. Up-front surgical option involved a large resection and reconstruction. After multidisciplinary discussion, we recommended and he opted for combined modality of vismodegib, radiotherapy, and local excision. The patient tolerated vismodegib well and his right cheek lesion decreased significantly in size. He was then treated with radiotherapy followed by local excision that revealed only focal residual BCC. Currently, he is without evidence of disease and has excellent cosmesis. *Conclusions.* We report a case of locally advanced BCC treated with trimodality therapy with vismodegib, radiotherapy, and local excision, resulting in excellent outcome and facial cosmesis, without requiring extensive resection or reconstructive surgery.

1. Introduction

For small, early stage, localized basal cell carcinoma (BCC) of the head and neck, primary surgical resection or primary radiation therapy is the mainstay of treatment [1, 2]. For more advanced and metastatic cases, however, the role of definitive surgery or radiation therapy alone is limited. Vismodegib, a small molecule inhibitor of the hedgehog pathway which is upregulated and causes uncontrolled proliferation of basal cells in BCC, has previously been shown to elicit response rates ranging from approximately 30% to 60% in advanced and metastatic cases, with a well-tolerated side effect profile [3–6]. Moreover, in a landmark phase 2 study, biopsies of

patients with locally advanced BCC treated with vismodegib alone revealed a complete pathologic response rate of 54% [4]. Based on these results, vismodegib became the first hedgehog signaling pathway targeted agent to gain US Food and Drug Administration (FDA) approval on January 30, 2012.

Several previous cases using vismodegib with combination therapy have been reported. In one such report, radiation therapy was used to treat squamous cell carcinoma of the skin while vismodegib was concurrently used for treatment of multiple BCC lesions [7]. In this single case, the authors demonstrated that radiation therapy for squamous cell carcinoma could be delivered safely and effectively at

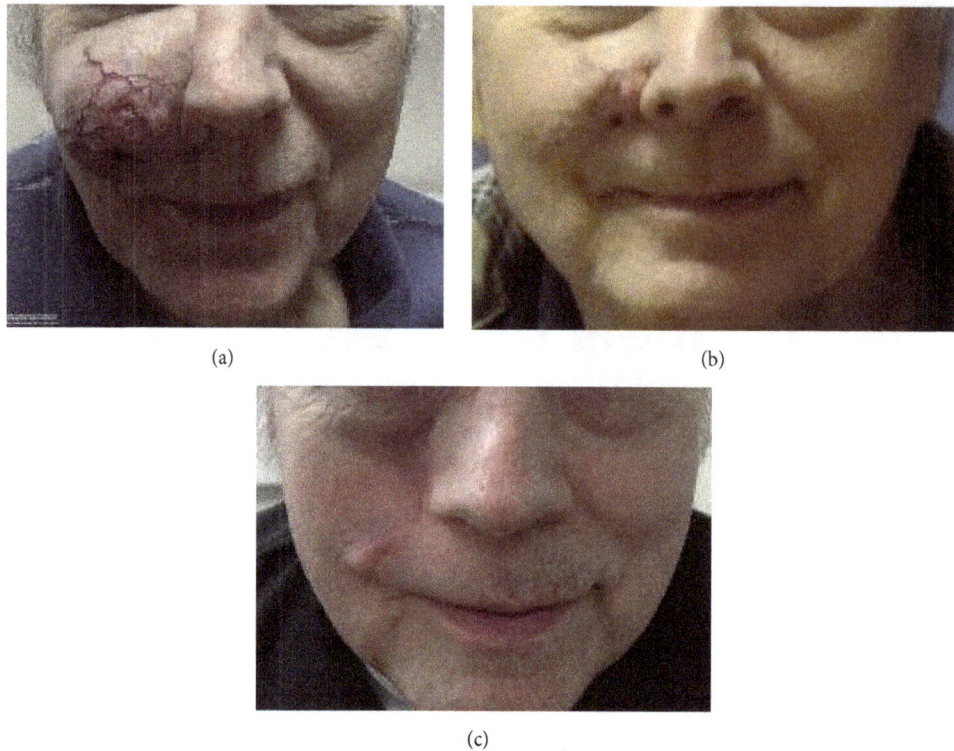

FIGURE 1: Clinical images. Photographs of the patient at the time of initial presentation (a), after 4 months of vismodegib therapy (b), and at first follow-up, 2 months after completion of trimodality therapy (c).

the same time as treatment with vismodegib [7]. Similarly, 2 cases were reported in which patients had an excellent clinical and radiographic response following completion of combination of vismodegib with concurrent radiation therapy for recurrent, locally advanced BCC [8]. For more advanced cases, potential use of vismodegib may include neoadjuvant treatment prior to a planned surgery, thus allowing for a smaller resection and subsequent reconstruction. A case utilizing this treatment paradigm has been reported with promising results [9]. Although vismodegib in combination with surgery alone or radiation therapy alone has been reported, to our knowledge, there have been no reports using all three modalities. Therefore, we present a case of locally advanced BCC of the face treated with vismodegib, radiation therapy, and ultimately local excision, without requiring a major resection or reconstruction and resulting in excellent function and cosmesis.

2. Case Report

A 64-year-old gentleman presented with a 5-year history of an enlarging right cheek mass. He reported that the lesion was not bothersome at first but that it had been growing slowly over time. He presented because the mass had grown so much in size that it was obscuring his inferior visual field to the point that he was unable to see beneath his cheek on the right side. He denied numbness or tingling of the face, facial pain, weight loss, or difficulty with chewing. He had no other bumps or masses and no other complaints.

His past medical history was significant for hypertension, hyperlipidemia, coronary artery disease with 3 myocardial infarctions and percutaneous coronary artery stenting, and an inguinal hernia repair. He walked with crutches for a left ankle fracture that he sustained as a youth. He was a previous cigar smoker but denied alcohol or illicit drug use. His father had BCC of the face, and his sister had breast cancer. Physical examination was significant for a 7 cm by 5 cm right cheek mass with extensive vascularization and central ulceration (see Figure 1(a)). The lesion involved the skin and soft tissues of the face and extended to the buccal mucosa of the right cheek but was mobile and did not appear fixed to the maxilla. He had numbness on the right side of his face in the distribution of cranial nerve V2. There was no palpable facial or cervical neck lymphadenopathy.

Noncontrast facial bone computed tomography (CT) scan revealed a mass-like subcutaneous lesion abutting the anterior aspect of the right maxilla, maxillary sinus, and inferior orbital rim and base of nasal bone, measuring about 5.5 cm in length by 5 cm in width by 4.5 cm in anterior to posterior dimension (see Figure 2(a)). No definite bone erosion or remodeling was demonstrated. No enlarged lymph nodes were evident in the field of view. Posterior-anterior and lateral 2-view chest X-ray was benign. Ultrasound guided fine needle aspiration of the mass revealed BCC of nodular type, staged as clinical T2N0M0, Stage II.

His case was discussed at multidisciplinary tumor board and the consensus was that up-front surgical monotherapy would involve a large full thickness resection of the skin of

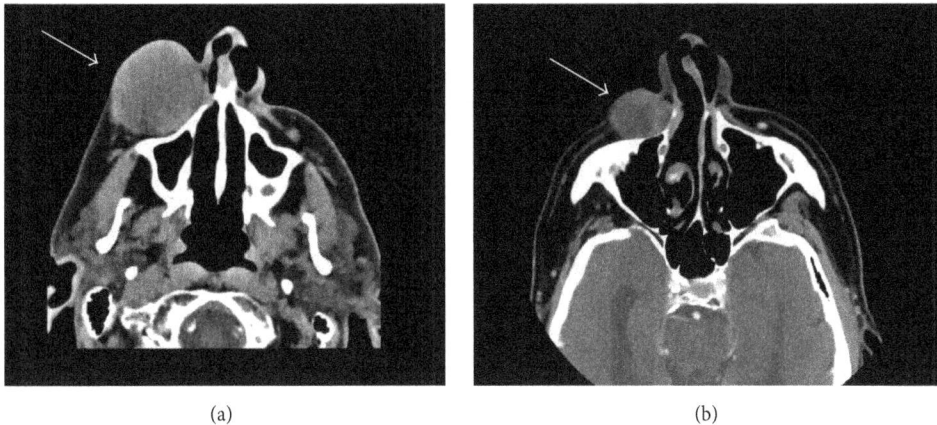

(a)   (b)

FIGURE 2: Radiographic images. Radiographic findings of facial bone computed tomography (CT) scan at time of initial presentation (a) and following 4 months of vismodegib therapy (b).

the face, likely with a frozen section of the infraorbital nerve, a full thickness resection through the cheek including removal of the buccal mucosa, and a radial forearm free flap reconstruction. Given his major medical comorbidity of coronary artery disease with multiple previous myocardial infarctions, there was concern that he may be medically unfit for such an extensive surgical procedure. Moreover, the patient was concerned about his postoperative recovery period and ultimate facial cosmesis following such an approach. Alternatively, he was offered combined modality therapy with once daily oral vismodegib 150 mg, followed by definitive radiation therapy once the response to vismodegib had either dramatically slowed or plateaued, reserving surgery for salvage. He was agreeable to this plan and vismodegib was initiated.

Overall, he tolerated the vismodegib very well and denied any muscle spasms, hair loss, weight loss, fatigue, nausea, decrease in appetite, or diarrhea. His only new complaint after 4 months of therapy was a minor decrease in taste which did not affect his appetite, ability to eat, or weight. Within 2 weeks of taking vismodegib, he noticed a decrease in the size of his lesion, and on physical exam it decreased to 6 cm by 4 cm. At 6-week follow-up, the lesion was 5 cm by 3 cm, and at 10-week follow-up it measured 4 cm by 3 cm. After approximately 14 weeks of vismodegib, the rate of reduction in the size of the lesion decreased, so the decision was made to proceed with definitive radiation therapy. The patient was maintained on vismodegib until the initiation of radiation therapy, resulting in approximately 4 months of drug therapy in total that resulted in an objective clinical response of greater than 50% reduction in the size of the lesion (see Figure 1(b)). Prior to starting radiation therapy, he underwent repeat facial bone CT scan which revealed that the lesion had decreased in size to 2.7 cm in largest dimension (see Figure 2(b)).

He then underwent CT simulation, in which he was positioned supine with a head and neck thermoplastic immobilization mask with a radioopaque wire placed around his residual lesion. His radiation therapy prescription was 50 Gy in 20 fractions of 2.5 Gy per fraction to the gross residual lesion (gross tumor volume, GTV) plus margin accounting for both local microscopic spread (clinical target volume,

TABLE 1: Dose-volume histogram data.

Dosimetric characteristic	Achieved
GTV, $D_{95\%}$	100%
CTV, $D_{95\%}$	99%
PTV, $D_{95\%}$	97%
Right eye, D_{max}	44 Gy
Right eye, mean	27 Gy
Right lacrimal gland, D_{max}	31 Gy
Right lacrimal gland, mean	24 Gy
Right optic nerve, D_{max}	30 Gy
Right optic nerve, mean	20 Gy

GTV: gross tumor volume; $D_{x\%}$: percent of prescribed dose delivered to $x\%$ of volume; D_{max}: maximum dose; Gy: Gray; CTV: clinical target volume; PTV: planning target volume.

CTV) and interfraction setup variability (planning target volume, PTV) delivered daily, Monday through Friday, for a total of 4 weeks. He was treated with a 0.5 cm daily skin bolus using 3-dimensional conformal radiation therapy (3DCRT) with a 4-field technique involving right anterior oblique, left anterior oblique, anterior superior oblique, and anterior inferior oblique field arrangements. Figure 3 shows representative views and dose distributions of the radiation therapy plan on his CT simulation scan. Table 1 relates target volumes to dose coverage and also shows representative doses to nearby critical structures. He tolerated radiation therapy very well with the expected toxicities of grade 1 fatigue that did not limit his daily activities and grade 2 moist skin desquamation in the area of the nasolabial fold that was improved with over-the-counter moisturizer and topical antibiotic cream.

At 3-month follow-up after the completion of radiation therapy, it was noted that he had a persistent 1.5 cm firm nodule in the right nasal-alar groove with overlying vasculature. Based on physical exam alone, it was difficult to determine if this nodule was scarring versus residual malignancy. Due to its firmness, size, and location, it was not amenable to

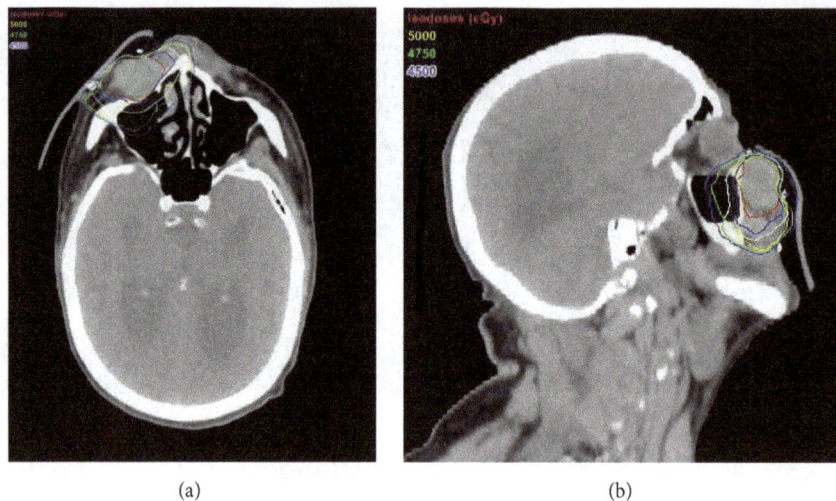

(a) (b)

FIGURE 3: Radiation therapy treatment plan. Axial (a) and sagittal (b) views of the radiation therapy treatment plan with target volumes and representative dose distributions: gross tumor volume (GTV) in red, clinical target volume (CTV) in blue, planning target volume (PTV) in cyan, and 45 Gy (blue), 47.5 Gy (light green), and 50 Gy (yellow) isodose lines.

fine needle aspiration, so the patient was taken for wide local excision, 2.5 cm by 5 cm, with intermediate closure. During the procedure, an elliptical incision was performed in the right cheek and the BCC in the right nasolabial fold was excised, resulting in a 2.5 cm by 5 cm defect which was then closed. He did not require reconstruction. Pathology from the wide local excision revealed only focal residual BCC with negative surgical margins. Overall, he tolerated the treatment very well and complained only of minor skin tightness and nasal congestion following his surgery. At 2-month follow-up after his surgery, he was doing very well, was clinically without evidence of disease, and had excellent facial cosmesis and functional capacity (see Figure 1(c)).

3. Conclusions

Mutations in hedgehog pathway genes have been implicated in several malignancies, including BCC [3–6]. Vismodegib, a first in class small molecule inhibitor of smoothened homologue, a key component of the hedgehog pathway, has been shown to be effective in the treatment of advanced and metastatic BCC [3–5]. In the setting of such promising results, particularly in a disease in which other systemic options are limited, there will be continued interest in utilizing vismodegib in combination with local therapy, surgery, and/or radiation therapy, for treatment of locally advanced nonmetastatic BCC, thus allowing for a smaller surgical procedure or smaller radiation therapy field.

Cases of combination of vismodegib with surgery alone or radiation therapy alone have been reported [7–9]. To our knowledge, this is the first case in which trimodality therapy—vismodegib, radiation therapy, and outpatient local excision—was used to treat locally advanced facial BCC that otherwise would have required a larger surgical resection, free flap reconstruction, overnight hospitalization, and overall significantly longer recovery time. Particularly in our

patient's case, in which there was concern that he might be medically unfit for such a large procedure because of his significant cardiac comorbidities, this trimodality approach presented an excellent option for oncologic control while maintaining facial cosmesis. Moreover, this report offers an example of the tolerability and safety of such an approach. Other than mild dysgeusia associated with vismodegib, he did not experience other previously reported toxicities, such as hair loss, muscle spasms, weight loss, nausea, decreased appetite, and diarrhea [4]. Following vismodegib, his radiation therapy was also well tolerated, and he did not have any perioperative surgical complications even after undergoing treatment with both vismodegib and radiation therapy. Similar to all patients treated with vismodegib, he will continue to be monitored closely, particularly for emergence of secondary squamous cell carcinoma lesions that may arise as sequelae from small molecule hedgehog pathway inhibitor therapy, which has been well documented previously [10–12].

Given the promising results of vismodegib in advanced and metastatic BCC, there will undoubtedly be growing popularity in a similar approach to that used in our patient in which vismodegib is combined with local therapy for locally advanced BCC. Although there are now several reported cases using vismodegib with surgery or radiation therapy, the most appropriate timing and sequencing of these modalities in order to provide the best outcomes with the least toxicity are widely unknown. A recent clinical trial, NCT01543581: Placebo-controlled, Double Blind Study to Assess Efficacy and Safety of Oral Vismodegib for the Treatment of BCC Preceding Excision by Mohs Micrographic Surgery (MMS), used vismodegib as neoadjuvant therapy prior to surgical resection in order to assess the efficacy and safety of vismodegib compared to placebo in the oral adjunctive presurgical treatment of BCC [13]. This study has closed to accrual and results are pending. Similarly, another trial, NCT01201915: A Phase II, Multicenter, Open-label, Three-cohort Trial Evaluating the

Efficacy and Safety of Vismodegib (GDC-0449) in Operable BCC, is evaluating the pathologic complete response rate in patients with operable BCC undergoing vismodegib therapy [14]. This study has also closed to accrual and results are pending. Finally, another trial, NCT01835626: A Phase II Study of Radiation Therapy and Vismodegib, for the Treatment of Locally Advanced BCC of the Head and Neck, is currently open to accrual and aims to assess the safety and tolerability of combined radiation therapy and concurrent vismodegib [15].

We await the results of these trials, which will shed more light on the role of vismodegib in combination with local therapy for the treatment of locally advanced BCC. In our patient, we found that combination of vismodegib, radiation therapy, and outpatient local excision for locally advanced BCC of the face was safe and well tolerated, allowed for a less extensive recovery that otherwise may have been unfavorable in a patient with severe cardiac comorbidities, and resulted in excellent oncologic control while maintaining function and cosmesis. Long-term follow-up of our patient is needed to determine long-term response to treatment.

Abbreviations

BCC: Basal cell carcinoma
CT: Computed tomography
GTV: Gross tumor volume
CTV: Clinical target volume
PTV: Planning target volume
3DCRT: 3-Dimensional conformal radiation therapy
MMS: Mohs micrographic surgery.

Consent

Written informed consent was obtained from the patient for publication of this case report and any accompanying images.

Disclosure

Alec M. Block and Fiori Alite are radiation oncology residents. Aidnag Z. Diaz is an attending radiation oncologist specializing in head and neck oncology. Richard W. Borrowdale is an attending head and neck surgical oncologist. Joseph I. Clark is an attending medical oncologist specializing in head and neck oncology. Mehee Choi is an attending radiation oncologist specializing in head and neck oncology.

Authors' Contribution

Alec M. Block participated in the planning and treatment of the patient in this case report, participated in the design of this treatment plan and case report, and drafted the paper. Fiori Alite participated in the planning and treatment of the patient in this case report, participated in the design of this treatment plan and case report, and assisted in drafting the paper. Aidnag Z. Diaz conceived of this case report and

assisted in drafting the paper. Richard W. Borrowdale and Joseph I. Clark participated in the treatment of the patient in this case report, participated in the design of this treatment plan and case report, and assisted in drafting the paper. Mehee Choi participated in the planning and treatment of the patient in this case report, participated in the design of this treatment plan and case report, assisted in drafting the paper, and oversaw the entirety of this project. All authors read and approved the final paper.

Acknowledgment

The authors thank their patient for allowing them to write about his case for the benefit of the academic community and future patients.

References

[1] M.-F. Avril, A. Auperin, A. Margulis et al., "Basal cell carcinoma of the face: surgery or radiotherapy? Results of a randomized study," *British Journal of Cancer*, vol. 76, no. 1, pp. 100–106, 1997.

[2] C. M. Chahbazian and G. S. Brown, "Radiation therapy for carcinoma of the skin of the face and neck. Special considerations," *The Journal of the American Medical Association*, vol. 244, no. 10, pp. 1135–1137, 1980.

[3] D. D. Von Hoff, P. M. LoRusso, C. M. Rudin et al., "Inhibition of the hedgehog pathway in advanced basal-cell carcinoma," *The New England Journal of Medicine*, vol. 361, no. 12, pp. 1164–1172, 2009.

[4] A. Sekulic, M. R. Migden, A. E. Oro et al., "Efficacy and safety of vismodegib in advanced basal-cell carcinoma," *The New England Journal of Medicine*, vol. 366, no. 23, pp. 2171–2179, 2012.

[5] A. L. S. Chang, J. A. Solomon, J. D. Hainsworth et al., "Expanded access study of patients with advanced basal cell carcinoma treated with the Hedgehog pathway inhibitor, vismodegib," *Journal of the American Academy of Dermatology*, vol. 70, no. 1, pp. 60–69, 2014.

[6] P. M. LoRusso, C. M. Rudin, J. C. Reddy et al., "Phase I trial of hedgehog pathway inhibitor vismodegib (GDC-0449) in patients with refractory, locally advanced or metastatic solid tumors," *Clinical Cancer Research*, vol. 17, no. 8, pp. 2502–2511, 2011.

[7] R. M. Gathings, C. S. Orscheln, and W. W. Huang, "Compassionate use of vismodegib and adjuvant radiotherapy in the treatment of multiple locally advanced and inoperable basal cell carcinomas and squamous cell carcinomas of the skin," *Journal of the American Academy of Dermatology*, vol. 70, no. 4, pp. e88–e89, 2014.

[8] E. L. Pollom, T. T. Bui, A. L. Chang, A. D. Colevas, and W. Y. Hara, "Concurrent vismodegib and radiotherapy for recurrent, advanced basal cell carcinoma," *JAMA Dermatology*, vol. 151, no. 9, pp. 998–1001, 2015.

[9] A. L. S. Chang, S. X. Atwood, D. M. Tartar, and A. E. Oro, "Surgical excision after neoadjuvant therapy with vismodegib for a locally advanced basal cell carcinoma and resistant basal carcinomas in Gorlin syndrome," *JAMA Dermatology*, vol. 149, no. 5, pp. 639–641, 2013.

[10] G. A. Zhu, U. Sundram, and A. L. S. Chang, "Two different scenarios of squamous cell carcinoma within advanced basal cell carcinomas: cases illustrating the importance of serial biopsy during vismodegib usage," *JAMA Dermatology*, vol. 150, no. 9, pp. 970–973, 2014.

[11] A. Iarrobino, J. L. Messina, R. Kudchadkar, and V. K. Sondak, "Emergence of a squamous cell carcinoma phenotype following treatment of metastatic basal cell carcinoma with vismodegib," *Journal of the American Academy of Dermatology*, vol. 69, no. 1, pp. e33–e34, 2013.

[12] A. Orouji, S. Goerdt, J. Utikal, and M. Leverkus, "Multiple highly and moderately differentiated squamous cell carcinomas of the skin during vismodegib treatment of inoperable basal cell carcinoma," *British Journal of Dermatology*, vol. 171, no. 2, pp. 431–433, 2014.

[13] ClinicalTrials.gov, "Placebo-controlled, Double Blind Study to Assess Efficacy and Safety of Oral Vismodegib for the Treatment of Basal Cell Carcinoma Preceding Excision by Mohs Micrographic Surgery (MMS)," NCT01543581, 2015.

[14] ClinicalTrials.gov, "A Phase II, Multicenter, Open-label, Three-cohort Trial Evaluating the Efficacy and Safety of Vismodegib (GDC-0449) in Operable BCC," NCT01201915, 2015.

[15] ClinicalTrials.gov, "A Phase II Study of Radiation Therapy and Vismodegib, for the Treatment of Locally Advanced BCC of the Head and Neck," NCT01835626, 2015.

13

Diagnostic Challenges in Primary Hepatocellular Carcinoma: Case Reports and Review of the Literature

Monika Pazgan-Simon,[1] **Sylwia Serafinska,**[2] **Justyna Janocha-Litwin,**[1] **Krzysztof Simon,**[2] **and Jolanta Zuwala-Jagiello**[3]

[1]*Infectious Disease Department, Wroclaw Medical University, Wroclaw, Poland*
[2]*Infectious Disease Department, Division of Infectious Disease and Hepatology, Wroclaw Medical University, Wroclaw, Poland*
[3]*Department of Pharmaceutical Biochemistry, Wroclaw Medical University, Wroclaw, Poland*

Correspondence should be addressed to Monika Pazgan-Simon; monika.pazgan.simon@gmail.com

Academic Editor: Raffaele Palmirotta

Hepatocellular carcinoma is the fifth most common malignancy and the third leading mortality cause worldwide. It typically develops secondarily to liver cirrhosis, due to hepatitis B or C infection, alcohol abuse, metabolic disease, and so forth. According to the American Association for the Study of Liver Diseases (AASLD) guidelines, which constitute diagnostic standards, the diagnosis of primary hepatocellular carcinoma (HCC) should be based on contrast-enhanced imaging. Lesion hyperenhancement should be observed throughout the arterial phase, followed by the washout during the venous phase. The diagnosis can also be based on the histopathological evaluation of liver biopsy specimen. Although the standards are clear, we often see patients with advanced HCC in clinical practice, who cannot be offered any effective treatment. Patients with chronic liver disease, presenting with inconclusive and changeable test results, constitute a separate problem. In such cases the diagnostic process is typically long-term and delayed. In this paper we present three case reports where the diagnosis could not be made promptly and the patients died as a result of a delayed diagnostic process.

1. Introduction

Hepatocellular carcinoma is the fifth most common malignancy (5% of all cancer cases) and the third leading cancer-associated mortality cause worldwide. It is also the most common primary hepatic malignancy (80% of liver cancer cases in adults and 35% in children) [1]. In almost all cases it is secondary to cirrhosis or other chronic liver damage. However, it may also develop without significant liver damage in children with HBV infection. HCC is the leading mortality cause in patients with cirrhosis. It is estimated that the main causes of liver disease leading to cirrhosis and/or HCC in Europe include hepatitis C (HCV) infection in 60% of patients, hepatitis B (HBV) infection in 15% of patients, and alcohol abuse in 10% of patients. The rest are attributed to metabolic liver diseases: nonalcoholic hepatic steatosis, alpha-1AT deficiency, hemochromatosis, and congenital tyrosinemia; carcinogens: aflatoxin B1, thorotrast, and dimethylaminoazobenzene; and some medications: anabolic hormones, estrogens, methyldopa, and methotrexate. The risk of HCC development increases with risk factor and cofactor accumulation; for example, cirrhosis concomitant with HBV infection increases this risk 1000-fold. The HBV/HCV, HBV/HIV, or HCV/HIV coinfection (or coinfection with all three types of a virus), alcohol abuse, long-term tobacco use, and other factors promote HCC development [2].

2. Primary Hepatocellular Carcinoma: Diagnostic Recommendations

The diagnostic management algorithms concerning cases of suspected cancerous lesions within the liver are (or at least should be) commonly known. They were developed and recently also updated by the European Association for the Study of the Liver (EASL) and the AASLD [3]. These are based (regardless of uncharacteristic clinical symptoms or their absence) on the findings of diagnostic imaging and histopathological assessment and in some cases on the serum alpha-fetoprotein (AFP) or des-gamma carboxyprothrombin (DCP) levels. The basis for an early diagnosis of HCC is regular screening of selected high-risk groups of patients. Patients with liver cirrhosis of variable etiology and Child-Pugh scores A and B as well as individuals with HBV infection and a family history of HCC need rigorous monitoring every 6 months. Liver ultrasound evaluation is recommended as a part of this monitoring. If the suspected focal lesion is 1-2 cm in diameter, 2 separate contrast-enhanced diagnostic imaging procedures must be performed (e.g., contrast-enhanced ultrasound, done relatively infrequently these days, contrast-enhanced computed tomography (CT) or triphasic, and contrast-enhanced magnetic resonance imaging (MRI) scans). If the findings are still inconclusive, the diagnosis should be confirmed with a cytological or histopathological evaluation. According to the international diagnostic guidelines, if the lesion is larger than 2 cm, HCC can be diagnosed based on contrast-enhanced imaging, confirming hypervascularization during the arterial phase and quick washout during the venous phase. If the histopathological evaluation fails to confirm cancerous lesion, diagnostic imaging should be performed repeatedly every 3–6 months.

The diagnosis of HCC can be based on AFP level, once the concentration exceeds 350 mg/dL. This parameter, however, was not included in the current screening programmes due to its low sensitivity in patients with smaller-size lesions. However, the consecutive increase of AFP level in a patient with liver cirrhosis should always raise the suspicion of hepatocellular carcinoma. The algorithms for HCC diagnosis are virtually unambiguous. Even though, due to the challenges faced in clinical practice, the diagnostic process is often delayed, which precludes early treatment and is reflected in the decreased survival.

3. Treatment Options

Until recently, there were no effective treatment methods available for HCC patients. However, a significant progress has been made in this respect in recent years. Complex management of HCC includes radical (surgery), conservative (medical), palliative, causal, and supplementary treatment. Psychological counselling, dietary interventions, and medical nutrition therapy belong to the supplementary treatment category. HCC can be treated successfully only if diagnosed early enough.

3.1. Radical Treatment. The only radical treatment offering some curative potential is complete surgical removal of cancerous lesion, that is, tumour excision with the adjacent liver tissue (partial hepatectomy and lobectomy—although these procedures do not address the underlying liver disease) or liver transplant surgery. Unfortunately, due to the advanced stages of HCC at the moment of diagnosis, only <20–30% of patients can benefit from surgical treatment. Surgery is possible in patients staged according to BCLC as very early

(<2 cm) or early HCC, provided that the lesion is limited to 1 lobe only (i.e., liver function is normal and no signs of portal hypertension are observed). Small lesions are excised with 1 cm surgical margin. If the lesions are more extensive but no major vessel involvement is present, liver transplant surgery is indicated.

The alternatives to tumour resection are radiofrequency ablation (RFA), laser photoablation, microwave ablation (MWA), cryoablation, and percutaneous ethanol injection (PEI). Each procedure must be repeated several times, and treatment outcomes in small tumours (up to 2 cm) are comparable to those of surgical treatment.

3.2. Medical (Conservative)/Palliative Therapy. If a patient cannot be treated surgically, medical (conservative)/palliative therapy is used (stages A–C according to BCLC), which includes the following.

(1) Transcatheter procedures are as follows: transarterial embolization (TAE), transarterial chemoembolization (TACE) (performed if resection cannot be performed or as a "bridging" procedure prior to liver transplant surgery), and radioembolization.

However, portal vein thrombosis or tumour infiltrating blood vessels preclude such interventions. The patient requires appropriate preparation and supplementary treatment during the perioperative period. These are high-risk procedures and 60–80% of patients develop some complications, which lead to death in 3% of cases. The estimated efficacy of such treatment ranges between 35 and 40%. However, a complete response can be achieved in less than 2% of cases [4].

(2) Intraoperative radiation therapy: brachytherapy and external beam radiation therapy (teletherapy): the available external beam techniques are intensity modulated radiation therapy (IMRT) and stereotactic radiation therapy; the efficacy is referred to as good local control and pain relief; treatment outcomes may be further improved by the simultaneous hepatic artery embolization [5].

(3) Neoadjuvant and adjuvant therapy: the beneficial effect of immune therapy or hormone replacement therapy on the efficacy of other HCC treatments has not been proved [6].

(4) Systemic treatment:

(a) Chemotherapy:

(i) Doxorubicin and cisplatin-based regimens, efficacy <10%.

(ii) Complex regimens: PIAF, XELOX, and GEMOX (gemcitabin plus oxiliplatin), efficacy <22%: chemotherapy of HCC is associated with high toxicity and numerous adverse effects, especially in patients with concomitant cirrhosis [7–10].

(b) Angiogenesis inhibitors and cellular signalling pathway blockers: sorafenib is the only approved drug in this group; it acts on a cancer cell level and inhibits multiple kinases: tyrosine kinases (VEGFR2, PDGFR, c-KIT, and receptor) and serine-threonine kinases (b-raf and p-38); at the same time sorafenib blocks the RAF/MEK/ERK signalling pathways, inhibits tumour angiogenesis, and induces tumour cell apoptosis; the inclusion criteria for sorafenib treatment are A–C, PS 0–2, and Child-Pugh A-B scores; the total survival median increased by approximately 11 months (6–14 months) in 40% of treated patients; even superior outcomes were achieved in patients on combination therapy based on sorafenib + daunorubicin/ capecitabine /oxaliplatin; the survival median was increased by additional 8 months; when TACE is combined with sorafenib, the results are not unambiguous.

(c) Hormone replacement therapy (androgenic and progesterone inhibitors): ineffective and not used.

(d) Octreotide: its efficacy has not been proven yet.

According to current opinions, supported by the published evidence, antiviral treatment is a crucial element of complex HCC treatment (although antiviral medications do not exert any proven delay effect on tumour growth) and plays an important role in tumour spread and/or recurrence prevention in patients with HBV or HCV infections (as they constitute the most numerous group of HCC patients from the epidemiology perspective) [11–13].

HCC diagnosis can be particularly challenging in some cases and the obtained results seem ambiguous, which is illustrated by the three cases we present below.

4. Case Reports

4.1. Case Report 1. A 33-year-old male is diagnosed with HCV infection, genotype 3, in 1993. In 2000 histopathological evaluation of liver biopsy specimen showed severe inflammation (G3 level) and fibrosis (S3 level) as well as steatosis. The patient underwent recombined interferon and ribavirin treatment twice in 2001 and 2003. Both attempts to treat him failed, although his HCV genotype typically has a good prognosis for treatment response. The patient regularly attended follow-up visits. In 2010 a gradual increase of AFP level was observed: August 2010, 35.77 ng/mL, May 2011, 189.1 ng/mL, and September 2011, 4062.36 ng/mL, whereas the general health status of the patient was good and he did not display any clinical symptoms of complete cirrhosis. The ultrasound scans performed regularly at 6-month intervals and the contrast-enhanced abdominal CT scan performed in May 2011 did not show any cancerous lesions within the cirrhotic liver. Due to very high AFP levels and negative results of already performed diagnostic imaging procedures, the patient was admitted to our department in September 2011. The contrast-enhanced MRI was performed, which showed a single focal lesion sized 80 × 50 × 80 mm located within the 6th and 7th segment and suggestive of HCC. A core needle biopsy confirmed the diagnosis of HCC. Due to

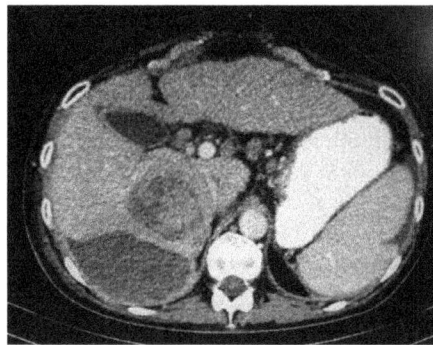

FIGURE 1: A three-phase CT of the abdomen. In a 4-segment focal lesion with typical enhancement in contrast phase and washout effect in a venous phase.

lesion size and patient's health which deteriorated rapidly, no conservative or antiviral treatment was commenced and the patient died two months later.

4.2. Case Report 2. The histopathological evaluation of liver biopsy specimen of a 50-year-old female diagnosed in 2001 with HCV infection (G1b genotype) and with the history of HBV infection (particularly unfavourable situation from the perspective of HCC pathogenesis) showed moderate inflammation and fibrosis (G2, S2). The patient underwent a 48-week therapy with peginterferon-alfa combined with ribavirin in 2004. However, the treatment did not lead to the sustained virologic response (SVR). The follow-up biopsy performed in 2006 showed slight disease progression (G2-3, S2-3). Due to the concomitant thrombocytopenia, the patient was subsequently treated with natural interferon and ribavirin. The therapy, however, was discontinued after 12 weeks because of lack of early virologic response. The patient remained under the care of Infectious Disease Outpatient Clinic and the follow-up ultrasound scans were performed on a regular basis. In May 2010 the patient was admitted to our department due to the deterioration of her general health status, including significant weight loss and clinical symptoms of complete, compensated, active cirrhosis. The triphasic CT scan showed a lesion suggestive of HCC located within the 4th segment; however, due to the size of the lesion the patient was not qualified for surgery (Figure 1). The targeted fine needle biopsy did not confirm the malignancy. The follow-up ultrasound scans did not show the progression of the described lesion; the AFP level did not increase, either, and remained within the range of 36.89 ng/mL to 44.6 ng/mL. Due to significant diagnostic uncertainties, another (core needle) biopsy of the tumour was performed in September 2011, which confirmed the presence of cirrhosis. The patient was readmitted to our department 3 months later due to liver decompensation and she died in a month. The final diagnosis of HCC was made during an autopsy.

4.3. Case Report 3. A 65-year-old female with liver cirrhosis of mixed-aetiology (alcohol abuse + HCV G1b infection), confirmed in 1993 with histopathological findings in the biopsy specimen, was admitted to our department in June

2010 for the extensive diagnosis of a hepatic focal lesion revealed within the 6th segment in a CT performed in February 2008. For the undetermined reason the patient had not attended the recommended follow-up consults and imaging procedures for 2 years. At admission the Child-Pugh score was A5; the patient had concomitant COPD and was an active tobacco user. The ultrasound scan showed a normoechogenic focal lesion sized 21×12 mm, which had no distinct margins accompanied by the peripheral hypoechoic halo zone. The patient's serum AFP level was 10.96 ng/mL. For the abovementioned reasons, the patient was not immediately qualified for causal treatment of HCV infection (such patients are included in the antiviral treatment scheme at the moment). The contrast-enhanced abdominal CT scan performed 3 months later showed a heterogeneous abnormal focus sized 42×27 mm, localized within the 6th segment, which compressed the right portal vein branch. Two new lesions sized 8 mm each were additionally revealed within the 8th segment. Moreover, signs of portal hypertension were shown. As the findings were ambiguous, in order to distinguish cancerous lesion from the intrahepatic arterioportal venous malformation abdominal angio-CT scan was performed, as recommended by the radiologist. However, the findings were still inconclusive, so the diagnosis could not be made. At that time the patient did not give her consent to invasive diagnostic procedures. The patient was hospitalized for the second time in March 2011. This time her Child-Pugh score was 6 and the AFP level remained stable at 11.5 ng/mL. The contrast-enhanced MRI revealed a focal lesion of poorly defined polycystic margins within the 6th segment, sized $4.5 \times 2.7 \times 3.5$ cm, and hepatic angioma and focal hepatic steatosis were excluded. The ultrasound-guided core needle biopsy did not confirm neoplastic malignant lesions or their precursors (dysplastic focal lesions). The image was typical of complete inflammatory cirrhosis, concomitant with alcoholic steatohepatitis and steatosis. The patient was readmitted to our department for follow-up imaging in October 2011. The AFP level decreased to 6.71 ng/mL. The ultrasound scan revealed a lesion sized $51 \times 65 \times 69$ mm within the 6th segment. The lesion infiltrated the right hepatic vein, which was an explicit confirmation of its malignant nature. With clinical diagnosis of HCC the patient was referred to the Organ Transplant Surgery Outpatient Clinic. Unfortunately, the tumour had already spread to the abdominal blood vessels, so she could not be approved as a liver recipient. A subsequent CT-guided core needle biopsy and histopathological evaluation of the biopsy specimen were performed as a part of qualification for treatment with sorafenib. The evaluation did not show any areas of neoplasia or dysplasia. The patient died a few months later due to the generalized cancer.

5. Discussion

Early diagnosis of HCC is an obvious key to potential good treatment outcomes. But, unfortunately, 70%–80% of patients cannot benefit from radical treatment (i.e., liver resection and liver transplant) due to being diagnosed too late. The delayed diagnosis results in most cases from the lack of proper follow-up and regular diagnostic imaging. This can be jointly attributed to the low awareness of the disease among the GPs, high costs, and patients' neglect. Other reasons include old diagnostic equipment, inexperienced clinicians assessing the obtained scans, choice of improper imaging technique (e.g., plain CT/MRI), relying on normal AFP levels, and the lack of histopathological confirmation of the diagnosis. Unfortunately, mostly for technical reasons, histopathological diagnosis is not always possible. The abovementioned problems caused the delay or lack of in vivo diagnosis of HCC in the discussed cases precluding early therapeutic interventions. Diagnostic imaging constitutes the main category of diagnostic tools used in HCC. Ultrasound evaluation used to be and still remains the standard screening technique in primary hepatocellular carcinoma. If performed every 6 months by an experienced radiologist/clinician, the ultrasound scan enables detection of smaller-size lesions and, in turn, faster diagnosis and effective treatment [14]. Computed tomography is a very good diagnostic tool for HCC patients. However, in order to be useful it must be contrast-enhanced, four-phase scan (precontrast phase, arterial phase, portal venous phase, and delayed phase), which requires well-trained, experienced healthcare personnel. The abdominal, contrast-enhanced MRI offers superior sensitivity, if performed and interpreted by an experienced radiologist. Two types of contrast media are used for MRI: manganese- or gadolinium-based agents characterised by hepatocyte affinity or agents captured by the mononuclear phagocyte system. The main advantage of the discussed diagnostic methods includes the possibility to differentiate between hepatocellular and nonhepatocellular malignancies [15].

Liver biopsy with the subsequent histopathological evaluation of specimen still remains the diagnostic standard for chronic hepatitis and HCC. However, the efficacy of different types of biopsy in HCC differs; the targeted fine needle biopsy is estimated to be effective in 10–30% of cases, whereas the estimated efficacy of core needle biopsy is approximately 50%. Such low efficacy is caused not only by the improper biopsy technique, but rather by the tumour itself, which can be highly differentiated and may even contain the intact hepatic parenchyma. In order to improve the efficacy of biopsy the use of newer systems (e.g., Tru-Cut biopsy) seems to be reasonable.

The AFP level measurement has been used as a diagnostic marker of primary hepatocellular carcinoma since 1970s. The elevated AFP levels correlate with large lesions, over 5 cm in diameter. However, the AFP concentration typically remains normal if the lesion is small (<2 cm). The primary hepatocellular carcinoma, not associated with AFP level elevation throughout its entire course, constitutes a separate diagnostic challenge. That is why the EASL no longer recommends the use of AFP in patient screening for HCC. This biomarker is actually useful in the assessment of tumour reoccurrence, which is a separate topic for discussion.

Liver elastography appears to be an interesting diagnostic tool, although its use is limited; the researchers from Japan and the United Kingdom showed a high risk of HCC in patients with liver stiffness over 20 kPa [16] and the risk of postoperative tumour reoccurrence in patients with liver stiffness over 13.4 kPa [17].

6. Summary

(1) Low sensitivity of ultrasound imaging and poor quality CT preclude early diagnosis of HCC and proper interventions, especially in smaller-size tumours.

(2) The technical difficulties in obtaining specimens for histopathological evaluation (e.g., too small specimens obtained during the targeted fine needle biopsy, subdiaphragmatic or periportal lesions, significant comorbidities, etc.) preclude early histopathological diagnosis in many cases, thus delaying or precluding treatment.

(3) The ambiguity of diagnostic imaging findings as well as long waiting time for hospital admission end imaging reports deprives many patients of their chance for an early, effective treatment.

References

[1] F. X. Bosch, J. Ribes, R. Cléries, and M. Díaz, "Epidemiology of hepatocellular carcinoma," *Clinics in Liver Disease*, vol. 9, no. 2, pp. 191–211, 2005.

[2] H. B. El-Serag and K. L. Rudolph, "Hepatocellular carcinoma: epidemiology and molecular carcinogenesis," *Gastroenterology*, vol. 132, no. 7, pp. 2557–2576, 2007.

[3] European Association for the Study of the Liver and European Organization for Research and Treatment of Cancer, "EASL-EORTC clinical practice guidelines: management of hepatocellular carcinoma," *Journal of Hepatology*, vol. 56, no. 4, pp. 908–943, 2012.

[4] J. W. Park, H. B. Kim, and I. J. Lee, "Transarterial therapies for hepatocellular carcinoma (HCC): a long way towards standardization," *Journal of Hepatology*, vol. 58, no. 1, p. 195, 2013.

[5] B. J. Debenham, K. S. Hu, and L. B. Harrison, "Present status and future directions of intraoperative radiotherapy," *The Lancet Oncology*, vol. 14, no. 11, pp. e457–e464, 2013.

[6] C. Verslype, O. Rosmorduc, and P. Rougier, "Hepatocellular carcinoma: ESMO-ESDO clinical practice guidelines for diagnosis, treatment and follow-up," *Annals of Oncology*, vol. 23, supplement 7, pp. vii41–vii48, 2012.

[7] S. Louafi, V. Boige, M. Ducreux et al., "Gemcitabine plus oxaliplatin (GEMOX) in patients with advanced hepatocellular carcinoma (HCC): results of a phase II study," *Cancer*, vol. 109, no. 7, pp. 1384–1390, 2007.

[8] U. Asghar and T. Meyer, "Are there opportunities for chemotherapy in the treatment of hepatocellular cancer?" *Journal of Hepatology*, vol. 56, no. 3, pp. 686–695, 2012.

[9] L. Rossi, F. Zoratto, A. Papa et al., "Current approach in the treatment of hepatocellular carcinoma," *World Journal of Gastrointestinal Oncology*, vol. 2, no. 9, pp. 348–359, 2010.

[10] A. Zaanan, N. Williet, M. Hebbar et al., "Gemcitabine plus oxaliplatin in advanced hepatocellular carcinoma: a large multicenter AGEO study," *Journal of Hepatology*, vol. 58, no. 1, pp. 81–88, 2013.

[11] European Association for the Study of the Liver, "EASL clinical practice guidelines: management of chronic hepatitis B virus infection," *Journal of Hepatology*, vol. 57, no. 1, pp. 167–185, 2012.

[12] P. Arends, M. J. Sonneveld, R. Zoutendijk et al., "Entecavir treatment does not eliminate the risk of hepatocellular carcinoma in chronic hepatitis B: limited role for risk scores in Caucasians," *Gut*, 2014.

[13] R. Zoutendijk, J. G. Reijnders, F. Zoulim et al., "Virological response to entecavir is associated with a better clinical outcome in chronic hepatitis B patients with cirrhosis," *Gut*, vol. 62, no. 5, pp. 760–765, 2013.

[14] American Association for the Study of Liver Diseases (AASLD), *Practice Guidelines*, American Association for the Study of Liver Diseases, 2012.

[15] T. A. Hope, M. A. Ohliger, and A. Qayyum, "MR imaging of diffuse liver disease: from technique to diagnosis," *Radiologic Clinics of North America*, vol. 52, no. 4, pp. 709–724, 2014.

[16] R. Masuzaki, R. Tateishi, H. Yoshida et al., "Assessment of disease progression in patients with transfusion-associated chronic hepatitis C using transient elastography," *World Journal of Gastroenterology*, vol. 18, no. 12, pp. 1385–1390, 2012.

[17] K. S. Jung, S. U. Kim, G. H. Choi et al., "Prediction of recurrence after curative resection of hepatocellular carcinoma using liver stiffness measurement (FibroScan)," *Annals of Surgical Oncology*, vol. 19, no. 13, pp. 4278–4286, 2012.

14

Metastatic Breast Carcinoma to the Prostate Gland

Meghan E. Kapp, Giovanna A. Giannico, and Mohamed Mokhtar Desouki

Department of Pathology, Microbiology and Immunology, Vanderbilt University Medical Center, Nashville, TN 37232, USA

Correspondence should be addressed to Mohamed Mokhtar Desouki; mokhtar.desouki@vanderbilt.edu

Academic Editor: Ossama W. Tawfik

Cancer of the male breast is an uncommon event with metastases to the breast occurring even less frequently. Prostate carcinoma has been reported as the most frequent primary to metastasize to the breast; however, the reverse has not been previously reported. Herein, we present, for the first time, a case of breast carcinoma metastasizing to the prostate gland. Prostate needle core biopsy revealed infiltrative nests of neoplastic epithelioid cells, demonstrated by immunohistochemistry (IHC) to be positive for GATA3 and ER and negative for PSA and P501S. A prostate cocktail by IHC study demonstrated lack of basal cells (p63 and CK903) and no expression of P501S. The patient's previous breast needle core biopsy showed strong ER positivity and negative staining for PR and HER2. Similar to the prostate, the breast was negative for CK5/6, p63, and p40. This case demonstrates the importance of considering a broad differential diagnosis and comparing histology and IHC to prior known malignancies in the setting of atypical presentation or rare tumors.

1. Introduction

Cancer of the male breast represents less than 1% of all breast cancers in the United States and incidence is increasing with recent approximations of 1.3/100,000 [1, 2]. While most men who develop breast cancer have no recognized risk factors, a minor subset have testicular damage (mumps, undescended testes, and high ambient working temperature). Risk has also been associated with increased body mass index, gynecomastia, increased serum estradiol level, and diabetes [3, 4]. Though formal screening programs are not established for men, most present with early stage I or II. Stage at diagnosis is a strong prognostic factor and men with triple-negative breast cancer have a worse prognosis [5].

Interestingly, men with ER-positive cancer are reported to have a 30% reduction in risk of death compared with ER-negative breast cancer; however, that benefit applies only to the first 5 years from diagnosis, at which time ER positive and negative have a similar prognosis [5]. Therapy for male breast cancer has mostly been extrapolated from treatment trials for female breast cancer, which has been shown to be ineffective. Important differences have emerged, including that male breast cancer prognosis is significantly better after adjuvant treatment with tamoxifen compared to an aromatase inhibitor, and that male breast cancer is not congruent with female breast cancer [6].

While primary carcinoma of the male breast is infrequent, metastatic carcinoma to the breast from distant organs is also very rare comprising approximately 1.2–2.7% of all malignant breast tumors [7] with the prostate being the most common primary site [8]. While breast is an exceptional site of prostatic carcinoma metastasis, it is a documented phenomenon, whereas the reverse has not been described. Herein, we present a case of metastatic breast carcinoma to the prostate of a 63-year-old male. To the best of our knowledge, this is the first-case report of breast carcinoma metastatic to the prostate.

2. Case Report

2.1. Clinical Presentation. The patient is a 63-year-old male who presented with a newly diagnosed neoplasm of the prostate. His past medical history was significant for Bowen's disease status after excision, and breast cancer status post-mastectomy and axillary dissection. The patient began to experience increasing lower urinary tract symptoms, manifested as urinary hesitancy, weak force of stream, and subjective sensation of incomplete bladder emptying. A rectal

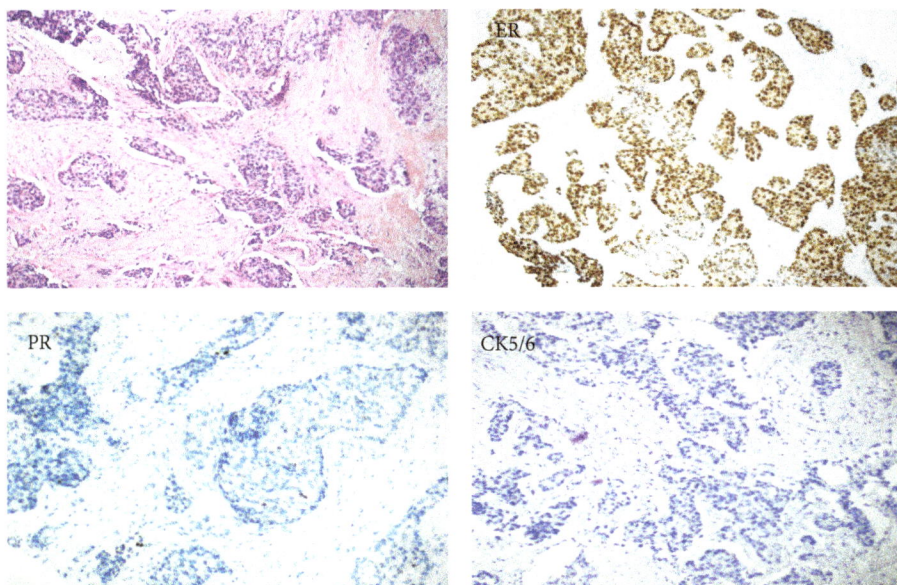

FIGURE 1: Breast core biopsy shows infiltrative nests of epithelioid cells with small ovoid hyperchromatic nuclei and modest eosinophilic cytoplasm separated by fibrous stroma with a desmoplastic reaction on H&E. Immunohistochemical stains show nuclear staining for ER and negative staining for PR and CK5/6.

examination revealed a firm prostatic nodule in the context of a PSA of 0.88.

2.2. Radiological Findings. CT scan with contrast of the chest demonstrated mediastinal and bilateral hilar lymphadenopathy, the dominant lymph node measuring 1.8 cm in greatest dimension. Multiple bilateral pulmonary masses, some of which appeared spiculated were identified. The dominant spiculated mass of the left lower lobe measured 2.4 cm in greatest dimension. The CT of the abdomen and pelvis identified two metastatic nodules in the omentum (1.6 cm in greatest dimension). The prostate was notably enlarged, heterogeneously enhancing, and bulging into the bladder base, which demonstrated mild thickening of its wall.

2.3. Surgery. Following needle core biopsies of his prostate, and due to high tumor density reported within the prostate, the patient was scheduled for a transurethral resection of prostate (TURP). and started on tamoxifen hormone therapy. Urinary retention was managed with self-catheterization; however, he experienced frequent inability to fully empty his bladder due to clots. Gross hematuria developed and TURP procedure was performed.

2.4. Pathology

2.4.1. Breast. Ultrasound guided needle core biopsy and simple mastectomy showed invasive mammary carcinoma, no special type, with high combined histologic grade and intermediate proliferative rate. The mass was 2.6 cm in greatest extent and margins on the mastectomy were negative for malignancy. Submitted immunohistochemistry (IHC) stains (Figure 1) showed the tumor cells to be ER positive (strong,

98% of neoplastic nuclei) and negative for progesterone and HER2.

2.4.2. Prostate Biopsies. Microscopic examination of the needle core biopsies from the prostate gland demonstrated a high burden of infiltrating neoplastic cells. IHC studies (Figure 2) showed the tumor cells to be positive for GATA-3 and to have strong positive ER nuclear staining in 100% of neoplastic nuclei. PSA and P501S were negative. A prostate immunohistochemical cocktail demonstrated a lack of basal cells (P63 and CK903) and no expression of P504S. In the setting of the patient's history and the characteristic morphology and immunoprofile, metastatic breast cancer was favored; however, urothelial carcinoma could not be entirely excluded [9]. IHC stains performed on both the breast and prostate biopsies showed a similar pattern of staining: negative CK5/6, p63, and p40.

2.4.3. Prostate Transurethral Resection. Grossly, the specimen consisted of multiple soft, pink-tan fragments of tissue admixed with blood clot weighing 9.2 grams and measuring 3.9 × 3.4 × 0.9 cm in aggregate. The specimen was entirely submitted for histopathologic review. Light microscopic evaluation demonstrated metastatic carcinoma, morphologically consistent with breast primary, similar to previous prostate biopsies and breast excision.

2.5. Management and Follow-Up. The patient received tamoxifen therapy, but his disease progressed rapidly. Brain metastases evidenced by 1.1 cm homogeneously T2 hyperintense rounded focus at the gray-white junction within the left frontal lobe and a second more ill-defined focus in the right paramidline parietal lobe posteriorly clinically

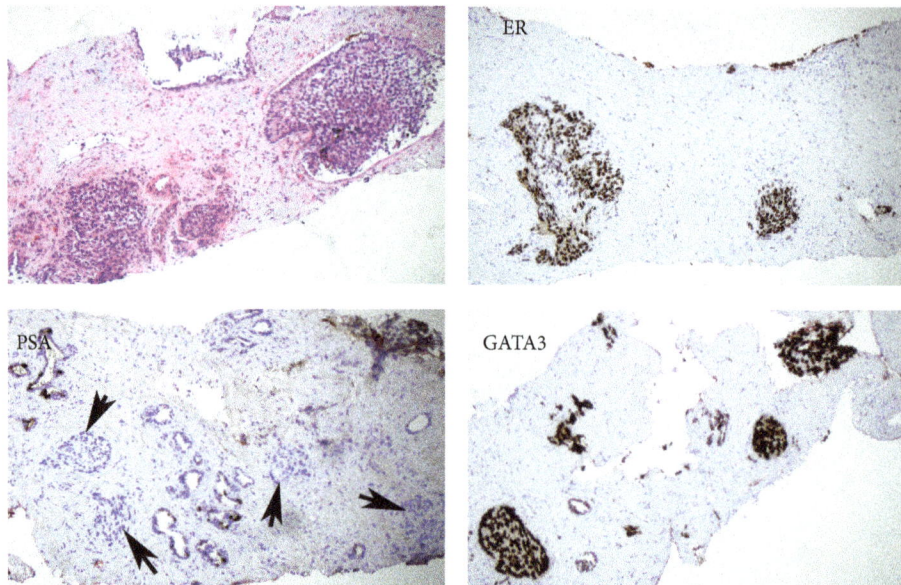

FIGURE 2: Prostate needle core biopsy shows infiltrative nests of hyperchromatic nuclei with modest eosinophilic cytoplasm separated by fibrous stroma with a desmoplastic reaction on H&E. Immunohistochemical stains show nuclear staining for ER and GATA3 and negative staining by PSA.

manifested with headache. Ophthalmologic evaluation of the patient's endorsement of blurry vision in the right eye, in addition to multiple new floaters and persistent flashing lights revealed creamy-white subretinal placoid lesions in association with serous exudative retinal detachment inferiorly concerning for metastatic disease. The patient's last hospitalization for diabetic ketoacidosis, septicemia, and urinary tract infection secondary to *E. faecalis* and fungemia was complicated by cardiopulmonary arrest secondary to thromboemboli, confirmed by postmortem examination.

3. Discussion

The involvement of the prostate gland by metastasis from noncontiguous tumors is a rare occurrence reported in <1% of surgical specimens and 3% of postmortem examinations [10, 11]. Secondary tumors of the prostate have been noted with most frequency from the digestive tract [12, 13], lung [14, 15], and kidney [16, 17]. Up to 20% of patients with secondary tumors of the prostate have no evidence of metastatic disease in additional sites [11].

Urothelial carcinoma may be a secondary tumor of the prostate and is a relatively common finding in advanced-stage bladder disease [10]. GATA-binding protein 3 (GATA3) is a highly sensitive and reproducible biomarker of urothelial differentiation; however, breast epithelial cells have also been shown to stain with GATA-3, rendering this IHC stain incapable of deciphering the two differentials in our case [18]. As morphology and initial IHC evaluation (GATA-3 and ER positivity) could not completely exclude urothelial primary with prostatic duct involvement, morphologic, and IHC comparison of the patient's primary breast cancer and current prostatic neoplasm was necessary [9, 18]. The comparison showed similar morphology and pattern of staining, thereby concluding prostatic involvement by metastatic breast carcinoma.

In the reported case, the correct diagnosis of metastatic breast cancer was important given the significant difference in management between patients with primary prostatic carcinoma, metastatic urothelial carcinoma, and breast cancer. For example, hormone therapy (tamoxifen) can be utilized as the first-round therapy for metastatic breast carcinoma with ER positivity [6]. In conclusion, this is the first reported case of metastatic breast cancer resulting in high disease burden of the prostate, and it demonstrates the importance of a broad differential diagnosis, patient history, and access to previous material for comparison in the setting of rare tumor or atypical presentation.

Abbreviations

IHC: Immunohistochemistry
ER: Estrogen receptor
PR: Progesterone receptor
TURP: Transurethral resection of the prostate.

Disclosure

The authors of this paper have no relevant financial relationships with commercial interests to disclose.

References

[1] W. F. Anderson, I. Jatoi, J. Tse, and P. S. Rosenberg, "Male breast cancer: a population-based comparison with female breast cancer," *Journal of Clinical Oncology*, vol. 28, no. 2, pp. 232–239, 2010.

[2] American Cancer Society, *Cancer Facts & Figures 2014*, 2014.

[3] L. A. Brinton, M. B. Cook, V. McCormack et al., "Anthropometric and hormonal risk factors for male breast cancer: male breast cancer pooling project results," *Journal of the National Cancer Institute*, vol. 106, no. 3, Article ID djt465, 2014.

[4] L. A. Brinton, T. J. Key, L. N. Kolonel et al., "Prediagnostic sex steroid hormones in relation to male breast cancer risk," *Journal of Clinical Oncology*, vol. 33, no. 18, pp. 2041–2050, 2015.

[5] J. P. Leone, A. O. Zwenger, J. Iturbe et al., "Prognostic factors in male breast cancer: a population-based study," *Breast Cancer Research and Treatment*, vol. 156, no. 3, pp. 539–548, 2016.

[6] H. Eggemann, A. Ignatov, B. J. Smith et al., "Adjuvant therapy with tamoxifen compared to aromatase inhibitors for 257 male breast cancer patients," *Breast Cancer Research and Treatment*, vol. 137, no. 2, pp. 465–470, 2013.

[7] I. Alvarado Cabrero, M. Carrera Álvarez, D. Pérez Montiel, and F. A. Tavassoli, "Metastases to the breast," *European Journal of Surgical Oncology*, vol. 29, no. 10, pp. 854–855, 2003.

[8] P. J. Carder, V. Speirs, J. Ramsdale, and M. R. J. Lansdown, "Expression of prostate specific antigen in male breast cancer," *Journal of Clinical Pathology*, vol. 58, no. 1, pp. 69–71, 2005.

[9] P. R. Croft, S. L. Lathrop, R. M. Feddersen, and N. E. Joste, "Estrogen receptor expression in papillary urothelial carcinoma of the bladder and ovarian transitional cell carcinoma," *Archives of Pathology and Laboratory Medicine*, vol. 129, no. 2, pp. 194–199, 2005.

[10] T. A. Zein, R. Huben, W. Lane, J. E. Pontes, and L. S. Englander, "Secondary tumors of the prostate," *Journal of Urology*, vol. 133, no. 4, pp. 615–616, 1985.

[11] A. W. Bates and S. I. Baithun, "Secondary solid neoplasms of the prostate: a clinico-pathological series of 51 cases," *Virchows Archiv*, vol. 440, no. 4, pp. 392–396, 2002.

[12] S. Roshni, T. M. Anoop, T. R. Preethi, G. Shubanshu, and A. L. Lijeesh, "Gastric adenocarcinoma with prostatic metastasis," *Journal of Gastric Cancer*, vol. 14, no. 2, pp. 135–137, 2014.

[13] F. R. Youssef, L. Hunt, P. D. Meiring, D. R. Taraporewalla, R. Gupta, and M. J. James, "Metastasis of a cecal adenocarcinoma to the prostate five years after a right hemicolectomy: a case report," *Journal of Medical Case Reports*, vol. 5, article 223, 2011.

[14] J. H. Yoo, J. H. Lee, E. K. Kim, Y. K. Hong, Y. Lee, and H. C. Jeong, "Prostatic metastasis of large cell neuroendocrine carcinoma of the lung," *Respirology*, vol. 14, no. 5, pp. 772–775, 2009.

[15] S. Madersbacher, G. Schatzl, M. Susani, and U. Maier, "Prostatic metastasis of a small cell lung cancer in a young male," *European Urology*, vol. 26, no. 3, pp. 267–269, 1994.

[16] R.-M. Fokt, A. Templeton, S. Gillessen, C. Öhlschlegel, and H.-P. Schmid, "Prostatic metastasis of renal cell carcinoma successfully treated with sunitinib," *Urologia Internationalis*, vol. 83, no. 1, pp. 122–124, 2009.

[17] O. C. Guler, N. Bal, and C. Onal, "Metachronous prostate metastasis of renal cell carcinoma: case report and review of the literature," *Clinical Genitourinary Cancer*, vol. 14, no. 2, pp. e211–e213, 2016.

[18] B. Z. Clark, S. Beriwal, D. J. Dabbs, and R. Bhargava, "Semiquantitative GATA-3 immunoreactivity in breast, bladder, gynecologic tract, and other cytokeratin 7-positive carcinomas," *American Journal of Clinical Pathology*, vol. 142, no. 1, pp. 64–71, 2014.

15

Diaphragmatic Amyloidosis Causing Respiratory Failure: A Case Report and Review of Literature

Aleksey Novikov,[1] Horatio Holzer,[1] Robert A. DeSimone,[2] Ghaith Abu-Zeinah,[1] David J. Pisapia,[2] Tomer M. Mark,[1] and Raymond D. Pastore[1]

[1]Department of Internal Medicine, New York Presbyterian Hospital, Weill Cornell Medical College, New York, NY 10065-4897, USA
[2]Department of Pathology and Laboratory Medicine, New York Presbyterian Hospital, Weill Cornell Medical College, New York, NY 10065-4897, USA

Correspondence should be addressed to Ghaith Abu-Zeinah; ghaith.azeinah@gmail.com

Academic Editor: Josep M. Ribera

Neuromuscular respiratory failure is a rare complication of systemic immunoglobulin light chain amyloidosis. We describe a case of a 70-year-old Caucasian man with multiple myeloma who presented with worsening dyspnea. The patient was diagnosed with and treated for congestive heart failure but continued to suffer from hypercapnic respiratory insufficiency. He had restrictive physiology on pulmonary function tests and abnormal phrenic nerve conduction studies, consistent with neuromuscular respiratory failure. The diagnosis of systemic immunoglobulin light chain amyloidosis was made based on the clinical context and a cardiac biopsy. Despite treatment attempts, the patient passed away in the intensive care unit from hypercapnic respiratory failure. Autopsy revealed dense diaphragmatic amyloid deposits without phrenic nerve infiltration or demyelination or lung parenchymal involvement. Only 5 cases of neuromuscular respiratory failure due to amyloid infiltration of the diaphragm have been described. All cases, including this, were characterized by rapid progression and high mortality. Therefore, diaphragmatic amyloidosis should be on the differential for progressive neuromuscular respiratory failure in patients with multiple myeloma or any other monoclonal gammopathy. Given its poor prognosis, early recognition of this condition is essential in order to address goals of care and encourage pursuit of palliative measures.

1. Case Report

A 70-year-old Caucasian man with a previously diagnosed, IgG-kappa multiple myeloma presented with a 3-month history of worsening dyspnea, dysphagia, and weight loss. The diagnosis of multiple myeloma was established one year prior to presentation with a serum kappa free light chain (K-FLC) level of 685 mg/dL and a lambda FLC level of 0.13 mg/dL (kappa/lambda (K/L) ratio of 5269). The patient had no lytic bone lesions or liver or heart involvement and had a normocellular bone marrow with 70% plasma cells. He was never noted to have macroglossia or albuminuria. His past medical history was otherwise notable for hypertension, type II diabetes mellitus, atrial fibrillation, and chronic kidney disease with Bence Jones proteinuria (K-FLC proteinuria of 691 mg/dL). Upon initial evaluation, the patient was hypoxic to 78% in room air. He appeared tachypneic,

with an increased work of breathing and accessory muscle use. Auscultation revealed overall reduced breath sounds, bibasilar crackles, and an irregular cardiac rhythm with a holosystolic grade III/VI murmur loudest at the cardiac apex.

The patient's arterial blood gas revealed a pH of 7.31, a pCO_2 of 60, and a pO_2 of 60 mmHg. His labs otherwise revealed an bicarbonate of 33 mmol/L, a creatinine of 2.55 mg/dL (increased from a baseline of 1.2 mg/dL), a hemoglobin of 10.3 g/dL, and a white blood cell count of 7.4×10^3 per μL. The patient also had a B-type natriuretic peptide level of 572 pg/mL and serial cardiac troponin I levels of 0.22, 0.22, and 0.21 ng/mL drawn 6 to 8 hours apart. His K-FLC level was 1379 mg/dL with L-FLC of 0.65 mg/dL (K/L-FLC ratio of 2121).

A chest radiograph showed mild pulmonary vascular congestion with small bilateral pleural effusions. His echocardiogram was notable for elevated pulmonary artery systolic

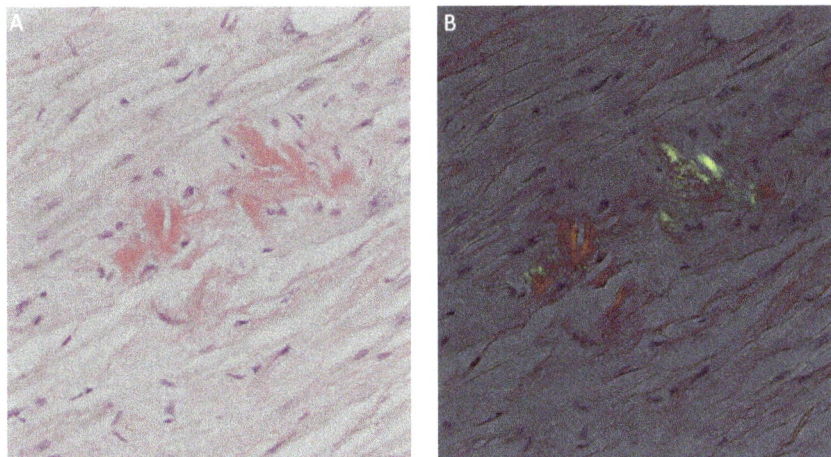

FIGURE 1: Cardiac amyloidosis. (A) Congo red stain of left ventricle showing focal positive staining (red-orange) of amorphous extracellular material, 400x. (B) Congo red stain of left ventricle showing apple-green birefringence under polarized light, diagnostic of amyloid, 400x.

pressure of 64 mmHg, biatrial dilatation with normal sized ventricles, and a preserved ejection fraction. A ventilation-perfusion scan was negative for acute or chronic pulmonary embolus.

Subsequently, the patient was admitted to the cardiac stepdown unit for inotropic diuresis and noninvasive positive pressure ventilation (NIPPV). After diuresis, a right heart catheterization (RHC) revealed PA pressure of 34/9/18 mmHg (systolic/diastolic/mean) and a pulmonary capillary wedge pressure of 10 mmHg.

Despite effective diuresis, the patient went into a worsening hypercapnic respiratory failure with almost continuous dependence on NIPPV. His pulmonary function tests revealed restrictive physiology with FEV1 of 61%, FVC of 58%, and FEV/FVC of 104%. A subsequent nerve conduction study was suggestive of bilateral phrenic axonal neuropathy.

With his worsening dysphagia and respiratory muscle weakness, the course was further complicated by aspiration pneumonitis. A barium swallow esophagram showed narrowing of the gastroesophageal junction and tertiary contractions in the esophagus. An upper endoscopy was unrevealing and biopsy samples were negative for amyloidosis, confirmed by lack of Congo red staining (not shown). A fat pad biopsy was also negative for amyloid.

Due to deteriorating cardiopulmonary and renal status, the patient was transferred to our cardiac intensive care unit. A repeat RHC was performed and a right ventricular biopsy was diagnostic of cardiac amyloidosis. The patient subsequently received 3 doses of bortezomib and dexamethasone but passed away soon after from the multiorgan system failure, approximately 5 weeks after admission.

Autopsy revealed IgG-kappa amyloid deposits in the left and right ventricles (Figure 1), the diaphragm (Figure 2), and the gastroesophageal junction (Figure 3). There was no demyelination, amyloid deposition, or other abnormalities of the phrenic nerves (Figure 4), nor was there amyloid infiltration of the lung parenchyma.

2. Discussion

The differential diagnosis of hypercapnic respiratory failure is extremely broad. It is ultimately the result of inadequate ventilation, which leads to an increase of the partial pressure of carbon dioxide in the blood. This subsequently leads to acidemia and concurrent hyperkalemia, both of which promote arrhythmias, muscle weakness, and CNS depression leading to death. This failure can be caused by disease in any organ system that is essential to the initiation and propagation of breathing including the airways, alveoli, central nervous system, peripheral nervous system, respiratory muscles including diaphragm, and chest wall. We propose that in this case the failure was caused by a mechanical defect in diaphragmatic function secondary to light chain amyloid infiltration of the diaphragm. We demonstrate sparing of the phrenic nerve and lung parenchyma on pathology, further supporting the hypothesis that diaphragmatic infiltration is the primary cause of respiratory failure in this reported case.

This rapidly progressive hypercapnic respiratory failure secondary to infiltration of the diaphragm by amyloid is only the fifth such case described in the literature. We have conducted an extensive search using National Library of Medicine database, looking for the words "amyloid", "amyloidosis", and "diaphragm". We were able to find only 4 other relevant cases in the literature. The first published article describes a 56-year-old black man with multiple myeloma [1]. Autopsy from this case showed amyloid infiltration of the diaphragm, without mention of amyloid infiltration of the phrenic nerves or lung parenchyma. Two other articles describe single cases of a 55-year-old man and a 73-year-old woman with a primary hypercapnic respiratory failure, both found to have amyloid infiltration of the diaphragm with sparing of the lungs and phrenic nerves [2, 3]. Postmortem investigation suggested the pathophysiology of hypercapnic respiratory failure was attributable to amyloid infiltration of the diaphragm, in the absence of lung and phrenic nerve involvement.

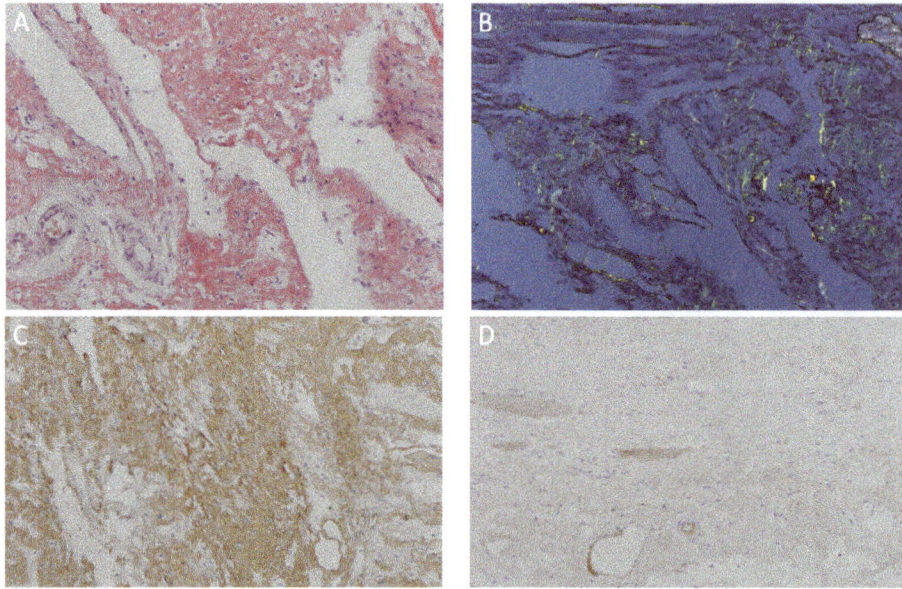

FIGURE 2: Diaphragmatic amyloidosis. (A) Congo red stain of diaphragm showing diffuse positive staining (red-orange) of amorphous extracellular material, 200x. (B) Congo red stain of diaphragm showing apple-green birefringence under polarized light, 200x. (C) Kappa light chain immunostain of diaphragm showing diffuse positivity, diagnostic of kappa amyloid light chain amyloidosis, 20x. (D) Negative lambda light chain immunostain of diaphragm, 20x.

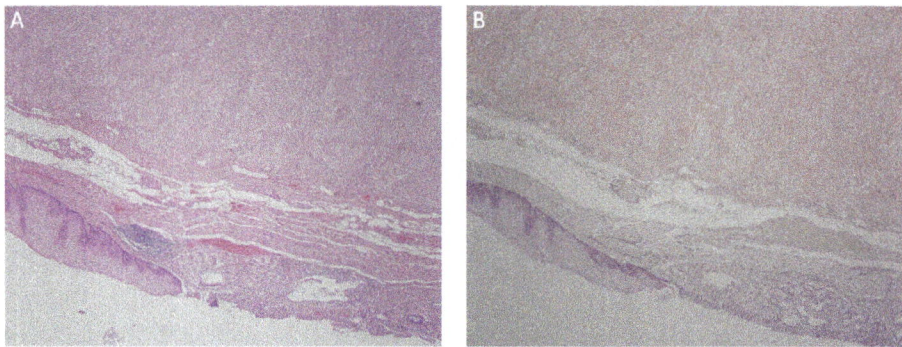

FIGURE 3: Gastroesophageal junction amyloidosis. (A) Hematoxylin and eosin stain of gastroesophageal junction showing a thickened muscularis propria, 20x. (B) Congo red stain showing diffuse extracellular positive staining (red-orange) restricted to the muscularis propria, 20x.

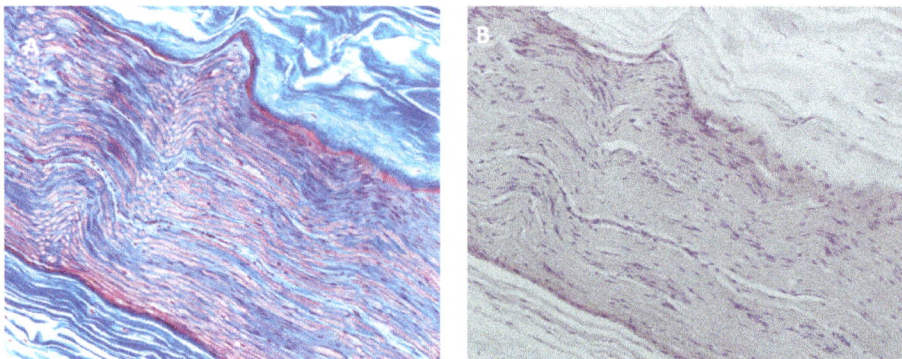

FIGURE 4: Phrenic nerve. (A) Trichrome staining of right phrenic nerve showing preservation of myelin sheath, 400x. (B) Congo red stain of right phrenic nerve, negative for amyloidosis, 400x.

To our knowledge, there is only one case report that proposes an alternative theory of respiratory failure driven by a peripheral nerve infiltration with amyloid [4]. This conclusion is based on the results of the abnormal neural conduction studies and fluoroscopy and spirometry studies. It is important to note that this report does not demonstrate a primary pathology of the phrenic nerves. On the other hand, autopsy results from all the other studies have shown amyloid infiltration only in the diaphragm, supporting the notion that diaphragmatic amyloidosis is the more likely etiology of respiratory failure.

Both our case and that by Berk et al. show abnormal nerve conduction studies. However, in the absence of pathology to suggest nervous system involvement or demyelination, it is very unlikely for phrenic nerve neuropathy to be the cause of respiratory failure in such patients. Therefore, nerve conduction studies should not be considered diagnostic. This becomes important when measures such as diaphragmatic pacing are considered, as it may be of benefit when the nervous system is involved but unlikely to benefit a diaphragm infiltrated by amyloid.

This case report highlights a rare but a rapidly fatal complication of systemic amyloidosis. The reported cases over the past 30 years show a 100% association between amyloid infiltration of the diaphragm and respiratory failure. In 4 out of the 5 cases of diaphragmatic amyloidosis reviewed, the diagnosis of respiratory failure carried an 80% mortality rate within 1 month. Only in 1 case did the patient survive hospitalization [4]. Given its high case mortality, findings of progressive respiratory failure in the setting of systemic amyloidosis should trigger goals of care discussions. While we have found no evidence to support the notion that amyloidosis of the phrenic nerves causes respiratory failure, we do think that the amyloid-induced respiratory failure should continue to be studied as diaphragmatic pacing could be considered in certain cases of phrenic nerve damage.

References

[1] R. M. Santiago, D. Scharnhorst, G. Ratkin, and E. C. Crouch, "Respiratory muscle weakness and ventilatory failure in AL amyloidosis with muscular pseudohypertrophy," *The American Journal of Medicine*, vol. 83, no. 1, pp. 175–178, 1987.

[2] E. A. Streeten, S. M. de la Monte, and T. P. Kennedy, "Amyloid infiltration of the diaphragm as a cause of respiratory failure," *Chest*, vol. 89, no. 5, pp. 760–762, 1986.

[3] J. Ashe, C. O. Borel, G. Hart, R. L. Humphrey, D. A. Derrick, and R. W. Kuncl, "Amyloid myopathy presenting with respiratory failure," *Journal of Neurology Neurosurgery and Psychiatry*, vol. 55, no. 2, pp. 162–165, 1992.

[4] J. L. Berk, J. F. Wiesman, M. Skinner, and V. Sanchorawala, "Diaphragm paralysis in primary systemic amyloidosis," *Amyloid*, vol. 12, no. 3, pp. 193–196, 2005.

16

A Rare Case of Metastatic Desmoplastic Small Round Cell Tumour: Diagnosis and Management

Shahzaib Nabi,[1] Abhijit Saste,[2] and Rohit Gulati[3]

[1]Department of Internal Medicine, Henry Ford Health System, 2799 W. Grand Boulevard, Detroit, MI 48202, USA
[2]Department of Hematology-Oncology, Henry Ford Health System, 2799 W. Grand Boulevard, Detroit, MI 48202, USA
[3]Department of Pathology, Henry Ford Health System, 2799 W. Grand Boulevard, Detroit, MI 48202, USA

Correspondence should be addressed to Shahzaib Nabi; snabi1@hfhs.org

Academic Editor: Jose I. Mayordomo

A 26-year-old male without any significant past medical history presented to the hospital with shortness of breath, cough, pleuritic chest pain, and weight loss for the past 3 months. On chest CT, he was found to have extensive mediastinal and hilar lymphadenopathy and multiple pulmonary nodules. On physical examination, a right groin mass was noted which had been slowly growing for the past 2 years. Ultrasound of the groin showed complex solid mass with internal vascular channels. CT guided biopsy of the mass showed desmoplastic small round cell tumour. His hospital course was complicated by hypoxic respiratory failure requiring emergent intubation and ICU admission where he completed one cycle of vincristine, cyclophosphamide, and doxorubicin with subsequent improvement, followed by extubation. His condition continued to improve after second cycle of chemotherapy and he was ultimately discharged in a stable condition to continue outpatient chemotherapy after a 2-month inpatient stay.

1. Introduction

This case report describes our clinical experience in the diagnosis and management of a rather uncommon malignancy. Given the rarity of this condition, with less than 200 cases reported to date, every case experience such as ours adds to the understanding of how varying clinical scenarios can be successfully managed and what the responses looked like. Additionally, a pool of such cases with information on progression free survivals and response rates may then help future investigators gain a better understanding of the efficacy of such a regimen, safety signals of its components, and management of any complications that clinicians may have encountered. More importantly, we successfully investigated and treated an intubated patient with chemotherapy to then discharge him in an ambulatory condition. He maintains an ECOG performance status of 0.

2. Case Presentation

Our patient is a 26-year-old male with no significant past medical history. He presented to the hospital with a 3-month history of shortness of breath, dry cough, and pleuritic chest pain. His symptoms started gradually but started to worsen about a week before presenting to the hospital. The shortness of breath was mainly exertional. Patient was also experiencing a dry cough related to this difficulty of breathing. He also complained of pleuritic chest pain, bilaterally in both lower chest fields, 5/10 in intensity, dull in nature without any radiation. Aggravating factor included bouts of cough but there were no specific relieving factors. The patient had also noticed some unintentional weight loss but was unsure about the amount of lost weight. Review of systems was negative for fever or any exposure to sick contacts. There was no history of night sweats. He did not have any risk factors for tuberculosis. There was no history of any recent travel and the patient did not complain of any leg swelling.

Physical examination showed a thin and lean male in slight respiratory distress. Patient was found to be tachypneic with a respiratory rate of 34 breaths per minute and tachycardic with a heart rate of 118 beats per minute. He was afebrile and normotensive. Auscultation of the lungs revealed diffuse bilateral wheezing. Chest palpation was negative for chest wall tenderness. Auscultation of the heart revealed

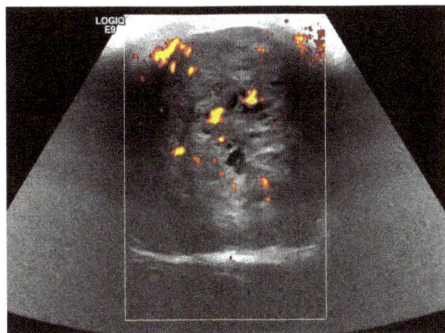

FIGURE 1: Ultrasound of groin showing complex vascular mass.

normal S1 and S2 with no added sounds. Neurologically, the patient was alert and oriented to time, place, and person. He was able to follow commands with no focal neurological deficits. Abdominal examination showed a soft, nontender abdomen with no organomegaly and normal bowel sounds. A large, firm, nontender mass, with poorly defined margins was palpated in the right groin. It was not reducible and there were no signs of infection (no redness, tenderness, or warmth). There was no change in the size or shape of the mass when the patient was asked to perform the valsalva maneuver. According to the patient, the mass had been slowly growing in his groin for the past 2 years. Penile examination was negative for any ulcers or discharge. Scrotal examination did not show any apparent testicular masses.

The patient's family history was negative for any significant problems. The patient did not smoke or drink alcohol and had no risk factors for sexually transmitted diseases. He was not taking any medications at the time of admission.

3. Investigations

Complete Blood Count (CBC) and basic metabolic panel were normal.

Ultrasound of the pelvis and scrotum showed a $7.5 \times 5.5 \times 5.9$ cm complex vascular mass in the rightward mons pubis with unremarkable sonographic appearance of the testicles (Figure 1). MRI of the pelvis showed mass lesions involving the right inguinal canal extending to the distal right iliac chain likely consistent with enlarged lymph nodes. Significant effacement and mass effect was seen upon the right corpora cavernosa of the penis without definite evidence of soft tissue or osseous invasion (Figure 2). Significant narrowing and effacement of the right external iliac vein were seen at the level of mass lesions.

Chest X-ray showed extensive parenchymal opacities throughout both lungs with mediastinal fullness (Figure 3). CT scan of the chest showed extensive mediastinal and hilar lymphadenopathy with prominent interstitial changes throughout both lungs and multiple diffuse pulmonary nodules (Figure 4).

Ultrasound guided biopsy of the inguinal mass was carried out and pathology results were consistent with desmoplastic small round cell tumour (DSRCT) (Figure 5). Immunohistochemical staining showed desmin and cytokeratin

(CAM 5.2) positivity (Figure 6). CD56 immunostain and leukocyte common antigen were negative. A fluorescent in situ hybridization (FISH) assay was positive for EWSR1 break apart (Figure 7). RT-PCR was negative for EWS-Fli1 and EWS-ERG rearrangements, indicating absence of t(11;22) and t(21;22), respectively, of Ewing's sarcoma/PNET. Endobronchial ultrasound (EBUS) guided biopsies of the lymph nodes and pulmonary masses were performed. The pathology was consistent with desmoplastic small round cell tumor.

4. Treatment

The patient's hospital course was complicated by respiratory distress and hypoxia resulting in admission to the intensive care unit where he was intubated for hypoxic respiratory failure. The etiology was believed to be resorption atelectasis secondary to the bronchial compression from metastatic lesions and a pneumothorax from his malignancy. He had a chest tube placed which successfully treated his pneumothorax. While on the ventilator, he was initiated on and completed cycle 1 of vincristine, cyclophosphamide, and doxorubicin as a part of the Memorial Sloan Kettering Cancer Center P6 chemotherapy protocol of VAC/IE (vincristine, adriamycin, and cyclophosphamide alternating with ifosfamide and etoposide). This resulted in significant regression in his pulmonary tumour burden and subsequent extubation. His course was also complicated by febrile neutropenia which were managed with intravenous antibiotics, transfusions, and growth factor support. He was eventually discharged from the hospital in a stable condition after a 2-month-long inpatient stay.

The patient continues to follow up with the oncology clinic as an outpatient and gets electively admitted for his chemotherapy. He is occupationally functional and maintains a good appetite. He maintains an ECOG performance status of 0. He has completed 3 cycles of vincristine, cyclophosphamide, and doxorubicin followed by two cycles of ifosfamide and etoposide. A restaging CT scan of the chest and abdomen done after completion of radiation and cycle 4 of VAC/IE has shown significant reduction in the size of his groin mass and pulmonary metastases (Figures 3 and 4). He has completed radiation therapy to the right groin mass for a total of 37.5 Gray given as 2.5 Gray daily for a total of 15 fractions. He is currently scheduled to undergo autologous stem cell transplant.

5. Discussion

Desmoplastic small round cell tumours (DSRCT) are a rare group of sarcomas found in almost all age groups. Like all other sarcomas, they are of mesenchymal origin. They occur more commonly in adolescents and young adults. They were first described in 1989 by Gerald and Rosai as small round blue cell tumours with predilection for serosal surfaces and occurring predominantly in young Caucasian males with predominantly intra-abdominal locations with focal rhabdoid pattern with an intense desmoplastic reaction [1, 2]. Up till 2013, less than 200 cases had been reported in the world literature [3].

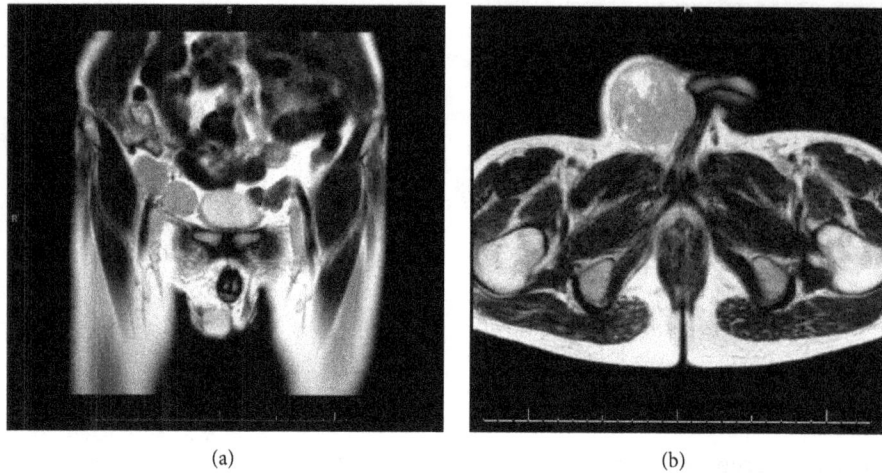

(a)

(b)

FIGURE 2: MRI coronal (a) and transverse (b) section showing mass lesion in the right inguinal region with mass effect on the corpora cavernosa of the penis.

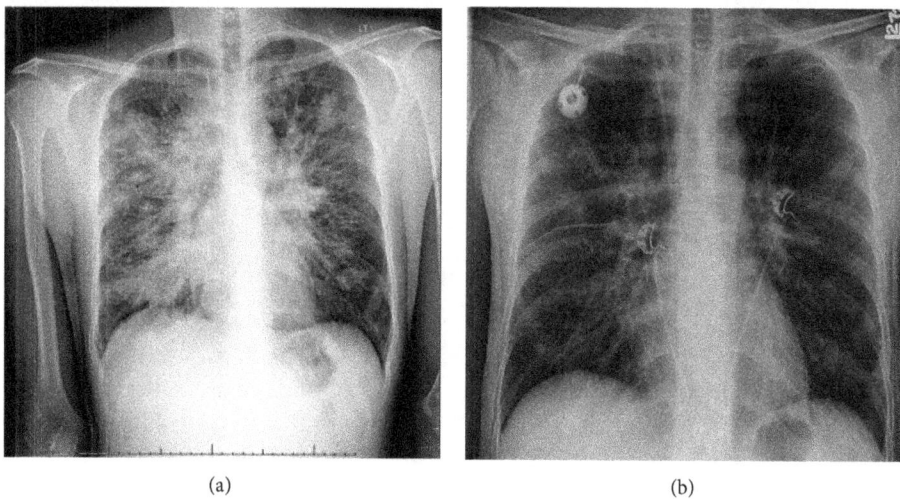

(a)

(b)

FIGURE 3: Chest X-ray with evidence of bilateral pulmonary opacities and hilar fullness on presentation (a) and after 4 cycles of VAC/IE chemotherapy (b).

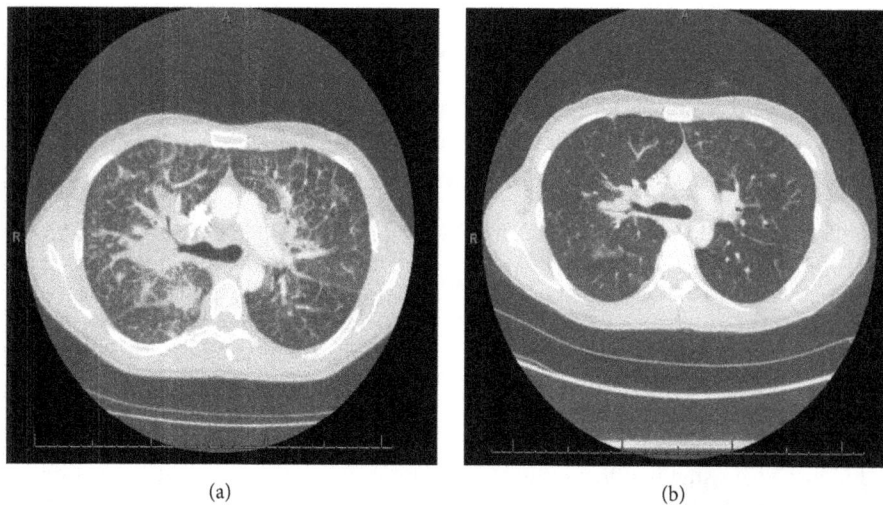

(a)

(b)

FIGURE 4: CT chest with large masses bilaterally at level of bifurcation of trachea (a) and after 4 cycles of VAC/IE chemotherapy (b).

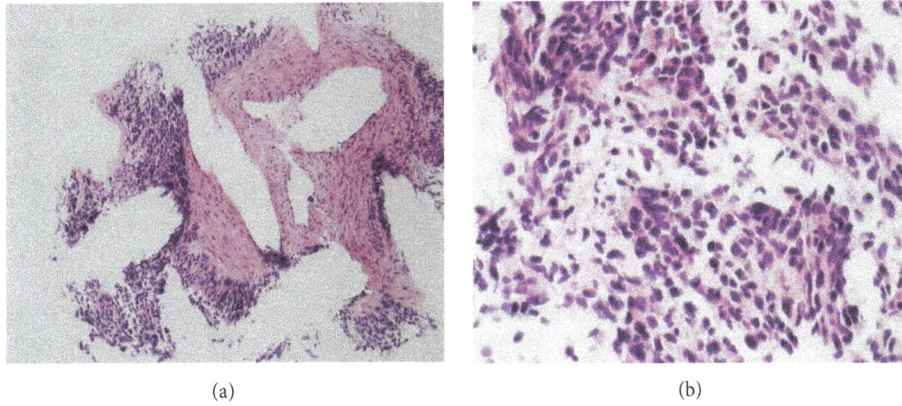

(a)

(b)

FIGURE 5: H&E stain (×200 on (a)) showing nests and sheets of small round blue cells infiltrating desmoplastic stroma. Tumour cells (×600 on (b)) with round to oval, hyperchromatic, mitotically active nuclei with scant cytoplasm.

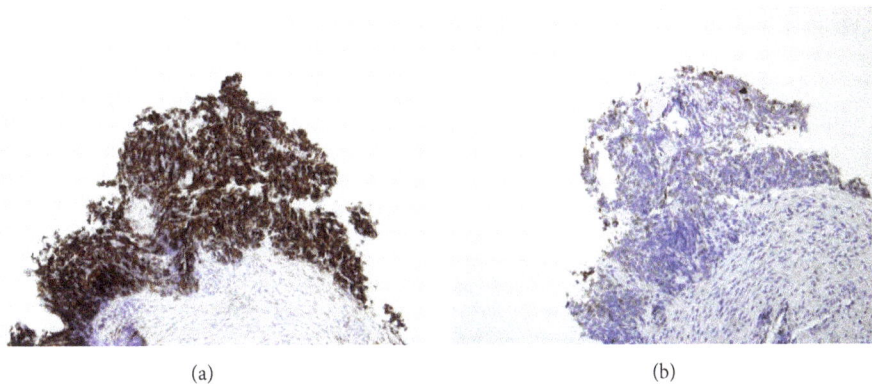

(a)

(b)

FIGURE 6: Immunohistochemical staining showing strong positivity for desmin (a) and focal positivity for cytokeratin (b).

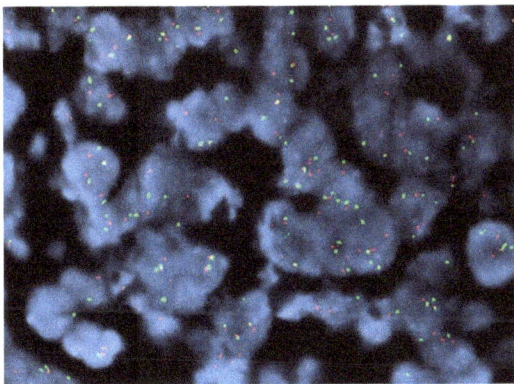

FIGURE 7: FISH assay showing positivity for EWSR1 gene rearrangement. Sixty five percent of the interphase cells showed separation of EWSR1.

Histologically, the tumour consists of poorly differentiated round cells with cytoplasmic densities and connective tissue stroma. They typically show immunohistochemical positivity for desmin, cytokeratin, vimentin, and CAM5.2 [4]. The peculiar perinuclear dot-like staining pattern for vimentin and desmin is characteristic for DSRCT. These tumours arise from a reciprocal translocation, t(11;22)(p13;q12), which results from fusion of Ewing's sarcoma (EWS) and Wilms' tumour (WT1) genes [5–8]. Histopathology is not sufficient to diagnose DRSCT as certain other tumours such as primitive neuroectodermal tumour can mimic DRSCT under the microscope. Molecular analysis is required for a final diagnosis [9].

The majority of the cases of DRSCT occur in the abdomen; however, many case reports have described this tumour originating from different organs such as testis, extremities, salivary glands, and brain [10–13]. Clinical presentation depends on the primary location of the tumour as well as disease stage. Diagnosis typically requires a tissue biopsy with identification of histopathological features along with immunohistochemistry and molecular testing. Fine-needle aspiration has also been used for the diagnosis of DRSCT [14]. As previously mentioned, hallmark feature in molecular testing is the presence of WT1-EWS fusion; however, case reports with atypical molecular features have also been described [15].

Surgery, radiation therapy, and chemotherapy are modalities that are utilized for the treatment of DRSCT but given the rarity of the condition no large scale prospective trials exist for head to head comparisons. Hyperthermic intraperitoneal chemotherapy using Cisplatin has been utilized as a low morbidity treatment option for DSRCT patients [16–18]. The reported results have been variable with some studies showing survival benefit when used instead of traditional systemic chemotherapy [19–21]. Yttrium microspheres have been used successfully to treat liver metastasis from DSRCT [22]. For limited stage disease, complete surgical resection is the treatment of choice. Based on the tumour size and grade, neoadjuvant/adjuvant radiotherapy and chemotherapy can be utilized.

The Memorial Sloan Kettering Cancer Center P6 protocol is one of the most studied and therefore commonly used chemotherapy regimens for DSRCT. It consists of seven cycles of chemotherapy. Cycles 1, 2, 3, and 6 include high dose cyclophosphamide, doxorubicin, and vincristine (VAC). Cycles 4, 5, and 7 consist of ifosfamide and etoposide (IE). Myeloablative chemotherapy with etoposide and thiotepa, followed by allogeneic stem cell transplantation, has been tried. Studies have shown that intense multimodality approach is associated with better outcomes [23, 24]. Certain investigational drugs, such as temsirolimus, an antiangiogenic serine/threonine protein kinase inhibitor, are being considered for these tumours, but the data on these is very limited [25]. Another agent named pazopanib, a tyrosine kinase inhibitor, is also under investigation for the treatment of these tumours [26].

The 5-year survival rate of DRSCT is only approximately 15% [27]. The prognosis is generally poor as the majority of the patients have metastatic disease at the time of presentation. The median survival ranges from 17 to 25 months [28].

References

[1] W. L. Gerald, H. K. Miller, H. Battifora, M. Miettinen, E. G. Silva, and J. Rosai, "Intra-abdominal desmoplastic small round-cell tumor. Report of 19 cases of a distinctive type of high-grade polyphenotypic malignancy affecting young individuals," *The American Journal of Surgical Pathology*, vol. 15, no. 6, pp. 499–513, 1991.

[2] W. L. Gerald and J. Rosai, "Case 2. Desmoplastic small cell tumor with divergent differentiation," *Pediatric Pathology/affiliated with the International Paediatric Pathology Association*, vol. 9, no. 2, pp. 177–183, 1989.

[3] A. Abu-Zaid, A. Azzam, A. AlNajjar, H. Al-Hussaini, and T. Amin, "Desmoplastic small round cell tumor of stomach," *Case Reports in Gastrointestinal Medicine*, vol. 2013, Article ID 907136, 6 pages, 2013.

[4] M. Li, M. Y. Cai, J. B. Lu, J. H. Hou, Q. L. Wu, and R. Z. Luo, "Clinicopathological investigation of four cases of desmoplastic small round cell tumor," *Oncology Letters*, vol. 4, no. 3, pp. 423–428, 2012.

[5] W. L. Gerald, M. Ladanyi, E. de Alava et al., "Clinical, pathologic, and molecular spectrum of tumors associated with t(11;22)(p13;q12): desmoplastic small round-cell tumor and its variants," *Journal of Clinical Oncology*, vol. 16, no. 9, pp. 3028–3036, 1998.

[6] H. Kang, J. H. Park, W. Chen et al., "EWS-WT1 oncoprotein activates neuronal reprogramming factor ASCL1 and promotes neural differentiation," *Cancer Research*, vol. 74, no. 16, pp. 4526–4535, 2014.

[7] R. La Starza, G. Barba, V. Nofrini et al., "Multiple EWSR1-WT1 and WT1-EWSR1 copies in two cases of desmoplastic round cell tumor," *Cancer Genetics*, vol. 206, no. 11, pp. 387–392, 2013.

[8] W. L. Gerald and D. A. Haber, "The EWS-WT1 gene fusion in desmoplastic small round cell tumor," *Seminars in Cancer Biology*, vol. 15, no. 3, pp. 197–205, 2005.

[9] B. Rekhi, R. Basak, S. B. Desai, and N. A. Jambhekar, "A t (11; 22) (p13; q12) EWS-WT 1 positive desmoplastic small round cell tumor of the maxilla: an unusual case indicating the role of molecular diagnosis in round cell sarcomas," *Journal of Postgraduate Medicine*, vol. 56, no. 3, pp. 201–205, 2010.

[10] O. W. Cummings, T. M. Ulbright, R. H. Young, A. P. Dei Tos, C. D. Fletcher, and M. T. Hull, "Desmoplastic small round cell tumors of the paratesticular region. A report of six cases," *The American Journal of Surgical Pathology*, vol. 21, no. 2, pp. 219–225, 1997.

[11] V. Adsay, J. Cheng, E. Athanasian, W. Gerald, and J. Rosai, "Primary desmoplastic small cell tumor of soft tissues and bone of the hand," *The American Journal of Surgical Pathology*, vol. 23, no. 11, pp. 1408–1413, 1999.

[12] S. K. Thondam, D. D. Plessis, D. J. Cuthbertson et al., "Intracranial desmoplastic small round cell tumor presenting as a suprasellar mass," *Journal of Neurosurgery*, vol. 122, no. 4, pp. 773–777, 2015.

[13] B. Pang, C. C. Leong, M. Salto-Tellez, and F. Petersson, "Desmoplastic small round cell tumor of major salivary glands: report of 1 case and a review of the literature," *Applied Immunohistochemistry & Molecular Morphology*, vol. 19, no. 1, pp. 70–75, 2011.

[14] J. Klijanienko, P. Colin, J. Couturier et al., "Fine-needle aspiration in desmoplastic small round cell tumor: a report of 10 new tumors in 8 patients with clinicopathological and molecular correlations with review of the literature," *Cancer Cytopathology*, vol. 122, no. 5, pp. 386–393, 2014.

[15] L. Liang, N. Tatevian, M. Bhattacharjee, K. Tsao, and J. Hicks, "Desmoplastic small round cell tumor with atypical immunohistochemical profile and rhabdoid-like differentiation," *World Journal of Clinical Cases*, vol. 2, no. 8, pp. 367–372, 2014.

[16] H. S. Fan, B. I'Ons, R. McConnell, V. Kumar, S. Alzahrani, and D. L. Morris, "Peritonectomy and hyperthermic intraperitoneal chemotherapy as treatment for desmoplastic small round cell tumour," *International Journal of Surgery Case Reports*, vol. 7, pp. 85–88, 2015.

[17] A. Hayes-Jordan, H. Green, H. Lin et al., "Cytoreductive surgery and hyperthermic intraperitoneal chemotherapy (HIPEC) for children, adolescents, and young adults: the first 50 cases," *Annals of Surgical Oncology*, vol. 22, no. 5, pp. 1726–1732, 2015.

[18] C. Honoré, K. Amroun, L. Vilcot et al., "Abdominal desmoplastic small round cell tumor: multimodal treatment combining chemotherapy, surgery, and radiotherapy is the best option," *Annals of Surgical Oncology*, vol. 22, no. 4, pp. 1073–1079, 2015.

[19] A. Hayes-Jordan, H. Green, N. Fitzgerald, L. Xiao, and P. Anderson, "Novel treatment for desmoplastic small round cell tumor: hyperthermic intraperitoneal perfusion," *Journal of Pediatric Surgery*, vol. 45, no. 5, pp. 1000–1006, 2010.

[20] S. Msika, E. Gruden, S. Sarnacki et al., "Cytoreductive surgery associated to hyperthermic intraperitoneal chemoperfusion for

desmoplastic round small cell tumor with peritoneal carcinomatosis in young patients," *Journal of Pediatric Surgery*, vol. 45, no. 8, pp. 1617–1621, 2010.

[21] G. Lauridant-Philippin, N. Ledem, F. Lemoine et al., "Optimal treatment with systemic chemotherapy, complete surgical excison and hyperthermic intraperitoneal chemotherapy for a desmoplastic small round cell tumor in an adult male patient," *Gastroentérologie Clinique et Biologique*, vol. 34, no. 4-5, pp. 321–324, 2010.

[22] A. Hayes-Jordan and P. M. Anderson, "The diagnosis and management of desmoplastic small round cell tumor: a review," *Current Opinion in Oncology*, vol. 23, no. 4, pp. 385–389, 2011.

[23] B. H. Kushner, M. P. LaQuaglia, N. Wollner et al., "Desmoplastic small round-cell tumor: prolonged progression-free survival with aggressive multimodality therapy," *Journal of Clinical Oncology*, vol. 14, no. 5, pp. 1526–1531, 1996.

[24] A. A. Kallianpur, N. K. Shukla, S. V. Deo et al., "Updates on the multimodality management of desmoplastic small round cell tumor," *Journal of Surgical Oncology*, vol. 105, no. 6, pp. 617–621, 2012.

[25] A. M. Thijs, W. T. van der Graaf, and C. M. van Herpen, "Temsirolimus for metastatic desmoplastic small round cell tumor," *Pediatric Blood & Cancer*, vol. 55, no. 7, pp. 1431–1432, 2010.

[26] A. M. Frezza, C. Benson, I. R. Judson et al., "Pazopanib in advanced desmoplastic small round cell tumours: a multi-institutional experience," *Clinical Sarcoma Research*, vol. 4, article 7, 2014.

[27] D. R. Lal, W. T. Su, S. L. Wolden, K. C. Loh, S. Modak, and M. P. La Quaglia, "Results of multimodal treatment for desmoplastic small round cell tumors," *Journal of Pediatric Surgery*, vol. 40, no. 1, pp. 251–255, 2005.

[28] A. Dufresne, P. Cassier, L. Couraud et al., "Desmoplastic small round cell tumor: current management and recent findings," *Sarcoma*, vol. 2012, Article ID 714986, 5 pages, 2012.

17

A Case of Multiple Myeloma with Metachronous Chronic Myeloid Leukemia Treated Successfully with Bortezomib, Dexamethasone, and Dasatinib

Samer Alsidawi,[1] Abhimanyu Ghose,[2] Julianne Qualtieri,[3] and Neetu Radhakrishnan[2]

[1] Department of Internal Medicine, University of Cincinnati, Cincinnati, OH 45267, USA
[2] Division of Hematology-Oncology, Department of Medicine, University of Cincinnati, Cincinnati, OH 45267, USA
[3] Department of Pathology, University of Cincinnati, Cincinnati, OH 45267, USA

Correspondence should be addressed to Neetu Radhakrishnan; radhaknu@ucmail.uc.edu

Academic Editor: Josep M. Ribera

The coexistence of multiple myeloma and chronic myeloid leukemia in a single patient is a very rare event that has been reported very infrequently in the literature. We report a case of a patient who developed chronic myeloid leukemia four years after his diagnosis with multiple myeloma. Historically, no link between the two malignancies has been identified. This synchronous existence complicates the treatment plan for these patients, and there is a lack of evidence on the best therapeutic approach. Our patient was successfully treated with a combination of bortezomib, dexamethasone, and dasatinib, which he tolerated well for eleven months until he eventually succumbed to cardiac complications and pulmonary hypertension leading to his death.

1. Introduction

Multiple myeloma (MM) is a plasma cell dyscrasia characterized by an uncontrolled proliferation of a single plasma cell clone leading to overproduction of a monoclonal immunoglobulin. MM is an overall uncommon malignancy accounting for approximately 1% of all cancers in the Unites States [1]. Chronic myeloid leukemia (CML) is a myeloproliferative disorder characterized by uncontrolled proliferation of mature granulocytes. CML is associated with the fusion of two genes: BCR (on chromosome 22) and ABL1 (on chromosome 9) resulting in the BCR-ABL1 fusion gene which gives rise to an abnormal chromosome 22 known as the Philadelphia chromosome which is closely linked to the pathogenesis of this malignancy. CML is also considered an uncommon malignancy with an annual incidence of 1 to 2 cases per 100.000 [2]. About 10 to 15 percent of patients with CML initially present in the accelerated phase or blast phase of the disease which resembles an acute leukemia. The cooccurrence of MM and CML in one patient is an extremely rare incident that has been reported in less than 20 cases in the literature and their simultaneous presence or management

is not yet fully understood. Here we present the case of a patient who achieved good response to his MM treatment but presented with CML four years after his MM diagnosis which further complicated his treatment plan.

2. Case Presentation

A 60-year-old African American male with beta-thalassemia minor, diabetes mellitus, and hypertension was diagnosed with IgG Kappa multiple myeloma (MM) in 2008 after a minor mechanical fall resulted in a right femur fracture. His X-rays showed multiple lytic lesions of the right femur. Labs at diagnosis were significant for microcytic anemia with a hemoglobin of 12.3 g/dL and a mean corpuscular volume (MCV) of 67 fL, normal white blood cells (WBC) and platelet counts, an M-spike of 3.9 g/dL on his serum protein electrophoresis (SPEP) with the immunofixation significant for a monoclonal IgG Kappa, and a high Kappa/Lambda ratio. There was 70% involvement of the bone marrow with plasma cells and the cytogenetic analysis was significant for male karyotype with trisomy of chromosome 3 and deletion of Y

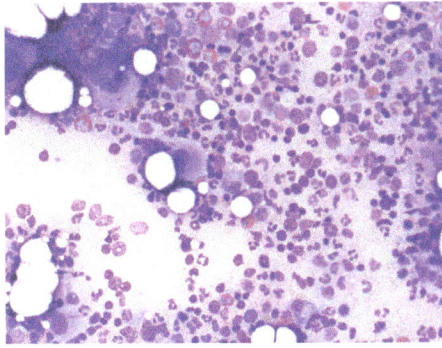

FIGURE 1: Bone marrow aspirate showing a hypercellular marrow with trilineage hematopoiesis and increased myeloid cell series (M : E ratio 4 : 1) with eosinophilia and plasmacytosis (approximately 15 to 20%).

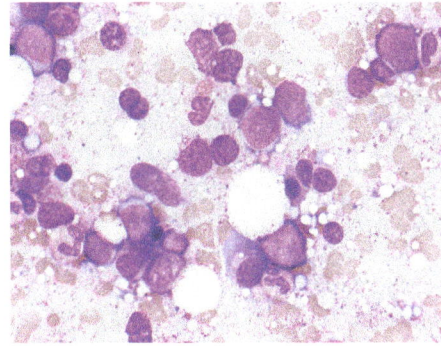

FIGURE 2: Bone marrow with markedly increased population of cells >20%, morphologically consistent with blasts.

chromosome in 4 out of 20 cells. The patient was treated with radiation to his femur after an orthopedic procedure and this was followed by five cycles of lenalidomide 25 mg daily on days 1–21 and dexamethasone 40 mg daily on days 1, 8, 15, and 22 every 4 weeks followed by bortezomib 1.3 mg/m^2 on days 1, 4, 8, and 11 every 3 weeks. The patient achieved stable disease with this regimen and he received no further treatment for almost four years. Meanwhile, he was being followed up regularly with clinical and laboratory assessments, serial serum protein electrophoresis with immunofixation, and free light chains. In 2012, four years after his initial diagnosis and treatment, the patient was found to have a relapse of his MM with an increase in his M-spike to >2 g/dL. Labs showed hemoglobin of 9.5 g/dL, WBC of 11.2 × 10^3/mm^3 with a normal differential except for slightly elevated eosinophils, and platelet count of 509 × 10^3/mm^3. Skeletal survey showed increase in his myeloma lytic bone lesions. A bone marrow aspirate and biopsy was done which demonstrated a hypercellular marrow with trilineage hematopoiesis, increased myeloid cell series (M : E ratio 4 : 1) with eosinophilia, and 15–20% monoclonal plasmacytosis based on CD138 immunostaining (Figure 1). The cytogenetics showed 46 XY t(9;22) (q34;q11.2) in 8 out of 15 cells and the fluorescent in situ hybridization (FISH) was consistent with BCR/ABL translocation in 72.8% of cells. Interestingly, no trisomy of chromosome 3 or deletion of Y chromosome was detected in the cells examined—which could be explained by their low levels and the small number of metaphases examined. It was decided to control the patient's myeloma first prior to starting a tyrosine kinase inhibitor (TKI) for his CML as there was evidence of an aggressive myeloma progression with the sudden increase in his bony lesions, while his WBC was normal at the time. He was started again on lenalidomide 25 mg every 3 weeks and dexamethasone 20 mg weekly. Three months later, the patient presented with symptoms of fatigue, malaise, abdominal discomfort, and generalized weakness. The M spike was 1.8 g/dL, WBC count 42.7 10^3/mm^3, and platelet count of 2472 10^3/mm^3. There was an increased number of myelocytes, metamyelocytes, bands, mature neutrophils with rare blasts (approximately 1% of

total cells), and increased basophils (4.2%). He underwent a bone marrow aspirate and biopsy that showed a hypercellular bone marrow with significantly increased myeloid progenitor population with a blast count of 37% in background of a myeloproliferative disorder, favoring transformation to acute myeloid leukemia (Figure 2). Unfortunately, the initial bone marrow biopsy from his MM diagnosis was not available to be examined for CML. A diagnosis of chronic myeloid leukemia in blast phase was made and cytoreductive treatment was started with hydration and hydroxyurea (up to 4 g/days) and subsequently he was started on dasatinib 140 mg daily. The patient reached major molecular response four months after treatment and complete molecular response four months after that. He was kept on maintenance treatment with dasatinib 100 mg daily. The treatment for the MM with lenalidomide was stopped when the patient presented in blast crisis. In 3 months, the patient had a quick progression of multiple myeloma with an increase of his M-spike to 2.5 g/dL and new diffuse lytic bone lesions. Treatment with weekly bortezomib 0.7 mg/m^2 which was later increased to 1.3 mg/m^2 weekly and dexamethasone 20 mg on days 1, 4, 8, and 11 of a 21-day cycle was restarted, concurrent with dasatinib. The patient tolerated the treatment combination of bortezomib and dasatinib well. He continued to show complete molecular response of his CML and he initially showed a good response of his MM as his M-spike stabilized around 1.9 g/dL transiently before increasing back to 2.3 g/dL again. One year from the start of dasatinib, the patient had an acute myocardial infarction. Dasatinib was continued while bortezomib and dexamethasone were discontinued which resulted in an improvement in his anemia while his M-spike remained stable. About five months later, he was admitted with pulmonary artery hypertension (PAH) with a mean pulmonary arterial pressure of 50–55 mm Hg on right heart catheterization. It was assumed that this was due to either the dasatinib or a diet pill that he admitted to taking over the counter or due to a combination of his comorbidities. Although dasatinib was stopped, he eventually succumbed to respiratory failure due to PAH 18 months after his CML diagnosis.

3. Discussion

The cooccurrence of MM and CML is a very rare entity that has been reported in less than twenty cases in the literature. There are only four reported cases where the diagnosis of MM preceded the diagnosis of CML [3–6]. Many of the reported cases in which the diagnosis of MM followed a long treatment course of CML [7–11] with the tyrosine kinase inhibitor, imatinib, suggested a link between this treatment and the development of MM. However, almost half of the reported cases of these two entities coexisting in a single patient are of patients who either developed MM first or were diagnosed with the two malignancies simultaneously [12–17]. This makes a link between imatinib and the development of MM very unlikely. Similarly, MM treatment does not seem to lead to the development of CML as the reported patients were treated for MM using regimens consisting of multiple different and unrelated agents. There is no evidence in the literature to suggest that either lenalidomide or bortezomib can lead to the development of CML. Lenalidomide is now known to be a risk factor for secondary malignancies, but it is usually nonmelanoma skin cancers and myelodysplastic syndromes [18]. The finding of Philadelphia chromosome in the bone marrow is an indicator of a myeloproliferative disease; however, there are reported cases of patients with MM with this translocation [19, 20]. The significance of such finding is unknown.

In the case presented above, we show that the combination of bortezomib and dasatinib was well tolerated. This represents the first case in which a patient with MM and CML received concurrent treatment with bortezomib, dexamethasone, and dasatinib. Pulmonary arterial hypertension is a known complication of dasatinib and is commonly seen after 8 to 48 months of treatment [21–24]. Although less common, pulmonary arterial hypertension has been reported with bortezomib as well [25, 26]. It was unclear if dasatinib was the only culprit in our patient's pulmonary hypertension as he also sustained a cardiac event and he later admitted to taking an unknown "diet pill" which might have all contributed to developing pulmonary hypertension. Most cases of pulmonary hypertension after dasatinib described near complete regression of this side effect after cessation of the drug. However, there are cases of refractory pulmonary hypertension that required treatment despite the withdrawal of dasatinib [27].

4. Conclusion

The cooccurrence of MM and CML is an extremely rare entity that creates dilemmas in the management of these two separate malignancies. We present our experience in a patient whose treatment of MM was complicated by the development of CML that quickly progressed into the blast phase. We found that the combination of bortezomib, dexamethasone, and dasatinib was well tolerated; however, special attention needs to be paid to the individual side effects of these medications.

Disclosure

This research received no specific grant from any funding agency in the public, commercial, or not-for-profit sectors.

References

[1] R. Siegel, J. Ma, Z. Zou, and A. Jemal, "Cancer statistics, 2014," *CA Cancer Journal for Clinicians*, vol. 64, no. 1, pp. 9–29, 2014.

[2] Y. Chen, H. Wang, H. Kantarjian, and J. Cortes, "Trends in chronic myeloid leukemia incidence and survival in the United States from 1975 to 2009," *Leukemia and Lymphoma*, vol. 54, no. 7, pp. 1411–1417, 2013.

[3] M. Nitta, K. Tsuboi, S. Yamashita et al., "Multiple myeloma preceding the development of chronic myelogenous leukemia," *International Journal of Hematology*, vol. 69, no. 3, pp. 170–173, 1999.

[4] P. J. Klenn, B. H. Hyun, Y. H. Lee, and W. Y. Zheng, "Multiple myeloma and chronic myelogenous leukemia: a case report with literature review," *Yonsei Medical Journal*, vol. 34, no. 3, pp. 293–300, 1993.

[5] L. Ragupathi, V. Najfeld, A. Chari, B. Petersen, S. Jagannath, and J. Mascarenhas, "A case report of chronic myelogenous leukemia in a patient with multiple myeloma and a review of the literature," *Clinical Lymphoma Myeloma and Leukemia*, vol. 13, no. 2, pp. 175–179, 2012.

[6] G. Caparrotti, D. Esposito, F. Graziani, F. G. De, and D. Pagiani, "Development of chronic myeloid leukemia in a patient with multiple myeloma: a case report," *Haematologica*, vol. 92, p. 183, 2007.

[7] C. Derghazarian and N. B. Whittemore, "Multiple myeloma superimposed on chronic myelocytic leukemia," *Canadian Medical Association Journal*, vol. 110, no. 9, pp. 1047–1050, 1974.

[8] M. Ide, N. Kuwahara, E. Matsuishi, S. Kimura, and H. Gondo, "Uncommon case of chronic myeloid leukemia with multiple myeloma," *International Journal of Hematology*, vol. 91, no. 4, pp. 699–704, 2010.

[9] M. Michael, M. Antoniades, E. Lemesiou, N. Papaminas, and F. Melanthiou, "Development of multiple myeloma in a patient with chronic myeloid leukemia while on treatment with imatinib mesylate for 65 months," *Oncologist*, vol. 14, no. 12, pp. 1198–1200, 2009.

[10] A. Galanopoulos, S. I. Papadhimitriou, E. Kritikou-Griva, M. Georgiakaki, and N. I. Anagnostopoulos, "Multiple myeloma developing after imatinib mesylate therapy for chronic myeloid leukemia," *Annals of Hematology*, vol. 88, no. 3, pp. 281–282, 2009.

[11] V. Garipidou, S. Vakalopoulou, and K. Tziomalos, "Development of multiple myeloma in a patient with chronic myeloid leukemia after treatment with imatinib mesylate," *The Oncologist*, vol. 10, no. 6, pp. 457–458, 2005.

[12] J. D. Schwarzmeier, M. Shehata, J. Ackermann, M. Hilgarth, H. Kaufmann, and J. Drach, "Simultaneous occurrence of chronic myeloid leukemia and multiple myeloma: evaluation by FISH analysis and in vitro expansion of bone marrow cells," *Leukemia*, vol. 17, no. 7, pp. 1426–1428, 2003.

[13] A. Alvarez-Larrán, M. Rozman, and F. Cervantes, "Simultaneous occurrence of multiple myeloma and chronic myeloid leukemia," *Haematologica*, vol. 86, no. 8, p. 894, 2001.

[14] M. Tanaka, R. Kimura, A. Matsutani, K. Zaitsu, Y. Oka, and K. Oizumi, "Coexistence of chronic myelogenous leukemia and multiple myeloma: case report and review of the literature," *Acta Haematologica*, vol. 99, no. 4, pp. 221–223, 1998.

[15] M. A. Boots and G. D. Pegrum, "Simultaneous presentation of chronic granulocytic leukaemia and multiple myeloma," *Journal of Clinical Pathology*, vol. 35, no. 3, pp. 364–365, 1982.

[16] C. Offiah, P. T. Murphy, J. P. Quinn, and P. Thornton, "Coexisting chronic myeloid leukaemia and multiple myeloma: rapid response to lenalidomide during imatinib treatment," *International Journal of Hematology*, vol. 95, no. 4, pp. 451–452, 2012.

[17] N. A. Romanenko, S. S. Bessmel'tsev, V. I. Udal'eva et al., "The combination of chronic myeloid leukemia and multiple myeloma in one patient," *Voprosy Onkologii*, vol. 59, no. 2, pp. 103–110, 2013.

[18] M. A. Dimopoulos, P. G. Richardson, N. Brandenburg et al., "A review of second primary malignancy in patients with relapsed or refractory multiple myeloma treated with lenalidomide," *Blood*, vol. 119, no. 12, pp. 2764–2767, 2012.

[19] N. S. Ranni, I. Slavutsky, A. Wechsler, and S. B. de Salum, "Chromosome findings in multiple myeloma," *Cancer Genetics and Cytogenetics*, vol. 25, no. 2, pp. 309–316, 1987.

[20] P. Martiat, C. Mecucci, Y. Nizet et al., "P190 *BCR/ABL* transcript in a case of Philadelphia-positive multiple myeloma," *Leukemia*, vol. 4, no. 11, pp. 751–754, 1990.

[21] D. Montani, E. Bergot, S. Günther et al., "Pulmonary arterial hypertension in patients treated by dasatinib," *Circulation*, vol. 125, no. 17, pp. 2128–2137, 2012.

[22] D. Mattei, M. Feola, F. Orzan, N. Mordini, D. Rapezzi, and A. Gallamini, "Reversible dasatinib-induced pulmonary arterial hypertension and right ventricle failure in a previously allografted CML patient," *Bone Marrow Transplantation*, vol. 43, no. 12, pp. 967–968, 2009.

[23] D. Dumitrescu, C. Seck, H. Ten Freyhaus, F. Gerhardt, E. Erdmann, and S. Rosenkranz, "Fully reversible pulmonary arterial hypertension associated with dasatinib treatment for chronic myeloid leukaemia," *European Respiratory Journal*, vol. 38, no. 1, pp. 218–220, 2011.

[24] W. Rasheed, B. Flaim, and J. F. Seymour, "Reversible severe pulmonary hypertension secondary to dasatinib in a patient with chronic myeloid leukemia," *Leukemia Research*, vol. 33, no. 6, pp. 861–864, 2009.

[25] A. Ghose, Z. Tariq, A. Taj, and R. Chaudhary, "Acute dyspnea from treatment of al amyloidisis with bortezomib," *The American Journal of Therapeutics*, vol. 18, no. 4, pp. e123–e125, 2011.

[26] C. Akosman, C. Ordu, E. Eroglu, and B. Oyan, "Development of acute pulmonary hypertension after bortezomib treatment in a patient with multiple myeloma: a case report and the review of the literature," *American Journal of Therapeutics*, 2013.

[27] J. A. Groeneveldt, S. J. M. Gans, H. J. Bogaard, and A. Vonk-Noordegraaf, "Dasatinib-induced pulmonary arterial hypertension unresponsive to PDE-5 inhibition," *European Respiratory Journal*, vol. 42, no. 3, pp. 869–870, 2013.

18

An Extremely Rare Case of Advanced Metastatic Small Cell Neuroendocrine Carcinoma of Sinonasal Tract

Yu Yu Thar,[1] Poras Patel,[2] Tiangui Huang,[3] and Elizabeth Guevara[1]

[1]Department of Medicine, Division of Hematology and Oncology, The Brooklyn Hospital Center, Brooklyn, NY 11201, USA
[2]Department of Medicine, The Brooklyn Hospital Center, Brooklyn, NY 11201, USA
[3]Department of Pathology, The Brooklyn Hospital Center, Brooklyn, NY 11201, USA

Correspondence should be addressed to Yu Yu Thar; dr.yuyuthar@gmail.com

Academic Editor: Su Ming Tan

Small cell neuroendocrine carcinoma (SNEC) is a rare form of malignancy. It mainly presents as bronchogenic neoplasm, and the extrapulmonary form accounts for only 0.1% to 0.4% of all cancers. These extrapulmonary tumors have been described most frequently in the urinary bladder, prostate, esophagus, stomach, colon and rectum, gall bladder, head and neck, cervix, and skin. Primary SNEC of the sinonasal tract is extremely rare with only less than 100 cases reported in the literature. Because of extreme rarity and aggressiveness of the tumor, the management for this entity varies considerably mandating multimodality approach. In this paper, we report a patient presented with left-sided facial swelling, and the histopathologic examination confirmed primary SNEC of left sinonasal tract. The tumor involved multiple paranasal sinuses with invasion into the left orbit and left infratemporal fossa and metastasized to cervical lymph nodes and bone. The patient encountered devastating outcome in spite of optimal medical management and treatment with palliative chemotherapy highlighting the necessity for further research of primary SNEC of head and neck.

1. Introduction

Neuroendocrine tumors constitute broad spectrum of malignant epithelial neuroendocrine neoplasms. They are further subdivided into typical carcinoid (well-differentiated), atypical carcinoid (moderately differentiated), and small cell carcinoma (poorly differentiated neuroendocrine carcinoma) [1]. Small cell neuroendocrine carcinoma (SNEC) was first described in the 19th century in the context of lung cancer. Head and neck SNEC have been described only since 1965 [2]. The most common site of head and neck neuroendocrine carcinoma is the larynx. Primary neuroendocrine carcinomas of nasal and paranasal cavities are extremely rare and less than 100 cases have been in the medical literature. It is a highly proliferative epithelial neuroendocrine tumor with an aggressive behavior that is characterized by early, widespread metastases via the lymphatic as well as the blood stream [2]. Because of the rarity of this neoplasm, there are no specific recommendations pertaining to the management and treatment options are generally extrapolated from similar tumors of pulmonary origin. In this case report, we have presented a patient who was diagnosed with an extremely rare poorly differentiated (small cell) neuroendocrine carcinoma of sinonasal tract with metastasis. We have also described the literature review of clinical presentation, imaging characteristics and pathologic features, and, most importantly, the management of SNEC of head and neck.

2. Case Report

A 54-year-old African-American chronic smoker woman presented to Emergency Department with worsening left-sided facial swelling and blurry vision for one week. Five months ago, the patient was evaluated for left neck mass with aspiration at the other facility. The pathology was benign and she was treated for infection with antibiotics. Then, the patient failed to follow up. Since then, the patient noted intermittent swelling of left neck mass for several months which for past one week has progressively gotten worse,

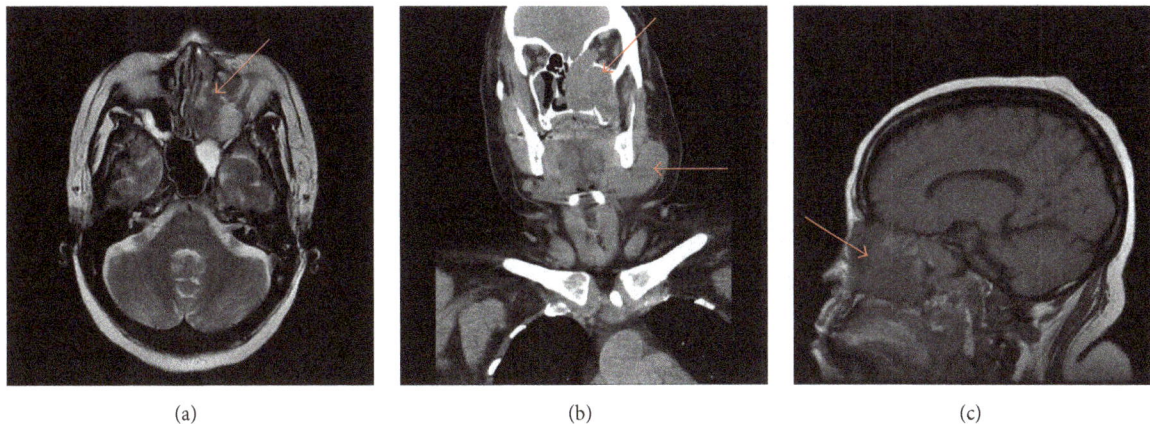

FIGURE 1: ((a) (axial), (b) (coronal), and (c) (sagittal)) CT scan of the neck showing extensive lymphadenopathy, left greater than right, and extensive soft tissue involving the left nasal cavity and multiple paranasal sinuses wit invasion into the left orbit and left infratemporal fossa.

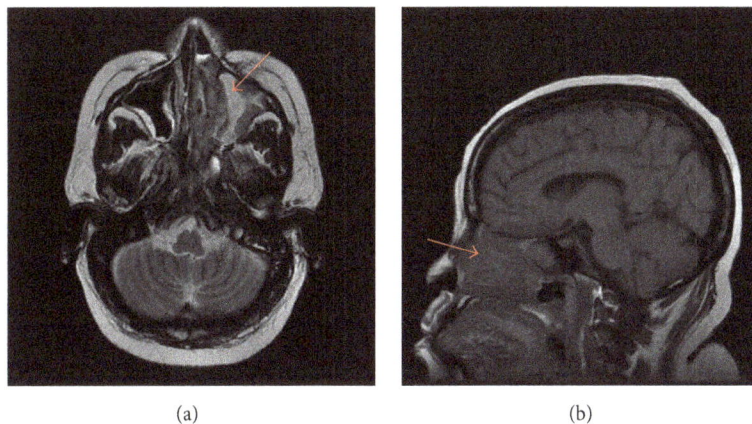

FIGURE 2: ((a) (axial) and (b) (sagittal)) MRI of the brain showing a soft tissue mass in the left maxillary sinus and left nasal cavity with extension to involve the medical left orbit.

associated with periorbital swelling, left-sided blurry vision, and left nasal congestion and epistaxis. She had 10–15 pounds of unintentional weight loss over last couple of months with increasing fatigue. She has a known history of HIV (noncomplaint with antiretroviral therapy), asymptomatic hepatitis B virus carrier, and chronic kidney disease.

Comprehensive physical examination revealed a nontendered, nonmobile, hard, large left-sided neck mass with left-sided facial and orbital swelling. She was also noted to have dry mouth, bilateral pale conjunctiva, mass in left nasal chamber, excessive lacrimation, intermittent alternating exotropia, and restricted left eye extraocular movement. Systemic review demonstrated no organomegaly and no other lymphadenopathy.

Laboratory results were significant for anemia, thrombocytopenia, elevated lactate dehydrogenase, and uric acid levels. Computerized tomography (CT) scan of neck showed extensive lymphadenopathies, left greater than right, and a soft tissue mass involving left nasal cavity and multiple paranasal sinuses with invasion into left orbit and left infratemporal fossa (Figures 1(a) and 1(b)). The patient proceeded incisional biopsy of the left nasal mass. Histopathology described the tumor cells were small with little cytoplasm

and a high nuclear/cytoplasmic ratio, arranged in sheets with both scattered and geographic necrosis. The nuclei were oval to spindle-shaped and pleomorphic with absent or indistinct nucleoli. Mitotic figures were numerous (Ki-67 is present). Immunohistochemical profile showed tumor cells positivity for cytokeratin AE1/AE3, Cam5.2, Epithelial Membrane Antigen (EMA) and positivity for neuroendocrine markers including CD56, chromogranin, synaptophysin, and neuron-specific enolase (NSE) (Figure 4). The tumor cells were also positive for Bcl-2 but were negative for lymphoid markers such as CD3, CD5, CD7, CD10, CD79a, CD20, and CD30. They were also negative for Thyroid Transcription Factor-1 (TTF-1), Napsin A, Epstein-Barr virus (EBV), Bcl-1, CD99, S100, and vimentin. The diagnosis of a small cell neuroendocrine carcinoma was made. Bone marrow biopsy disclosed infiltration of monomorphic small blue cells diffusely positive for CD56, consistent with bone marrow involvement of nasal small cell neuroendocrine carcinoma. CT scan of the chest, abdomen, and pelvis was unremarkable. Magnetic resonance imaging (MRI) study of the brain demonstrated soft tissue mass in the left maxillary sinus and left nasal cavity with extension to involve the medial left orbit. No intracranial mass lesion was found (Figures 2(a) and 2(b)). Positron

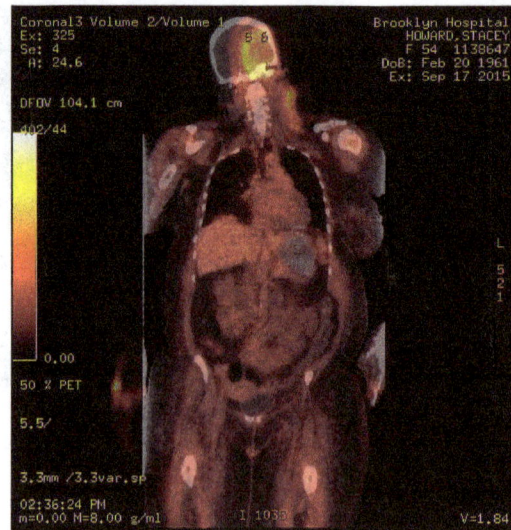

FIGURE 3: Positron Emission Tomography/Computed Tomography (PET/CT) showing minimal FDG uptake at the large mass lesion at the left ethmoid and maxillary sinuses, moderate to significant FDG uptake at bilateral cervical lymph nodes, and minimal heterogeneous FDG uptake along the thoracolumbar vertebra and pelvic bones.

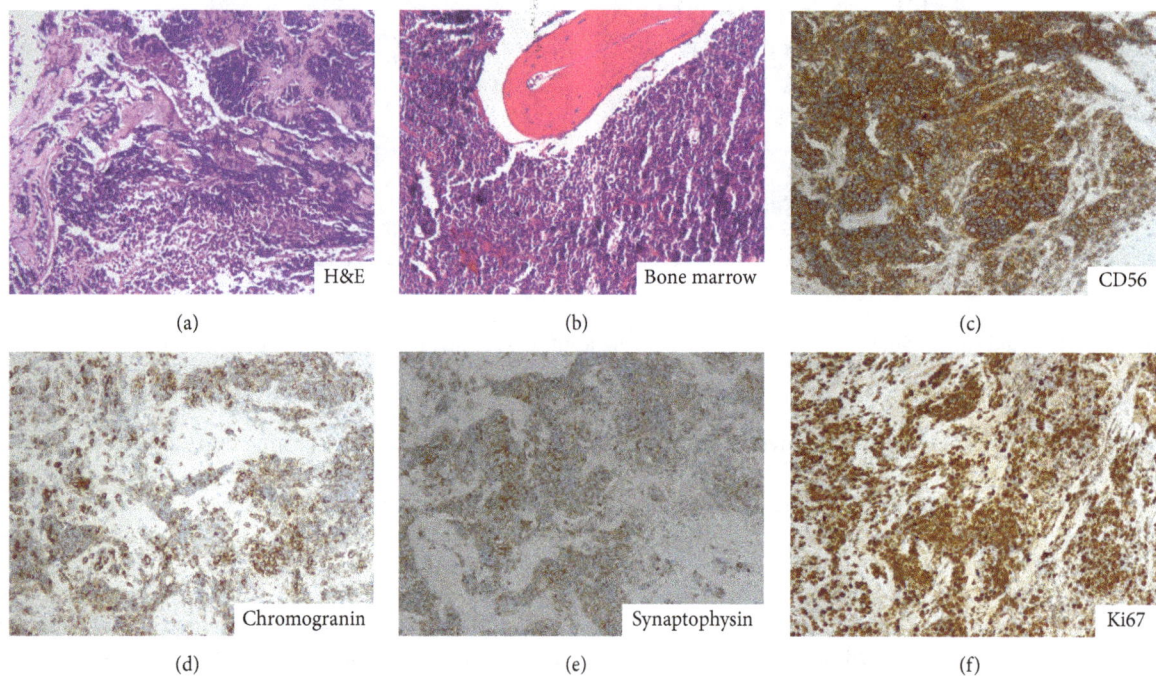

FIGURE 4: Pathology of the left nasal mass and bone marrow shows small cell undifferentiated (neuroendocrine) carcinoma. Light microscopy showed small round cells with scanty cytoplasm and hyperchromatic nuclei ((a) and (b)). Immunohistochemical staining showing tumor positivity for CD56 (c), chromogranin (d), and synaptophysin (e) (IHC ×100) and nuclear positivity to Ki-67 (f) (IHC ×100).

Emission Tomography/Computed Tomography (PET/CT) disclosed a large destructive mass involving the left nasal cavity, paranasal sinuses, and left orbit with extensive bilateral cervical adenopathy, all of which were hypermetabolic (Figure 3). The clinical TNM (tumor node metastasis) stage of the patient was T4N2M1 (stage IV) according to the American Joint Committee on Cancer (AJCC) [3].

During the course, the patient had acute chronic renal failure and worsening of hematological parameters requiring hemodialysis and blood products, respectively. Given the extent of her disease, the patient was started on palliative chemotherapy with carboplatin (etoposide was omitted due to thrombocytopenia) urgently as inpatient. The patient was not felt to be a candidate for cisplatin based chemotherapy due to her renal dysfunction. Treatment with combined carboplatin and etoposide was planned initially. But etoposide was omitted due to severe thrombocytopenia. There was a good clinical response after receiving the first cycle of chemotherapy; however, due to worsening anemia and thrombocytopenia, further chemotherapy was delayed. Unfortunately, the patient succumbed to the disease. The autopsy was performed and there was no definite mass found below the neck. Extensive sampling of lung, gastrointestinal tract including liver and spleen, and genitourinary tract were unremarkable. Only the vertebra showed small blue cells which was further confirmed by CD56 stain.

3. Discussion

Small cell undifferentiated neuroendocrine carcinomas of sinonasal tract, also known as poorly differentiated neuroendocrine carcinomas, are extremely rare and represent a histological spectrum of differentiation. It has been reported to be highly aggressive with very poor prognosis. Most prevailing malignancy of head and neck is squamous cell carcinoma, followed by adenocarcinoma [2]. Larynx is the most common site for neuroendocrine carcinoma in the head and neck, whereas paranasal sinuses accounts for approximately 0.3% of all cancers. The mean age at presentation is approximately 50 years (range: 26–77 years) and there is no predilection for race or sex reported in the literature. Distant metastases frequently occur in lungs, liver, and bone [4, 5].

Most frequent clinical features of patients with neuroendocrine carcinoma of the head and neck, which were also seen in our case, are recurrent epistaxis, nasal obstruction, nasal discharge, proptosis, paresthesia, and anosmia. Occasionally, the presenting symptoms may be exophthalmos, facial pain, and swelling [4]. These tumors may be associated with paraneoplastic syndrome that often manifests as the syndrome of inappropriate antidiuretic hormone secretion (SIADH). However, it is an uncommon presentation for SNEC of the head and neck [6, 7]. There is no distinctive computed tomography (CT) or magnetic resonance imaging (MRI) characteristics to diagnose or differentiate nonlaryngeal neuroendocrine carcinoma in the head and neck from the most common salivary gland neoplasms.

Microscopically, it is indistinguishable between SNEC of head and neck from those of bronchogenic origin. These cells are typically densely cellular, oval to spindle-shaped, and pleomorphic nuclei, frequent mitoses, and necrosis [5]. Cytokeratin (AE 1/3), chromogranin, and neuron-specific enolase, which were all positive in the immunohistochemical profile of our patient, are characteristic tumor markers of epithelial and neuroendocrine differentiation [8]. EBV RNA is negative by in situ hybridization [9]. Cytokeratin is the most useful marker to differentiate between neural and epithelial neuroendocrine tumors. The use of immunostains, electromicroscopy, and molecular genetics has helped to understand this lesion, but the mainstay of diagnosis of this tumor remains to be the light microscopy [4, 10]. SNEC is exceptionally rare and it is important to differentiate from sinonasal undifferentiated carcinoma (SNUC) which are distinctly larger, with more prominent eosinophilic cytoplasm and larger nuclei, often with prominent nucleoli by light miscopy

[11]. Immunohistochemistry is very useful in distinguishing small cell neuroendocrine carcinoma from basaloid squamous cell carcinoma and adenocystic carcinoma, which can be difficult to distinguish on small biopsy specimen. It is very important for management and prognosis to differentiate small cell neuroendocrine carcinoma from the more common nasopharyngeal squamous cell carcinoma [12, 13].

As witnessed in our case, tumors of this type are often disseminated at diagnosis; thus, it is essential to perform thorough metastatic workup before initiating the treatment. Multimodality therapy is increasingly used in small cell neuroendocrine carcinoma as it is an aggressive malignancy with high rates of local recurrence and metastases. Treatment modalities include chemotherapy, radiotherapy, and possibly surgery, depending on the extent of disease or the primary site. Surgical option is reserved for local relapse with no evidence of metastases because surgical results for this tumor have been disappointing. The combination of chemotherapy and radiation therapy, with or without surgery, has been recommended since late 1990s [9, 14]. Platinum-based chemotherapy followed by radiotherapy is a well known recommendation that has been tested in a large study. Due to high rates of intracranial metastases in patients with small cell neuroendocrine cancer of the nasal and paranasal sinuses, studies have suggested that it should be treated with systemic chemotherapy and radiotherapy and prophylactic cranial irradiation [7]. Prognosis remains poor despite combined modality treatment. More extensive studies are needed to assess the optimal management and development of standardized treatment protocols.

4. Conclusion

SNEC of sinonasal tract is an uncommon neoplasm with tendency toward recurrence and distant metastasis. Because of its rarity and aggressive nature, diagnosis and management of SNEC remain a challenge. Further research is needed to develop more specific, targeted approach of SNEC of head and neck in order to improve patient's survival and quality of life.

References

[1] J. L. Barker Jr., B. S. Glisson, A. S. Garden et al., "Management of nonsinonasal neuroendocrine carcinomas of the head and neck," *Cancer*, vol. 98, no. 11, pp. 2322–2328, 2003.

[2] R. N. Raychowdhuri, "Oat-cell carcinoma and paranasal sinuses," *The Journal of Laryngology and Otology*, vol. 79, pp. 253–255, 1965.

[3] S. Edge, D. Byrd, C. Compton et al., *AJCC Cancer Staging Manual*, Springer, New York, NY, USA, 7th edition, 2010.

[4] A. T. Monroe, C. G. Morris, E. Lee, and W. M. Mendenhall, "Small cell carcinoma of the head and neck: the University of Florida Experience," *Journal of the Hong Kong College of Radiologists*, vol. 8, no. 2, pp. 83–86, 2005.

[5] S.-F. Huang, W.-Y. Chuang, S.-D. Cheng, L.-J. Hsin, L.-Y. Lee, and H.-K. Kao, "A colliding maxillary sinus cancer of adenosquamous carcinoma and small cell neuroendocrine carcinoma—a case report with EGFR copy number analysis," *World Journal of Surgical Oncology*, vol. 8, article 92, 2010.

[6] S. Choe, R. S. Gill, E. Reiter, J. Myers, and F. S. Celi, "Syndrome of inappropriate antidiuretic hormone secretion associated with maxillary sinus small cell neuroendocrine tumor," in *Proceedings of the Endocrine Society's 98th Annual Meeting and Expo*, Boston, Mass, USA, April 2016.

[7] D. I. Rosenthal, J. L. Barker Jr., A. K. El-Naggar et al., "Sinonasal malignancies with neuroendocrine differentiation: patterns of failure according to histologic phenotype," *Cancer*, vol. 101, no. 11, pp. 2567–2573, 2004.

[8] J. M. Woodruff and R. T. Senie, "Atypical carcinoid tumor of the larynx. A critical review of the literature," *Journal for Otorhinolaryngology and Its Related Specialties*, vol. 53, no. 4, pp. 194–209, 1991.

[9] E. Babin, V. Rouleau, P. O. Vedrine et al., "Small cell neuroendocrine carcinoma of the nasal cavity and paranasal sinuses," *Journal of Laryngology and Otology*, vol. 120, no. 4, pp. 289–297, 2006.

[10] S. M. David and K. K. Haskins, "Pathological quiz case 2," *Archives of Otolaryngology—Head and Neck Surgery*, vol. 124, pp. 219–222, 1998.

[11] A. Ejaz and B. M. Wenig, "Sinonasal undifferentiated carcinoma: clinical and pathologic features and a discussion on classification, cellular differentiation, and differential diagnosis," *Advances in Anatomic Pathology*, vol. 12, no. 3, pp. 134–143, 2005.

[12] M. Capelli, G. Bertino, P. Morbini, C. Villa, S. Zorzi, and M. Benazzo, "Neuroendocrine carcinomas of the upper airways: a small case series with histopathological considerations," *Tumori*, vol. 93, no. 5, pp. 499–503, 2007.

[13] J. P. Klussmann and H. E. Eckel, "Small cell neuroendocrine carcinoma of the larynx," *Ear, Nose and Throat Journal*, vol. 78, no. 1, pp. 22–24, 1999.

[14] B. Perez-Ordonez, S. M. Caruana, A. G. Huvos, and J. P. Shah, "Small cell neuroendocrine carcinoma of the nasal cavity and paranasal sinuses," *Human Pathology*, vol. 29, no. 8, pp. 826–832, 1998.

19

Myofibroblastoma of the Breast: Literature Review and Case Report

Mario Metry, Mohamad Shaaban, Magdi Youssef, and Michael Carr

Breast Surgery Unit, Northumbria Healthcare NHS Foundation Trust, Woodhorn Lane, Ashington NE63 9JJ, UK

Correspondence should be addressed to Mohamad Shaaban; dr.mohamed.shaaban@gmail.com

Academic Editor: Jose I. Mayordomo

Myofibroblastoma of the breast is a rare benign spindle cell tumor. The main aim of this study is to review the literature of this rare tumor. We present a case of a mammary myofibroblastoma occurring in an 82-year-old man, emphasizing the clinical, radiological, and pathological features. The tumor was successfully identified and managed in our hospital. We would like to draw the attention of clinicians to myofibroblastoma as a rare possibility in the differential diagnosis of a breast mass.

1. Introduction

Recently, it has been confirmed that mammary myofibroblastoma belongs to the category of the benign mesenchymal tumors showing deletion of 13q14 region, together with spindle cell lipoma and cellular angiofibroma [1].

Myofibroblastoma was first reported by Wargotz et al. in 1987, as a benign spindle cell tumor of the breast with myofibroblastic features [2]. Only a few cases of this tumor have been reported in the English literature, so that the report of a new case gave us the opportunity to review the clinical management of myofibroblastoma.

2. Case Presentation

An 82-year-old man presented to the low-risk breast clinic with a few days' history of a tender lump in his left breast. He gave no family history of breast or ovarian cancer and was a nonsmoker. He suffered from ischemic heart disease and was on medications for benign prostatic hyperplasia.

Physical examination revealed a 20 mm smooth, mobile mass E2, situated asymmetrically behind the left areola at the 11 o'clock position, towards the upper inner quadrant of the breast tissue. This was nontender and there was no associated axillary lymphadenopathy. In addition, there was mild, diffuse, clinically benign gynecomastia on the right breast.

Ultrasound scan examination showed the symptomatic lesion of the left breast as a 16 × 15 mm rounded hypoechoic mass U3 (Figure 1). There was no evidence of gynecomastia.

A USS guided core biopsy was carried out from the mass. Histological examination confirmed a well-circumscribed mesenchymal lesion consisting of bland-looking spindle-shaped cells arranged in interlacing short bundles interrupted by keloidal-like, brightly eosinophilic collagen bands. No atypia or mitotic activity was seen.

Immunohistochemistry showed a positive reaction with alpha-smooth muscle actin (SMA), desmin, and CD34. Neoplastic cells were also positive for estrogen receptor (ER), but they were negative with MNF116, S100, and p63. Based on these morphological and immunohistochemical features, the diagnosis of "classic type myofibroblastoma of the breast was rendered".

Options of treatment were discussed with the patient; the patient opted for excision of the mass.

Uneventful excision was performed from which the patient made a rapid and uncomplicated recovery.

Macroscopic examination revealed a circumscribed tumor mass measuring 15 mm in greatest diameter, with a specimen weight of 2.75 grams.

Histological examination showed a well-circumscribed mesenchymal tumor with features similar to those of the relative core biopsy. It consisted of short fascicles of spindle cells with pale cytoplasm and oval nuclei, with interspersed

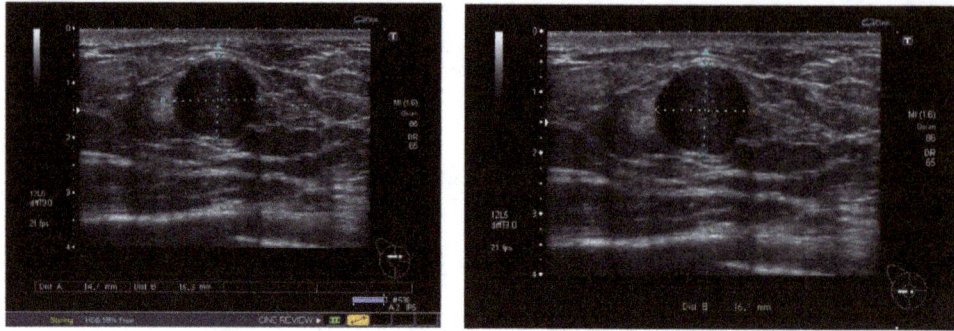

FIGURE 1: Ultrasound scan showing the lesion 15 × 16 mm mass (U3).

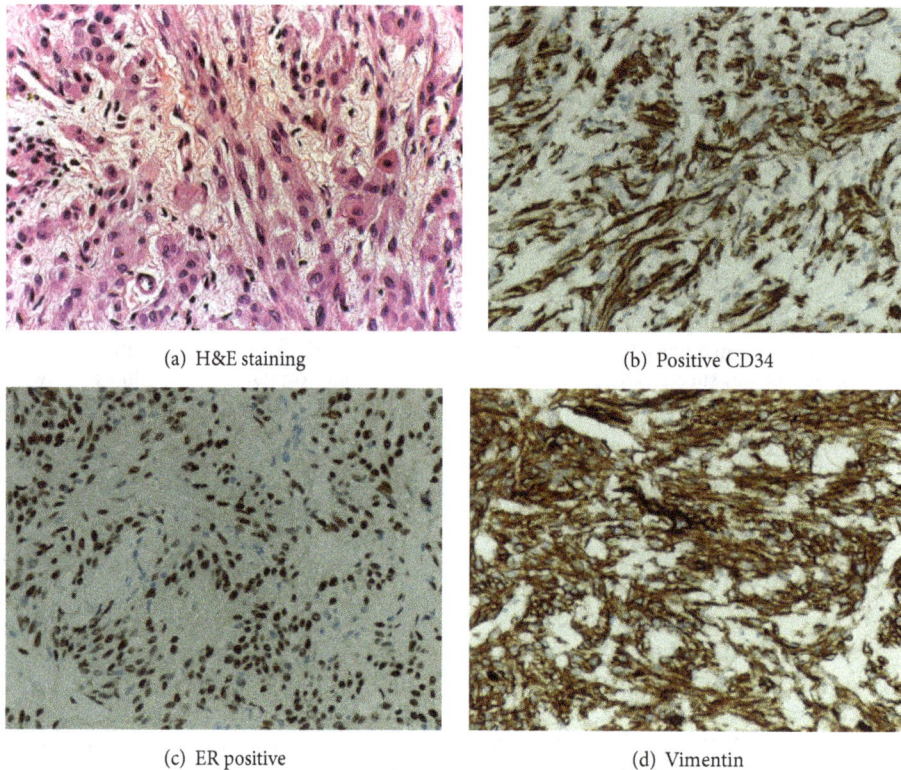

(a) H&E staining

(b) Positive CD34

(c) ER positive

(d) Vimentin

FIGURE 2: The histological pictures of the specimen as obtained from the histopathology department.

thick collagen bands. Although the tumor was moderately cellular, there was neither nuclear atypia nor mitoses (Figure 2(a)). Immunohistochemistry studies showed positive CD34 (Figure 2(b)), moderately positive for desmin, SMA, and ER (Figure 2(c)), and diffuse immunoreactivity for vimentin (Figure 2(d)). Pancytokeratin staining was negative, while CD31 highlighted intratumoral blood vessels.

3. Discussion and Literature Review

Myofibroblasts play an important role in the response to tissue injury. Damaged cells and some malignant tumor cells produce cytokines, particularly transforming growth factor $\beta1$, causing fibroblasts to migrate into the injured tissue. They begin to develop smooth muscle actin fibers, and they are transformed into myofibroblasts with contractile ability. Contraction of injured tissue speeds the processes of healing and repair [3].

Myofibroblastoma has recently been described as a rare benign mesenchymal tumor which usually occurs in the breast parenchyma of both females and males [4]. Most cases of myofibroblastoma occur most often in women and men aged 40–87 years. It tends to affect older men and postmenopausal women [5–8]. Characteristically, these lesions present as a solitary, painless, firm, and freely mobile mass which grows slowly for several months or years [8, 9]. It can exhibit a wide range of histological patterns including the following: collagenized/fibrous, cellular, lipomatous, infiltrative, myxoid, epithelioid, and deciduoid-like variant [10, 11].

Histologically, myofibroblastoma is composed of bipolar spindle-shaped cells arranged in short intersecting fascicles interrupted by keloidal-like eosinophilic collagen bands. Mammary ducts or lobules are characteristically absent. Macroscopically, the cut surface shows a well-demarcated pale pink or tan round mass [8–11]. Immunohistochemically, myofibroblastoma is positive for vimentin and CD34 and variably positive for desmin and SMA. It is also positive for CD10, CD99, estrogen, progesterone receptors, and bcl-2 protein and only focally positive for h-caldesmon. S100 protein, HMB-45, epithelial markers (EMA and pancytokeratins), and C-kit (CD117) are consistently negative. Immunohistochemical results are consistent with the fibroblastic/myofibroblastic nature of the neoplastic cells [1, 12–15]. Unlike mammary-type myofibroblastoma, myofibroblastoma that primarily arises in the lymph nodes exhibits nuclear palisading. Some reported cases represent a hitherto unreported variant of mammary-type myofibroblastoma closely mimicking schwannoma [16].

The appearances of myofibroblastoma on imaging are nonspecific. On sonography, it shows a homogeneously hypoechoic well-circumscribed solid mass which resembles fibroadenoma. The mammographic findings usually consist of a well-circumscribed round or oval dense and noncalcified mass [17]. The MRI finding (although not often done) shows a homogeneously enhanced mass with internal septations [18–22]. Most reported cases vary between 10 and 37 mm in size although much larger tumors have recently been described [23, 24].

Given the nonspecific radiological appearances, the final diagnosis of myofibroblastoma requires a needle core biopsy. Myofibroblastoma can be treated with local excision mainly for symptomatic relief; local recurrence is not a recognized feature of myofibroblastoma [8, 9].

4. Conclusion

Myofibroblastoma is a rare breast tumor occurring in both postmenopausal women and elderly men. Triple assessment by clinical examination, ultrasound scanning, and needle core biopsy will lead to an accurate diagnosis. Recurrence is unlikely following excision with clear resection margins.

We would like to draw the attention of clinicians to myofibroblastoma as a rare possibility in the differential diagnosis of a breast mass with well-circumscribed margins.

References

[1] G. Magro, A. Righi, L. Casorzo et al., "Mammary and vaginal myofibroblastomas are genetically related lesions: fluorescence in situ hybridization analysis shows deletion of 13q14 region," *Human Pathology*, vol. 43, no. 11, pp. 1887–1893, 2012.

[2] E. S. Wargotz, S. W. Weiss, and H. J. Norris, "Myofibroblastoma of the breast: sixteen cases of a distinctive benign mesenchymal tumor," *American Journal of Surgical Pathology*, vol. 11, no. 7, pp. 493–502, 1987.

[3] G. Magro, "Epithelioid-cell myofibroblastoma of the breast: expanding the morphologic spectrum," *The American Journal of Surgical Pathology*, vol. 33, no. 7, pp. 1085–1092, 2009.

[4] G. Magro, "Mammary myofibroblastoma: an update with emphasis on the most diagnostically challenging variants," *Histology and Histopathology*, vol. 31, no. 1, pp. 1–23, 2016.

[5] G. Magro, M. Bisceglia, M. Michal, and V. Eusebi, "Spindle cell lipoma-like tumor, solitary fibrous tumor and myofibroblastoma of the breast: a clinico-pathological analysis of 13 cases in favor of a unifying histogenetic concept," *Virchows Archiv*, vol. 440, no. 3, pp. 249–260, 2002.

[6] J. S. Reis-Filho, L. N. Faoro, E. L. Gasparetto, J. T. Totsugui, and F. C. Schmitt, "Mammary epithelioid myofibroblastoma arising in bilateral gynecomastia: case report with immunohistochemical profile," *International Journal of Surgical Pathology*, vol. 9, no. 4, pp. 331–334, 2001.

[7] G. Magro, "Mammary myofibroblastoma: a tumor with a wide morphologic spectrum," *Archives of Pathology and Laboratory Medicine*, vol. 132, no. 11, pp. 1813–1820, 2008.

[8] G. Magro, L. Salvatorelli, S. Spadola, and G. Angelico, "Mammary myofibroblastoma with extensive myxoedematous stromal changes: a potential diagnostic pitfall," *Pathology Research and Practice*, vol. 210, no. 12, pp. 1106–1111, 2014.

[9] G. Magro, A. Gurrera, and M. Bisceglia, "H-caldesmon expression in myofibroblastoma of the breast: evidence supporting the distinction from leiomyoma," *Histopathology*, vol. 42, no. 3, pp. 233–238, 2003.

[10] G. Magro, F. Fraggetta, A. Torrisi, C. Emmanuele, and S. Lanzafame, "Myofibroblastoma of the breast with hemangiopericytoma-like pattern and pleomorphic lipoma-like areas. Report of a case with diagnostic and histogenetic considerations," *Pathology Research and Practice*, vol. 195, no. 4, pp. 257–262, 1999.

[11] G. Magro, M. Michal, E. Vasquez, and M. Bisceglia, "Lipomatous myofibroblastoma: a potential diagnostic pitfall in the spectrum of the spindle cell lesions of the breast," *Virchows Archiv*, vol. 437, no. 5, pp. 540–544, 2000.

[12] A. Iglesias, M. Arias, P. Santiago, M. Rodríguez, J. Mañas, and C. Saborido, "Benign breast lesions that simulate malignancy: magnetic resonance imaging with radiologic-pathologic correlation," *Current Problems in Diagnostic Radiology*, vol. 36, no. 2, pp. 66–82, 2007.

[13] G. Magro, R. Caltabiano, A. Di Cataldo, and L. Puzzo, "CD10 is expressed by mammary myofibroblastoma and spindle cell lipoma of soft tissue: an additional evidence of their histogenetic linking," *Virchows Archiv*, vol. 450, no. 6, pp. 727–728, 2007.

[14] L. Pina, L. Apesteguía, R. Cojo et al., "Myofibroblastoma of male breast: report of three cases and review of the literature," *European Radiology*, vol. 7, no. 6, pp. 931–934, 1997.

[15] B. Hinz, S. H. Phan, V. J. Thannickal, A. Galli, M.-L. Bochaton-Piallat, and G. Gabbiani, "The myofibroblast: one function, multiple origins," *The American Journal of Pathology*, vol. 170, no. 6, pp. 1807–1816, 2007.

[16] G. Magro, M. P. Foschini, and V. Eusebi, "Palisaded myofibroblastoma of the breast: a tumor closely mimicking schwannoma: report of 2 cases," *Human Pathology*, vol. 44, no. 9, pp. 1941–1946, 2013.

[17] J. S. Greenberg, S. S. Kaplan, and C. Grady, "Myofibroblastoma of the breast in women: imaging appearances," *American Journal of Roentgenology*, vol. 171, no. 1, pp. 71–72, 1998.

[18] G. Magro, M. Michal, and M. Bisceglia, "Benign spindle cell tumors of the mammary stroma: diagnostic criteria, classification, and histogenesis," *Pathology Research and Practice*, vol. 197, no. 7, pp. 453–466, 2001.

[19] G. Magro, P. Amico, and A. Gurrera, "Myxoid myofibroblastoma of the breast with atypical cells: a potential diagnostic pitfall," *Virchows Archiv*, vol. 450, no. 4, pp. 483–485, 2007.

[20] W. D. Dockery, H. R. Singh, and R. E. Wilentz, "Myofibroblastoma of the male breast: imaging appearance and ultrasound-guided core biopsy diagnosis," *The Breast Journal*, vol. 7, no. 3, pp. 192–194, 2001.

[21] G. Magro, M. Bisceglia, and M. Michal, "Expression of steroid hormone receptors, their regulated proteins, and bcl-2 protein in myofibroblastoma of the breast," *Histopathology*, vol. 36, no. 6, pp. 515–521, 2000.

[22] G. Magro, G. M. Vecchio, M. Michal, and V. Eusebi, "Atypical epithelioid cell myofibroblastoma of the breast with multinodular growth pattern: a potential pitfall of malignancy," *Pathology Research and Practice*, vol. 209, no. 7, pp. 463–466, 2013.

[23] F. A. Tavassoli and P. Devilee, *WHO Classification of Tumors. Pathology and Genetics of Tumors of the Breast and Female Genital Body*, IARC Press, Lyon, France, 2003.

[24] G. Magro, F. R. Longo, L. Salvatorelli, E. Vasquez, and G. M. Vecchio, "Lipomatous myofibroblastoma of the breast: case report with diagnostic and histogenetic considerations," *Pathologica*, vol. 106, no. 2, pp. 36–40, 2014.

20

EGFR T790M-Positive Lung Adenocarcinoma Metastases to the Pituitary Gland Causing Adrenal Insufficiency: A Case Report

Michael L. Adashek [1], **Kenneth Miller,** [2] **and Arit A. Silpasuvan** [3]

[1]*Department of Internal Medicine, Sinai Hospital, Baltimore, MD, USA*
[2]*University of Maryland Marlene & Stewart Greenebaum Comprehensive Cancer Center, Baltimore, MD, USA*
[3]*Department of Endocrinology, Sinai Hospital, Baltimore, MD, USA*

Correspondence should be addressed to Michael L. Adashek; madashek@osteo.wvsom.edu

Academic Editor: Giovanni Tallini

A 64-year-old man, with history of micropapillary thyroid cancer and epidermal growth factor receptor-positive lung adenocarcinoma with no evidence of active disease for 3 years after chemotherapy and radiation on erlotinib, presented with fatigue, nausea, lack of appetite, and xeroderma. A screening magnetic resonance image of the patient's head demonstrated a new bilateral pituitary mass. Initial evaluation revealed low morning cortisol, and the patient was diagnosed with adrenal insufficiency. His symptoms rapidly improved with maintenance glucocorticoids. Soon thereafter, the patient developed an acute visual deficit secondary to enlargement of the pituitary mass, and biopsy revealed EGFR T790M positive metastatic lung adenocarcinoma. Hence, we present a rare case of metastatic lung adenocarcinoma to the pituitary causing secondary adrenal insufficiency.

1. Introduction

Adrenal insufficiency (AI) is a broadly encompassing term for inadequate physiologic corticosteroid production. Primary AI is due to adrenal gland inadequacy, whereas secondary AI is due to disruption of the hypothalamus or pituitary in the hypothalamus-pituitary-adrenal (HPA) axis. We present a case of a man who presented with new fatigue, nausea, lack of appetite, and xeroderma who was found to have a new pituitary mass resulting in secondary AI.

2. Case Presentation

2.1. Presentation. A 64-year-old man with a medical history of micropapillary thyroid cancer and stage IIIb lung adenocarcinoma with no evidence of active disease for 3 years after chemotherapy and radiation presented with subjective complaints of new onset fatigue, nausea, scalp tenderness, and xeroderma. His medications included gabapentin 300 mg four times a day for chemotherapy-induced neuropathy, erlotinib 150 mg once daily for epidermal growth factor receptor- (EGFR-) positive lung adenocarcinoma, and omeprazole 40 mg once daily for subjective gastroesophageal reflux disease. A screening magnetic resonance image of the head revealed a new hypovascular pituitary mass measuring approximately 1 cm by 0.8 cm (Figure 1(a)).

2.2. Assessment. On examination, the patient's vital signs were within normal limits. On physical exam, xeroderma was appreciated in all extremities. Finger size was proportional and no prognathism, acromegaly, or Cushingoid features were appreciated. The cardiopulmonary exam was normal.

Initial lab values demonstrated normal free triiodothyronine (T3) of 2.4 pg/mL (normal range (NR) 1.8–4.2 pg/mL), normal T3 of 86 ng/dL (NR 70–172 ng/dL), and normal free thyroxine of 1.00 ng/dL (NR 0.84–1.68 ng/dL). Prolactin was elevated at 28.9 ng/mL (NR 2.5–17.0 ng/mL). The patient's morning cortisol was immeasurably low at <1.0 mcg/dL (NR > 10 mcg/dL) as was the patient's testosterone level at <20 ng/dL (280–1100 ng/dL). Luteinizing hormone was low at 0.05 mIU/mL (NR 1.8–12.0 mIU/L).

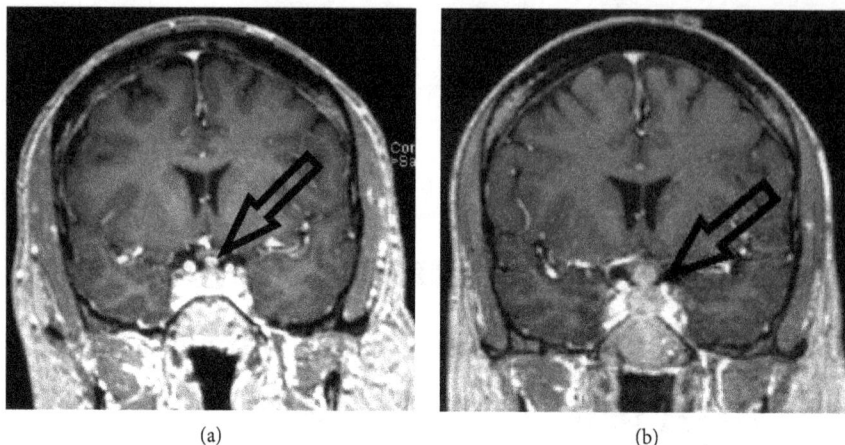

(a)   (b)

FIGURE 1: Brain magnetic resonance imaging demonstrating enlarging pituitary mass. (a) T1-weighted MRI demonstrating enlarged pituitary gland containing a hypovascular 10.5 × 7.5 mm mass lesion with thickening of the pituitary infundibulum without intracranial hemorrhage or extra-axial fluid collection. (b) Imaging one month later with T1-weighted MRI demonstrating a 22.0 × 12.0 mm bilobed mass with 8 mm suprasellar extension exerting mass effect on overlying optic chiasm.

The patient was started on prednisone 20 mg by mouth daily, at which point he noticed immediate improvement in his energy and appetite as well as decrease in his nausea. For chronic steroid replacement therapy, the patient's treatment was changed from prednisone to hydrocortisone 20 mg of hydrocortisone in the morning and 10 mg in the evening. The patient was additionally instructed about the dangers of adrenal crisis and told to increase his hydrocortisone to 90 mg daily if acutely ill.

2.3. Diagnosis. Within a month of initial diagnoses, the patient suffered acute visual bilateral field cut and loss of peripheral vision. A repeat MRI demonstrated rapid enlargement of his pituitary mass, nearly doubled in size and described as a 2.2 cm by 1.2 cm mass impinging on the overlying optic chiasm (Figure 1(b)).

The patient subsequently underwent transsphenoidal resection of his pituitary mass. Gross histology characterized the mass as firm and fibrous. Macroscopic analysis revealed metastatic lung adenocarcinoma described as adenohypophysis fibrosis. Further histologic analysis revealed positive identification of cytokeratin 7, TTF-1, Ki-67, and epidermal growth factor receptor (EGFR) positive with EGFR gene nucleotide change demonstrating T790M and L858R positivity. This histopathology demonstrated further EGFR mutation of the patient's known history of lung adenocarcinoma which initially was only positive for EGFR mutation L585R.

After transsphenoidal resection and subsequent whole-brain radiation, further results demonstrated a continued low morning cortisol at <1.0 mcg/dL (NR > 10 mcg/dL) and testosterone level at <20 ng/dL (280–1100 ng/dL). Luteinizing hormone was low at <0.1 mIU/mL (NR 1.8–12.0 mIU/L) as was follicle-stimulating hormone 0.8 mIU/mL (NR 1.5–12.4 mIU/mL). Free T4 was low at 0.65 ng/dL (NR 0.84–1.68 ng/dL) and thyroid-stimulating hormone was low at 0.019 MCI/mL (NR 0.4–4.0 MCI/mL). Prolactin was lower than previous but still elevated at 14.9 ng/mL (NR 2.5–17.0 ng/mL).

3. Discussion

Annually, 200,000 new patients are diagnosed with brain metastasis (BM), making BM the most frequent cause of intercranial neoplasm in adults in the United States. An estimated 20–40% of adult patients with systemic malignancies will develop BM, and of those, a further 20% will become symptomatic over the course of their disease. Lung cancer comprises the majority of these BM cases (50%), followed by breast cancer (20–30%) and melanoma (5–10%) [1]. Complications of brain metastases are one of the chief causes of mortality and morbidity in patients with non-small cell lung cancer [2]. Adrenal insufficiency (AI) secondary to metastatic malignancy is highly unusual and has been reported in under 100 cases in English literature [3].

Adrenal insufficiency (AI) stems from inadequate physiologic steroid production and is most commonly a result of discontinuation of long-term glucocorticoid treatment. The signs of adrenal insufficiency are wide and varied including orthostatic hypotension, altered mental status, nausea and vomiting, abdominal pain, weight loss, and salt craving, many of which can be attributed to fluid losses from reduced mineralocorticoid function [4]. Physical signs of AI can include Cushingoid appearance: thinning skin, striae, obesity, muscle wasting, and psychiatric disturbance, all of which may indicate prior chronic iatrogenic steroid exposure. The treatment is physiologic replacement, with hydrocortisone demonstrating decreased LDL levels compared to prednisone making hydrocortisone the replacement therapy of choice [5]. The patient demonstrated initial rapid symptomatic improvement with physiologic corticosteroid replacement. Of note, AI develops only in patients with bilateral hypothalamic-pituitary-adrenal (HPA) axis involvement. However, HPA metastasis typically results in an excitation of the HPA system leading to increased cortisol levels, making our patient's presentation of AI secondary to pituitary metastases an unusual one [6].

TABLE 1: Laboratory results before and after transsphenoidal pituitary metastases resection.

Hormone	Normal limit	Preresection	Postresection
Thyroxine	0.84–1.68 ng/dL	1.00 ng/dL	0.65 ng/dL
Thyroid-stimulating hormone	0.3–4.0 mIU/L	0.016 MCI/mL	0.019 MCI/mL
Follicle-stimulating hormone	1.6–17.8 mIU/mL	2.4 mIU/mL	0.8 mIU/mL
Luteinizing hormone	NR 1.8–12.0 mIU/L	0.05 mIU/mL	<0.1 mIU/mL
Testosterone	280–1100 ng/dL	<20 ng/dL	<20 ng/dL
Adrenocorticotropic hormone	9–52 pg/mL (2.0–11.0 pmol/L)	6.0 pg/mL	<5.0 pg/mL
Morning cortisol	>10 mcg/dL	<1.0 mcg/dL	<1.0 mcg/dL
Prolactin	<12.3 ng/mL (<0.55 nmol/L)	**28.9 ng/mL**	**14.9 ng/mL**

Radiologically, it is difficult to differentiate BM from primary intercranial malignancies. BM is typically found in the cerebral hemispheres (80%), followed by the cerebellum (15%) and brainstem (5%) [7]. Unfortunately, the lifetime risk of BM in non-small cell lung cancer has been estimated at 40% [2], making clinical history one of the greatest prognosticators for BM. Had the patient not been undergoing regular surveillance magnetic resonance imaging of the head, his clinical diagnoses of BM may have been significantly delayed. Symptomatic presence of pituitary BM often presents as medial visual field cut secondary to cranial nerve impingement as seen in this patient.

Chemical indications of pituitary BM are severely limited. Pituitary stalk compression, a common side effect of pituitary metastases, may lead to elevated prolactin. Prolactinomas are well known to produce prolactin levels > 200 ng/mL, whereas pituitary stalk compression may present with a prolactin level between the upper limit of normal (13 ng/mL) and <200 ng/mL [8]. Table 1 demonstrates the decrease in prolactin production with relief of pituitary stalk compression after resection of the lung adenocarcinoma metastasis. Values between 20–200 ng/mL may be artificially low due to prolactin levels > 5000 ng/mL resulting in saturation and incorrect analyses of both capture and signal assay antibodies. This "hook effect" can be addressed with 1/100 dilution of the sample [9]. BM can additionally present with central diabetes insipidus with symptoms of both polyuria and hypernatremia, neither of which was seen in this patient.

The patient's bilateral medial visual field cut indicated acutely symptomatic BM. Initial treatment is both dexamethasone 4–8 mg/day and alleviation of the mass effect through surgical or stereotactic radiotherapy if feasible. The current literature does not recommend prophylactic anticonvulsant therapy [7]. The brain is a singularly difficult target for medical treatment as the blood-brain barrier (BBB) limits the efficacy of many types of chemotherapy, often creating a haven for metastases. However, there is ongoing debate in literature suggesting that the integrity of this BBB is compromised in the setting of these lesions. This patient's symptoms successfully resolved with surgery; however, further positron emission tomography revealed uptake in the area indicative of returning metastatic disease. Although treatments for BM are both variable and highly dependent on tumor type, it has been noted that donepezil has demonstrated

to improve cognition, mood, and quality of life in these patients [7].

The patient demonstrated progression of disease on erlotinib, a 1st-generation EGFR tyrosine kinase inhibitor (TKI). Response rates of EGFR TKIs generally range from 70–80% with longer progression-free survival than previous standard chemotherapy regimens [7]. On average, the progression of disease occurs in 10–14 months due to new resistance mutations associated with EGFR-positive lung adenocarcinoma [10]. Initial screening for EGFR mutation from the lung core needle biopsies was performed with high-affinity class ribonucleotide analogs termed "locked nucleic acid probes" to identify wild-type EGFR and T790M mutations. However, this technique has a minimum sensitivity of 3% for T790M and 10–15% for L585R mutations [11]. There is emerging evidence to suggest that T790M mutation singularly develops during erlotinib treatment of EGFR-positive malignancies [12], and it is unlikely that the initial lung adenocarcinoma expressed T790M as the doubling time of the pituitary tumor was approximately 1 month and would have been visible far sooner on regular screening CT/MRI imaging. The patient's symptomatic pituitary mass was tested for T790M mutation through real-time PCR analysis [13] via the cobas EGFR Mutation Test P120019 (Roche Molecular Systems Inc., CA, USA) [14]. The patient's initial lung biopsy demonstrated the L858R EGFR mutation on exon 21 and when recurred was additionally identified with the T790M mutation on exon 20. This T790M mutation resulted in conformational change, sterically hindering erlotinib from binding to the adenosine triphosphate kinase pocket. Current EGFR TKIs include second-generation agents such as afatinib, dacomitinib, and neratinib or third-generation agents such as osimertinib, rociletinib, or olmutinib. Osimertinib in particular has been approved in T790M-positive non-small cell lung cancers (NSCLC), penetrates the BBB [15], and may offer this patient future benefit.

Unfortunately, neurosurgery could not be delayed due to mass effect of the underlying lung adenocarcinoma metastases on the pituitary and overlying optic chiasm. Had surgery been delayable, a far less invasive diagnostic test for T790M mutation could have been performed. The FDA has approved "liquid biopsy" [13] for EGFR mutations, which involves the testing of circulating cell-free tumor DNA (cfDNA) and has been demonstrated to reveal EGFR mutations not previously detected by biopsy in up to 34% of patients [16]. Moreover, this test can be performed on serum, rather than tumor tissue as previous ribonucleotide analogues have required. Given the rate of disease advancement on erlotinib [10], serial screens of cfDNA may play a future role in preempting changes in TKI treatment regimens before radiologic imaging reflects tumor progression. However, osimertinib has been associated with "pseudoprogression" or temporary paradoxical enlargement of EGFR T790M adenocarcinomas and may have worsened this patient's mass effect rather than relieved it [17].

In conclusion, physicians caring for patients with prior history of breast or lung cancer should remain vigilant in their history and physical exam for underlying signs of metastatic disease. AI is a rare complication of metastatic disease to the HPA axis and requires physiologic steroid replacement, ideally with hydrocortisone due to its lower LDL profile. Patients should be instructed to assess for signs of adrenal crises as soon as a diagnosis of AI is made as it can be life-threatening. Prolactin elevation < 200 ng/mL may be the first sign of pituitary stalk compression, and when an alarming clinical sign such as medial visual field cuts presents itself, patients should be started on dexamethasone dosing of 4–8 mg daily. The relief of mass effect is key in symptomatic pituitary BM and includes multidisciplinary involvement from specialties such as neurosurgery, as well as both medical oncology and radiation oncology. Given the recent advancements in tumor genomics and genetically targeted treatment modalities, BM pathology should be obtained via minimally invasive techniques provided the BM is not exerting mass effect on adjacent structures and requires surgical intervention. Finally, serum cfDNA may offer accurate nonsurgical screening for EGFR TKI resistance mutations and in turn facilitate changes in therapy to improve long-term patient outcomes.

Ethical Approval

This paper has been written in keeping with the principles of the Declaration of Helsinki.

Consent

Informed consent was obtained from the patient for educational use of the abovementioned data and no personal patient information has been disclosed.

References

[1] G. Rahmathulla, S. A. Toms, and R. J. Weil, "The molecular biology of brain metastasis," *Journal of Oncology*, vol. 2012, Article ID 723541, 16 pages, 2012.

[2] H. Li, J. Lian, S. Han et al., "Applicability of graded prognostic assessment of lung cancer using molecular markers to lung adenocarcinoma patients with brain metastases," *Oncotarget*, vol. 8, no. 41, pp. 70727–70735, 2017.

[3] Y. Imaoka, F. Kuranishi, Y. Ogawa, H. Okuda, and M. Nakahara, "Adrenal failure due to bilateral adrenal metastasis of rectal cancer: a case report," *International Journal of Surgery Case Reports*, vol. 31, pp. 1–4, 2017.

[4] M. R. Huecker and E. Dominique, "Adrenal, insufficiency," in *StatPearls*, StatPearls Publishing LLC, Treasure Island, FL, USA, 2017, NBK441832 [bookaccession].

[5] M. Quinkler, B. Ekman, C. Marelli et al., "Prednisolone is associated with a worse lipid profile than hydrocortisone in patients with adrenal insufficiency," *Endocrine Connections*, vol. 6, no. 1, pp. 1–8, 2017.

[6] A. Lutz, M. Stojkovic, M. Schmidt, W. Arlt, B. Allolio, and M. Reincke, "Adrenocortical function in patients with macrometastases of the adrenal gland," *European Journal of Endocrinology*, vol. 143, no. 1, pp. 91–97, 2000.

[7] C. D'Antonio, A. Passaro, B. Gori et al., "Bone and brain metastasis in lung cancer: recent advances in therapeutic strategies," *Therapeutic Advances in Medical Oncology*, vol. 6, no. 3, pp. 101–114, 2014.

[8] J. Komninos, V. Vlassopoulou, D. Protopapa et al., "Tumors metastatic to the pituitary gland: case report and literature review," *The Journal of Clinical Endocrinology & Metabolism*, vol. 89, no. 2, pp. 574–580, 2004.

[9] S. Melmed, F. F. Casanueva, A. R. Hoffman et al., "Diagnosis and treatment of hyperprolactinemia: an endocrine society clinical practice guideline," *The Journal of Clinical Endocrinology & Metabolism*, vol. 96, no. 2, pp. 273–288, 2011.

[10] S. G. Wu and J. Y. Shih, "Management of acquired resistance to EGFR TKI-targeted therapy in advanced non-small cell lung cancer," *Molecular Cancer*, vol. 17, no. 1, p. 38, 2018.

[11] NeoGenomics, "EGFR T790M germline mutation analysis," 2018, May 2018, https://neogenomics.com/test-menu/egfr-t790m-germline-mutation-analysis.

[12] C. Demuth, A. T. Madsen, B. Weber, L. Wu, P. Meldgaard, and B. S. Sorensen, "The T790M resistance mutation in EGFR is only found in cfDNA from erlotinib-treated NSCLC patients that harbored an activating EGFR mutation before treatment," *BMC Cancer*, vol. 18, no. 1, p. 191, 2018.

[13] "FDA approves first blood test to detect gene mutations associated with non-small cell lung cancer," June 2016, https://www.fda.gov/NewsEvents/Newsroom/PressAnnouncements/ucm504488.htm.

[14] B. Weber, P. Meldgaard, H. Hager et al., "Detection of EGFR mutations in plasma and biopsies from non-small cell lung cancer patients by allele-specific PCR assays," *BMC Cancer*, vol. 14, no. 1, pp. 294–2407, 2014.

[15] P. Ballard, J. W. T. Yates, Z. Yang et al., "Preclinical comparison of osimertinib with other EGFR-TKIs in EGFR-mutant NSCLC brain metastases models, and early evidence of clinical brain metastases activity," *Clinical Cancer Research*, vol. 22, no. 20, pp. 5130–5140, 2016.

[16] E. Alegre, J. P. Fusco, P. Restituto et al., "Total and mutated EGFR quantification in cell-free DNA from non-small cell lung cancer patients detects tumor heterogeneity and presents prognostic value," *Tumor Biology*, vol. 37, no. 10, pp. 13687–13694, 2016.

[17] S. Okauchi, H. Osawa, K. Miyazaki, M. Kawaguchi, and H. Satoh, "Paradoxical response to osimertinib therapy in a patient with T790M-mutated lung adenocarcinoma," *Molecular and Clinical Oncology*, vol. 8, no. 1, pp. 175–177, 2017.

21

A Rare Case of Glioblastoma Multiforme with Osseous Metastases

Rubens Barros Costa, Ricardo Costa, Jason Kaplan, Marcelo Rocha Cruz, Hiral Shah, Maria Matsangou, and Benedito Carneiro

Developmental Therapeutics Program, Feinberg School of Medicine and Robert H. Lurie Comprehensive Cancer Center of Northwestern University, 233 East Superior Street, Chicago, IL 60611, USA

Correspondence should be addressed to Rubens Barros Costa; rubens.filho@northwestern.edu

Academic Editor: Guido Fadda

Glioblastoma multiforme is the most common malignant primary central nervous system neoplasm in adults. It has a very aggressive natural history with a median overall survival estimated at 14.6 months despite multimodality treatment. Extracranial metastases are very rare with few case reports published to date. We report the case of a 65-year-old male who underwent maximal safe resection for a newly diagnosed brain mass after presentation with new neurologic symptoms. He then received standard postsurgical adjuvant treatment for glioblastoma. Subsequently, he underwent another resection for early progressive disease. Several months later, he was hospitalized for new-onset musculoskeletal complaints. Additional investigation revealed new metastatic osseous lesions which were initially felt to be a new malignancy. The patient opted for supportive care and died 12 days later. Despite choosing no treatment, he elected to undergo a bone biopsy to understand the new underlying process. Results were that of metastatic GBM and were reported after the patient expired. Physicians caring for patients with GBM and new non-neurologic symptoms may contemplate body imaging.

1. Introduction

Glioblastoma multiforme (GBM) is a common primary central nervous system (CNS) neoplasm in adults with a very aggressive natural history and grim prognosis [1, 2]. For fit patients, the standard treatment approach is maximal safe resection with adjuvant brain radiation and temozolomide. Important prognostic factors are age and performance status. The median overall survival is estimated at 14.6 months with combined therapy [3]. The cause of death is usually related to local progression and its complications. Extracranial metastases are rare, with reports scarcely available. Possible explanations for the lack of metastatic dissemination are short survival time and the presence of the blood brain barrier. For these reasons, screening for metastases is not a common practice. The median survival time from metastasis diagnosis is short (~14 months) [3–5]. Herein, we report a case of glioblastoma multiforme with metastases to the bones and a poor outcome.

2. Case Report

The patient was a 65-year-old gentleman with a past medical history of hypertension and diabetes mellitus type 2 who was admitted to the hospital with progressive weakness, headache, dizziness, and confusion. His general and neurologic exam was grossly normal. Blood laboratory data were within normal limits. A nonenhanced computed tomography (CT) of the brain showed a large mass within the right parietal lobe with surrounding vasogenic edema. A brain magnetic resonance imaging (MRI) showed an irregularly enhancing mass measuring 5.8 cm anteroposterior × 3.2 cm transverse × 4.4 cm craniocaudal within the right parieto-occipital lobe, with significant vasogenic edema (Figures 1 and 2). He then underwent a right parietal craniotomy with maximal safe resection of the tumor.

The surgical pathology report showed a high-grade glioma with foci of necrosis and microvascular proliferation consistent with GBM (WHO Grade IV) (Figure 3). His postsurgical course unfolded without complications.

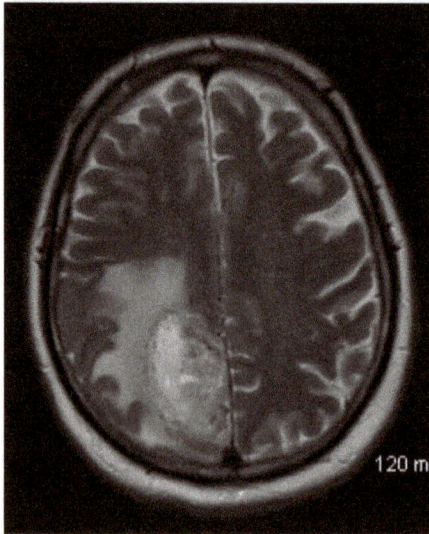

FIGURE 1: Axial T2-weighted image demonstrating heterogeneous mass in the right parasagittal parietal lobe with extensive surrounding vasogenic edema.

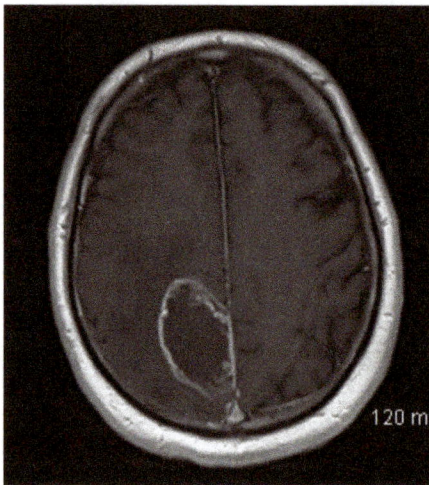

FIGURE 2: Axial T1-weighted image after administration of gadolinium demonstrating peripheral nodular enhancement of right parietal mass.

He then went on to receive adjuvant radiation therapy with a total of 60 Grays divided into 30 fractions during the course of 44 days. He additionally received temozolomide at $75 \, mg/m^2$ daily while on radiation therapy, with essentially no toxicity. Temozolomide was subsequently continued at $150 \, mg/m^2$ daily five days out of a 28-day cycle.

A follow-up MRI of the brain approximately 5 weeks post completion of combined therapy showed increased enhancement and diameter of the parietal mass, mass effect on the adjacent right occipital horn of the right ventricle, and diffuse vasogenic edema on the right cerebral hemisphere.

Subsequently, the patient was transferred to an outlying institution for additional management where he underwent reopening craniotomy with microsurgical resection of the tumor with Gliadel wafer placement approximately 17 weeks

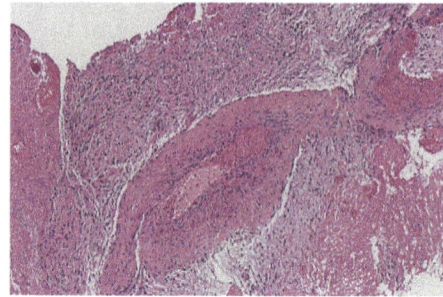

FIGURE 3: Brain surgical specimen. High-grade glioma with foci of necrosis and microvascular proliferation consistent with glioblastoma multiforme (WHO Grade IV).

from his initial resection. The surgical specimen showed progressive glioblastoma. His postsurgical recovery was complicated by hydrocephalus, hemiparesis, and an acute non-segment elevated myocardial infarction. He returned to the operating room for a right ventriculoperitoneal shunt placement on postoperative day 12.

About 4 weeks after the procedure, the patient was started on bevacizumab every 3 weeks. He received 5 treatments with this agent which had to be discontinued due to proteinuria and hypertension. A follow-up brain MRI five months post second resection showed postoperative changes without evidence of recurrent and/or progressive disease.

Approximately five weeks after his most recent follow-up MRI, he was hospitalized with excruciating lower back pain radiating to his right hip and anterior thigh. MRI of the pelvis showed extensive lesions with involvement of femurs, iliac bones, and sacrum (Figure 4). A CT chest, abdomen, and pelvis was negative for visceral metastatic disease. Bone scan (Tc 99m) showed subtle uptake in the bilateral humeri and increased uptake in the region of the greater trochanter on the right. Subtle increased uptake in the trochanteric region on the left was also reported. A biopsy of a right femoral lesion showed numerous tumor cells in a reactive stroma replacing much of the bone marrow (Figure 5). The tumor cells stained positive for glial fibrillary acidic protein (GFAP) (Figure 6). The conclusion was that it was representative of a high-grade astrocytoma (i.e., glioblastoma). Given the limited therapeutic options and poor performance status, the patient elected for supportive care only and died 12 days after the biopsy. No brain imaging was performed during the hospitalization.

3. Discussion

GBM is a very common and aggressive malignant neoplasm of the CNS in adults. In the seminal paper by Stupp et al., the median overall survival was roughly 14.6 months for patients who underwent resection, followed by adjuvant chemoradiotherapy [3]. With an estimated 5-year survival rate of less than 5%, the cause of death is almost always related to local progression and its complication. Osseous and visceral metastases are a rare phenomenon in the natural history of GBM with incidences reported anywhere from 0.4 to 2% [4]. Possible explanations for the low occurrence

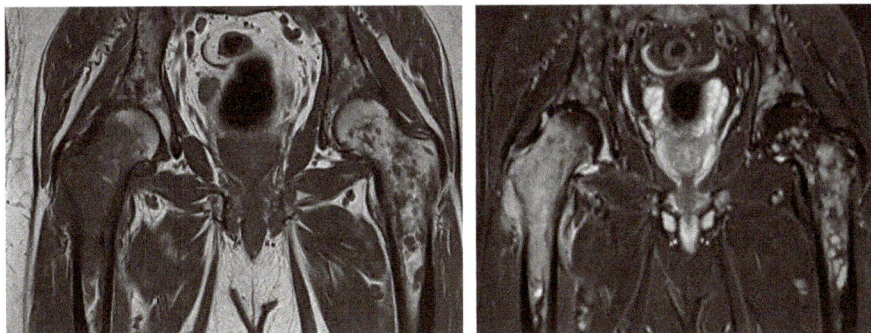

FIGURE 4: Coronal T1- (left) and T2- (right) weighted images approximately 6 months following resection demonstrating extensive neoplastic lesions throughout both femurs, iliac bones, and the sacrum.

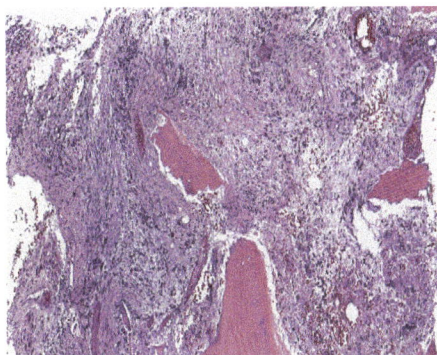

FIGURE 5: GBM osseous metastasis (higher power). Microscopic sections showing a destructive cellular neoplasm with highly atypical and hyperchromatic tumor cells, abundant necrosis, and vascular proliferation.

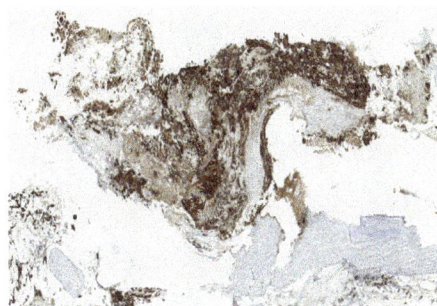

FIGURE 6: GBM with GFAP stain. GFAP (glial fibrillary acidic protein) immunohistochemical stain showing strong staining within the fibrillary cytoplasmic processes of the viable tumor cells.

or detection of extracranial dissemination are short survival and the blood brain barrier [4]. It is possible that metastasis is not a rare occurrence, but for most patients it will never represent a life-threatening event in light of almost universal early progression in the CNS. For this reason, clinicians usually do not screen for disease spread outside of the brain. Indeed, the most recent version of the National Comprehensive Cancer Network Guidelines does not have a formal recommendation to screen for metastases in patients with high-grade gliomas after maximal safe resection [6].

A recent review by Kalokhe et al. found 79 cases with extracranial disease for patients who were 18 years or older, proven by either biopsy or autopsy. The most common sites of metastases were the bone (38%), lymph nodes (37%), lungs (32%), and liver (18%). Other organs included the eyes, spleen, liver, parotid and adrenal glands, and subcutaneous tissues [4]. Malignant effusion may also be the initial presentation of GBM in patients without evidence of brain pathology on brain imaging after solid organ allografting from a previous donor with GBM found on autopsy [7]. In this analysis, the median survival in their analysis was 13 months compared to 14 months in the seminal trial by Stupp. The median survival from the time of diagnosis of metastatic disease was 5 months. Chemotherapy but not surgery and/or radiation was the only therapeutic modality that possibly lengthened survival and time to metastases, barring the limitations of their report [4].

More recently, Fonkem et al. have pointed out that GBM cells may be present in the circulation as there is evidence that the blood brain barrier may be disrupted in GBM [8, 9]. Furthermore, another report by Franceschi et al. showed mutations in patient blood germinal DNA that matched that of a primary GBM with biopsy-proven metastasis to the sternum [10]. This is important in that it could allow for accrual of patients with very few treatment options into multiple-histology basket trials while circumventing the need for invasive biopsies. Nonetheless, they also postulated that the immune system may suppress the growth of GBM cells in the circulation, preventing its seeding in other organs. Building upon this concept, other cases of extracranial GBM metastases in recipients of donors of solid organ with previously treated GBM have been described [8, 11–13]. Further understanding of mechanisms of immune evasion leading to disease progression could allow for possible use of cytotoxic immune stimulation with checkpoint inhibitors as is in other solid tumors.

This report adds to others of previous metastatic GBM [4, 10, 11, 14, 15]. Our patient faired very poorly, in keeping with the other cases in the literature. His survival post diagnosis was approximately 8 months. We cannot be certain of his cranial disease status at time of diagnosis of metastatic disease. We could possibly speculate that the placement of the ventriculoperitoneal shunt may have contributed to disseminated metastasis as others have previously as a mechanism of spread of a primary CNS tumor [16].

In summary, this case illustrates that extracranial metastatic disease may be an event in the natural course of the patient's GBM.

References

[1] W. J. Curran Jr., C. B. Scott, J. Horton et al., "Recursive partitioning analysis of prognostic factors in three Radiation Therapy Oncology Group malignant glioma trials," *Journal of the National Cancer Institute*, vol. 85, no. 9, pp. 704–710, 1993.

[2] Q. T. Ostrom, H. Gittleman, P. Farah et al., "CBTRUS statistical report: primary brain and central nervous system tumors diagnosed in the United States in 2006-2010," *Neuro-Oncology*, vol. 15, no. 2, pp. ii1–ii56, 2013.

[3] R. Stupp, W. P. Mason, M. J. van den Bent et al., "Radiotherapy plus concomitant and adjuvant temozolomide for glioblastoma," *New England Journal of Medicine*, vol. 352, no. 10, pp. 987–996, 2005.

[4] G. Kalokhe, S. A. Grimm, J. P. Chandler, I. Helenowski, A. Rademaker, and J. J. Raizer, "Metastatic glioblastoma: case presentations and a review of the literature," *Journal of Neuro-Oncology*, vol. 107, no. 1, pp. 21–27, 2012.

[5] K. J. Waite, S. B. Wharton, S. E. Old, and N. G. Burnet, "Systemic metastases of glioblastoma multiforme," *Clinical Oncology*, vol. 11, no. 3, pp. 205–207, 1999.

[6] Network, N.C.C, "Central Nervous System Cancers (Version 1.2016)," June 2017, https://www.nccn.org/professionals/physician_gls/pdf/cns.pdf.

[7] D. W. Nauen and Q. K. Li, "Cytological diagnosis of metastatic glioblastoma in the pleural effusion of a lung transplant patient," *Diagnostic Cytopathology*, vol. 42, no. 7, pp. 619–623, 2014.

[8] E. Fonkem, M. Lun, and E. T. Wong, "Rare phenomenon of extracranial metastasis of glioblastoma," *Journal of Clinical Oncology*, vol. 29, no. 34, pp. 4594-4595, 2011.

[9] Y. Rong, D. L. Durden, E. G. van Meir, and D. J. Brat, "'Pseudopalisading' necrosis in glioblastoma: a familiar morphologic feature that links vascular pathology, hypoxia, and angiogenesis," *Journal of Neuropathology and Experimental Neurology*, vol. 65, no. 6, pp. 529–539, 2006.

[10] S. Franceschi, F. Lessi, and P. Aretini, "Molecular portrait of a rare case of metastatic glioblastoma: somatic and germline mutations using whole-exome sequencing," *Neuro-Oncology*, vol. 18, no. 2, pp. 298–300, 2016.

[11] F. Val-Bernal, J. C. Ruiz, J. G. Cotorruelo, and M. Arias, "Glioblastoma multiforme of donor origin after renal transplantation: report of a case," *Human Pathology*, vol. 24, no. 11, pp. 1256–1259, 1993.

[12] M. Y. Armanios, S. A. Grossman, S. C. Yang et al., "Transmission of glioblastoma multiforme following bilateral lung transplantation from an affected donor: case study and review of the literature," *Neuro-Oncology*, vol. 6, no. 3, pp. 259–263, 2004.

[13] H. Chen, A. S. Shah, R. E. Girgis, and S. A. Grossman, "Transmission of glioblastoma multiforme after bilateral lung transplantation," *Journal of Clinical Oncology*, vol. 26, no. 19, pp. 3284-3285, 2008.

[14] J. H. Morse, J. G. Turcotte, R. M. Merion et al., "Development of a malignant tumor in a liver transplant graft procured from a donor with a cerebral neoplasm," *Transplantation*, vol. 50, no. 5, pp. 875-876, 1990.

[15] S. S. Mujtaba, S. Haroon, and N. Faridi, "Cervical metastatic glioblastoma multiforme," *Journal of the College of Physicians and Surgeons–Pakistan*, vol. 23, no. 2, pp. 160-161, 2013.

[16] J. H. Ko, P. H. Lu, T. C. Tang, and Y. H. Hsu, "Metastasis of primary CNS lymphoma along a ventriculoperitoneal shunt," *Journal of Clinical Oncology*, vol. 29, no. 34, pp. e823–e824, 2011.

22

Histiocytic Sarcoma Associated with Coombs Negative Acute Hemolytic Anemia: A Rare Presentation

Sandeep Batra,[1] **Stephen C. Martin,**[1] **Mehdi Nassiri,**[2] **Amna Qureshi,**[2] **and Troy A. Markel**[3]

[1]*Department of Pediatrics, Section of Pediatric Hematology and Oncology, Riley Hospital for Children at Indiana University Health, Indiana University School of Medicine, Indianapolis, IN 46202, USA*

[2]*Department of Pathology and Laboratory Medicine, Indiana University School of Medicine, Indianapolis, IN 46202, USA*

[3]*Department of Surgery, Section of Pediatric Surgery, Riley Hospital for Children at Indiana University Health, Indiana University School of Medicine, Indianapolis, IN 46202, USA*

Correspondence should be addressed to Sandeep Batra; batras@iu.edu

Academic Editor: Jose I. Mayordomo

Histiocytic sarcoma (HS) rarely involves extranodal sites, such as the spleen. We report a unique pediatric case of massive splenomegaly and refractory Coombs negative hemolytic anemia (CNHA) secondary to HS. The CNHA resolved completely after an emergent splenectomy. Next generation sequencing (NGS) revealed novel ASXL1, PTPN11, KIT, and TP53 mutations, unmasking a clonal heterogeneity within the same neoplasm.

1. Introduction

Malignant histiocytic disorders such as histiocytic sarcoma (HS) are rare in the pediatric population [1]. HS commonly presents with fever, malaise, weight loss, and abdominal pain, but clinical manifestations are varied. HS can be localized or fulminant and uncommonly involves extranodal sites such as skin, bone marrow, soft tissue, and spleen [2]. Fulminant or disseminated HS is often associated with a poor outcome [2].

HS may occur before or after mature B cell lymphomas, acute lymphoblastic, and hairy cell leukemia, suggesting that a common oncogenic cellular origin may exist in some patients [3, 4]. HS can also be associated with autoimmune lymphoproliferative syndrome [5]. The majority of HS express macrophage or histiocytic markers such as lysozyme, alpha-antitrypsin, CD68 (KP1 and PGM1), CD163, CD11c, and CD14 but typically lack Langerhans cell (CD1a and langerin), follicular dendritic cell (CD21 and CD35), and myeloid cell (CD33, CD13, and myeloperoxidase) markers. CD34, CD3, and CD20 (T and B lymphocyte markers, resp.), melanoma (Melan-A, human melanoma black-45, and tyrosinase), and carcinoma (cytokeratin) markers are typically absent [6]. Rarely lineage infidelity may be present and could lead to misdiagnosis of a lymphoma [7].

We report a case of a 17-year-old who presented with massive splenomegaly and severe Coombs negative hemolytic anemia (CNHA). The diagnosis of histiocytic sarcoma (HS) was established after an emergent splenectomy. To our knowledge, HS associated with CNHA in the pediatric population has not been previously reported.

2. Case Report

A 17-year-old African American male presented to the local emergency department with fatigue, abdominal pain, jaundice, and worsening pallor, for 2 weeks. On exam, he was pale and icteric and had tender splenomegaly (spleen was palpable 5-6 cm below costal margin). Labs revealed a hematocrit equal to 17%, serum bilirubin equal to 3 mg/dL, a negative Coombs test (direct and indirect), and a platelet count of 39,000. The peripheral smear showed anisopoikilocytosis, abundant spherocytes, tear drop cells, polychromatophilia, with normal appearing granulocytes, and decreased platelets (Figure 2(a)). A bone marrow aspirate revealed a hypercellular marrow, negative for blasts, dysplasia, or hemophagocytosis. The local hematologist initiated treatment with oral prednisone (2 mg/kg/day) and weekly rituximab (375 mg/m^2 for 4 total doses) and administered 2 doses of intravenous

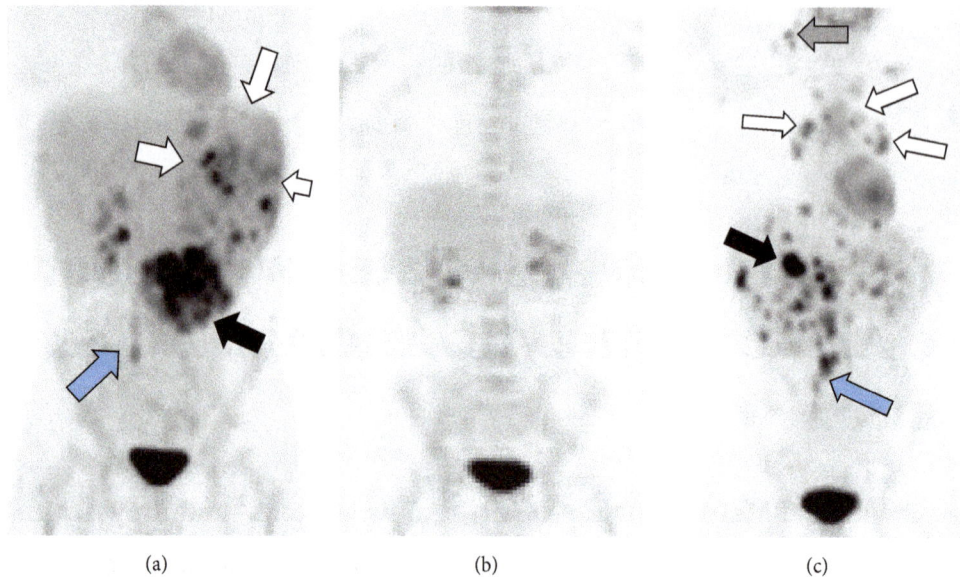

FIGURE 1: PET scans. (a) Prechemotherapy PET-CT scan (anterior view) demonstrates marked splenomegaly (white arrows), with multiple hypermetabolic foci scattered throughout the spleen and in the retroperitoneum (blue arrow). There was a large aggregate of abnormal foci at the lower edge of the spleen that measured $7 \times 6 \times 5$ cm (black arrow); (b) PET-CT after 6 cycles of CHOP chemotherapy shows no evidence of disease; (c) recurrent hypermetabolic foci and lymphadenopathy involving multiple sites within the liver (black arrow), peritoneum (blue arrow), mediastinum (white arrows), and neck (gray arrow).

immunoglobulin (1 gram/kilogram body weight given a week apart), based on the presumptive diagnosis of a Coombs negative Evans Syndrome.

However, the hemolytic anemia persisted, and the patient continued to require 2–4 units of packed RBC transfusions to keep the hematocrit >25%. The spleen (now below umbilicus) continued to increase in size and was associated with severe abdominal pain and distension. He was then referred to our hematology service for further evaluation. We obtained additional labs as follows: ALPS panel (negative), cold agglutinins (negative), reticulocyte count (10%), indirect and direct Coombs testing (negative), bilirubin (5 mg/dL, mostly indirect), and serum haptoglobin (undetectable). Flow cytometry on peripheral blood failed to reveal an abnormal blast population and demonstrated a normal RBC expression pattern for CD55 or CD59, excluding acute leukemia or PNH, respectively, as the probable cause of the presentation. The urinalysis was negative for hemosiderin or blood. Infectious work-up for *Bartonella*, brucellosis, tuberculosis, and malaria was negative. We obtained an abdominal PET-CT which demonstrated marked splenomegaly, with multiple areas of heterogeneous and hypermetabolic enhancing foci/masses that were scattered throughout the spleen and also in the retroperitoneum (Figure 1(a)). These findings were suggestive of a lymphoproliferative and neoplastic process.

An urgent open splenectomy was performed. The surgically removed spleen (Figure 2(b)) was massively enlarged (weight = 1770 grams, $24 \times 14 \times 11$ cm in size) and very firm in consistency. There were several hypertrophied vessels noted in the splenic hilum. Serial sections revealed a red-brown, congested parenchyma, with numerous gray-yellow nodules (0.1–2 cm in size), concentrated at the lower edge of

the spleen. A repeat bone marrow aspirate demonstrated a hypercellular marrow, with trilineage maturation and devoid of HS or hemophagocytosis.

Histological sections of the spleen revealed sheets of atypical multinucleated cells with a high nuclear to cytoplasmic ratio, irregular to round nuclear contour, prominent nucleoli, and an abundant eosinophilic cytoplasm (Figure 2(c)), with varying degrees of apoptosis. These neoplastic cells stained positively for CD45, CD68 PGM and Kp1 (Figures 2(d) and 2(e), resp.), CD14, CD23, fascin, and lysozyme (Figure 2(f)) and were negative for CD34, myeloperoxidase, and S100 protein, confirming the diagnosis of HS [7]. CD20, Pax-5, CD3, CD30, keratin cocktail, desmin, factor VIII, factor XIIIa, CD163, CD1a, CD21, CD35, CD123 immunostains, and BRAF^{V600E} mutation were negative.

We also performed hotspot mutation detection by high-throughput next generation sequencing (NGS), using optimized oligonucleotide probes [8]. Specimens were reviewed by a pathologist before processing. Formalin-fixed paraffin-embedded splenic tissue obtained at the time of diagnosis was used to isolate DNA. Fifteen full genes (exons only) as well as additional 39 oncogenic hotspots were analyzed with highly multiplexed next generation sequencing (Illumina TruSight Myeloid Sequencing Panel) (Supplemental Table 1 in Supplementary Material available online at http://dx.doi.org/10.1155/2016/3179147) [8]. Limit of detection of this assay as established by our laboratory is 1-2% mutant alleles. The variants were classified according to previously published guidelines and databases. Low prevalence (<10% of allele frequency) mutations were detected in the ASLX1, KIT, PTPN11, and TP53 genes (Supplemental Table 2), along with multiple variants of unknown significance (not included in

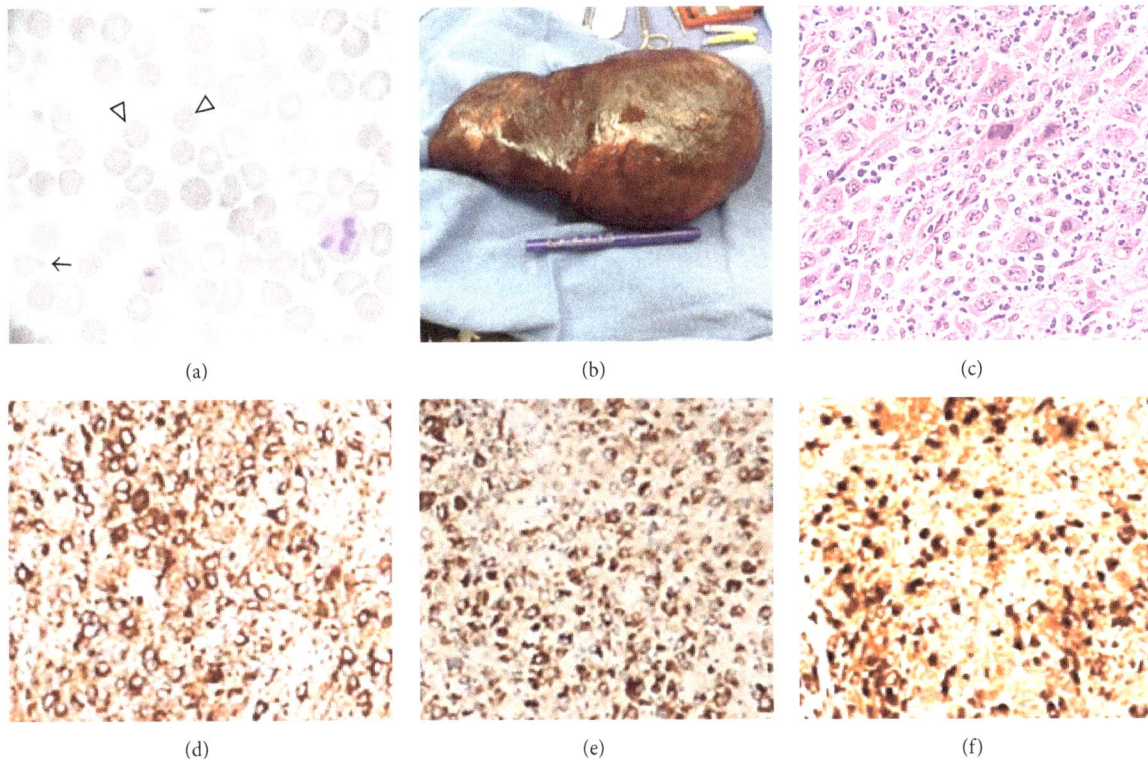

FIGURE 2: Peripheral blood smear and histopathology of the spleen. (a) Prechemotherapy peripheral blood smear with anisopoikilocytosis, numerous spherocytes (white arrows), tear drop cell (black arrow), and decreased platelets; (b) massively enlarged, surgically removed spleen (weight = 1770 grams; 24 × 14 × 11 cm in size); (c) histological sections of the spleen revealed sheets of atypical cells with a high nuclear to cytoplasmic ratio, prominent nucleoli, and an abundant eosinophilic cytoplasm (400x magnification); (d, e, and f) areas of spleen involved with HS demonstrated strong and diffuse immunoreactivity with macrophage-specific markers (CD68 PGM (d), CD68 KP1 (e), and lysozyme (f)) [7].

supplemental data), suggesting that mutated or variant tumor cells comprised only a minor portion of the malignant clone.

Importantly, the hemolytic anemia and thrombocytopenia resolved rapidly and completely after splenectomy. We then elected to treat our patient with adjuvant CHOP chemotherapy (cyclophosphamide, doxorubicin, vincristine, and oral prednisone) [9, 10]. The PET-CT scans after 3 cycles of CHOP and at the end of therapy (Figure 1(b)) demonstrated no residual or recurrent FDG avid lesions. However, the remission only lasted 3-4 months; recurrent disease was identified in the liver and abdominal lymph nodes (Figure 1(c)) on a PET scan and confirmed with a supraclavicular (neck) lymph node and CT guided liver needle biopsy. Interestingly, the CNHA did not recur with the relapse.

The relapsed disease was treated with 4 cycles of ICE (ifosfamide, carboplatin, and etoposide) chemotherapy [11] followed by an autologous stem cell transplant (using BEAM, carmustine, etoposide, cytarabine, and melphalan, as a conditioning regimen) for consolidation [12]. Unfortunately, our patient remained in remission only for 5-6 months, after transplant, and elected for palliative care.

3. Discussion

Acquired Coombs negative hemolytic anemia (CNHA) is rare in the adolescent age group. The differential diagnosis of CNHA (nonimmune hemolysis) associated with splenomegaly, in pediatric patients, includes both inherited and acquired causes such as hemoglobinopathies, RBC enzyme or membrane defects, infections, toxins, HLH, immunodeficiencies, microangiopathies, and uncommonly neoplasms [13, 14]. Splenectomy is rarely performed in these patients but may be indicated in severe refractory immune mediated hemolysis, recurrent splenic sequestration, or hypersplenism [15].

Our patient presented with a Coombs negative hemolytic anemia (CNHA), associated with massive splenic involvement by HS. To our knowledge, this is the first pediatric report describing this atypical presentation. The CNHA could have resulted from the altered circulation, hypoxia, and acidification in the massive spleen. An emergent total splenectomy led to a rapid resolution of CNHA, supporting that notion.

Treatment with rituximab, IVIG, and steroids did not improve the CNHA. This initial lack of response to rituximab is, most likely, due to lack of CD20 expression or the existence of a nonimmune mechanism, such as the extravascular destruction of RBCs in the spleen, or direct cell mediated cytotoxicity [16, 17]. There was no lab evidence of significant microangiopathy (no RBC fragments or schistocytosis) or hemophagocytic lymphohistiocytosis (HLH) (hemophagocytosis, hypertriglyceridemia, low NK activity, or hypofibrinogenemia) [18]. In addition, NGS failed to identify high prevalence (>10%) oncogenic mutations that could explain the pathogenesis or the unique presentation of this HS.

Interestingly, the HS infiltrated spleen harbored mutations in the ASLX1, KIT, PTPN11, and TP53 genes (Supplemental Table 2). Mutations in ASXL1 have been observed frequently in acute myelogenous leukemia and myelodysplastic syndromes and are associated with a worse outcome due to an aberrant hematopoiesis [19]. Genomic profiling of acute myelogenous leukemia has identified somatic variants in both PTPN11 and KIT genes [20] and TP53 mutations [21], implicating resistant pathways that require further investigation [22]. It is plausible that these cooperating mutations contributed to HS relapse, in our patient.

4. Conclusion

This case report underscores the importance of ruling out an occult malignancy as a rare cause of refractory CNHA. Splenectomy is an effective option to treat CNHA due to splenic involvement by HS.

Abbreviations

HS: Histiocytic sarcoma
CNHA: Coombs negative hemolytic anemia
PET-CT: Positron emission tomography-computed
          tomography
ALPS: Autoimmune lymphoproliferative
          syndrome
CHOP: Cyclophosphamide, doxorubicin,
          vincristine, and prednisone
ICE: Ifosfamide, carboplatin, and etoposide
BEAM: Carmustine, etoposide, cytarabine, and
          melphalan
CD: Cluster of differentiation
BRAF: Serine/threonine-protein kinase B-Raf
HLH: Hemophagocytic lymphohistiocytosis
NGS: Next generation sequencing.

References

[1] J. L. Heath, S. E. Burgett, A. M. Gaca, R. Jaffe, and D. S. Wechsler, "Successful treatment of pediatric histiocytic sarcoma using abbreviated high-risk leukemia chemotherapy," *Pediatric Blood and Cancer*, vol. 61, no. 10, pp. 1874–1876, 2014.

[2] J. L. Hornick, E. S. Jaffe, and C. D. M. Fletcher, "Extranodal histiocytic sarcoma: clinicopathologic analysis of 14 cases of a rare epithelioid malignancy," *American Journal of Surgical Pathology*, vol. 28, no. 9, pp. 1133–1144, 2004.

[3] P. Brunner, A. Rufle, S. Dirnhofer et al., "Follicular lymphoma transformation into histiocytic sarcoma: indications for a common neoplastic progenitor," *Leukemia*, vol. 28, no. 9, pp. 1937–1940, 2014.

[4] E. C. C. Castro, C. Blazquez, J. Boyd et al., "Clinicopathologic features of histiocytic lesions following ALL, with a review of

the literature," *Pediatric and Developmental Pathology*, vol. 13, no. 3, pp. 225–237, 2010.

[5] C. Guitton, F. Le Deist, and B. Bader-Meunier, "Coombs' negative haemolytic anaemia as a first manifestation of autoimmune lymphoproliferative disease," *British Journal of Haematology*, vol. 129, no. 3, pp. 442–443, 2005.

[6] E. Takahashi and S. Nakamura, "Histiocytic sarcoma: an updated literature review based on the 2008 WHO classification," *Journal of Clinical and Experimental Hematopathology*, vol. 53, no. 1, pp. 1–8, 2013.

[7] S. A. Pileri, T. M. Grogan, N. L. Harris et al., "Tumours of histiocytes and accessory dendritic cells: an immunohistochemical approach to classification from the international lymphoma study group based on 61 cases," *Histopathology*, vol. 41, no. 1, pp. 1–29, 2002.

[8] C. H. Au, A. Wa, D. N. Ho, T. L. Chan, and E. S. K. Ma, "Clinical evaluation of panel testing by next-generation sequencing (NGS) for gene mutations in myeloid neoplasms," *Diagnostic Pathology*, vol. 11, no. 1, article 11, 2016.

[9] H. Tsujimura, T. Miyaki, S. Yamada et al., "Successful treatment of histiocytic sarcoma with induction chemotherapy consisting of dose-escalated CHOP plus etoposide and upfront consolidation auto-transplantation," *International Journal of Hematology*, vol. 100, no. 5, pp. 507–510, 2014.

[10] Y. Kitano, M. Nakagawa, M. Kojima et al., "Case of malignant histiocytosis treated with chop therapy and splenectomy," *Nihon Naika Gakkai Zasshi*, vol. 83, no. 6, pp. 990–992, 1994.

[11] J. Tomlin, R. K. Orosco, S. Boles et al., "Successful treatment of multifocal histiocytic sarcoma occurring after renal transplantation with cladribine, high-dose cytarabine, G-CSF, and mitoxantrone (CLAG-M) followed by allogeneic hematopoietic stem cell transplantation," *Case Reports in Hematology*, vol. 2015, Article ID 728260, 6 pages, 2015.

[12] B. Cazin, N. C. Gorin, J. P. Jouet et al., "Successful autologous bone marrow transplantation in second remission of malignant histiocytosis," *Bone Marrow Transplantation*, vol. 5, no. 6, pp. 431–433, 1990.

[13] V. Cecinati, F. Brugnoletti, M. D'Angiò et al., "Autoimmune hemolytic anemia and immune thrombocytopenia as unusual presentations of childhood hodgkin lymphoma: a case report and review of the literature," *Journal of Pediatric Hematology/Oncology*, vol. 34, no. 4, pp. 280–282, 2012.

[14] L. Uzunova, C. E. Hook, M. Gattens, and G. A. Burke, "Cold antibody autoimmune haemolytic anaemia in a child with diffuse large B cell lymphoma," *Annals of Hematology*, vol. 95, no. 1, pp. 151–152, 2016.

[15] S. Patel, J. Said, S. Song, W. Nishimoto, and R. Paquette, "A case of hemolytic anemia and severe thrombocytopenia related to histiocytic sarcoma," *Leukemia Research*, vol. 34, no. 9, pp. e257–e258, 2010.

[16] E. Biagi, G. Assali, F. Rossi, M. Jankovic, B. Nicolini, and A. Balduzzi, "A persistent severe autoimmune hemolytic anemia despite apparent direct antiglobulin test negativization," *Haematologica*, vol. 84, no. 11, pp. 1043–1045, 1999.

[17] A. Fujimi, Y. Kamihara, Y. Kanisawa et al., "Anti-erythropoietin receptor antibody-associated pure red cell aplasia accompanied by Coombs-negative autoimmune hemolytic anemia in a patient with T cell/histiocyte-rich large B cell lymphoma," *International Journal of Hematology*, vol. 100, no. 5, pp. 490–493, 2014.

[18] M. B. Jordan, C. E. Allen, S. Weitzman, A. H. Filipovich, and K. L. McClain, "How I treat hemophagocytic lymphohistiocytosis," *Blood*, vol. 118, no. 15, pp. 4041–4052, 2011.

[19] J. E. Churpek, K. Pyrtel, K.-L. Kanchi et al., "Genomic analysis of germ line and somatic variants in familial myelodysplasia/acute myeloid leukemia," *Blood*, vol. 126, no. 22, pp. 2484–2490, 2015.

[20] C. C. Coombs, M. S. Tallman, and R. L. Levine, "Molecular therapy for acute myeloid leukaemia," *Nature Reviews Clinical Oncology*, vol. 13, no. 5, pp. 305–318, 2016.

[21] C. Y. Ok, K. P. Patel, G. Garcia-Manero et al., "TP53 mutation characteristics in therapy-related myelodysplastic syndromes and acute myeloid leukemia is similar to de novo diseases," *Journal of Hematology and Oncology*, vol. 8, no. 1, article 139, 2015.

[22] M. Tokumasu, C. Murata, A. Shimada et al., "Adverse prognostic impact of KIT mutations in childhood CBF-AML: the results of the Japanese Pediatric Leukemia/Lymphoma Study Group AML-05 trial," *Leukemia*, vol. 29, no. 12, pp. 2438–2441, 2015.

23

Cutaneous Basal Cell Carcinoma with Lymph Node and Pulmonary Metastases

Renate U. Wahl ⓘ,[1] Claudio Cacchi,[2] and Albert Rübben ⓘ[1]

[1]Department of Dermatology, Euregional Skin Cancer Center, University Hospital of the RWTH-Aachen, Aachen, Germany
[2]Department of Pathology, University Hospital of the RWTH-Aachen, Aachen, Germany

Correspondence should be addressed to Renate U. Wahl; rwahl@ukaachen.de

Academic Editor: Constantine Gennatas

Basal cell carcinoma (BCC) is the most common skin cancer. Metastatic BCC is an extraordinary rare finding observed in only 0.5% of all cases. Until the introduction of the small molecule hedgehog inhibitor vismodegib, patients with metastatic BCC were treated with chemotherapy, most frequently platinum-based with mixed responses to therapy. We present the case of a 55-year-old Caucasian man who suffered from BCC on his left arm with lymph node and pulmonary metastases. Sonic hedgehog blockade with vismodegib only induced a short remission, and the patient succumbed to the cancer.

1. Introduction

Basal cell carcinoma (BCC) of the skin is the most common human cancer in Caucasians. Its high incidence can be explained by genetics as inactivation of only one-signal transduction pathway; that is, the sonic hedgehog (SHH) signaling, either by one activating mutation in the *SMO gene* or by two inactivating mutational events targeting the *PTCH1 gene*, seems to be sufficient for cancer formation. Consequently, blockade of SHH signaling has been developed as systemic treatment of advanced BCC [1]. Although BCC can induce extensive and lethal local tissue destruction, formation of metastases is exceedingly rare. Metastasis frequency is estimated to range from 0.003% to 0.5% [2]. Low frequency of metastases of BCC stands in contrast to the very high mutation load demonstrated in sporadic BCC and to a lesser extent also in syndromic BCC [3–5]. On the other hand, most mutations demonstrate an UV-signature and one might speculate that a cancer driven mostly by exogenous UV-induced mutations might be less prone to acquire the additional mutations necessary for the metastatic process than a cancer evolving primarily through a mutator phenotype or through marked aneuploidy. Nevertheless, genetic instability in BCC is not excluded, and

mutations of the caretaker gene P53 and chromosomal instability have been observed frequently in BCC [3].

We would like to present an additional case of metastatic and fatal BCC in a surprisingly young male patient.

2. Case Presentation

In January 2015, a 55-year-old Caucasian man was admitted to our department with a 12-year history of a slow-growing ulcerating tumor of the left forearm. The patient had no comorbidities and no prior skin cancer history but a 40-year history of cigarette smoking. The only skin cancer risk factor was a Fitzpatrick skin type II. The patient had avoided medical care due to diffuse fear and distrust in the health care system, but within the last couple of months, the patient developed an ulceration of the left axilla which ultimately forced him to seek medical advice.

On initial presentation, we observed an 8×15 cm measuring wound on the left forearm and a 5×8 cm measuring and 3-4 cm deep ulceration of the left axilla (Figure 1). Several dark brown papules were seen on the left thoracic wall. We performed biopsies from the lesion on the left forearm, the axillary ulcers, and the papules on the thoracic wall with the histopathological finding of a basal cell

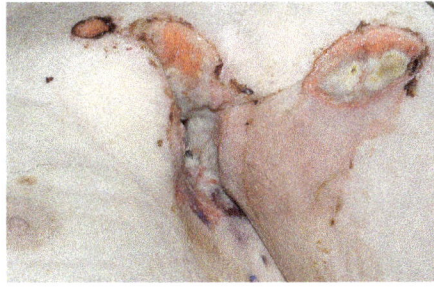

FIGURE 1: Axillary ulcerating lymph node metastases of cutaneous basal cell carcinoma located on the left forearm.

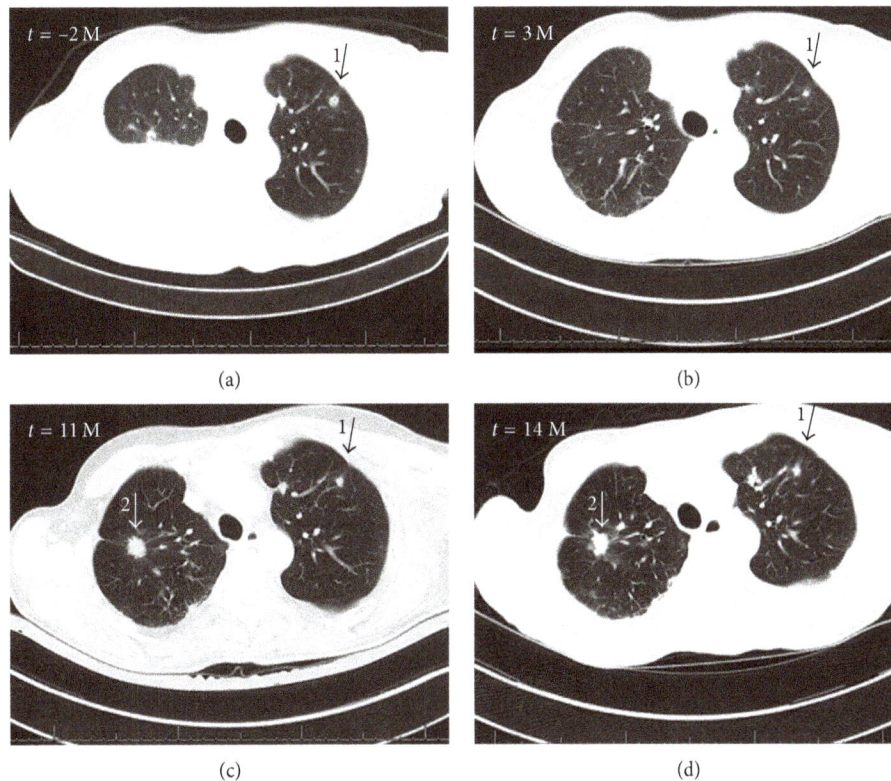

(a)

(b)

(c)

(d)

FIGURE 2: Computer tomography demonstrating pulmonary metastases two months before treatment ($t = -2$ M), with partial regression after 3 months of vismodegib treatment ($t = 3$ M, arrow 1) and with progressive disease after 11 and 14 months (arrow 1). Arrow 2 indicates new metastasis first visible on the CT scan after 11 months of treatment.

carcinoma (BCC) in all lesions. A metastasized BCC was diagnosed, and subsequent radiographic diagnostics revealed a pleural effusion in the right lung and multiple suspicious lesions in both lungs (Figure 2). Lung metastases of the BCC were confirmed by bronchoscopy and pleural biopsy. The carcinomatous pulmonary tissue matched to the lesion on the patient's left forearm by histology and immunohistochemistry with strong marking of CK 5/6 and a positive reaction to BerEP4 (Figure 3).

An oral medication with the SHH pathway inhibitor vismodegib, 150 mg/day, was started, and the patient's health state improved temporarily. The patient suffered from therapy-induced alopecia as well as from mild muscle spasms and mild dysgeusia which were first reported after 5 months of treatment, but vismodegib dosage does not need to be reduced. Initially, the cutaneous and pulmonary metastases decreased in size (Figure 2, arrow 1), but 6 months after starting vismodegib, radiotherapy of refractory and slowly progressive ulcerations of the left axilla and the forearm had to be performed. Pulmonary metastases demonstrated progression 9 months after starting vismodegib (Figure 2). In order to rule out a secondary pulmonary neoplasm, an additional metastatic pulmonary lesion was excised and histopathology again confirmed metastatic BCC.

Therapy with vismodegib was discontinued 11 months after initiation of treatment in order to switch to chemotherapy. However, the patient soon developed pneumonia and died of septic infection 4 months after vismodegib discontinuation and before chemotherapy could be initiated.

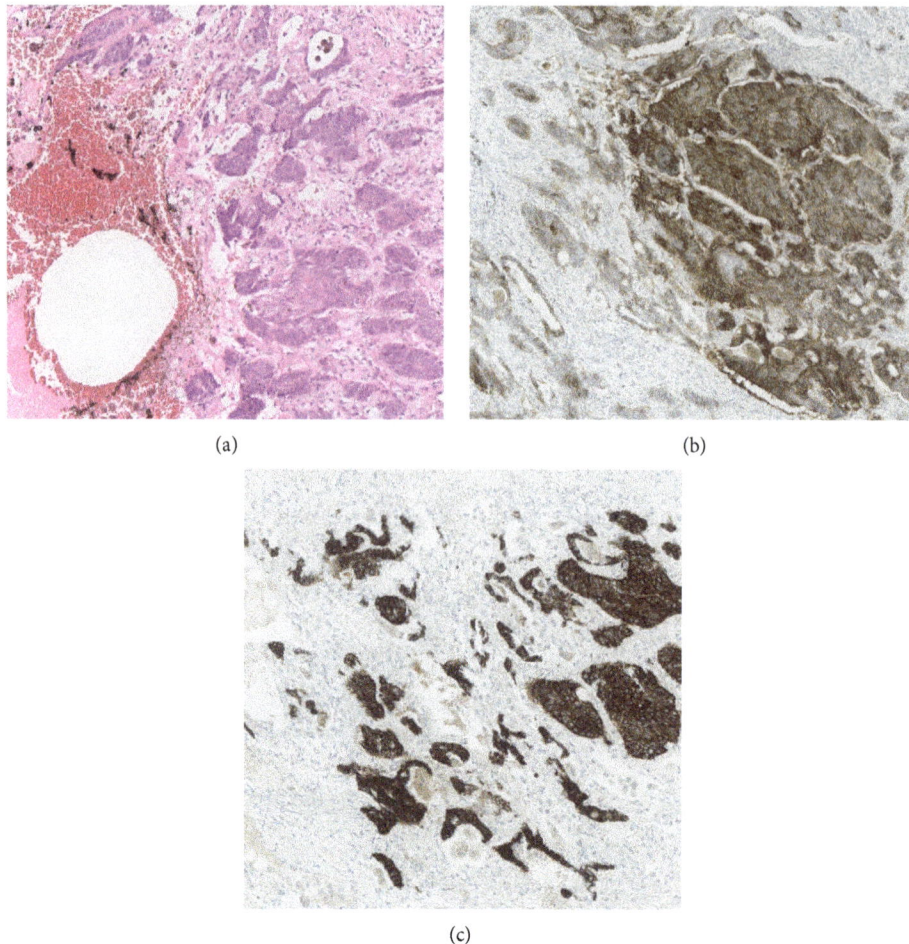

(a)

(b)

(c)

FIGURE 3: (a) H&E staining of pulmonary metastatic tissue demonstrating typical hyperchromatic basaloid cells (×200). (b) Positive BerEP4 staining of tumor tissue (×200). (c) Positive CK 5/6 staining of tumor tissue (×200).

3. Discussion

Basal cell carcinoma (BCC) is the most commonly diagnosed skin cancer, but metastatic BCC is an extraordinary rare finding. Metastatic BCC was first described by Beadles in 1894 [6]. In 1951, Lattes and Kessler provided narrow criteria for the definition of true metastatic BCC cases [7]. Less than 400 cases of true metastatic BCCs have been described till now [2].

Metastatic BCC spreads into lymph nodes by hematogenous dissemination, with the lung being the most often affected organ [2, 8, 9]. Metastatic BCC has a poor prognosis with mean survival rates of 3 years in cases of locoregional lymphatic metastases and of 8 months in patients with distant metastases. Large primary tumors, invasion of blood vessels or of perineural spaces, location in the head and neck region, multiple recurring or primary tumors, condition after radiotherapy, immunosuppression, and fair skin as well as male gender have been described as risk factors for developing a metastatic BCC [2, 9].

Immunohistochemistry should be performed additionally to routine histopathology in order to differentiate basal cell carcinoma from squamous cell carcinoma (SCC) of the skin or from basosquamous carcinoma, which presents a mixture of squamous and basaloid components. In our case, a strong reaction to CK 5/6 and a weaker reaction to BerEP4 were found. Cytokeratin 5/6 antibodies frequently show immunoreactivity in BCC as well as in squamous cell carcinoma of the skin [10]. However, pulmonary adenocarcinomas and pulmonary small cell cancers do not express CK 5/6, thereby allowing differentiation from primary pulmonary carcinoma [10]. BerEP4 is an antibody to the transmembrane epithelial adhesion molecule EpCAM. EpCAM is present on all nonsquamous epithelial cells [11]. Accordingly, BerEP4 is a sensitive marker of BCC but does not stain cutaneous SCC [12]. Clinics as well as the BerEP4 staining in our patient's cutaneous and pulmonary biopsies supported the diagnosis of a metastatic BCC.

Therapeutic standard for localized BCC is micrographic controlled surgery. Topical treatment with 5-FU or imiquimod, photodynamic therapy, cryotherapy, or laser therapy can be considered for superficial BCC. In cases of inoperable BCCs due to size, location, age, or medical history of the patient, radiotherapy is a palliative option. Until January 2012, no specific systemic therapy was available for patients with locally advanced or metastatic BCC. Patients were treated with chemotherapy, most frequently platinum-based or with more than one chemotherapy agent with mixed responses [1, 2, 8].

In the US, vismodegib was introduced as the first targeted therapy for BCC on January 30, 2012. Locally advanced BCCs showed a complete response to vismodegib in 21% and an assessed response rate of 43%, whereas the assessed response rate in patients with metastatic BCC was only 30% [13]. Muscle spasm, alopecia, dysgeusia, weight loss, and fatigue are the most common adverse side effects of vismodegib. Similar to other targeted therapeutic agents, development of resistance to vismodegib can be observed during treatment or after therapy-free periods. The mean response duration is 7.6 months [13]. Unfortunately, with loss of efficacy, the disease progresses rapidly causing the patients' death in short term as mirrored by our case report.

Activation of the RAS-MAPK pathway has been identified as one mechanism of resistance to SSH blockade [14] which is in line with the observation that some BCC have responded to EGFR blockade of the RAS-MAPK pathway [15]. Ongoing studies are exploring the immunologic approach by PDL1 blockade in advanced BCC, and preliminary results have demonstrated some efficacy in metastatic BCC [16]. A strong medical need persists to develop effective treatments for advanced and metastatic cutaneous basal cell carcinoma.

References

[1] R. Danhof, K. Lewis, and M. Brown, "Small molecule inhibitors of the hedgehog pathway in the treatment of basal cell carcinoma of the skin," *American Journal of Clinical Dermatology*, vol. 19, no. 2, pp. 195–207, 2018.

[2] M. McCusker, N. Basset-Seguin, R. Dummer et al., "Metastatic basal cell carcinoma: prognosis dependent on anatomic site and spread of disease," *European Journal of Cancer*, vol. 50, no. 4, pp. 774–783, 2014.

[3] S. S. Jayaraman, D. J. Rayhan, S. Hazany, and M. S. Kolodney, "Mutational landscape of basal cell carcinomas by whole-exome sequencing," *Journal of Investigative Dermatology*, vol. 134, no. 1, pp. 213–220, 2014.

[4] X. Bonilla, L. Parmentier, B. King et al., "Genomic analysis identifies new drivers and progression pathways in skin basal cell carcinoma," *Nature Genetics*, vol. 48, no. 4, pp. 398–406, 2016.

[5] A. Chiang, P. D. Jaju, P. Batra et al., "Genomic stability in syndromic basal cell carcinoma," *Journal of Investigative Dermatology*, vol. 138, no. 5, pp. 1044–1051, 2018.

[6] C. F. Beadles, "Rodent ulcer," *Transactions of the Pathological Society of London*, vol. 45, pp. 176–181, 1894.

[7] R. Lattes and R. W. Kessler, "Metastasizing basal-cell epithelioma of the skin: report of two cases," *Cancer*, vol. 4, no. 4, pp. 866–878, 1951.

[8] A. Weissferdt, N. Kalhor, and C. A. Moran, "Cutaneous basal cell carcinoma with distant metastasis to thorax and bone: a clinicopathological and immunohistochemical study of 15 cases," *Virchows Archiv*, vol. 470, no. 6, pp. 687–694, 2017.

[9] V. Di Lernia, C. Ricci, I. Zalaudek, and G. Argenziano, "Metastasizing basal cell carcinoma," *Cutis*, vol. 92, pp. 244–246, 2013.

[10] P. G. Chu and L. M. Weiss, "Expression of cytokeratin 5/6 in epithelial neoplasms: an immunohistochemical study of 509 cases," *Modern Pathology*, vol. 15, no. 1, pp. 6–10, 2002.

[11] K. Sheibani, S. S. Shin, J. Kezirian, and L. M. Weiss, "Ber-EP4 antibody as a discriminant in the differential diagnosis of malignant mesothelioma versus adenocarcinoma," *American Journal of Surgical Pathology*, vol. 15, no. 8, pp. 779–784, 1991.

[12] B. Dasgeb, T. M. Mohammadi, and D. R. Mehregan, "Use of Ber-EP4 and epithelial specific antigen to differentiate clinical simulators of basal cell carcinoma," *Biomarkers in Cancer*, vol. 5, pp. 7–11, 2013.

[13] A. Sekulic, M. R. Migden, A. E. Oro et al., "Efficacy and safety of vismodegib in advanced basal-cell carcinoma," *New England Journal of Medicine*, vol. 366, no. 23, pp. 2171–2179, 2012.

[14] X. Zhao, T. Ponomaryov, K. J. Ornell et al., "RAS/MAPK activation drives resistance to Smo inhibition, metastasis, and tumor evolution in Shh pathway-dependent tumors," *Cancer Research*, vol. 75, no. 17, pp. 3623–3635, 2015.

[15] J. Caron, O. Dereure, D. Kerob, C. Lebbe, and B. Guillot, "Metastatic basal cell carcinoma: report of two cases treated with cetuximab," *British Journal of Dermatology*, vol. 161, no. 3, pp. 702-703, 2009.

[16] G. S. Falchook, R. Leidner, E. Stankevich et al., "Responses of metastatic basal cell and cutaneous squamous cell carcinomas to anti-PD1 monoclonal antibody REGN2810," *Journal for ImmunoTherapy of Cancer*, vol. 4, no. 1, p. 70, 2016.

24

Advanced Alveolar Soft Part Sarcoma Treated with Pazopanib over Three Years

Yoji Shido and Yukihiro Matsuyama

Department of Orthopaedic Surgery, Hamamatsu University School of Medicine, 1-20-1 Handayama, Higashi-ku, Hamamatsu, Shizuoka 431-3192, Japan

Correspondence should be addressed to Yoji Shido; shido@hama-med.ac.jp

Academic Editor: Jeanine M. Buchanich

Alveolar soft part sarcoma (ASPS) is a rare malignant tumor that generally occurs in adolescents and young adults. It progresses slowly, but lung and brain metastases often occur in the early phase of the clinical course, and chemotherapy has been reported as not being effective for ASPS. Pazopanib is a multitargeted tyrosine kinase inhibitor that has been clinically available from November 2012 in Japan. This is a case report of a patient presented with multiple lung metastases and unresectable primary abdominal ASPS. We initially treated this patient by systemic chemotherapy with combination use of ifosfamide and doxorubicin. Stable disease was observed without any objective response. Then, we finally started to administrate pazopanib 800 mg/day. After 25 months of pazopanib administration, slight tumor reduction and a decrease of enhancement were observed. Objective responses were achieved for both the primary tumor and metastatic lung tumor; however, a newly developed brain metastasis was subsequently identified. Based on this case, pazopanib appears effective against ASPS, except for brain metastases. This case suggests that pazopanib may be useful as a first-line drug against unresectable ASPS and that longitudinal assessment of brain metastasis should be performed in similar cases.

1. Introduction

Alveolar soft part sarcoma (ASPS) is a rare malignant tumor that generally occurs in adolescents and young adults [1]. ASPS progresses slowly, but lung and brain metastases often occur in the early phase of the clinical course [2], and chemotherapy has been reported as not being effective for ASPS [3].

Pazopanib is a multitargeted tyrosine kinase inhibitor [4] that has been clinically available from November 2012 in Japan. Objective responses were achieved for both the primary tumor and metastatic lung tumor; however, a newly developed brain metastasis was subsequently identified. Based on this case, pazopanib appears effective against ASPS, except for brain metastases. For unresectable ASPS patients, systemic treatment using pazopanib with longitudinal assessment against brain metastasis may be feasible.

2. Case Report

A 37-year-old female presented with multiple lung and abdominal masses. She had no past medical history. She had noticed an abdominal mass gradually enlarging over 10 years but had not visited a hospital. She was shown to have multiple lung masses by routine chest X-ray at a medical checkup. As a result, she visited her local hospital, where multiple lung tumors and a large abdominal tumor were found. These tumors were pathologically diagnosed as ASPS, and she was consequently referred to our hospital. At the initial visit to our hospital, a palpable soft mass in her left lower abdomen was observed. No abnormality was identified in the hematological examination, while chest X-ray showed multiple round shadows at the bilateral lung fields. Computed tomography (CT) of the chest revealed multiple lung metastases. Magnetic resonance image (MRI) showed a lobulated lesion with strong enhancement (Figure 1(a)), and, in part of the lesion, low signal intensity was noted on T1- and T2-weighted images, suggesting flow void. The tumor was located at the abdominal wall, bulging to the lumbar spine (Figure 1(b)). Enhanced CT revealed marked dot-like enhancement at the arterial phase, suggesting abundant vascular formation (Figure 2). Brain MRI at first presentation showed no brain metastasis. Needle biopsy was

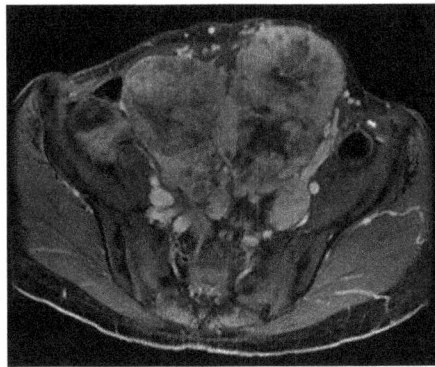

(a)

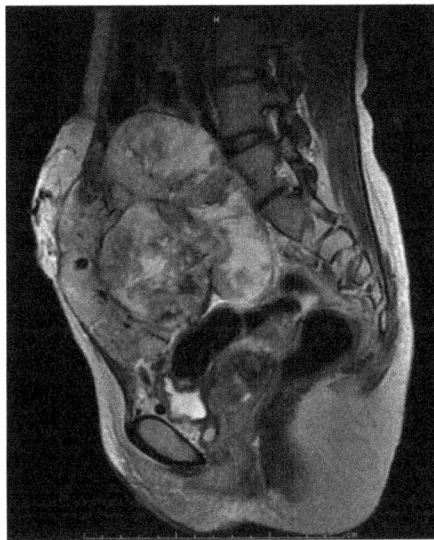

(b)

FIGURE 1: Magnetic resonance imaging findings at the initial visit. (a) T1-weighted fat suppression gadolinium-enhanced image (axial view). (b) T1-weighted fat suppression gadolinium-enhanced image (sagittal view). This MRI showed a large lobulated lesion with strong enhancement. The tumor was located at the abdominal wall, bulging to the lumbar spine.

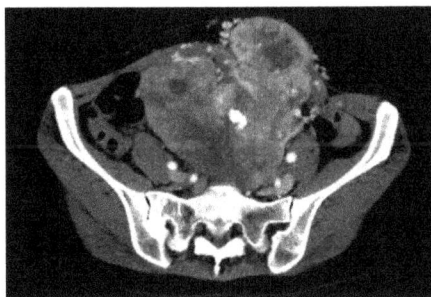

FIGURE 2: Enhanced computed tomography findings at the initial visit. CT revealed marked dot-like enhancement at the arterial phase, suggesting abundant vascular formation.

performed, and the specimen showed a nesting pattern, along with positive immunostaining of transcription factor E3 (TFE3). Moreover, fluorescence in situ hybridization examination revealed *ASPL-TFE3* gene fusion. Accordingly,

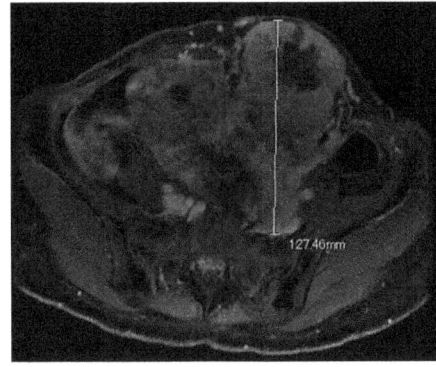

(a)

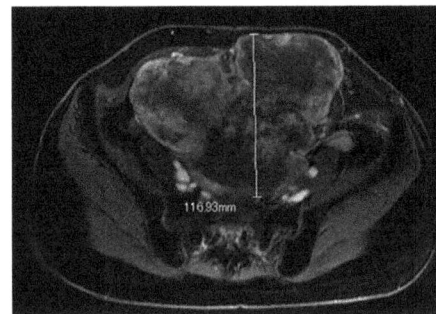

(b)

FIGURE 3: Magnetic resonance imaging findings (T1-weighted fat suppression gadolinium-enhanced image). (a) After four courses of IFM/DXR. (b) After 31 months of pazopanib administration. It was classified as no change by the RECIST criteria; however, slight tumor reduction and a decrease of enhancement were observed after 31 months of pazopanib administration.

the tumor was diagnosed as typical ASPS with multiple lung metastases. At this time, it was announced that pazopanib would become clinically available in the near future for second-line chemotherapy against advanced soft tissue sarcoma. Hence, we decided to initially treat this patient by systemic chemotherapy with combination use of ifosfamide ($10\,g/m^2$/cycle) and doxorubicin ($75\,mg/m^2$/cycle) (IFM/DXR) and to switch to pazopanib once it became commercially available. After four courses of chemotherapy, the response was defined as stable disease by the RECIST criteria; however, a slight enlargement of the tumor and increased enhancement effect were observed. After the four courses of combination treatment with IFM/DXR and one course of single DXR, we finally started to administrate pazopanib 800 mg/day. After 25 months of administration, a slight diminishment of the enhancement was observed. In comparison with the MRI obtained after the initial chemotherapy regimen, the response was defined as stable disease by the RECIST criteria; however, slight tumor reduction and a decrease of enhancement were observed after 31 months of pazopanib administration (Figures 3(a) and 3(b)). Chest CT also showed slight reduction of the lung metastases after 34 months of pazopanib administration (Figures 4(a) and 4(b)). However, after 35 months of administration, speech impairment and consciousness disturbance occurred. At this time, brain CT and MRI revealed multiple brain metastases, with surrounding edema and a midline shift (Figure 5).

(a)

(b)

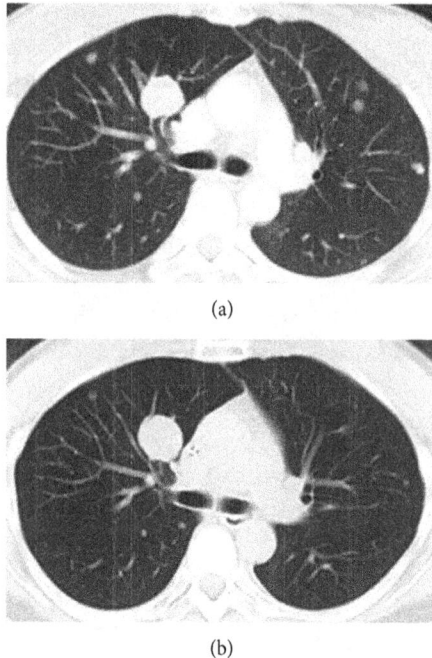

FIGURE 4: Computed tomography findings. (a) After four courses of IFM/DXR. (b) After 31 months of pazopanib administration. It was classified as no change by the RECIST criteria; however, slight tumor reduction was observed after 31 months of pazopanib administration.

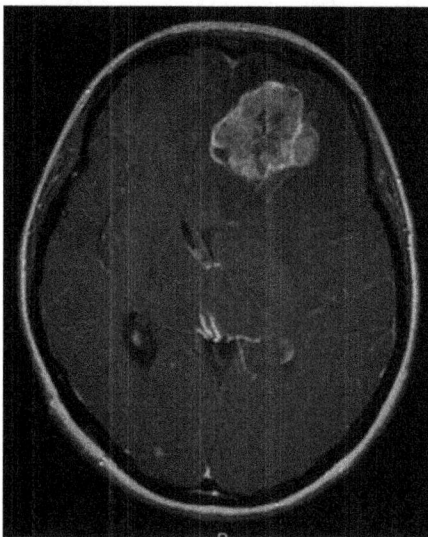

FIGURE 5: Head magnetic resonance imaging findings (T1-weighted fat suppression gadolinium-enhanced image) after 35 months of pazopanib administration. This MRI showed brain metastases with surrounding edema and a midline shift.

As a result, decompression surgery and stereotactic radiation therapy were planned, and we hence had to discontinue the administration of pazopanib to avoid incomplete wound healing. After the decompression surgery, the speech impairment was recovered. A drug holiday for six weeks was needed, after which tumor regrowth was observed (Figure 6). Similarly, regrowth of the lung metastases was also observed. Currently, the patient is taking pazopanib 800 mg/day again.

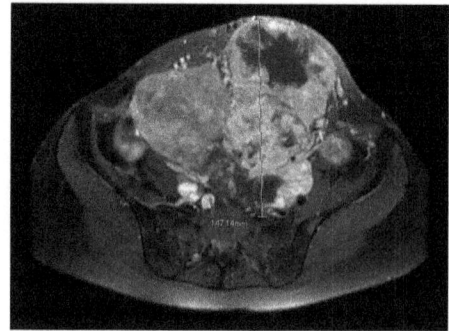

FIGURE 6: Magnetic resonance imaging findings (T1-weighted fat suppression gadolinium-enhanced image) after a drug holiday for six weeks. Tumor regrowth with increased enhancement was observed.

At the latest follow-up, six months after restarting pazopanib, no brain bleeding and stable disease of the abdominal tumor were observed. Informed consent for publication has been obtained from the patients.

3. Discussion

ASPS is a rare type of sarcoma, comprising 0.5–1% of all soft tissue sarcomas, and generally occurs in teenagers and young adults aged <40 years [1]. In almost all cases, ASPS is characterized by a tumor-specific der(17)t(X;17)(p11;q25) mutation that fuses the *TFE3* gene at Xp11 to the *ASPL* gene at 17q25, creating an ASPL-TFE3 fusion protein [5]. Radical surgery is the only known cure, and standard cytotoxic chemotherapy regimens used for these soft tissue sarcomas are ineffective [2, 3, 6, 7]. Patients with localized disease at first presentation have a 71% five-year survival rate, as compared with 20% for patients with metastatic disease at the time of diagnosis [7]. In one previous study, more than half of all patients had metastasis at the time of initial clinical presentation [7], indicating a poor prognosis of ASPS patients.

ASPS is a vascular tumor, as visualized on angiography [8], and gene expression profiling studies have revealed upregulation of genes associated with angiogenesis [9, 10]. Pazopanib is a multitargeted tyrosine kinase inhibitor that targets vascular endothelial growth factor receptor, platelet-derived growth factor receptor, and c-Kit, among others [11]. The antiangiogenic activity of pazopanib through inhibition of the vascular endothelial growth factor receptor pathway might be effective against ASPS. And other tyrosine kinase inhibitors that target vascular endothelial growth factor receptors such as sunitinib and bevacizumab might be the treatment option. [12].

ASPS shows a high incidence of brain metastasis, at least 3 times higher than that of other soft tissue sarcomas [6]. In this case, a partial response was observed for the primary tumor and metastatic lung tumors, but brain metastasis occurred nevertheless. A previous animal study reported that the brain delivery of pazopanib was severely restricted [13], and it is possible that pazopanib might not pass through the blood-brain barrier in sufficient amounts. Importantly, antiangiogenic drugs such as pazopanib are supposed to be discontinued in the perioperative period to avoid wound breakage. If we had detected the brain metastasis earlier in the present case, we could have treated the patient with radiosurgery without surgical intervention. Accordingly, it is important to make a longitudinal evaluation against brain metastasis. One case report about pazopanib against ASPS was published [12], but its follow-up period was relatively short. One of the considerations for using pazopanib was high drug cost. Although it was covered by universal self-healthcare insurance in Japan, it costs over 54000 US dollars per year. In summary, to our knowledge, this is the first case report of advanced ASPS treated with pazopanib over three years. Objective responses were achieved for the primary tumor and metastatic lung tumors; however, a newly developed brain metastasis was identified. This case suggests that pazopanib may be useful as a first-line drug against unresectable ASPS and that longitudinal assessment of brain metastasis should be performed in similar cases.

References

[1] P. H. Lieberman, M. F. Brennan, M. Kimmel, R. A. Erlandson, P. Garin-Chesa, and B. Y. Flehinger, "Alveolar soft-part sarcoma. A clinico-pathologic study of half a century," *Cancer*, vol. 63, no. 1, pp. 1–13, 1989.

[2] A. Ogose, Y. Yazawa, T. Ueda et al., "Alveolar soft part sarcoma in Japan: multi-institutional study of 57 patients from the Japanese Musculoskeletal Oncology Group," *Oncology*, vol. 65, no. 1, pp. 7–13, 2003.

[3] S. Kummar, D. Allen, A. Monks et al., "Cediranib for metastatic alveolar soft part sarcoma," *Journal of Clinical Oncology*, vol. 31, no. 18, pp. 2296–2302, 2013.

[4] W. T. van der Graaf, J. Y. Blay, S. P. Chawla et al., "Pazopanib for metastatic soft-tissue sarcoma (PALETTE): a randomised, double-blind, placebo-controlled phase 3 trial," *The Lancet*, vol. 379, no. 9829, pp. 1879–1886, 2012.

[5] M. Ladanyi, M. Y. Lui, C. R. Antonescu et al., "The der(17)t(X;17)(p11;q25) of human alveolar soft part sarcoma fuses the TFE3 transcription factor gene to ASPL, a novel gene at 17q25," *Oncogene*, vol. 20, no. 1, pp. 48–57, 2001.

[6] P. Reichardt, T. Lindner, D. Pink, P. C. Thuss-Patience, A. Kretzschmar, and B. Dörken, "Chemotherapy in alveolar soft part sarcomas. What do we know?," *European Journal of Cancer*, vol. 39, no. 11, pp. 1511–1516, 2003.

[7] C. A. Portera Jr., V. Ho, S. R. Patel et al., "Alveolar soft part sarcoma: clinical course and patterns of metastasis in 70 patients treated at a single institution," *Cancer*, vol. 91, no. 3, pp. 585–591, 2001.

[8] J. G. Lorigan, F. N. O'Keeffe, H. L. Evans, and S. Wallace, "The radiologic manifestations of alveolar soft-part sarcoma," *American Journal of Roentgenology*, vol. 153, no. 2, pp. 335–339, 1989.

[9] A. J. Lazar, P. Das, D. Tuvin et al., "Angiogenesis-promoting gene patterns in alveolar soft part sarcoma," *Clinical Cancer Research*, vol. 13, no. 24, pp. 7314–7321, 2007.

[10] L. H. Stockwin, D. T. Vistica, S. Kenney et al., "Gene expression profiling of alveolar soft-part sarcoma (ASPS)," *BMC Cancer*, vol. 9, p. 22, 2009.

[11] G. Sonpavde and T. E. Hutson, "Pazopanib: a novel multi-targeted tyrosine kinase inhibitor," *Current Oncology Reports*, vol. 9, no. 2, pp. 115–119, 2007.

[12] W. L. Read and F. Williams, "Metastatic alveolar soft part sarcoma responsive to pazopanib after progression through sunitinib and bevacizumab: two cases," *Case Reports in Oncology*, vol. 9, no. 3, pp. 639–643, 2016.

[13] M. Minocha, V. Khurana, and A. K. Mitra, "Determination of pazopanib (GW-786034) in mouse plasma and brain tissue by liquid chromatography-tandem mass spectrometry (LC/MS-MS)," *Journal of Chromatography B*, vol. 901, pp. 85–92, 2012.

25

Beyond the Dual Paraneoplastic Syndromes of Small-Cell Lung Cancer with ADH and ACTH Secretion: A Case Report with Literature Review and Future Implications

Krishna Adit Agarwal[ID] **and Myat Han Soe**[ID]

Department of Medicine, Baystate Medical Center, University of Massachusetts Medical School, Springfield, MA, USA

Correspondence should be addressed to Myat Han Soe; myathansoe@gmail.com

Academic Editor: Jeanine M. Buchanich

We present a case of small-cell lung cancer (SCLC) with syndrome of inappropriate antidiuretic hormone secretion (SIADH) in which serum sodium gradually normalized with the onset of hypertension, refractory hypokalemia, and chloride-resistant metabolic alkalosis due to ectopic adrenocorticotrophic hormone (ACTH) secretion (EAS). In this case report, we discuss the diagnostic challenges of dual paraneoplastic syndromes with SIADH and EAS, management of SCLC with paraneoplastic endocrinopathies, and their prognostic impact on SCLC. In addition, we discuss neuroendocrine differentiation and ectopic hormone production in relation to intratumoral heterogeneity in SCLC and propose tumor microenvironment and hormonal and metabolic dependence as important determinants of tumor growth and survival.

1. Introduction

Small-cell lung cancer (SCLC) is an aggressive neuroendocrine subtype of lung cancer and is associated with paraneoplastic syndromes in about 20 to 40% of cases [1, 2]. SIADH and EAS are the most common paraneoplastic endocrinopathies associated with SCLC. The Notch signaling pathway, which mediates cell fate decisions, plays an important role in tumor biology of SCLC. Notch pathway activation inhibits differentiation of SCLC tumor cells into neuroendocrine fate. When the Notch signaling pathway is suppressed, tumor cells remain in neuroendocrine phenotypes and have the potential to secrete various hormones and peptides leading to paraneoplastic syndromes [3, 4].

The association of SCLC with SIADH is well known, with up to 15% of SCLC exhibiting SIADH [5], while 1% to 5% of SCLC has ectopic ACTH secretion resulting in paraneoplastic Cushing syndrome (pCS) [1, 6]. It is very rare to have SCLC with dual ectopic SIADH and ACTH secretion. Only eight cases have been reported in literature [7–14]. Though hyponatremia in SCLC is relatively easy to recognize, EAS can be easily overlooked due to lack of typical Cushingoid picture. Instead, it presents with muscle wasting, weakness, and syndrome of apparent mineralocorticoid excess (SAME), manifesting as resistant hypertension and hypokalemic metabolic alkalosis. In SCLCs with dual SIADH and EAS, the opposing effects of cortisol and ADH on renal sodium excretion can make diagnosis even more challenging. In addition, the presence of these paraneoplastic syndromes is indicative of poor prognosis in SCLC patients, especially EAS carrying the worst prognosis [6]. We present a case of SCLC with hyponatremia at presentation which normalized with the onset of ectopic ACTH secretion.

2. Case Description

A 55-year-old female was evaluated for persistent hyponatremia of one-month duration. The physical exam was unremarkable for volume overload or depletion. The workup (Table 1) revealed a sodium level of 126 mmol/l without other electrolyte abnormalities, serum osmolality of 260 mOsm/kg, serum uric acid level of 2.0 mg/dl, normal cortisol, normal TSH, urine sodium of 45 mmol/l, and urine osmolality of 274 mOsm/kg, consistent with SIADH.

TABLE 1: Some important laboratory results. D stands for day. *Patient passed away on D78.

Test	Initial office visit (D0)	After the onset of EAS (D47)	Chemotherapy day 1 of 3 (D53)	Postchemo day 8 (D63)	MICU admission (D72)	Comfort measures initiated (D77) *
Hemoglobin (g/dl)	12.7	12.9	8.6	8.5	8.2	6.7
Hematocrit (%)	35.1	37.9	25.4	24.4	24.3	20.1
WBC ($10^3/mm^3$)	7.4	19.4	14.7	0.3	20.6	16.3
Platelet count ($10^3/mm^3$)	255	200	168	23	366	379
Sodium (mEq/l)	126	135	128	134	139	138
Potassium (mEq/l)	4.3	2.8	4.4	3.3	4.1	5.3
Chloride (mEq/l)	83	76	84	87	92	97
Bicarbonate (mEq/l)	28	45	34	34	37	29
Anion gap (mEq/l)	15	14	10	13	10	12
Glucose (mg/dl)	82	98	111	118	127	131
BUN (mg/dl)	11	11	27	9	11	10
Creatinine (mg/dl)	0.6	0.5	0.6	0.5	0.5	0.5
S. osm (mOsm/kg)	260					
Calcium (mEq/l)	9	9				Ical—1.27
AST (U/l)	25			17	14	
ALT (U/l)	18			33	20	
T. bilirubin (mg/dl)	0.3			0.4	0.1	
Troponin (ng/ml)	0.01					
ACTH (pg/ml)		319	265	399		
Cortisol (μg/dl)	7.1	131.5		164.4	138.5	134.7
TSH (mIU/l)	0.88					
PRA		<0.15				
Aldosterone (ng/dl)		<1.0				
Epinephrine (pg/ml)					47	
Norepinephrine (pg/ml)					1004	
Dopamine (pg/ml)					126	
DHEA sulfate (μg/dl)			60			

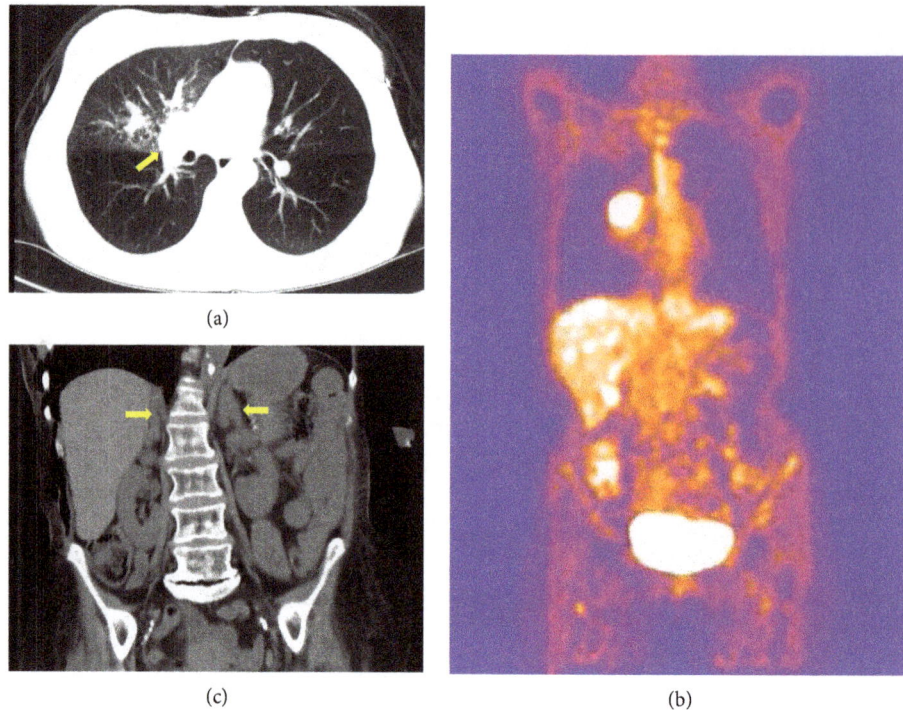

FIGURE 1: (a) Chest CT (lung window) with a yellow arrow pointing to the right hilar lung primary. (b) PET-CT scan showing an FDG-avid primary tumor in the right lung and metastasis in the liver. (c) Abdomen CT showing bilateral adrenal hypertrophy (yellow arrows).

Citalopram was thought to be the cause of SIADH and stopped. However, persistent hyponatremia prompted a further workup, especially with extensive smoking history and weight loss. Computed tomography showed right hilar mass with metastasis to the liver, right femur, and ribs (Figures 1(a) and 1(b)) with biopsy revealing SCLC.

Despite SCLC diagnosis, the patient continued to smoke cigarettes. Approximately two weeks later, the patient was admitted for acute hypoxic and hypercapnic respiratory failure due to postobstructive pneumonia, COPD exacerbation, and secondary pneumothorax, which were managed with improvement in her respiratory status. However, $PaCO_2$ and serum bicarbonate began to increase with the bicarbonate level approaching up to 45 mEq/dl, associated with refractory hypokalemia and uncontrolled hypertension. Metabolic alkalosis was noted to be chloride resistant (urine chloride of >20 mEq/dl). Additionally, hyponatremia which responded moderately to fluid restriction gradually normalized after the onset of metabolic alkalosis (Figure 2). Uncontrolled hypertension, chloride-resistant metabolic alkalosis, and hypokalemia prompted the workup for hyperaldosteronism. Serum aldosterone and plasma renin activity were within normal limits. A high-dose dexamethasone suppression test revealed elevations of ACTH (319 pg/ml) and cortisol (131.5 μg/dl), consistent with ACTH-dependent hypercortisolism and SAME (Table 1) from an ectopic nonsuppressible source of ACTH.

The patient also had significant weight loss of 28 pounds after diagnosis of SCLC, and profound muscle wasting. The second chest CT showed extensive local infiltration of the lung cancer with widespread hepatic metastasis and bilateral adrenal hypertrophy (Figure 1(c)). Palliative chemotherapy was commenced with carboplatin (target AUC—5, dose = 635 mg) and etoposide (100 mg/m^2 IV). But ACTH and cortisol levels remained elevated (Table 1) despite the first cycle of chemotherapy. Oral ketoconazole (200 mg two times a day) was subsequently started two weeks after chemotherapy. However, the patient did not tolerate the therapy well and continued to deteriorate rapidly with persistent hypercortisolism. Given end-stage disease with poor functional status, palliative care, and comfort measures were pursued as end-of-life care. The patient passed away within 2 months after diagnosis of EAS. Family did not want an autopsy.

3. Discussion

We described a case of SCLC with dual sequential paraneoplastic SIADH and EAS in which hyponatremia led to the diagnosis of SCLC, and it gradually faded with the onset of SAME from EAS. SIADH responded moderately to fluid restriction (Na of 126 mmol/l to 130 mmol/l) and the sodium level normalized to about 140 mmol/l after the onset of EAS (Figure 2). Interestingly, EAS may mask SIADH due to the antagonistic action of cortisol and ADH on renal sodium excretion. In EAS, hypercortisolism unmasks the mineralocorticoid action of cortisol due to saturation of 11-betahydroxysteroid dehydrogenase, leading to renal sodium retention. In addition, ADH has been shown to increase plasma ACTH and cortisol levels in patients with Cushing disease, although this relationship is only rarely described

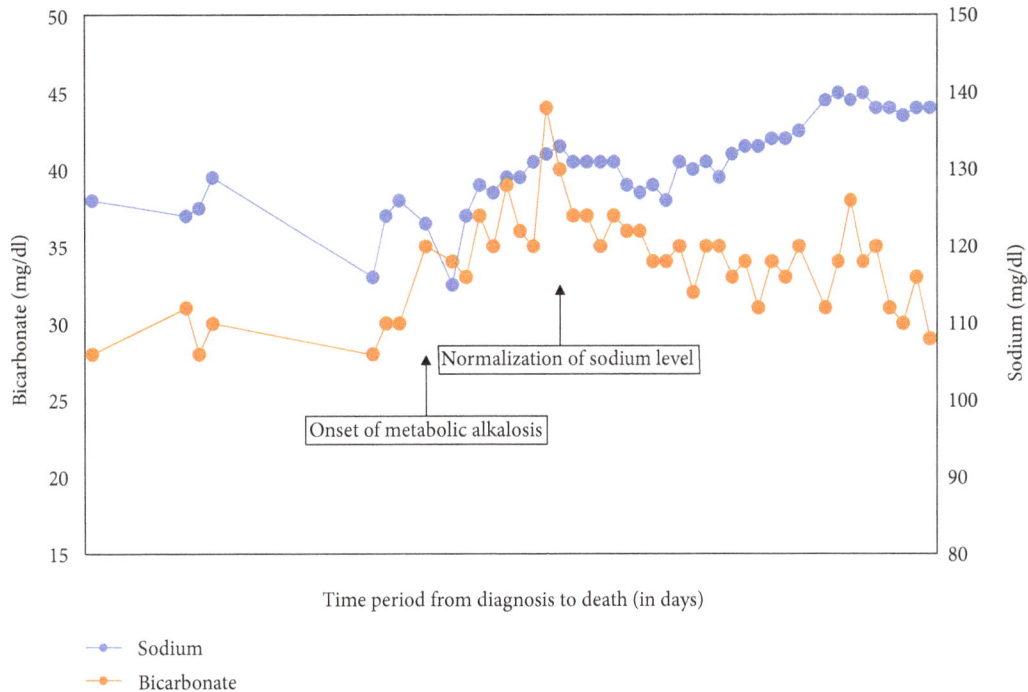

FIGURE 2: Graph showing serum sodium (blue) and bicarbonate levels (orange) from diagnosis to patient's demise. Note how serum sodium normalizes with onset of metabolic alkalosis.

in EAS. ACTH response to ADH in EAS appears to depend on vasopressin receptor subtype expression [15, 16].

Hyponatremia is present at presentation in about 15% of patients with SCLC in retrospective studies [17]. However, SIADH is not the only cause of paraneoplastic hyponatremia. Inappropriate secretion of atrial natriuretic peptide (SIANP) has also been documented, and it can also present with hyponatremia due to its pathologic natriuretic effect [18]. Fluid restriction of 1000 ml/day can be applied in SCLC patients newly diagnosed with hyponatremia to differentiate SIADH and SIANP. In our case, hyponatremia responded to fluid restriction, which favored the diagnosis of SIADH rather than SIANP, in which hyponatremia does not respond to 72 to 96 hours of 1000 ml/day fluid restriction and V2 receptor (V2R) antagonists [17].

Management of hyponatremia should be an integral part of SCLC treatment as hyponatremia is associated with a poorer prognosis regardless of an extensive or limited stage. SCLC patients with serum sodium less than 129 mmol/l had a median survival of only 8.63 months compared to 13.6 months in patients with normal sodium, and the degree of hyponatremia is a significant predictor for prognosis [19]. Demeclocycline, which inhibits the effect of ADH in collecting ducts, can be used at a dose of 100 to 300 mg for 3 to 4 times a day. However, its effect is delayed for 1 to 2 weeks. Tolvaptan is also effective in management of SIADH in SCLC patients with sodium level < 125 mmol/l [20]. In our patient, the V2R antagonist was not used as hyponatremia faded with the onset of EAS.

EAS occurs only in 1 to 5% of SCLC patients, and its presentation usually lacks typical Cushingoid features. Patients with EAS usually present with muscle wasting, proximal

muscle weakness, and SAME. Diagnosis is established by a high-dose dexamethasone suppression test with nonsuppressible ACTH and cortisol levels. The presence of EAS in SCLC patients confers a very poor prognosis, with a life expectancy of only three to six months [6, 21]. The magnitude of weight loss, rapid decline of performance status, and poor response to chemotherapy makes EAS the most severe of all paraneoplastic syndromes as EAS and SCLC reinforce each other's deleterious effects. The immunosuppression induced by SCLC itself is further amplified by that induced by hypercortisolism, leading to serious infectious complications. Metabolic disorders including steroid-induced hyperglycemia, hypokalemia, and metabolic alkalosis can also significantly worsen general health status [2].

Given its deleterious effects, many authors emphasize treating hypercortisolism before chemotherapy to prevent infectious complications which can be aggravated by cortisol-induced immunosuppression and chemotherapy-induced neutropenia despite the use of granulocyte colony-stimulating factors [1]. Control of severe hypercortisolism before administering chemotherapy may achieve longer survival. Ketoconazole, metyrapone, etomidate, mitotane, and mifepristone can be used to reduce the circulating cortisol level. Ketoconazole was said to have the best tolerance profile [22]. However, being a strong inhibitor of cytochrome P4503A4, ketoconazole may increase the risk of chemotherapy toxicity when used concurrently, and therefore, metyrapone has been reported as a better alternative [23]. For EAS, combinations of metyrapone and ketoconazole or of mitotane, metyrapone, and ketoconazole can be used to control hypercortisolism. If hypercortisolism is refractory to medical therapy, bilateral adrenalectomy might be considered [21, 24].

TABLE 2: Summary of previously published case reports of SCLC with dual ectopic ADH and ACTH secretion.

Liddle et al.	SCLC with SIADH and EAS. Chronology of SIADH and EAS was not mentioned. Na was 115 mmol/l. Clinical picture of EAS, management, and life expectancy were not described [7].
O'Neal et al.	Extensive SCLC with >3 organ metastases (liver, adrenals, brain, diaphragm, and retroperitoneal and mediastinal lymph nodes) and simultaneous SIADH and EAS, presenting with uncontrolled hypertension, puffy face, and hyponatremia (Na 121–125 mmol/l). The patient had a gradual development of hypokalemic metabolic alkalosis and Cushingoid picture in 2 months and died after 5 weeks of diagnosis of dual SIADH and EAS. Management was not described [8].
Coscia et al.	Extensive SCLC (3 cm in size) with >3 organ metastasis (adrenals, pancreas, mediastinal lymph nodes, bone marrow, liver, and spleen) and simultaneous SIADH and EAS presenting with symptomatic, profound hyponatremia (Na 103 mmol/l), hypertension, hemoptysis, and weight loss of 10 pounds without typical Cushingoid picture. The patient also had few weeks of nausea, vomiting, anorexia, and diarrhea before presentation. Hyponatremia was treated with 3% saline and fluid restriction. No antisteroid agent was used for EAS. The patient died on the 24th hospital day [9].
Suzuki et al.	Extensive SCLC with >3 organ metastasis (adrenals, contralateral lung, pleurae, liver, bone marrow, pancreas, spleen, thyroid, and multiple lymph nodes) and simultaneous SIADH and EAS presenting with significant weight loss in 6 weeks, cough, dyspnea, uncontrolled hypertension, hyperglycemia, muscle weakness, hypokalemic metabolic alkalosis, and hyponatremia (Na 126 mmol/l). The patient did not have typical Cushingoid picture. Treatment of SIADH and EAS was not mentioned. The patient was treated with nimustine without success. The patient died from severe pancytopenia and GI bleeding on the 42nd hospital day [10].
Pierce et al.	Extensive SCLC (2 cm in size) with 3 organ metastases (right adrenal gland, thyroid, and pancreas) and simultaneous SIADH and EAS, presenting with hyponatremia (Na 126 mmol/l), hypokalemia, metabolic alkalosis, hyperglycemia, hypertension, and 15-pound weight loss in one month. No typical Cushingoid picture was identified. SCLC was treated with cisplatin and etoposide; SIADH was treated with fluid restriction and demeclocycline; EAS was treated with aminoglutethimide. Despite all treatments, ADH and ACTH levels remained elevated. The patient died 127 days after diagnosis [11].
Shaker et al.	Metastatic extrapulmonary small-cell carcinoma in the bone marrow presenting with renal phosphate wasting and SIADH (Na 107 mmol/l). SIADH responded to fluid restriction and demeclocycline. There was a resolution of cancer with adriamycin, cyclophosphamide, cisplatin, and etoposide 5 months after diagnosis. Eight months after diagnosis, patient presented with bone pain, adenopathy, Cushingoid picture, hypokalemia, hypertension, and recurrent SIADH. No antisteroid agent was used for EAS. The patient died 2 months after the onset of EAS and SIADH, despite chemotherapy [12].
Mayer et al.	SCLC (3.5 cm in size) with dual sequential SIADH and EAS, initially presenting with limited-stage SCLC diagnosed from SIADH workup (Na 123 mmol/l). SIADH responded to fluid restriction, and SCLC achieved a complete remission after 4 cycles of carboplatin, etoposide, and concurrent radiation therapy. EAS occurred 8 months after diagnosis, presenting with weight loss of 20 pounds in 2 weeks, hypokalemia, muscle weakness, hyperglycemia, and hypertension. The patient had metastatic disease in the liver, pericardial lymph nodes, bilateral adrenal glands, and the mesenteric fat. The patient died 2 days after diagnosis of EAS [13].
Müssig et al.	Extensive SCLC (4.9 cm × 10.6 cm in size) with 2 organ metastases (liver and brain) and simultaneous SIADH and EAS, presenting with 28-pound weight loss over 6 months, persistent hypokalemia, and hyponatremia (Na of 116 mmol/l). EAS lacked typical Cushingoid picture. SIADH was treated with fluid restriction only. No antisteroid agent was used for EAS. A nearly complete radiological remission with resolution of SIADH and EAS was achieved after the fourth cycle of carboplatin and etoposide. Life expectancy was not mentioned [14].

The occurrence of paraneoplastic syndromes is directly related to the tumor bulk. According to one study, 72% of patients presenting with a paraneoplastic syndrome of any type had extensive disease at diagnosis [25]. EAS is often found when the tumor bulk is particularly large and heterogeneous with three or more organs affected by metastasis [2]. ACTH can be secreted either by the primary tumor or metastatic lesions, a condition referred to as spatial intratumoral heterogeneity. This could reflect an acquisition of new mutations during metastasis and the emergence of clones with secretory ability according to the branched clonal expansion hypothesis [2]. Different SCLC subclones might be able to secrete different ectopic hormones while one clonal type of SCLC cells might also be capable of secreting more than one hormone. Immunohistochemistry of specimens might be helpful to identify origins of ectopic hormones.

Eight cases of SCLC [7–14] with dual SIADH and EAS described in literature are summarized in Table 2. Six [7, 9–11, 13, 14] out of eight cases did not have typical Cushingoid picture and presented with weight loss and SAME. We notice that dual SIADH and EAS in SCLC can be simultaneous or sequential with the latter carrying worse prognosis and shorter life expectancy compared to simultaneous disease. Two reported cases [12, 13] of sequential SIADH and EAS occurred in recurrent disease diagnosed in about 8 months following resolution of the first cancer. Our case is the first reported case of SCLC with sequential SIADH followed by EAS within two months of diagnosis of SCLC with SIADH. All cases of dual sequential SIADH and EAS, including our case, were treatment refractory, and patients died within two months after diagnosis [12, 13].

4. Future Implications

Tumor microenvironment and hormonal and metabolic dependence of tumors are important determinants for tumor growth and survival in addition to oncogenic addiction fed by driver gene mutations [26]. SCLC cells can generate their own microenvironment and mediate chemoresistance by transforming a subset of tumor cells into a nonneuroendocrine phenotype via the activation of Notch signaling [3]. One study has shown that endogenous activation of the Notch pathway results in switching from a neuroendocrine to nonneuroendocrine fate in 10 to 50% of tumor cells, generating intratumoral heterogeneity. Nonneuroendocrine Notch-active SCLC cells are slow growing, but they are relatively chemoresistant and provide trophic support to neuroendocrine tumor cells [4, 27]. This finding may provide future implications for Notch status analysis and inhibition in SCLC treatment.

Regarding hormonal dependence, studies have shown that hypercortisolism might induce chemoresistance. In vitro experiments suggested that steroids protect cancer cells from cytotoxic effects of several chemotherapy agents including carboplatin, cisplatin, actinomycin D, and ionizing radiation [28]. This might explain why SCLC with EAS is chemoresistant, as seen in our case. It has been shown that glucocorticoids increase gene expression of several key mediators such as cellular glutathione, metallothionein synthesis, multidrug resistance efflux pump ABCB1 and ABCG2 expression and activity, and O6-methylguanine DNA methyltransferase activity [28, 29]. However, no study has evaluated if SCLC is a hormone-dependent tumor, feeding on its own ectopic hormones. It would be interesting to evaluate if these ectopic hormones, in addition to their target organ effects, also act in autocrine and paracrine fashions on the tumor itself and neighboring cells to influence tumor biology.

Regarding metabolic dependence, we hypothesize that SCLC might have metabolic benefits from hyponatremia and metabolic alkalosis in the tumor microenvironment, which might favor tumor growth and hinder antitumor immune response. The literature mostly describes the prevalence of hyponatremia in SCLC patients along with its poor prognosis. However, there is no study yet to evaluate the effect of hyponatremia on tumor growth, chemoresistance, and antitumor immune response. In the hyponatremic milieu, cells may leak out organic osmoles including glycine, glutamate, and inositol to maintain osmotic balance with extracellular fluid [30]. We hypothesize that hyponatremia might promote tumor growth by providing inositol and glutamate from neighboring cells in tumor microenvironment, and it might also impair cytotoxic activity of CD8+ T lymphocytes and NK cells via SGK signaling [31]. According to one recent study, glutamate inhibits the xCT glutamate-cystine antiporter, leading to intracellular cysteine depletion. EglN1, the main HIF1 prolyl hydroxylase, undergoes oxidative self-inactivation in the absence of cysteine, resulting in HIF1 accumulation and cellular proliferation via the pseudohypoxic pathway [32]. Further studies are needed to shed light into the effects of paraneoplastic endocrinopathies and their resultant metabolic effects on the tumor growth, metastasis, and immune response.

References

[1] F. A. Shepherd, J. Laskey, W. K. Evans, P. E. Goss, E. Johansen, and F. Khamsi, "Cushing's syndrome associated with ectopic corticotropin production and small-cell lung cancer," *Journal of Clinical Oncology*, vol. 10, no. 1, pp. 21–27, 1992.

[2] H. Nagy-Mignotte, O. Shestaeva, L. Vignoud et al., "Prognostic impact of paraneoplastic Cushing's syndrome in small-cell lung cancer," *Journal of Thoracic Oncology*, vol. 9, no. 4, pp. 497–505, 2014.

[3] T. Ito, S. Kudoh, T. Ichimura, K. Fujino, W. A. M. A. Hassan, and N. Udaka, "Small cell lung cancer, an epithelial to mesenchymal transition (EMT)-like cancer: significance of inactive Notch signaling and expression of achaete-scute complex homologue 1," *Human Cell*, vol. 30, no. 1, pp. 1–10, 2017.

[4] J. S. Lim, A. Ibaseta, M. M. Fischer et al., "Intratumoural heterogeneity generated by Notch signalling promotes small-cell lung cancer," *Nature*, vol. 545, no. 7654, pp. 360–364, 2017.

[5] O. Hansen, P. Sørensen, and K. H. Hansen, "The occurrence of hyponatremia in SCLC and the influence on prognosis," *Lung Cancer*, vol. 68, no. 1, pp. 111–114, 2010.

[6] L. Delisle, M. J. Boyer, D. Warr et al., "Ectopic corticotropin syndrome and small-cell carcinoma of the lung," *Archives of Internal Medicine*, vol. 153, no. 6, pp. 746–752, 1993.

[7] G. W. Liddle, J. R. Givens, W. E. Nicholson, and D. P. Island, "The ectopic ACTH syndrome," *Cancer Research*, vol. 25, no. 7, pp. 1057–1061, 1965.

[8] L. W. O'Neal, D. M. Kipnis, S. A. Luse, P. E. Lacy, and L. Jarett, "Secretion of various endocrine substances by ACTH-secreting tumors—gastrin, melanotropin, norepinephrine, serotonin, parathormone, vasopressin, glucagon," *Cancer*, vol. 21, no. 6, pp. 1219–1232, 1968.

[9] M. Coscia, R. D. Brown, M. Miller et al., "Ectopic production of antidiuretic hormone (ADH), adrenocorticotrophic hormone (ACTH) and beta-melanocyte stimulating hormone (β-MSH) by an oat cell carcinoma of the lung," *The American Journal of Medicine*, vol. 62, no. 2, pp. 303–307, 1977.

[10] H. Suzuki, Y. Tsutsumi, K. Yamaguchi, K. Abe, and T. Yokoyama, "Small cell lung carcinoma with ectopic adrenocorticotropic hormone and antidiuretic hormone syndromes: a case report," *Japanese Journal of Clinical Oncology*, vol. 14, no. 1, pp. 129–137, 1984.

[11] S. T. Pierce, M. Metcalfe, E. R. Banks, M. E. O'Daniel, and P. Desimone, "Small cell carcinoma with two paraendocrine syndromes," *Cancer*, vol. 69, no. 9, pp. 2258–2261, 1992.

[12] J. L. Shaker, R. C. Brickner, A. B. Divgi, H. Raff, and J. W. Findling, "Case report: renal phosphate wasting, syndrome of inappropriate antidiuretic hormone, and ectopic corticotropin production in small cell carcinoma," *The American Journal of the Medical Sciences*, vol. 310, no. 1, pp. 38–41, 1995.

[13] S. Mayer, A. M. Cypess, O. N. Kocher et al., "Uncommon presentations of some common malignancies," *Journal of Clinical Oncology*, vol. 23, no. 6, pp. 1312–1314, 2005.

[14] K. Müssig, M. Horger, H. U. Häring, and M. Wehrmann, "Syndrome of inappropriate antidiuretic hormone secretion

and ectopic ACTH production in small cell lung carcinoma," *Lung Cancer*, vol. 57, no. 1, pp. 120–122, 2007.

[15] P. Colombo, E. Passini, T. Re, G. Faglia, and B. Ambrosi, "Effect of desmopressin on ACTH and cortisol secretion in states of ACTH excess," *Clinical Endocrinology*, vol. 46, no. 6, pp. 661–668, 1997.

[16] W. Arlt, P. L. M. Dahia, F. Callies et al., "Ectopic ACTH production by a bronchial carcinoid tumour responsive to desmopressin in vivo and in vitro," *Clinical Endocrinology*, vol. 47, no. 5, pp. 623–627, 1997.

[17] J. P. Chute, "A metabolic study of patients with lung cancer and hyponatremia of malignancy," *Clinical Cancer Research*, vol. 12, no. 3, pp. 888–896, 2006.

[18] N. H. Sun, S. H. Wang, J. N. Liu et al., "The productions of atrial natriuretic peptide and arginine vasopressin in small cell lung cancer with brain metastases and their associations with hyponatremia," *European Review for Medical and Pharmacological Sciences*, vol. 21, no. 18, pp. 4104–4112, 2017.

[19] W. Wang, Z. Song, and Y. Zhang, "Hyponatremia in small cell lung cancer is associated with a poorer prognosis," *Translational Cancer Research*, vol. 5, no. 1, pp. 36–43, 2016.

[20] C. Petereit, O. Zaba, I. Teber, H. Lüders, and C. Grohé, "A rapid and efficient way to manage hyponatremia in patients with SIADH and small cell lung cancer: treatment with tolvaptan," *BMC Pulmonary Medicine*, vol. 13, no. 1, 2013.

[21] H. Zhang and J. Zhao, "Ectopic Cushing syndrome in small cell lung cancer: a case report and literature review," *Thoracic Cancer*, vol. 8, no. 2, pp. 114–117, 2017.

[22] A. Tabarin, A. Navarranne, J. Guérin, J. B. Corcuff, M. Parneix, and P. Roger, "Use of ketoconazole in the treatment of Cushing's disease and ectopic ACTH syndrome," *Clinical Endocrinology*, vol. 34, no. 1, pp. 63–70, 1991.

[23] S. I. Aziz, M. A. Khattak, Z. Usmani, N. Ladipeerla, and K. Pittman, "Metyrapone: a management option for ectopic ACTH syndrome in small cell lung cancer treated with intravenous etoposide," *Case Reports*, vol. 2011, 2011.

[24] N. Kanaji, N. Watanabe, N. Kita et al., "Paraneoplastic syndromes associated with lung cancer," *World Journal of Clinical Oncology*, vol. 5, no. 3, pp. 197–223, 2014.

[25] L. Gandhi and B. E. Johnson, "Paraneoplastic syndromes associated with small cell lung cancer," *Journal of the National Comprehensive Cancer Network*, vol. 4, no. 6, pp. 631–638, 2006.

[26] J. Luo, N. L. Solimini, and S. J. Elledge, "Principles of cancer therapy: oncogene and non-oncogene addiction," *Cell*, vol. 136, no. 5, pp. 823–837, 2009.

[27] W. A. Hassan, R. Yoshida, S. Kudoh et al., "Notch1 controls cell chemoresistance in small cell lung carcinoma cells," *Thoracic Cancer*, vol. 7, no. 1, pp. 123–128, 2016.

[28] I. Mitre-Aguilar, A. Cabrera-Quintero, and A. Zentella-Dehesa, "Genomic and non-genomic effects of glucocorticoids: implications for breast cancer," *International Journal of Clinical and Experimental Pathology*, vol. 8, no. 1, pp. 1–10, 2015.

[29] H. P. Rutz, "Effects of corticosteroid use on treatment of solid tumours," *The Lancet*, vol. 360, no. 9349, pp. 1969-1970, 2002.

[30] M. L. Mcmanus, K. B. Churchwell, and K. Strange, "Regulation of cell volume in health and disease," *New England Journal of Medicine*, vol. 333, no. 19, pp. 1260–1267, 1995.

[31] G. Shi, Q. Wang, X. Zhou et al., "Response of human non-small-cell lung cancer cells to the influence of Wogonin with SGK1 dynamics," *Acta Biochimica et Biophysica Sinica*, vol. 49, no. 4, pp. 302–310, 2017.

[32] K. J. Briggs, P. Koivunen, S. Cao et al., "Paracrine induction of HIF by glutamate in breast cancer: EglN1 senses cysteine," *Cell*, vol. 166, no. 1, pp. 126–139, 2016.

26

GNQ-209P Mutation in Metastatic Uveal Melanoma and Treatment Outcome

Nagla Abdel Karim,[1] **Ihab Eldessouki** ⓘ**,**[1] **Ahmad Taftaf** ⓘ**,**[1] **Deeb Ayham,**[1] **Ola Gaber** ⓘ**,**[1] **Abouelmagd Makramalla,**[2] **and Zelia M. Correa**[3]

[1]*Department of Hematology-Oncology, University of Cincinnati, Cincinnati, OH, USA*
[2]*Department of Interventional Radiology, University of Cincinnati, Cincinnati, OH, USA*
[3]*Department of Ophthalmology, University of Cincinnati, Cincinnati, OH, USA*

Correspondence should be addressed to Ihab Eldessouki; ihab_del@yahoo.com

Academic Editor: Raffaele Palmirotta

Metastatic prognosis in uveal melanoma is assessed by gene expression profiling (GEP) testing of the tumor cells, usually obtained by fine needle aspiration (FNA). GEP has demonstrated high accuracy in distinguishing class I and II tumors, both having different metastatic potential. Transcriptomic studies identified distinct mutations including somatic mutations in *GNAQ* and *GNA11*, detected in more than 80%, and contribute to the upregulation of the mitogen-activated protein kinase (MAPK) pathway and the development of uveal melanoma (UM). The role of these mutations in treatment selection and possible benefit from targeted therapy are somewhat unclear. However, until the discovery of novel agents, local versus systemic therapies remain options for treatment that can still be considered for disease control in certain cases. We report a series of patients with metastatic UM with distinct mutational profiles. One had significant liver metastases with proven *GNQ-209P* mutation on tissue biopsy while peripheral blood molecular profiling did not show these mutations. The other three cases had no *GNQ-209P* mutation. All cases received nab-paclitaxel (Abraxane) as a treatment drug, and we record their responses to treatment and their molecular-profiling results.

1. Introduction

Uveal melanoma (UM) is significantly less common than cutaneous melanoma and has a distinct molecular pathogenesis. Meanwhile, it is the most common primary intraocular tumor in adults [1]. Despite the high success rate of disease control with local therapy, the potential for developing metastases remains high even after a prolonged period of remission [2–4]. The predominant target organ for metastasis is the liver although disease involvement of the skin, bone, brain, and lungs has also been reported [5, 6]. Key mutations in the disease are *GNAQ* and *GNA11* mutations. It was reported that 83% of the cases have somatic mutations in *GNAQ* or *GNA11* [7]. *GNAQ* gene is the gene coding for the alpha subunit of heterotrimeric G proteins. The latter proteins couple seven-transmembrane domain receptors to intracellular signaling machinery [8], and they are composed of three subunits, namely, alpha, beta, and gamma. The alpha subunit is the G-protein molecular switch, activated when it is bound to guanosine triphosphate (GTP), and when GTP is hydrolyzed to guanosine diphosphate (GDP), it is deactivated [9]. The alpha subunit has a key glutamine that contacts the GTP molecule, located at position 209 (Q209) in Gαq and is substituted when mutated to either leucine or proline [10–13]. At this point, the alpha subunit is locked in a constitutively active state, and its GTPase activity is blocked [14–16]. Taxanes work by preventing microtubule disassembly, so the mitotic functions are inhibited, leading to cell death [17]. They have shown reasonable activity in several phase II studies [18]. Nab-paclitaxel is a solvent-free formula that renders the drug more competent in the treatment of UM. Multiple therapeutic

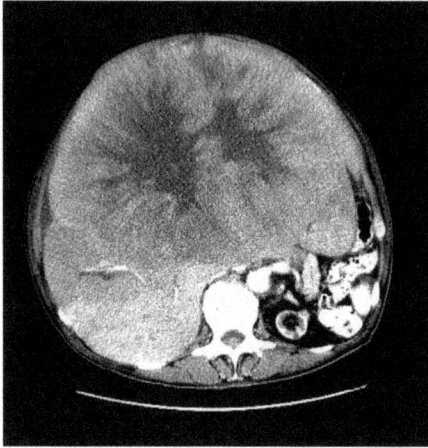

FIGURE 1: Abdominal CT scan at diagnosis.

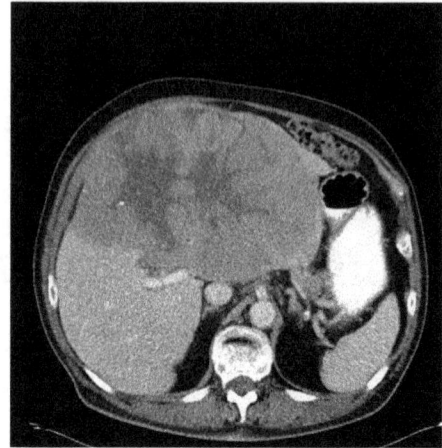

FIGURE 2: CT scan 24 months after the treatment.

approaches for metastatic UM have been studied although none has shown any impact on the overall survival, and thus standard of care has not yet been established for these patients. In our report, we present the case of a patient with metastatic uveal carcinoma to the liver who was successfully treated with nab-paclitaxel, allowing for recovery from life-threatening spontaneous tumor lysis.

2. Methods

GNAQ and GNA11 mutations were assessed by genomic hybridization on paraffin-embedded blocks obtained from the primary tumor tissue. Mutations were followed up by circulating tumor DNA in plasma using next-generation sequencing using serial blood samples.

3. Case Presentation

This is a 75-year-old man with a history of choroidal melanoma of the right eye diagnosed in 1984 and treated by radioactive Co-60 plaque. Thirty years later, he presented with progressive abdominal distention, early satiety, and weight loss of 20 pounds over a period of 6 months. He was seen by his primary care physician who requested a CT scan of the abdomen that showed a large hepatic mass measuring 34 cm by 26 cm, replacing the majority of the liver without retroperitoneal or mesenteric lymphadenopathy (Figure 1). Hepatic tumor biopsy revealed metastatic melanoma consistent with his primary choroidal melanoma. While completing his diagnostic workup, the patient developed generalized weakness prompting his hospital admission due to acute renal failure, hyperkalemia, and spontaneous tumor lysis. He started hemodialysis promptly followed by the administration of weekly nab-paclitaxel 150 mg/m^2 and then reduced to 75 mg/m^2 thereafter due to severe neutropenia. The patient recovered his renal function as serum creatinine improved from 4.93 mg/dl to 0.69 mg/dl (normal values 0.60–1.20 mg/dl) and demonstrated clinical improvement of his generalized weakness, abdominal distention, and edema of the legs after three doses of nab-paclitaxel. A repeat abdominal CT scan one month after the therapy revealed

a good response to treatment with significant decrease in tumor burden. This is donated by full clinical recovery and total resolution of tumor lysis manifestations. However, according to RECIST criteria, the response can be minimal followed by maintained stable disease. CT scan of the abdomen after 4 cycles of nab-paclitaxel revealed shrinkage of the hepatic lesion to 24 × 15 cm in maximum diameter (approximately 7% decrease in the largest lesion per RECIST criteria) (Figure 2). This patient is still alive and continues to have excellent functional status, ECOG performance status of I, and no signs or symptoms of disease progression for 32 months now.

Our patient with this metastatic uveal melanoma with extensive liver metastases with GNQ-209P mutation on the tissue biopsy (Figures 3 and 4) and undetectable mutations on the peripheral blood molecular profiling in serial follow-up samples suggests marked response to nab-paclitaxel. This can be understood by the dramatic tumor response on CT scans which was accompanied clinically by spontaneous tumor lysis syndrome followed by very prolonged disease control up to 30 months indicating nab-paclitaxel efficacy. All other patients with metastatic ocular melanoma, who did not have the GNQ-209P mutation, did not respond and did not have prolonged survival when treated with nab-paclitaxel.

Our patient has received 8 cycles of Abraxane with initial minimal response followed by no increase and stable tumor size in the following imaging scans. In an attempt to achieve further response, the patient received an anti-PD-L1 in a clinical trial for 9 cycles. No further reduction in tumor size was achieved, and the patient was disqualified from the study after he developed sarcoidosis/interstitial pneumonitis. He was then restarted on Abraxane, achieving clinical and radiological stabilization of his disease with no major toxicities, and remains fully functional. He has received to date 12 cycles of Abraxane (in addition to the prior cycles of Abraxane received initially).

4. Discussion

UM has a high potential for developing a rapidly progressive course despite local or systemic therapies [1]. Even with

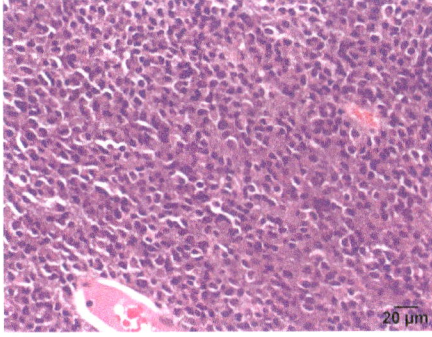

FIGURE 3: Liver biopsy (H&E).

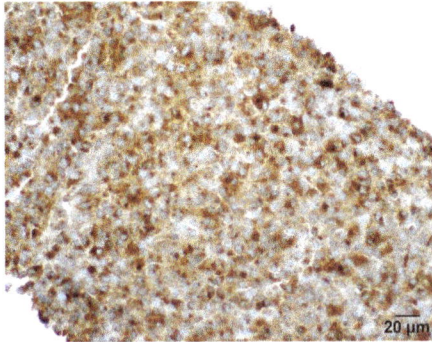

FIGURE 4: Liver biopsy (MART).

TABLE 1: Different types of genomic mutations in patients with metastatic melanoma of the liver.

Case number	Age (years)	Gender	Genomic mutation
1	75	Male	GNAQ-Q209P by tissue testing
2	77	Female	GNAQ-Q209L by peripheral circulating DNA
3	70	Female	GNAQ-Q209L
4	78	Female	Kit H580y

TABLE 2: Comparison between GNAQ-Q209P and GNAQ-Q209L.

Mutations	Location of mutation	Frequency of mutations among GNAQ-mutated primary uveal melanoma
GNAQ-Q209P	Exon 5	~64%
GNAQ-Q209L	Exon 5	~33%

several FDA-approved agents for advanced cutaneous melanoma, there is a lack of agents that show survival benefit in patients with advanced UM. This issue is likely twofold from the rare occurrence of the disease itself as well as a lack of complete understanding regarding the pathogenesis and immunobiology that underlies this disease process. Current studies are ongoing to uncover these uncertainties in hopes of ultimately identifying potentially treatable targets and more effective treatments [19, 20]. Until a standard of care is established, however, existing treatment options must be applied on a case-by-case basis [21, 22].

In metastatic disease, different approaches have been studied including surgical resection in suitable candidates in addition to local versus systemic infusion of cytotoxic agents. A comprehensive review of the role of metastectomy in selected surgical candidates showed improved survival in patients who had a complete liver metastases resection compared to patients for whom a complete resection was not feasible [23]. Local therapies including the hepatic arterial infusion of melphalan or fotemustine revealed in randomized trial, a significant improvement in progression-free survival (PFS) but not overall survival when compared to the systemic infusion of the same agents [24]. In contrast, a retrospective study from Mayo Clinic showed only improvement in overall survival among patients treated with different local therapies in comparison to different systemic agents including bevacizumab, ipilimumab, and kinase inhibitors [25]. Systemic chemotherapy options have shown minimal benefit in treatment. Single agents such as cisplatin or paclitaxel versus

combined agents such as the BOLD regimen (bleomycin + vincristine + lomustine + dacarbazine) plus recombinant interferon alpha 2-b have been studied with no more than 20% response rate (RR) and absence of survival advantages [7, 26]. A similar study to ours that was presented at the ASCO annual meeting shows clinically useful responses in two of four patients with metastatic ocular melanoma treated with nab-paclitaxel [27]. In terms of targeted therapy, the ability to understand the genetic characteristic of UM has helped in identifying different mutations and key signaling pathways that can permit therapeutic intervention at a site specific to the pathway abnormality. UM is genetically characterized by frequent, mutually exclusive mutations in guanine nucleotide-binding protein G(q) subunit alpha (GNAQ) and guanine nucleotide-binding protein subunit alpha-11 (GNA11) which can be detected in 83% of patients with UM [12]. GNAQ stimulates the mitogen-activated protein kinase (MAPK), which is parallel to the consequence of mutations in the BRAF or NRAS oncogenes in cutaneous melanomas. Furthermore, GNAQ stimulates the transcriptional coactivator YAP that is essential for UM cell proliferation. The aforementioned MAPK pathway is highly interconnected with the PI3K/ACT pathway, and both of them converge on the same downstream targets. MEK inhibitor, PI3K inhibitor, mTOR inhibitor, and YAP inhibitor each represent novel therapeutic target for UM, and studies are ongoing to uncover the role of these agents either as a single or dual inhibition approach in patients with advanced disease or early disease associated with high-risk features [10, 20, 28].

Our patient presented with acute renal failure secondary to spontaneous tumor lysis, and there was an urgent need for disease control, which was achieved by using systemic chemotherapy with nab-paclitaxel. The absence of standard of care in these patients and the extrapolated data from the phase III trial of nab-paclitaxel when compared to dacarbazine [29] in patients with cutaneous melanoma led to the use of this agent in our patient who was not a candidate for cisplatin. In his case, the tissue from the liver biopsy was insufficient to run molecular testing, so we used a liquid biopsy (circulating tumor DNA) obtained from the patient, to search for genomic alterations that came back negative for mutations; however, subsequent liver biopsy revealed *GNAQ* exon 5 Q209 mutation where the *GNA11* mutation or amplification was not detected.

In comparison to this case (Case 1), we had other patients (Case 2, 3, and 4) in our institution, in whom a diagnosis of metastatic UM was made. All patients started on treatment with nab-paclitaxel, but they had metastatic disease that continued to progress. In patients (Cases 2 and 3), a molecular testing of DNA circulating in the blood revealed *GNAQ*/Q209L mutation while our patient (Case 1) had *GNAQ*-Q209P (Tables 1 and 2). This might draw our attention that *GNQ-209P* might be a predictive marker of sensitivity to nab-paclitaxel in metastatic uveal melanoma.

5. Conclusion

Although our understanding of the molecular underpinnings of UM continues to improve and certain targeted agents are showing promise, genomic alteration studies might play a role in treatment selection. As we see from the cases we present, *GNAQ*-Q209P and not Q209L mutation could be associated with a considerable disease control when treated with nab-paclitaxel chemotherapy. We suggest the implication of molecular profiling with specific attention to the status of not only *GNAQ* but also the exon 209P or Q209L for personalized use of therapies in future clinical trials designed to treat patients with metastatic UM. Such clinical trials are needed to prove the efficacy and survival advantages of nab-paclitaxel in patients with metastatic UM and to study its role in comparison to the evolving targeted or immunotherapeutic agents. In general, reports of rare and less commonly encountered cases can have a pivotal effect on the collective clinical experience and drug research.

Acknowledgments

The authors thank their colleagues in the pathology department who helped with this work.

References

[1] A. D. Singh, L. Bergman, and S. Seregard, "Uveal melanoma: epidemiologic aspects," *Ophthalmology Clinics of North America*, vol. 18, no. 1, pp. 75–84, 2005.

[2] J. Scotto, J. F. Fraumeni, and J. A. Lee, "Melanomas of the eye and other noncutaneous sites: epidemiologic aspects," *Journal of the National Cancer Institute*, vol. 56, no. 3, pp. 489–491, 1976.

[3] E. Kujala, T. Ma¨kitie, and T. Kivela¨, "Very long-term prognosis of patients with malignant uveal melanoma," *Investigative Opthalmology and Visual Science*, vol. 44, no. 11, p. 4651, 2003.

[4] M. Diener-West, S. M. Reynolds, D. J. Agugliaro et al., "Development of metastatic disease after enrollment in the COMS trials for treatment of choroidal melanoma:

collaborative ocular melanoma study group report no. 26," *Archives of Ophthalmology*, vol. 123, no. 12, pp. 1639–1643, 2005.

[5] The Collaborative Ocular Melanoma Study Group, "Assessment of metastatic disease status at death in 435 patients with large choroidal melanoma in the Collaborative Ocular Melanoma Study (COMS): COMS report no. 15," *Archives of Ophthalmology*, vol. 119, no. 5, pp. 670–676, 2001.

[6] S. Bakalian, J. C. Marshall, P. Logan et al., "Molecular pathways mediating liver metastasis in patients with uveal melanoma," *Clinical Cancer Research*, vol. 14, no. 4, pp. 951–956, 2008.

[7] C. D. Van Raamsdonk, K. G. Griewank, M. B. Crosby et al., "Mutations in GNA11 in uveal melanoma," *New England Journal of Medicine*, vol. 363, no. 23, pp. 2191–2199, 2010.

[8] S. R. Neves, P. T. Ram, and R. Iyengar, "G protein pathways," *Science*, vol. 296, no. 5573, pp. 1636–1639, 2002.

[9] D. Markby, R. Onrust, and H. Bourne, "Separate GTP binding and GTPase activating domains of a G alpha subunit," *Science*, vol. 262, no. 5141, pp. 1895–1901, 1993.

[10] C. D. Van Raamsdonk, V. Bezrookove, G. Green et al., "Frequent somatic mutations of GNAQ in uveal melanoma and blue naevi," *Nature*, vol. 457, no. 7229, pp. 599–602, 2009.

[11] S. Lamba, L. Felicioni, F. Buttitta et al., "Mutational profile of GNAQQ209 in human tumors," *PLoS One*, vol. 4, no. 8, article e6833, 2009.

[12] M. D. Onken, L. A. Worley, M. D. Long et al., "Oncogenic mutations in GNAQ occur early in uveal melanoma," *Investigative Opthalmology and Visual Science*, vol. 49, no. 12, pp. 5230–5234, 2008.

[13] J. Bauer, E. Kilic, J. Vaarwater, B. C. Bastian, C. Garbe, and A. De Klein, "Oncogenic GNAQ mutations are not correlated with disease-free survival in uveal melanoma," *British Journal of Cancer*, vol. 101, no. 5, pp. 813–815, 2009.

[14] C. A. Landis, S. B. Masters, A. Spada, A. M. Pace, H. R. Bourne, and L. Vallar, "GTPase inhibiting mutations activate the alpha chain of Gs and stimulate adenylyl cyclase in human pituitary tumours," *Nature*, vol. 340, no. 6236, pp. 692–696, 1989.

[15] G. Kalinec, A. J. Nazarali, S. Hermouet, N. Xu, and J. S. Gutkind, "Mutated alpha subunit of the Gq protein induces malignant transformation in NIH 3T3 cells," *Molecular and Cellular Biology*, vol. 12, no. 10, pp. 4687–4693, 1992.

[16] J. Sondek, D. G. Lambright, J. P. Noel, H. E. Hamm, and P. B. Sigler, "GTPase mechanism of Gproteins from the 1.7-Å crystal structure of transducin α - GDP AIF–4," *Nature*, vol. 372, no. 6503, pp. 276–279, 1994.

[17] P. B. Schiff and S. B. Horwitz, "Taxol stabilizes microtubules in mouse fibroblast cells," *Proceedings of the National Academy of Sciences*, vol. 77, no. 3, pp. 1561–1565, 1980.

[18] R. A. Leon-Ferre and S. N. Markovic, "Nab-paclitaxel in patients with metastatic melanoma," *Expert Review of Anticancer Therapy*, vol. 15, no. 12, pp. 1371–1377, 2015.

[19] J. J. Luke, P. L. Triozzi, K. C. McKenna et al., "Biology of advanced uveal melanoma and next steps for clinical therapeutics," *Pigment Cell and Melanoma Research*, vol. 28, no. 2, pp. 135–147, 2015.

[20] S. S. Agarwala, A. M. M. Eggermont, S. O'Day, and J. S. Zager, "Metastatic melanoma to the liver: a contemporary and comprehensive review of surgical, systemic, and regional therapeutic options," *Cancer*, vol. 120, no. 6, pp. 781–789, 2014.

[21] N. A. Karim, J. Schuster, I. Eldessouki et al., "Pulmonary sarcomatoid carcinoma: University of Cincinnati experience," *Oncotarget*, vol. 9, no. 3, 2018.

[22] N. Karim, I. Eldessouki, M. Yellu, T. Namad, J. Wang, and O. Gaber, "A case study in advanced lung cancer patients with vimentin over expression," *Clinical Laboratory*, vol. 63, no. 10, 2017.

[23] J. F. Pingpank, M. S. Hughes, H. R. Alexander et al., "A phase III random assignment trial comparing percutaneous hepatic perfusion with melphalan (PHP-mel) to standard of care for patients with hepatic metastases from metastatic ocular or cutaneous melanoma," *Journal of Clinical Oncology*, vol. 28, no. 18, p. LBA8512, 2010.

[24] J. C. Moser, J. S. Pulido, R. S. Dronca, R. R. McWilliams, S. N. Markovic, and A. S. Mansfield, "The Mayo Clinic experience with the use of kinase inhibitors, ipilimumab, bevacizumab, and local therapies in the treatment of metastatic uveal melanoma," *Melanoma Research*, vol. 25, no. 1, pp. 59–63, 2015.

[25] L. E. Flaherty, J. M. Unger, P. Y. Liu, W. C. Mertens, and V. K. Sondak, "Metastatic melanoma from intraocular primary tumors," *American Journal of Clinical Oncology*, vol. 21, no. 6, pp. 568–572, 1998.

[26] T. Kivelä, S. Suciu, J. Hansson et al., "Bleomycin, vincristine, lomustine and dacarbazine (BOLD) in combination with recombinant interferon alpha-2b for metastatic uveal melanoma," *European Journal of Cancer*, vol. 39, no. 8, pp. 1115–1120, 2003.

[27] T. J. Smith, S. Temin, E. R. Alesi et al., "American Society of Clinical Oncology provisional clinical opinion: the integration of palliative care into standard oncology care," *Journal of Clinical Oncology*, vol. 30, no. 8, pp. 880–887, 2012.

[28] E. M. Hersh, M. Del Vecchio, M. P. Brown, and R. F. Kefford, "Phase 3, randomized, open-label, multicenter trial of nab-paclitaxel (nab-P) vs dacarbazine (DTIC) in previously untreated patients with metastatic malignant melanoma (MMM)," *Pigment Cell & Melanoma Research*, vol. 25, p. 863, 2012.

[29] P. J. Hesketh, M. G. Kris, E. Basch et al., "Antiemetics: American Society of Clinical Oncology clinical practice guideline update," *Journal of Clinical Oncology*, vol. 35, no. 28, pp. 3240–3261, 2017.

27

Squamous Cell Carcinoma of the Thyroid as a Result of Anaplastic Transformation from BRAF-Positive Papillary Thyroid Cancer

Alina Basnet,[1] **Aakriti Pandita,**[2] **Joseph Fullmer,**[3] **and Abirami Sivapiragasam**[1]

[1]*Department of Hematology Oncology, SUNY Upstate Medical University, Syracuse, NY 13205, USA*
[2]*Department of Medicine, SUNY Upstate Medical University, Syracuse, NY 13205, USA*
[3]*Department of Pathology, SUNY Upstate Medical University, Syracuse, NY 13205, USA*

Correspondence should be addressed to Alina Basnet; basnetalina@hotmail.com

Academic Editor: Jose I. Mayordomo

Papillary thyroid carcinoma (PTC) is the most common malignant neoplasm of the thyroid. Majority of the PTC carries an excellent prognosis. However, patients with tall cell variant (TCV) of papillary thyroid carcinoma have a worse prognosis than those with the classic variant. On the other hand, squamous cell carcinoma of the thyroid (SCT) is an unusual neoplasm thought to arise as a primary tumor or as a component of an anaplastic or undifferentiated carcinoma. We report a patient with TCV of PTC presenting years later with squamous transformation. In addition, the patient was found to have BRAF mutation. Such dedifferentiation is considered to be a rare phenomenon and has been reported only in the form of case reports in the literature. The relationship between BRAFV600E mutation and squamous cell transformation of papillary thyroid cancer is unknown at this time. Meticulous pathology is needed to identify such variants. Our patient responded to treatment with concurrent chemotherapy with carboplatin and paclitaxel along with radiation.

1. Introduction

Papillary thyroid carcinoma (PTC) is the most common malignant neoplasm of the thyroid [1]. Tall cell variant (TCV) of PTC was originally defined by Hawk and Hazard, and this group is recognized by cells with height that is at least two times the width [2]. The incidence of papillary thyroid cancer varies between 3.2 and 19% [2–5]. However, patients with TCV of papillary thyroid carcinoma have a worse prognosis than those with the classic variant [6]. On the other hand, squamous cell carcinoma of the thyroid (SCT) is an unusual neoplasm thought to arise as a primary tumor or as a component of an anaplastic or undifferentiated carcinoma [7]. It is often mixed with heterogeneous elements and is usually associated with areas of well-differentiated papillary or follicular carcinoma [7]. We report a patient with TCV of PTC presenting years later with squamous transformation. In addition, the patient was found to have BRAF mutation which confers a very poor prognosis.

2. Case Report

Our patient is a 56-year-old male who was diagnosed with TCV of PTC in 2011 when he presented with multiple enlarged cervical lymph nodes. He underwent total thyroidectomy with central compartment neck dissection followed by radioactive iodine (RAI) therapy. His tumor was pTNM (pathologic primary tumor, regional node, and distant metastasis) pT2N1bM0-stage I. Six months later, he had an early local recurrence in the left neck, for which he underwent a left neck dissection. After about a year, he had a positron emission tomography (PET) scan that showed activity in the right neck, and he underwent a right neck dissection. Then, he was followed up with surveillance scans. Three years later, a PET scan showed uptake suggestive of recurrence along the left thyroid bed as well as activity along the right paratracheal region. Fine-needle aspiration of the left thyroid bed as well as a right paratracheal node came back positive for recurrent papillary thyroid carcinoma. At that time, he was symptomatic with more fatigue and weight loss. He then underwent revision

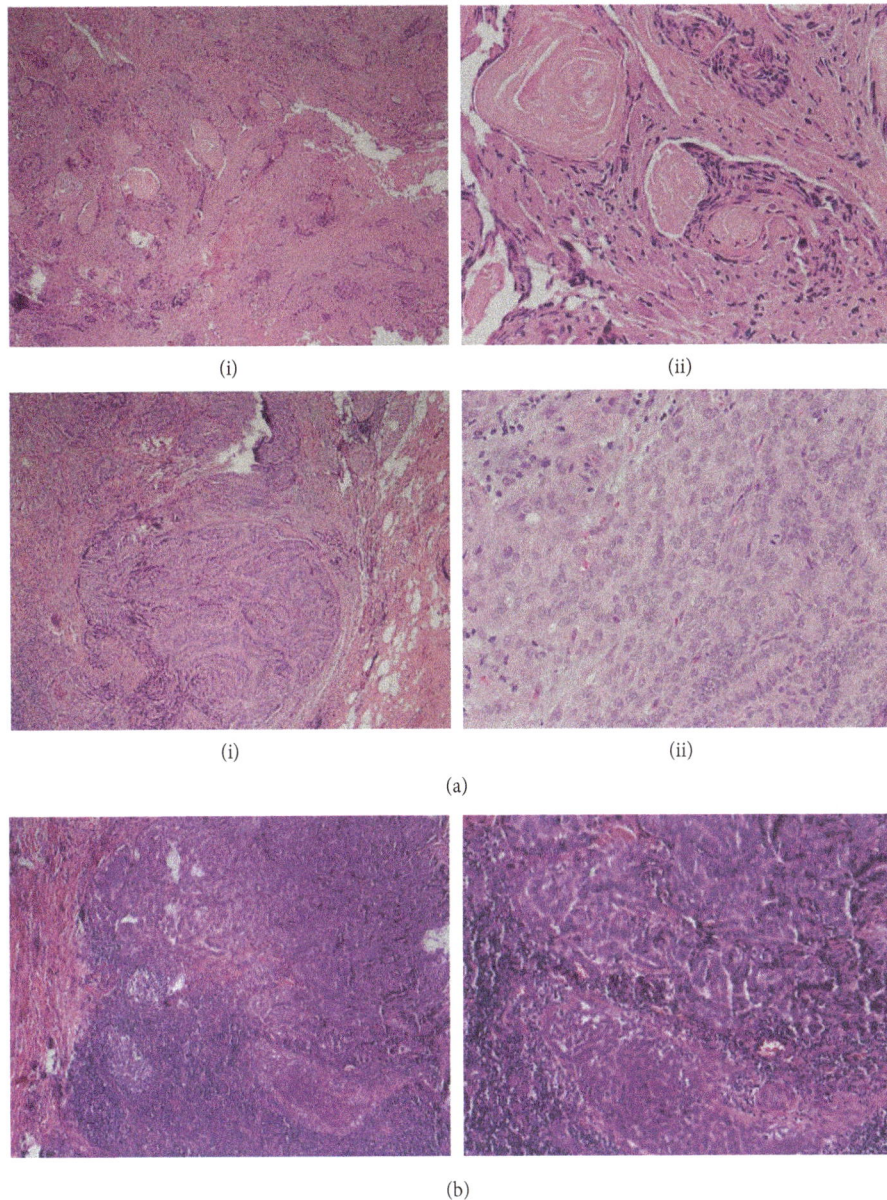

FIGURE 1: (a) H&E staining of the thyroid bed and paratracheal lymph node. Top row, from left to right: (i) squamous cell carcinoma in the thyroid bed; (ii) keratin pearls of squamous cell carcinoma in higher power. Bottom row, from left to right: (i) paratracheal lymph node showing papillary feature of thyroid cancer; (ii) tall cell areas showing mitotic figure in higher power. (b) From left to right, low power showing papillary thyroid cancer and squamous cell cancer in the same field adjacent to each other.

of left paratracheal and central neck dissection with right paratracheal and mediastinal lymph node dissection along with shave biopsy of the right neck lesion. Histopathology of one of the right paratracheal lymph nodes showed metastatic poorly differentiated thyroid carcinoma composed of papillary tall cell phenotype involving one lymph node. In addition, the left thyroid bed and a second right paratracheal lymph node demonstrated squamous cell carcinoma (Figures 1(a) and 1(b)). The poorly differentiated papillary thyroid carcinoma component was positive for TTF-1, thyroglobulin, and PAX8 while the squamous cell carcinoma was positive for p63, PAX8 (focally), and TTF-1 (very focally positive) and negative for thyroglobulin (Figures 2(a) and 2(b)). This pattern

of immunohistochemistry suggests that the squamous variant seen was actually a transformation from papillary cancer unlike the primary squamous cancer which stains negative for TTF-1 and PAX8. The specimen also tested positive for BRAF mutation via immunohistochemistry (IHC). We then retrospectively analyzed his primary tumor for BRAF, and his primary tumor was positive for BRAF as well. He was started on concurrent radiation and chemotherapy with weekly dosing of carboplatin and Taxol. He went on to complete that over the course of 6 weeks. PET-CT was done after 12 weeks of completion of therapy and suggested near-complete resolution of metabolic activity in the thyroid bed and regional lymph node areas.

(a)

(b)

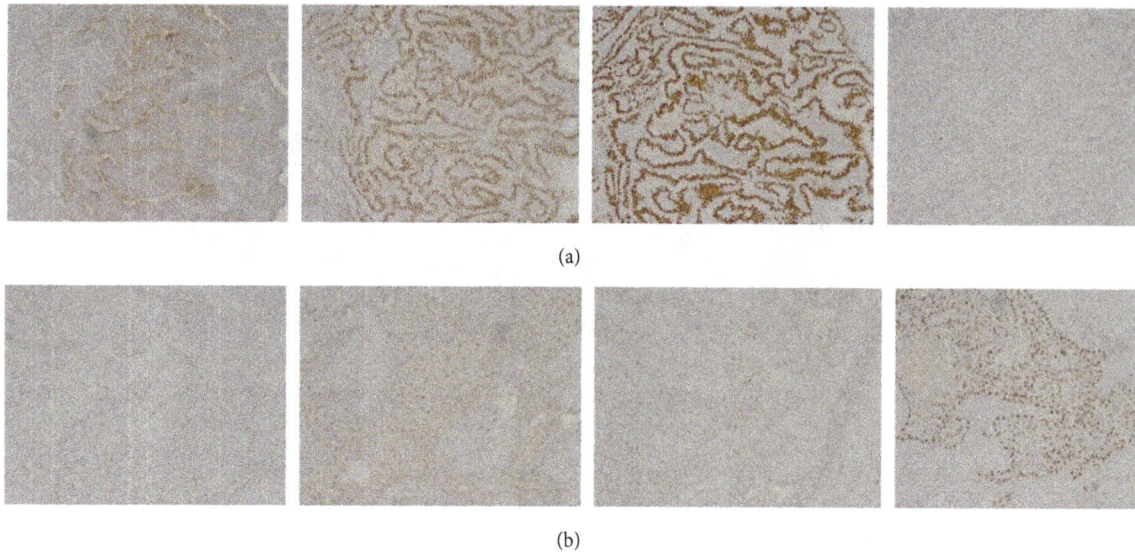

FIGURE 2: (a) From left to right are the papillary tall cell variant portion of thyroid cancer staining positive for thyroglobulin, PAX8, and TTF-1 and negative for p63. (b) From left to right are squamous cell area of thyroid cancer staining negative for thyroglobulin, weakly positive for PAX8 and TTF-1, and strongly positive for p63.

3. Discussion

Several investigators found that the TCV of PTC was more aggressive than ordinary well-differentiated papillary carcinoma [8]. Tall cell variant tends to have more frequent extrathyroidal extension with higher recurrence and mortality rate [9]. Papillary carcinomas are also described with several other variants like focal insular component, spindle and giant cell carcinoma, squamous cell carcinoma, and mucoepidermoid carcinoma [10]. It is not rare to find papillary carcinoma showing characteristics of more than one variant [1]. Squamous transformation, however, is usually rare and has been described only in the form of case reports in the literature [11–13]. It is also suggested that the tall cell variant can evolve into the spindle cell type of squamous cell carcinoma [4, 14]. LiVolsi and Merino suggested that, in most cases, squamous cell carcinomas appear as a result of metaplasia of follicular epithelial cells [15].

Bronner and LiVolsi described five tumors which were composed of squamous cell carcinoma of thyroid (SCT) and TCV [14]. These tumors behaved in an aggressive fashion [14]. LiVolsi and Merino described eight cases of primary SCT with extension in perithyroidal soft tissues of the neck, with prominent vascular invasion (two cases) and perineural invasion (one case) [15]. Kleer et al. found 4 out of 8 cases of SCT to be associated with tall cell variant. p53 expression and high MIB1 labeling index conferred a worse prognosis [7] with frequent capsular and vascular invasion as well as tumor recurrence even after excision.

When histological biopsy from any head and neck yields SCC, it is integral to consider if transformation has occurred [12]. Squamous cells can be found in the thyroid from persistence of thyroglossal ducts or brachial pouch–derived structures or from squamous metaplasia in Hashimoto's thyroiditis. In the presence of squamous cell carcinoma involving the thyroid, direct involvement from the tumor of the larynx or trachea should be ruled out in addition to metastasis from the lungs.

While there is no recognized pattern of progression from differentiated thyroid carcinoma to a particular form of anaplastic carcinoma, Bronner and LiVolsi reported significant risk factors for progression which include preexisting thyroid neoplasm, radiation therapy to the neck region, and I-131 therapy [4, 15].

Due to the rarity of this tumor variant, there is no consensus for its management. A case series has described surgery with re-resections, external beam radiation therapy, and chemotherapy as treatment options [12]. Chemotherapy concurrent with radiation has been described in the literature. We adopted the same approach for our patient, and he tolerated the treatment well.

BRAFV600E mutation has been found positive in the tall cell areas as well as squamous cell transformation, whereas in our patient tall cell portion was positive and squamous cell transformation was only focally positive [16]. Other high-risk factors are male gender, tumor size >5 mm, bilateral/multifocal location, lower third of the thyroid lobe location, lymph node metastasis at presentation, superficial tumor location, capsule invasion/extrathyroidal extension, and stromal fibrosis [10].

Our patient had recurrence with BRAF mutation, which is closely associated with aggressive clinic pathological characteristics that led to poorer outcome in papillary thyroid cancer. Accordingly, aggressive treatment should be considered for papillary thyroid cancer patients with BRAF mutation [17]. A meta-analysis of 20,764 patients suggested that the BRAFV600E mutation is associated with several high-risk clinical variables used in prognostic staging systems, including extrathyroidal invasion, high TNM stage, lymph node metastasis, recurrence, and overall survival. However, distant metastasis occurrence was less in tumors with BRAF mutation. Thus, the overall survival effect of BRAFV600E mutation on PTC tumor remains to be determined.

References

[1] S. Dizbay Sak, "Variants of papillary thyroid carcinoma: multiple faces of a familiar tumor," *Turkish Journal of Pathology*, vol. 31, pp. 34–47, 2015.

[2] A. Machens, H.-J. Holzhausen, C. Lautenschläger, and H. Dralle, "The tall-cell variant of papillary thyroid carcinoma: a multivariate analysis of clinical risk factors," *Langenbeck's Archives of Surgery*, vol. 389, no. 4, pp. 278–282, 2004.

[3] K.-C. Loh, F. S. Greenspan, L. Gee, T. R. Miller, and P. P. B. Yeo, "Pathological tumor-node-metastasis (pTNM) staging for papillary and follicular thyroid carcinomas: a retrospective analysis of 700 patients," *Journal of Clinical Endocrinology & Metabolism*, vol. 82, no. 11, pp. 3553–3562, 1997.

[4] C. A. Saunders and R. Nayar, "Anaplastic spindle-cell squamous carcinoma arising in association with tall-cell papillary cancer of the thyroid: a potential pitfall," *Diagnostic Cytopathology*, vol. 21, no. 6, pp. 413–418, 1999.

[5] M. Xing, "Molecular pathogenesis and mechanisms of thyroid cancer," *Nature Reviews Cancer*, vol. 13, no. 3, pp. 184–199, 2013.

[6] W. A. Hawk and J. B. Hazard, "The many appearances of papillary carcinoma of the thyroid," *Cleveland Clinic Quarterly*, vol. 43, no. 4, pp. 207–215, 1976.

[7] C. G. Kleer, T. J. Giordano, and M. J. Merino, "Squamous cell carcinoma of the thyroid: an aggressive tumor associated with tall cell variant of papillary thyroid carcinoma," *Modern Pathology*, vol. 13, no. 7, pp. 742–746, 2000.

[8] T. L. Johnson, R. V. Lloyd, N. W. Thompson, W. H. Beierwaltes, and J. C. Sisson, "Prognostic implications of the tall cell variant of papillary thyroid carcinoma," *American Journal of Surgical Pathology*, vol. 12, no. 1, pp. 22–27, 1988.

[9] R. A. Ghossein, R. Leboeuf, K. N. Patel et al., "Tall cell variant of papillary thyroid carcinoma without extrathyroid extension: biologic behavior and clinical implications," *Thyroid*, vol. 17, no. 7, pp. 655–661, 2007.

[10] E. Roti, E. C. degli Uberti, M. Bondanelli, and L. E. Braverman, "Thyroid papillary microcarcinoma: a descriptive and meta-analysis study," *European Journal of Endocrinology*, vol. 159, no. 6, pp. 659–673, 2008.

[11] V. A. LiVolsi, "Papillary thyroid carcinoma: an update," *Modern Pathology*, vol. 24, no. 2, pp. S1–S9, 2011.

[12] W. D. G. Evans, "De-differentiation of papillary thyroid carcinoma into squamous cell carcinoma. A case of co-existence within an excised neck lesion," *BMJ Case Reports*, vol. 2012, 2012.

[13] M. K. Hararah, R. J. Gertz, R. S. Sippel, and A. M. Wieland, "De-differentiation of conventional papillary thyroid carcinoma into squamous cell carcinoma," *Journal of Thyroid Disorders & Therapy*, vol. 4, no. 192, p. 3, 2015.

[14] M. Bronner and V. LiVolsi, "Spindle cell squamous carcinoma of the thyroid: an unusual anaplastic tumor associated with tall cell papillary cancer," *Modern Pathology*, vol. 4, no. 5, pp. 637–643, 1991.

[15] V. A. LiVolsi and M. J. Merino, "Squamous cells in the human thyroid gland," *American Journal of Surgical Pathology*, vol. 2, no. 2, pp. 133–140, 1978.

[16] J. H. Lee, E. S. Lee, and Y. S. Kim, "Clinicopathologic significance of BRAF V600E mutation in papillary carcinomas of the thyroid," *Cancer*, vol. 110, no. 1, pp. 38–46, 2007.

[17] C. Liu, T. Chen, and Z. Liu, "Associations between BRAF V600E and prognostic factors and poor outcomes in papillary thyroid carcinoma: a meta-analysis," *World Journal of Surgical Oncology*, vol. 14, no. 1, p. 241, 2016.

28

Retroperitoneal Solitary Fibrous Tumor: A "Patternless" Tumor

D. Myoteri,[1] **D. Dellaportas,**[2] **C. Nastos,**[2] **I. Gioti,**[1] **G. Gkiokas,**[2] **E. Carvounis,**[1] **and T. Theodosopoulos**[2]

[1]*Pathology Department, Aretaieion University Hospital, Medical School of Athens, Athens, Greece*
[2]*2nd Department of Surgery, Aretaieion University Hospital, Medical School of Athens, Athens, Greece*

Correspondence should be addressed to D. Myoteri; dmyoteri@gmail.com

Academic Editor: Raffaele Palmirotta

Introduction. Solitary fibrous tumor is a rare type of mesenchymal, spindle-cell tumor reported mostly in the pleura. Retroperitoneal occurrence is rare and histopathological diagnosis is challenging. *Case Presentation.* A 55-year-old woman with nonspecific abdominal pain was found to have a retroperitoneal/pelvic mass adjacent to the upper rectum. The patient underwent surgical resection in clear margins of this pelvic tumor, entering the total mesenteric excision surgical plane. Final histopathology revealed a solitary fibrous tumor and the case is presented herein. *Discussion.* Solitary fibrous tumor in the retroperitoneum is rarely found in the literature and to the best of our knowledge less than a hundred cases are described so far. Histopathological diagnosis is mostly based on a "patternless pattern" on microscopic examination, which is a storiform arrangement of spindle cells combined with a "hemangiopericytoma-like appearance" and increased vascularity of the lesion. Surgery is the mainstay of treatment and recurrence rates are generally low.

1. Introduction

Solitary fibrous tumor (SFT) is a rare type of mesenchymal, spindle-cell tumor and includes heterogenous variety of neoplasms, both benign and malignant. They are mostly reported arising in the pleura, and about 30% develop in extrapleural tissues, including the retroperitoneal space [1]. Surgical resection in clear margins is the mainstay of treatment, alike all retroperitoneal sarcomas. Histopathological diagnosis is very interesting and stepwise, based on exclusion criteria and on a characteristic "patternless pattern" of the spindle cells. A rare case of a retroperitoneal SFT is presented herein, along with the histopathological and oncological challenges of this seldom found tumor [2].

2. Case Presentation

A 55-year-old woman was investigated for nonspecific lower abdominal and back pain. The patient's past medical and surgical history was clear and physical examination as well as routine haematological and biochemical laboratory investigations were unremarkable. Computed tomography (CT) of the abdomen and pelvis revealed an approximately 10×10 cm tumor in the retroperitoneal space, immediately anterior to the aortic bifurcation, high in the pelvis, and posteriorly to the upper third of the rectum (Figure 1(a)). Magnetic resonance imaging (MRI) of the pelvis followed and confirmed the solid nature of this mass, showing that it was independent from the bowel/rectum, featuring a retroperitoneal sarcoma type of mass rather than a lymph nodal bloc (Figure 1(b)).

After multidisciplinary team (MDT) meeting discussion, surgical exploration was decided and performed via midline laparotomy. Bilateral ureter guidewires were inserted intraoperatively, to facilitate identification of the ureters. The left colon was mobilized and the total mesorectal excision (TME) surgical plane was entered; the tumor was mobilized and excised in clear margins macroscopically without any intraoperative adverse events (Figures 2(a) and 2(b)). There was no close relation of the tumor to any adjacent anatomical structure, having its blood supply from small arterial branches originating from the common iliac arteries and the mesentery of the rectum. The mass was resected without compromising the integrity of the rectum or the sigmoid colon, excluding any relationship with the uterus as well.

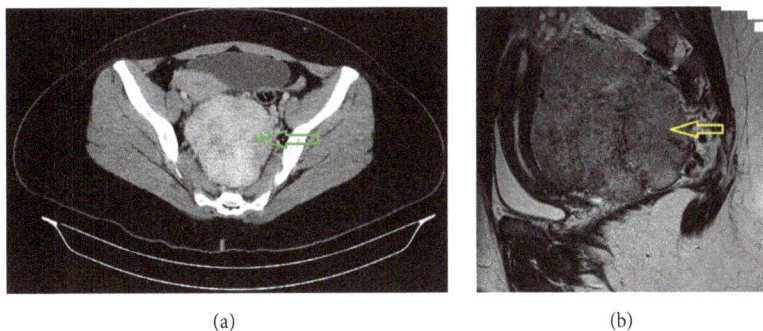

FIGURE 1: (a) Computed tomography (CT) of the abdomen. Green arrow showing the large pelvic mass. (b) Sagittal view-Magnetic Resonance Imaging (MRI). Yellow arrow showing the tumor.

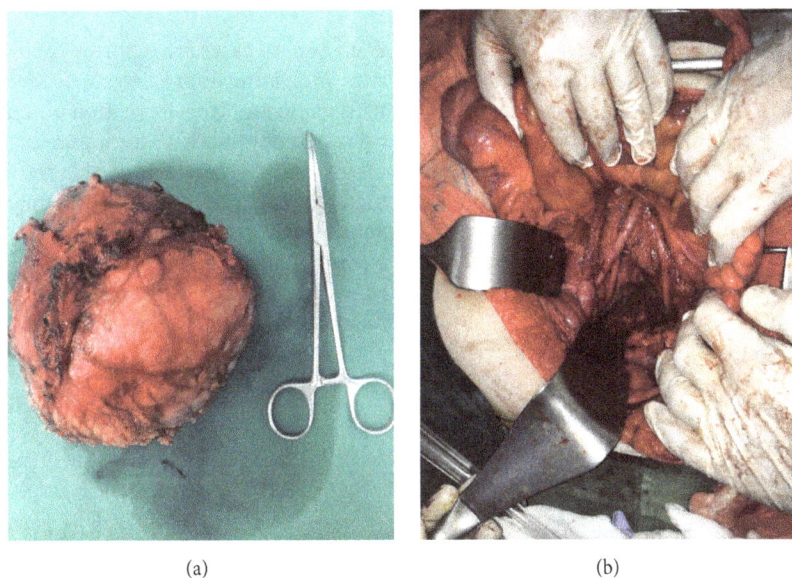

FIGURE 2: (a) Macroscopic view of the surgical specimen. (b) Intraoperative view of the pelvis, after tumor resection. Total mesenteric excision plane was entered.

The patient had an uneventful postoperative course and was discharged on the 7th day postop.

Histopathological examination showed a neoplasm composed of bland and uniform oval to spindle cells with minimal cytoplasm, small elongated nuclei, and indistinct nucleoli (Figure 3(a)). The tumor exhibited an overall patternless architecture of hypo- and hypercellular areas separated by thick, hyalinized collagen with cracking artifact and staghorn vessels. The neoplasm had minimal pleomorphism, no atypia, and rare mitotic figures (<1 mitoses per 10 High Power Fields). Neither necrosis nor hemorrhagic alterations were observed. Immunohistochemical examination showed positive staining for Bcl-2, CD34 (Figure 3(b)), vimentin, and CD99 while desmin and S-100 were negative. The Ki-67 index was 7%, confirming the overall indolent nature of this tumor. Final diagnosis was retroperitoneal solitary fibrous tumor.

No adjuvant treatment was decided on the MDT and the patient remains asymptomatic and tumor free on follow-up visits one year later.

3. Discussion

SFTs are soft tissue spindle-cell neoplasms, first described by Klemperer and Rabin in 1931 [3]. World Health Organization (WHO) classifies SFT as intermediate fibroblastic or myofibroblastic tumors along with hemangiopericytomas, which means that SFTs are considered tumors that rarely if ever metastasize [4]. These neoplasms usually affect the pleura, while extrapleural sites are reported in about 30% of cases. The latter include the nasal cavity, salivary glands, orbit, upper respiratory tract, thyroid, peritoneum, genitourinary system, and retroperitoneum and pelvis [5].

SFT in the retroperitoneum, as in the case reported above, is rarely found in the literature and to the best of our knowledge less than 100 cases are described so far [6]. The main characteristic of these is the large size they can reach due to the lack of specific symptoms, leading to the need for major surgical resections of the primary tumor along with adjacent structures.

(a)   (b)

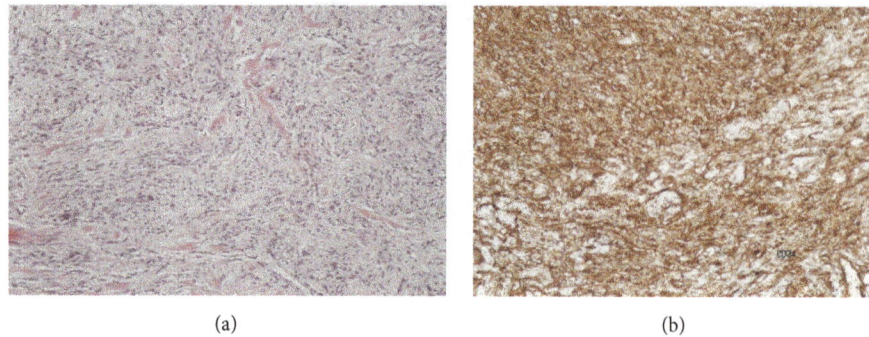

FIGURE 3: (a) Microscopic view (H-E ×100) of bland and uniform oval to spindle cells with minimal cytoplasm, small elongated nuclei, and indistinct nucleoli. (b) Immunohistochemical examination with positive staining for CD34.

Histopathological diagnosis is challenging and mostly based on a "patternless pattern" on microscopic examination. This pattern is a storiform arrangement of spindle cells combined with a "hemangiopericytoma-like appearance" and increased vascularity of the lesion [7]. Differential diagnosis includes other spindle-cell neoplasms such as leiomyoma, inflammatory myofibroblastic tumor, angiomyolipoma, and gastrointestinal stromal tumor. Immunohistochemistry is very helpful, and SFTs are positive for Bcl-2, vimentin, and CD99, as well as CD34 [8]. Negative expression of S100, cytokeratin, EMA, SMA, CD117, CD31, and desmin is the norm and adds to the correct diagnosis. The combination of positive Bcl-2 and CD34 is guiding histopathologically towards the diagnosis of SFT, since 75% of extrapleural SFTs positively express these two markers [5].

SFTs are considered malignant when histopathological examination shows high cellularity, high mitotic activity (more than 4 mitoses per 10 HPF), pleomorphism, necrosis, and hemorrhagic changes [9].

Moreover, SFTs can cause paraneoplastic syndromes and mainly hypoglycemia, which is thought to arise due to the production of Insulin like Growth Factor-2 (IGF-2) from the tumor. Such a condition may be the presenting symptom for these cases [10]. When complete resection is feasible these syndromes subside. This was not the case for the patient presented above.

Tomographic imaging cannot differentiate retroperitoneal SFT from other solid retroperitoneal sarcomas [11, 12]; however it is invaluable to guide the surgical team to the right approach and strategy for radical excision in clear margins. As with most of the sarcoma-like tumors, surgery is the main and usually the only effective treatment of SFTs. In the whole, recurrence rates are low and positive resection margins seem to affect these rates [13], underlying the importance of a sound surgical excision.

Due to the rarity of SFTs, especially in the retroperitoneum, studies to define the best management approach are lacking and adjuvant treatment options are based on case reports and observational studies. Interestingly, antiangiogenic drugs, as bevacizumab, based on the high vascularity of the lesion are used initially and conventional chemotherapy to keep the disease stable is a strategy proposed in an important study on the matter, treating advanced disease [14].

Even benign cases are reported recurring locally or at distant sites, indicating unpredictable behavior of this rare neoplasm, with malignant transformation potential [15]. The latter is the basis of follow-up with tomographic imaging.

In conclusion, SFT in the retroperitoneum should be managed aggressively with primary surgery and has a good prognosis. Histopathological diagnosis is stepwise and immunohistochemistry can guide towards the right direction in equivocal cases. Uncertain clinical behavior and lack of management guidelines confuse clinicians and multidisciplinary team approach is of paramount importance.

References

[1] K. Kunieda, Y. Tanaka, N. Nagao et al., "Large solitary fibrous tumor of the retroperitoneum: report of a case," *Surgery Today*, vol. 34, no. 1, pp. 90–93, 2004.

[2] J. S. Gold, C. R. Antonescu, C. Hajdu et al., "Clinicopathologic correlates of solitary fibrous tumors," *Cancer*, vol. 94, no. 4, pp. 1057–1068, 2002.

[3] P. Klemperer and B. R. Coleman, "Primary neoplasms of the pleura. A report of five cases," *American Journal of Industrial Medicine*, vol. 22, no. 1, pp. 1–31, 1992.

[4] C. D. Fletcher, "The evolving classification of soft tissue tumours—an update based on the new 2013 WHO classification," *Histopathology*, vol. 64, pp. 2–11, 2014.

[5] T. Hasegawa, Y. Matsuno, T. Shimoda, F. Hasegawa, T. Sano, and S. Hirohashi, "Extrathoracic solitary fibrous tumors: their histological variability and potentially aggressive behavior," *Human Pathology*, vol. 30, no. 12, pp. 1464–1473, 1999.

[6] R. Rajeev, M. Patel, T. T. Jayakrishnan et al., "Retroperitoneal solitary fibrous tumor: surgery as first line therapy," *Clinical Sarcoma Research*, vol. 5, no. 1, 2015.

[7] C. Gengler and L. Guillou, "Solitary fibrous tumour and haemangiopericytoma: evolution of a concept," *Histopathology*, vol. 48, no. 1, pp. 63–74, 2006.

[8] W. Ge, D.-C. Yu, G. Chen, and Y.-T. Ding, "Clinical analysis of 47 cases of solitary fibrous tumor," *Oncology Letters*, vol. 12, no. 4, pp. 2475–2480, 2016.

[9] D. M. England, L. Hochholzer, and M. J. McCarthy, "Localized benign and malignant fibrous tumors of the pleura. A clinico-pathologic review of 223 cases," *American Journal of Surgical Pathology*, vol. 13, pp. 640–658, 1989.

[10] S. Otake, T. Kikkawa, M. Takizawa et al., "Hypoglycemia observed on continuous glucose monitoring associated with IGF-2-producing solitary fibrous tumor," *Journal of Clinical Endocrinology and Metabolism*, vol. 100, no. 7, pp. 2519–2524, 2015.

[11] A. K. Shanbhogue, S. R. Prasad, N. Takahashi, R. Vikram, A. Zaheer, and K. Sandrasegaran, "Somatic and visceral solitary fibrous tumors in the abdomen and pelvis: cross-sectional imaging spectrum," *Radiographics*, vol. 31, no. 2, pp. 393–408, 2011.

[12] A. B. Rosenkrantz, N. Hindman, and J. Melamed, "Imaging appearance of solitary fibrous tumor of the abdominopelvic cavity," *Journal of Computer Assisted Tomography*, vol. 34, no. 2, pp. 201–205, 2010.

[13] W. J. Van Houdt, C. M. A. Westerveld, J. E. P. Vrijenhoek et al., "Prognosis of solitary fibrous tumors: A multicenter study," *Annals of Surgical Oncology*, vol. 20, no. 13, pp. 4090–4095, 2013.

[14] M. S. Park, V. Ravi, A. Conley et al., "The role of chemotherapy in advanced solitary fibrous tumors: a retrospective analysis," *Clinical Sarcoma Research*, vol. 3, no. 1, article 7, 2013.

[15] M.-K. Law, Y.-W. Tung, and J.-S. Jinc, "Malignant transformation in solitary fibrous tumor of the pleura," *Asian Cardiovascular and Thoracic Annals*, vol. 22, no. 8, pp. 981–983, 2014.

29

Giant Cystic Pheochromocytoma with Low Risk of Malignancy: A Case Report and Literature Review

Ravi Maharaj,[1] Sangeeta Parbhu,[1] Wesley Ramcharan,[1] Shanta Baijoo,[1] Wesley Greaves,[1] Dave Harnanan,[1] and Wayne A. Warner[2,3]

[1]Department of Clinical Surgical Sciences, University of the West Indies, Eric Williams Medical Sciences Complex, Champ Fleurs, Trinidad and Tobago
[2]Division of Oncology, Siteman Cancer Center, Washington University School of Medicine, St. Louis, MO 63110, USA
[3]Department of Cell Biology and Physiology, Washington University School of Medicine, St. Louis, MO 63110, USA

Correspondence should be addressed to Sangeeta Parbhu; sangeenator@gmail.com

Academic Editor: Jose I. Mayordomo

Giant pheochromocytomas are rare silent entities that do not present with the classical symptoms commonly seen in catecholamine-secreting tumors. In many cases they are accidentally discovered. The algorithm to diagnose a pheochromocytoma consists of biochemical evaluation and imaging of a retroperitoneal mass. The female patient in this case report presented with a palpable abdominal mass and was cured with surgical resection. She suffered no recurrence or complications on follow-up. The left retroperitoneal mass measured 27 × 18 × 12 cm and weighed 3,315 grams. Biochemical, radiological, and pathological examinations confirmed the diagnosis of a pheochromocytoma. In this paper, we report on our experience treating this patient and provide a summary of all giant pheochromocytomas greater than 10 cm reported to date in English language medical journals. Our patient's giant cystic pheochromocytoma was the fourth heaviest and fifth largest maximal diameter identified using our literature search criteria. Additionally, this tumor had the largest maximal diameter of all histologically confirmed benign/low metastatic risk pheochromocytomas. Giant cystic pheochromocytomas are rare entities requiring clinical suspicion coupled with strategic diagnostic evaluation to confirm the diagnosis.

1. Introduction

A pheochromocytoma (PCC) is a rare catecholamine-secreting tumor that originates from the chromaffin cells of the adrenal medulla. First described by Frankel [1] in 1886, the estimated worldwide incidence of these tumors is 2 to 8 per million persons per year [2]. Classical symptoms at presentation include severe hypertension with associated headaches, sweating, and palpitations; however, 20–30% of patients remain asymptomatic. Asymptomatic PCCs are typically detected as an incidental adrenal mass on routine screening. Biochemical evidence of elevated plasma free metanephrines provides the highest sensitivity for PCC diagnosis [3]. Most of these lesions are benign/low metastatic potential but histopathological characteristics defined by the pheochromocytoma of the adrenal gland scaled score (PASS) can identify tumors with potentially more aggressive

biological behavior such as the presence of chromaffin tissue at extra adrenal sites. Giant PCCs are generally classified as those with maximal diameter greater than 10 cm. They are commonly asymptomatic and are diagnosed incidentally on imaging. Surgical resection is the standard treatment option and is usually curative, preventing future potentially lethal complications of these lesions. We present the case of a 50-year-old female patient with a left side adrenal PCC which was treated successfully with open surgical resection in the surgical unit of Eric Williams Medical Sciences Complex, Trinidad and Tobago.

2. Case Presentation

A 50-year-old East Indian woman with a 6-month history of lower back pain, fatigue, and unintentional weight loss was referred to our surgical outpatient clinic upon detection

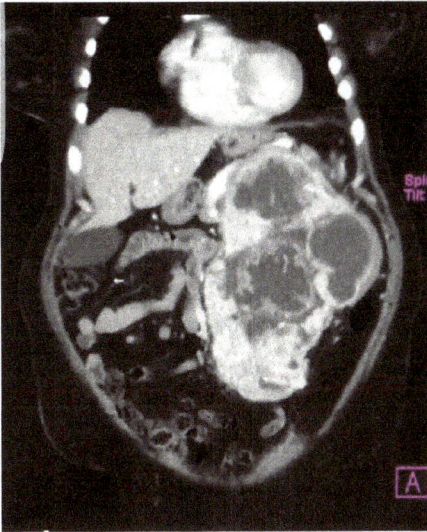

FIGURE 1: CT scan showing a 23 cm, thick-walled, multicystic mass occupying most of the left upper quadrant of the abdomen.

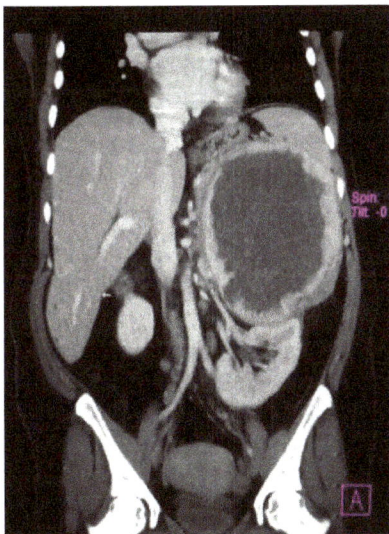

FIGURE 2: Coronal CT image demonstrating the mass displacing the left kidney inferiorly. Evidence of locally invasive disease was not present.

TABLE 1: Biochemical investigations confirming the pheochromocytoma diagnosis.

	Patient values	Normal values
Test (fractionated plasma)		
Metanephrine	259 pg/mL	<58 pg/mL
Normetanephrine	4603 pg/mL	<149 pg/mL
Total metanephrine	4862 pg/mL	<206 pg/mL
Epinephrine	16 pg/mL	<84 pg/mL
Norepinephrine	509 pg/mL	<420 pg/mL
Dopamine	<30 pg/mL	<60 pg/mL
Total catecholamines	525 pg/mL	<504 pg/mL
Test (24-hour urine values)		
Total catecholamines	131 ug/24 hr	<100 ug/24 hr
Norepinephrine	120 ug/24 hr	<80 ug/24 hr
Epinephrine	11 ug/24 hr	<20 ug/24 hr
Dopamine	466 ug/24 hr	<500 ug/24 hr
Vanillylmandelate (VMA)	88.3 ug/24 hr	3.8–6.7 mg/24 hr
Creatinine	1.47 ug/24 hr	0.63–2.50 g/24 hr

of a large abdominal mass during an abdominal ultrasound. The mass was located in the left upper quadrant and thought to be possibly splenic or renal in origin. Physical examination revealed a large nontender lump arising from the left upper quadrant and crossing the midline. Initial laboratory investigations were unremarkable except for microcytic anemia with a mean corpuscular hemoglobin concentration (MCHC) of 7.3 g/dL. The patient had no history of hypertension, headache, palpitations, or excessive sweating and no family history of cancer.

Computed tomography (CT) revealed a 23.2 × 17.6 × 13.6 cm mass with predominant areas of necrosis, punctate areas of calcification, and irregular contours superior to the left kidney (Figures 1 and 2). The mass displaced the

pancreas anteriorly and compressed the left kidney inferiorly. The nonvisualization of a normal left adrenal gland strongly suggested an adrenocortical carcinoma. The liver, spleen, right adrenal gland, and right kidney were normal. Despite mesenteric and para-aortic lymphadenopathy there was no evidence of distant metastasis. Preoperative biopsy was not performed, due to the risk of tumor seeding along the biopsy path.

The tumor markers carcinoembryonic antigen, carbohydrate antigen (CA) 15-3, CA 19-9, and CA 125 were normal. The differential diagnosis included adrenocortical carcinoma, pheochromocytoma, myelolipoma, metastasis from an unidentified primary tumor, sarcoma, and lymphoma. Biochemical investigations were performed to exclude a functional adrenal mass, and the diagnosis of pheochromocytoma was made upon observation of elevated plasma free metanephrines, urine catecholamines, and their metabolites (Table 1).

Preoperatively, the patient was transfused with packed red blood cells to stable hemoglobin of 10 g/dL. Adequate catecholamine blockade was achieved, after medical consultation using the alpha adrenergic blocker, terazosin (Hytrin). An open left adrenalectomy was performed through a Chevron incision extending to the left flank. The mass was completely resected en bloc with the spleen, distal pancreas, left kidney, and a 2 cm area of the left hemidiaphragm (Figure 3). Intraoperatively, there were significant fluctuations in the patient's blood pressure, which was well managed by the surgical team. There were no other significant surgical complications and the patient made an uneventful recovery prior to discharge on postoperative day 11. Three months later, at the time of this report, the patient remains stable and disease-free. Given that there is recurrence in approximately 10% of these cases, long-term follow-up with CT scans and hematologic monitoring is warranted.

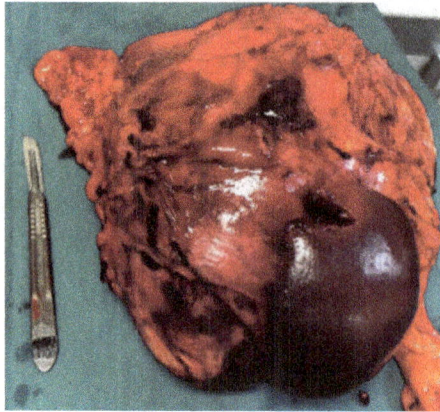

FIGURE 3: En bloc resection of the left adrenal mass, pancreatic tail, spleen, and left kidney.

Pathological examination of the surgical specimen revealed a circumscribed mass, surrounded by a variably thick fibrous capsule/pseudocapsule with relatively scantly attached fat, measuring $27 \times 18 \times 12$ cm and weighing 3,315 g (Figure 3). Residual normal-appearing adrenal gland parenchyma was present, while neither infiltration of the surrounding fat, vascular invasion, nor confluent tumor necrosis was identified. Mitoses were rare (<1 per high-power field). Histological sections revealed typical morphological features of PCC predominantly characterized by nests of plump tumor cells with abundant basophilic granular cytoplasm surrounded by sustentacular cells (Figure 4(a)). No unfavorable features such as diffuse growth pattern, increased cellularity, or increased pleomorphism were observed. The spleen, distal pancreas, and kidney did not show any pathologic abnormalities. Immunohistochemical staining revealed that the tumor cells were diffusely positive for chromogranin A (Figure 4(b)), while there was no significant highlighting of sustentacular cells by S-100. Of note, the lack of prominent staining of sustentacular cells by S-100 has been suggested to be predictive of nonfamilial sporadic PCC [38].

To determine the clinicopathological features of giant PCCs, an extensive literature search of the PubMed/MEDLINE and Embase databases was conducted. Search terms included "giant pheochromocytoma", "cystic giant pheochromocytoma", "English language" and "case reports". One case in which the tumor lacked dimensions but was found to be one of the heaviest PCCs recorded was included. Full texts were accessed to confirm eligibility for inclusion. A summary of the 36 final cases are presented in Table 2. Relative to the others, our patient's tumor was the fourth heaviest with the fifth greatest maximal diameter and the largest histologically confirmed pheochromocytoma with a low risk of malignancy/benign classification. Unlike patients with classical symptoms, those with giant PCCs may be asymptomatic as occurred in 31% (=11) of the cases. Twenty-two % (=8) and 17% (=6) of the cases presented with hypertension and back/abdominal pain, respectively. Only one case had evidence of metastasis at the time of diagnosis, characterized by invasion of the right lobe of the liver [5].

Twenty-two percent (=8) of the cases presented at similar locations, commonly in the left abdomen. The mean age at diagnosis was 49.46 years (range 12–85 years) which was the age of our patient.

3. Discussion

Pheochromocytomas are neoplasms that arise from the chromaffin cells of the sympathoadrenal system [39]. Eighty-five percent of these lesions arise in the adrenal medulla [40]. Sporadic cases of PCC usually present in the fourth to fifth decades of life. Various hereditary conditions such as multiple endocrine neoplasia 2A and 2B, Von Hippel-Lindau syndrome, and neurofibromatosis 1 are associated with increased risk for PCC [41]. There are no known environmental, dietary, or lifestyle risk factors that impact the risk of developing PCC. The classic tetrad of symptoms consists of palpitations, headaches, sweating, and hypertension. However, approximately 49–57% of PCC patients are asymptomatic with an adrenal mass being detected incidentally during unrelated imaging.

The malignant potential of a PCC cannot be determined preoperatively unless there is evidence of local invasion or metastases at the time of diagnosis. Previously, it was believed that size was a predictor of malignant potential; however, with numerous case reports of giant benign PCCs, size can no longer be used as a definitive indicator of aggressive disease [42]. Histologically, the PASS is referenced to distinguish tumors of high from those with a low risk of malignancy [43]. This scoring system assesses vascular invasion, capsular invasion, extension into the periadrenal adipose tissue, the presence of focal or confluent necrosis, high cellularity, tumor cell spindling, cellular monotony, >3 mitoses per high-power field, atypical mitotic figures, profound nuclear pleomorphism, and increased tumor cell hyperchromasia [43]. Biologically aggressive tumors have been found to have a PASS ≥ 4 whereas lesions with a low risk of malignancy have a PASS < 4. Our patient harbored a giant PCC with a low risk of malignancy as noted by the PASS of 2.

Approximately 20 to 30% of all PCCs are clinically silent [12]. Factors that contribute to the lack of symptoms include extensive necrosis of the adrenal gland, decreasing the production of catecholamines and the retention of these hormones within the capsular mass after secretion. Consequently, the time to diagnosis is delayed and tumor size tends to be larger once it is detected. A recent report that reviewed 20 cases of PCCs larger than 10 cm reported that 13 presented with abdominal pain with only 5 presenting with any of the classical symptoms of PCCs [16].

Surgical resection is the only curative option for these giant lesions. Laparoscopic adrenalectomy is considered safe and effective for tumors up to 12 cm in its greatest dimensions. However, in the realm of these giant PCCs, open en bloc resection is required. Intraoperative manipulation of these tumors is frequently associated with profound hypertension. However, early isolation of the tumor's venous drainage decreases the risk of intraoperative hypertensive crises [36]. This must be coupled with catecholamine blockade and

TABLE 2: A summary of reported giant pheochromocytomas with maximal diameter greater than 10 cm, arranged by largest to smallest maximum diameter. The weight was not recorded in many of the papers.

Author/year	Sex/age	Country	Size (cm)/weight (g)	Location	Presentation	Histopathological evaluation	Metastasis
Grissom et al./1979 [4]	F/54	USA	45 × 25/3000+	Left abdomen	Asymptomatic	Unknown	None
Costa et al./2008 [5]	M/46	Brazil	30/unknown	Right adrenal	Abdominal pain	Malignant	Liver
Basso et al./1996 [6]	M/47	Italy	29 × 21 × 12/4050	Left abdomen	Asymptomatic	Malignant	None
Karumanchery et al./2012 [7]	F/85	England	28 × 16 × 13/2300	Left abdomen	Lower back pain	Unknown	None
Current case	F/50	Trinidad & Tobago	27 × 18 × 12/3315	Left abdomen	Lower back pain	Low risk of malignancy	None
Gupta et al./2016 [8]	F/65	India	25 × 17 × 15/2750	Left abdomen	Asymptomatic	Benign	None
Okuda et al./2013 [9]	F/43	Japan	24 × 23 × 16/5900	Abdomen	Vulva edema	Unknown	None
Suga et al./2000 [10]	M/48	Japan	21 × 13 × 21/3900	Left abdomen	Asymptomatic	Unknown	None
Terk et al./1993 [11]	M/35	USA	21 × 20 × 11/2870	Organ of Zuckerkandl	Disproportionate abdominal girth, hypertension	Unknown	None
Soufi et al./2012 [12]	F/17	India	21 × 15	Right upper abdomen	Asymptomatic	Malignant	None
Arcos et al./2009 [13]	F/36	Canada	21 × 17 × 11	Left abdomen	Lower back pain	Malignant	Lymph node
Melegh et al./2002 [14]	M/55	Hungary	20/unknown	Left renal hilus	Asymptomatic	Unknown	None
Korgali et al./2014 [15]	M/63	Turkey	20 × 17 × 9/1736	Left adrenal gland	Chest pain, sweating, nausea	Malignant	Rib
Ambati et al./2014 [16]	F/77	Canada	19 × 18 × 12/2460	Right retroperitoneum	Dyspnea	Benign	None
Pan et al./2008 [17]	M/46	USA	18 × 14 × 13/1450	Left abdomen	Episodic hypertension and headache	Unknown	Unknown
Uysal et al./2015 [18]	M/37	Turkey	18 × 8 × 13	Left abdomen	Hypertension	Malignant	Multiorgan*
Sharma/2006 [19]	M/55	India	17 × 12/850	Right adrenal gland	Asymptomatic	Benign	None
Daughtry et al./1977 [20]	M/53	USA	17/1150	Unknown	Mild hypertension	Unknown	Unknown
Gupta et al./2016 [8]	M/40	India	16.4 × 14/1836	Left thyroid gland	Severe hypertension	Unknown	Unknown
Costa et al./2008 [5]	F/43	Brazil	16	Right upper abdomen	Abdominal pain	Malignant	Unknown

TABLE 2: Continued.

Author/year	Sex/age	Country	Size (cm)/weight (g)	Location	Presentation	Histopathological evaluation	Metastasis
Jain and Agarwal /2002 [21]	F/26	India	16 × 11	Left abdomen	Asymptomatic	Malignant	Unknown
Wu et al./2000 [22]	F/49	USA	15 × 12 × 12	Right upper abdomen	Asymptomatic	Unknown	Unknown
Santarone et al./2008 [23]	F/81	Italy	13	Right upper abdomen	Hypertension, palpitation, sweating	Unknown	Unknown
Sundahl et al./2016 [24]	F/54	Sweden	12.5 × 10 × 3/204	Right adrenal gland	Asymptomatic	Benign	None
Zhu et al./2014 [25]	F/67	Japan	12.1 × 10.8	Left adrenal gland	Dizziness, vomiting, and stomachache	Unknown	None
Ikegami et al./2009 [26]	M/47	Japan	12 × 10	Abdomen	Back pain	Unknown	Unknown
Li et al./2012 [27]	M/56	Canada	12 × 11 × 11	Right upper abdomen	Progressive weight loss and nausea	Benign	None
Kakoki et al./2015 [28]	M/70	Japan	12 × 11 × 8/530	Left adrenal gland	Ileus after hypertension medication	Benign	None
Schnakenburg et al./1976 [29]	M/12	Ukraine	12 × 10 × 9/1100	Right abdomen	Hemihypertrophy	Malignant	Lung, brain
Filippou et al./2003 [30]	M/70	Greece	12 × 8 × 10	Left abdomen	Asymptomatic	Malignant	None
Sarveswaran et al./2015 [31]	F/59	India	11.2 × 9.6 × 9.8	Right suprarenal region	Upper right abdominal discomfort	Unknown	Unknown
Chan et al./2000 [32]	M/63	China	11 × 6.6 × 11	Right suprarenal region	Asymptomatic	Malignant	Bone, lung
Awada et al./2003 [33]	F/26	USA	11 × 10 × 9	Right adrenal gland	Dyspnea, paresthesia, chest pain, palpitation	Unknown	Unknown
Goldberg et al./2011 [34]	F/27	Canada	10.5 × 10.6	Right adrenal gland region	Headaches, episodic palpitations, pallor	Unknown	Unknown
Antedomenico and Wascher/2005 [35]	F/39	USA	10.5/782	Left upper abdomen	Abdominal pain	Unknown	Unknown
Wang et al./2015 [36]	F/36	China	10.3 × 9.3	Left upper abdomen	Abdominal pain	Unknown	Unknown
Basiri and Radfar/2010 [37]	M/53	Iran	Unknown/3150	Left abdomen	Abdominal pain	Benign	None

M, male; F, female. * Liver, lymph nodes, right adrenal gland, lungs, and bones.

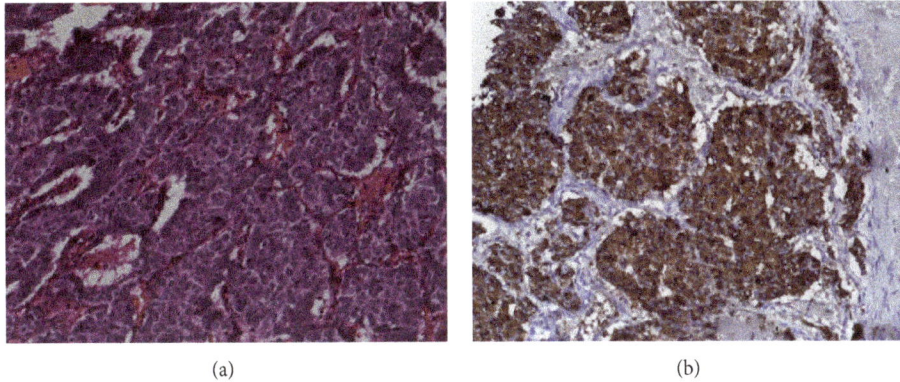

(a) (b)

FIGURE 4: Microscopic images of pheochromocytoma. (a) Routine hematoxylin and eosin (H&E) staining at low magnification (20x) highlights the typical "Zellballen" growth pattern characterized by nests of tumor cells surrounded by delicate fibrovascular stroma. (b) Immunohistochemistry for the neuroendocrine marker chromogranin A shows strong, diffuse staining in the tumor cells.

intravenous fluids to diminish the risk of postoperative hypotension. It is therefore critical to have good coordination between the anesthesiologist and surgeon before and during surgery. Intensive care monitoring is crucial for at least 24 hours postoperatively as it is common for patients to experience fluctuations in blood pressure and heart rate as well as hypoglycemia. Pheochromocytomas have an excellent prognosis, with 5-year survival exceeding 95% in benign tumors and a recurrence rate of less than 10% [44]. Statistical data are not available for malignant PCCs due to their low incidence.

4. Conclusion

In this report, we presented the case of a 50-year-old female with a giant PCC that was the fourth heaviest and had the fifth largest maximal diameter of all reported PCCs. Additionally, using our search criteria, the tumor had the largest maximal diameter of reported, histologically confirmed PCCs with a low risk of malignancy. Our patient, 3 months after resection of the tumor, remains stable and disease-free. Giant PCCs do not present with the classical symptoms associated with smaller PCCs and are usually associated with a lower risk of malignancy. Previously, larger size was believed to be an indicator of malignancy in these adrenal lesions; however, upon review of the 10 largest known PCCs, this belief was unsubstantiated.

Acknowledgments

Wayne A. Warner was supported by Washington University School of Medicine, St. Louis (Grant no. GSAS/CGFP, Fund 94028C).

References

[1] E. L. Bravo and R. W. Gifford Jr., "Pheochromocytoma: diagnosis, localization and management," *The New England Journal of Medicine*, vol. 311, no. 20, pp. 1298–1303, 1984.

[2] M. Lefebvre and W. D. Foulkes, "Pheochromocytoma and paraganglioma syndromes: genetics and management update," *Current Oncology*, vol. 21, no. 1, pp. e8–e17, 2014.

[3] M. A. Nguyen-Martin and G. D. Hammer, "Pheochromocytoma: an update on risk groups, diagnosis, and management," *Hospital Physician*, vol. 42, no. 2, pp. 17–24, 2006.

[4] J. R. Grissom, H. T. Yamase, and P. R. Prosser, "Giant pheochromocytoma with sarcoidosis," *Southern Medical Journal*, vol. 72, no. 12, pp. 1605–1607, 1979.

[5] S. R. P. Costa, N. M. Cabral, A. T. Abhrão, R. B. da Costa, L. M. da Silva, and R. A. Lupinacci, "Giant cystic malignant pheochromocytoma invading right hepatic lobe: report on two cases," *Sao Paulo Medical Journal*, vol. 126, no. 4, pp. 229–231, 2008.

[6] L. Basso, L. Lepre, M. Melillo, F. Fora, P. L. Mingazzini, and A. Tocchi, "Giant phaeochromocytoma: case report," *Irish Journal of Medical Science*, vol. 165, no. 1, pp. 57–59, 1996.

[7] R. Karumanchery, J. R. Nair, A. Hakeem, and R. Hardy, "An unusual case of back pain: a large Pheochromocytoma in an 85 year old woman," *International Journal of Surgery Case Reports*, vol. 3, no. 1, pp. 16–18, 2012.

[8] A. Gupta, L. Bains, M. K. Agarwal, and R. Gupta, "Giant cystic pheochromocytoma: a silent entity," *Urology Annals*, vol. 8, no. 3, pp. 384–386, 2016.

[9] K. Okuda, T. Nishizawa, T. Oshima, and K. Misawa, "A case of cystic pheochromocytoma weighing 5,900 g," *Nihon Rinsho Geka Gakkai Zasshi*, vol. 74, no. 4, pp. 1075–1080, 2013.

[10] K. Suga, K. Motoyama, A. Hara, N. Kume, M. Ariga, and N. Matsunaga, "Tc-99m MIBG imaging in a huge clinically silent pheochromocytoma with cystic degeneration and massive hemorrhage," *Clinical Nuclear Medicine*, vol. 25, no. 10, pp. 796–800, 2000.

[11] M. R. Terk, H. de Verdier, and P. M. Colletti, "Giant extra-adrenal pheochromocytoma: magnetic resonance imaging with

gadolinium-DTPA enhancement," *Magnetic Resonance Imaging*, vol. 11, no. 1, pp. 47–50, 1993.

[12] M. Soufi, M. K. Lahlou, S. Benamr et al., "Giant malignant cystic pheochromocytoma: a case report," *Indian Journal of Surgery*, vol. 74, no. 6, pp. 504–506, 2012.

[13] C. T. Arcos, V. R. Luque, J. A. Luque, P. M. García, A. B. Jiménez, and M. M. Muñoz, "Malignant giant pheochromocytoma: a case report and review of the literature," *Journal of the Canadian Urological Association*, vol. 3, no. 6, pp. E89–E91, 2009.

[14] Z. Melegh, F. Rényi-Vámos, Z. Tanyay, I. Köves, and Z. Orosz, "Giant cystic pheochromocytoma located in the renal hilus," *Pathology Research and Practice*, vol. 198, no. 2, pp. 103–106, 2002.

[15] E. Korgali, G. Dundar, G. Gokce et al., "Giant malignant pheochromocytoma with palpable rib metastases," *Case Reports in Urology*, vol. 2014, Article ID 354687, 4 pages, 2014.

[16] D. Ambati, K. Jana, and T. Domes, "Largest pheochromocytoma reported in Canada: a case study and literature review," *Canadian Urological Association Journal*, vol. 8, no. 5-6, pp. E374–E377, 2014.

[17] Z. Pan, S. Repertinger, C. Deng, and P. Sharma, "A giant cystic pheochromocytoma of the adrenal gland," *Endocrine Pathology*, vol. 19, no. 2, pp. 133–138, 2008.

[18] E. Uysal, T. Kirdak, A. O. Gürer, and M. A. İkidağ, "Giant multicystic malignant pheochromocytoma," *Turkish Journal of Surgery*, 2015.

[19] P. P. Sharma, "Pheochromocytoma: a composite resection," *Indian Journal of Surgery*, vol. 68, no. 3, pp. 163–164, 2006.

[20] J. D. Daughtry, L. P. Susan, R. A. Straffon, and B. H. Stewart, "A case of a giant pheochromocytoma," *Journal of Urology*, vol. 118, no. 5, pp. 840–842, 1977.

[21] S. K. Jain and N. Agarwal, "Asymptomatic giant pheochromocytoma," *Journal of Association of Physicians of India*, vol. 50, no. 6, pp. 842–844, 2002.

[22] J. Wu, S. N. Ahya, M. D. Reploeg et al., "Pheochromocytoma presenting as a giant cystic tumor of the liver," *Surgery*, vol. 128, no. 3, pp. 482–484, 2000.

[23] M. Santarone, C. Borghi, E. Miglierina, S. Senatore, and G. Corrado, "Giant cystic pheochromocytoma," *Journal of Cardiovascular Medicine*, vol. 9, no. 9, pp. 971–972, 2008.

[24] N. Sundahl, S. Van Slycke, and N. Brusselaers, "A rare case of clinically and biochemically silent giant right pheochromocytoma: case report and review of literature," *Acta Chirurgica Belgica*, vol. 116, no. 4, pp. 239–242, 2016.

[25] D. Zhu, J. Yu, X. Li, X. Jiang, and C. Zhuang, "Takotsubo-like cardiomyopathy in a giant pheochromocytoma," *International Journal of Cardiology*, vol. 176, no. 3, pp. e113–e116, 2014.

[26] Y. Ikegami, Y. Tsukada, M. Abe, Y. Abe, and C. Tase, "Delayed shock after minor blunt trauma due to myocarditis caused by occult giant pheochromocytoma," *The Journal of Trauma: Injury, Infection, and Critical Care*, vol. 67, no. 3, pp. E65–E68, 2009.

[27] C. Li, Y. Chen, W. Wang, and L. Teng, "A case of clinically silent giant right pheochromocytoma and review of literature," *Canadian Urological Association Journal*, vol. 6, no. 6, pp. E267–E269, 2012.

[28] K. Kakoki, Y. Miyata, Y. Shida et al., "Pheochromocytoma multisystem crisis treated with emergency surgery: a case report and literature review Case Reports," *BMC Research Notes*, vol. 8, no. 1, article 758, 2015.

[29] K. V. Schnakenburg, M. Müller, K. Dörner et al., "Congenital hemihypertrophy and malignant giant pheochromocytoma— a previously undescribed coincidence," *European Journal of Pediatrics*, vol. 122, no. 4, pp. 263–273, 1976.

[30] D. C. Filippou, S. Rizos, A. Nissiotis, and V. Papadopoulos, "A rare case of clinically silent giant pheochromocytoma," *The Internet Journal of Oncology*, vol. 2, no. 1, 2003.

[31] V. Sarveswaran, S. Kumar, A. Kumar, and M. Vamseedharan, "A giant cystic pheochromocytoma mimicking liver abscess an unusual presentation—a case report," *Clinical Case Reports*, vol. 3, no. 1, pp. 64–68, 2015.

[32] F. K. W. Chan, K. L. Choi, S. C. Tiu, C. C. Shek, and T. K. Au Yong, "A case of giant malignant phaeochromocytoma," *Hong Kong Medical Journal*, vol. 6, no. 3, pp. 325–328, 2000.

[33] S. H. Awada, A. Grisham, and S. E. Woods, "Large dopamine-secreting pheochromocytoma: case report," *Southern Medical Journal*, vol. 96, no. 9, pp. 914–917, 2003.

[34] A. Goldberg, S. E. Pautler, C. Harle et al., "Giant cystic pheochromocytoma containing high concentrations of catecholamines and metanephrines," *The Journal of Clinical Endocrinology & Metabolism*, vol. 96, no. 8, pp. 2308–2309, 2011.

[35] E. Antedomenico and R. A. Wascher, "A case of mistaken identity: giant cystic pheochromocytoma," *Current Surgery*, vol. 62, no. 2, pp. 193–198, 2005.

[36] H.-L. Wang, B.-Z. Sun, Z.-J. Xu, W.-F. Lei, and X.-S. Wang, "Undiagnosed giant cystic pheochromocytoma: a case report," *Oncology Letters*, vol. 10, no. 3, pp. 1444–1446, 2015.

[37] A. Basiri and M. H. Radfar, "Giant cystic pheochromocytoma," *Urology Journal*, vol. 7, no. 1, p. 16, 2010.

[38] R. V. Lloyd, M. Blaivas, and B. S. Wilson, "Distribution of chromogranin and S100 protein in normal and abnormal adrenal medullary tissues," *Archives of Pathology & Laboratory Medicine*, vol. 109, no. 7, pp. 633–635, 1985.

[39] L. C. Pederson and J. E. Lee, "Pheochromocytoma," *Current Treatment Options in Oncology*, vol. 4, no. 4, pp. 329–337, 2003.

[40] P. L. M. Dahia, "Evolving concepts in pheochromocytoma and paraganglioma," *Current Opinion in Oncology*, vol. 18, no. 1, pp. 1–8, 2006.

[41] L. Fishbein and K. L. Nathanson, "Pheochromocytoma and paraganglioma: understanding the complexities of the genetic background," *Cancer Genetics*, vol. 205, no. 1-2, pp. 1–11, 2012.

[42] J. Park, C. Song, M. Park et al., "Predictive characteristics of malignant pheochromocytoma," *Korean Journal of Urology*, vol. 52, no. 4, pp. 241–246, 2011.

[43] G. Eisenhofer, S. R. Bornstein, F. M. Brouwers et al., "Malignant pheochromocytoma: current status and initiatives for future progress," *Endocrine-Related Cancer*, vol. 11, no. 3, pp. 423–436, 2004.

[44] N. Reisch, M. Peczkowska, A. Januszewicz, and H. P. H. Neumann, "Pheochromocytoma: presentation, diagnosis and treatment," *Journal of Hypertension*, vol. 24, no. 12, pp. 2331–2339, 2006.

30

Gastric Linitis Plastica and Peritoneal Carcinomatosis as First Manifestations of Occult Breast Carcinoma: A Case Report and Literature Review

Mara Mantiero [1,2] Giovanni Faggioni,[1] Alice Menichetti,[1,2] Matteo Fassan,[3]
Valentina Guarneri,[1,2] and Pierfranco Conte[1,2]

[1]Medical Oncology Unit 2, Istituto Oncologico Veneto, IRCCS, Padova, Italy
[2]Department of Surgical, Oncological and Gastroenterological Sciences, University of Padova, Padova, Italy
[3]Department of Medicine, Surgical Pathology & Cytopathology Unit, University of Padova, Padova, Italy

Correspondence should be addressed to Mara Mantiero; mara.mantiero@hotmail.it

Academic Editor: Constantine Gennatas

Gastric linitis plastica is a diffuse involvement of the stomach walls by neoplastic cells. It represents about 3–19% of primitive gastric adenocarcinomas, but it can also be the manifestation of a metastatic disease. Breast cancer is the most frequent malignancy in women, and the metastatic spread to the stomach occurs in less than 10% of the cases. We present an unusual case of gastric linitis plastica and peritoneal carcinomatosis as manifestations of an occult breast cancer in a 53-year-old woman. Imaging and endoscopic evaluation were not able to discriminate a primary from a secondary gastric lesion. The histological evaluation excluded the diagnosis of a primary gastric neoplasia. The IHC profile was consistent with the diagnosis of metastases from the breast cancer. Due to the hormonal receptors' positivity, we started therapy with fulvestrant (500 mg, day 0, 14, and 28 and every 28 days thereafter by intramuscular injection). After 20 months, the same therapy is still ongoing and well tolerated, while the patient is in good condition with improvement of the dysphagia. Almost 2 years after the diagnosis of linitis plastica, the primitive breast lesion is still occult.

1. Introduction

Metastatic cancer of unknown primary (CUP site syndrome) is characterized by the presence of the metastatic lesion without the primitive carcinoma. It accounts for 3–5% of all solid malignant tumours, and the prognosis is generally poor [1]. Only microscopic analysis, with histological and immunohistochemical exam, can define the primary origin of the lesion, and it is fundamental for the clinician to define the correct treatment plan. The discussion with the pathologist is essential.

Metastasis from breast cancer to the gastrointestinal tract is rare, less than 10% [2], and typically occurs many years after the diagnosis.

We present an unusual case of gastric linitis plastica and peritoneal carcinomatosis as first manifestations of an occult breast cancer. The correct identification of the primary origin of the lesion was crucial to avoid a potentially useless gastric surgery.

2. Case Presentation

In March 2016, a 53-year-old premenopausal woman was admitted to our institute with the diagnosis of gastric linitis plastica and peritoneal carcinomatosis. She presented with upper abdominal pain, dyspepsia, nausea, and daily postprandial vomiting with weight loss of approximately 4 kilograms in 2 months. The Eastern Cooperative Oncology Group (ECOG) performance status (PS) was 2. Her medical history was negative for oncologic diseases, and she had no relevant comorbidities; no history of *Helicobacter pylori*-associated gastritis. At clinical examination, she presented with epigastric tenderness and no mass. Blood tests were within the normal values, with the exception of CA15.3

(211 U/ml) and CEA (11.1 ng/ml). Abdominal computed tomography (CT) revealed an increased wall thickness of the pyloric antrum along with mesenteric lymphadenopathy (20 mm) and peritoneal carcinomatosis. No liver metastases were detected. At esophagogastroduodenoscopy (EGDS), a severe pyloric stenosis was reported in the absence of mucosal lesions. The clinical manifestation was strongly suggestive of linitis plastica. Several gastric biopsies were performed, and histology concluded for a diffuse localization of epithelial cancer. Immunohistochemistry excluded gastrointestinal origin. There was a strong immunoreactivity for estrogen and progesterone receptors (ER-PgR: 80%-80%), GATA3 (3+), and cytokeratin (CK) 7, 8, 18, and 19; the human epithelial growth factor receptor 2 (HER2) was negative (1+) and the Ki67 index was <5%. Histological exam concluded for metastatic breast cancer with gastric linitis plastica.

A complete breast radiological investigation including bilateral ultrasound and mammography, and magnetic resonance imaging excluded the presence of breast abnormalities. Multiple bilateral suspicious axillary lymph nodes (maximum diameter of approximately 10 mm) were identified at ultrasonography and MRI. A fine-needle aspiration of a right axillary lymph node was performed, and cytology was positive for epithelial malignant cells.

To definitively exclude a gastrointestinal origin of the neoplasm, the patient also underwent laparoscopic peritoneal biopsy. Histological and immunohistochemical studies confirmed breast origin. After the multidisciplinary discussion, a surgical approach was excluded. A Witzel feeding jejunostomy was created.

All international breast cancer guidelines recommend endocrine therapy in luminal metastatic breast cancer without visceral crisis. Our patient, after jejunostomy creation and starting of enteral nutrition, was asymptomatic, and so, in April 2016, hormone therapy with fulvestrant was started (500 mg, day 0, 14, and 28 and every 28 days thereafter by intramuscular injection). We decided on intramuscular therapy to overcome the patient's dysphagia.

After four months of hormone therapy, CT scan was performed and reported stable disease. The patient also experienced clinical improvement with weight increase (1 kg) and palliation of dysphagia. Sporadic postprandial vomiting was still present.

In January 2017, CA15.3 was normalized (3.8 U/ml) and a new EGDS with biopsies was performed. Histology confirmed localization of adenocarcinoma with immunohistochemistry ER 90%, PgR 35%, CK7 3+, gross cystic disease fluid protein 15 (GCDFP-15) 3+, and HER2 1+ (Figure 1).

The patient is still in a good clinical condition with ECOG PS 1 up to this day. Supportive enteral nutrition is still ongoing, but dysphagia has significantly improved. Hormone therapy with fulvestrant is still ongoing and well tolerated. The last radiological evaluation was performed in February 2018, and it showed a stable disease.

Additionally, because of a potential genetic correlation between diffuse gastric carcinoma and early-onset lobular breast carcinoma [3], we also performed a genetic evaluation and searched for CDH1 germline mutations, but no genetic abnormalities were identified. In our case, the absence of

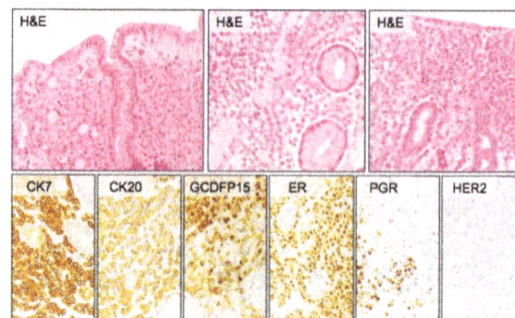

FIGURE 1: Histology confirmed localization of adenocarcinoma with immunohistochemistry: ER 90%, PgR 35%, CK7 3+, GCDFP-15 3+, and HER2 1+.

primitive lesion prevented any possibility of the histological subdefinition, although the lobular histological subtype is the most common cause of metastatic gastric linitis plastica caused by breast cancer [4].

3. Discussion

Breast cancer is the most common malignancy in women, accounting for about 30% of new diagnosis. Approximately 6–10% of new breast cancer cases are initially metastatic, and the most common sites of metastatization are the liver, lung, brain, and bone [5]. Metastases from breast cancer to the gastrointestinal tract are rare. Harris et al. published in 1984 the data about an autopsy series of 109 patients who died from breast cancer: 84% of them were metastatic and only 8.8% had gastric involvement [2].

Typically, metastatic spread to the gastrointestinal tract occurs many years after the diagnosis of breast cancer. In our case, it was at the onset of the disease. Gastric metastatization can have two different patterns of manifestation: nodular pattern with ulcerative masses, typical of invasive ductal carcinoma (IDC), or a diffuse mural involvement, typical of invasive lobular carcinoma (ILC). In the latter case, multiple and deep biopsies are recommended for the diagnosis because sometimes the scirrhous and fibrotic reaction can invade the gastric wall without mucosal involvement.

Although the cases described are not many, the lobular histological subtype is the most common cause of metastatic gastric linitis plastica caused by breast cancer [4]. Taal et al. performed a retrospective analysis in a 15-year period showing that 83% of patients with breast cancer and gastric metastasis have lobular histological subtype [6]. Rare cases of linitis plastica of the rectum as a possible clinical presentation of lobular breast carcinoma are also described [7–10]. However, the biological mechanism underlying this unusual correlation is not yet clear.

The presence of the metastatic lesion without primitive carcinoma represents a heterogeneous group defined as "carcinoma of unknown primary" (CUP). They account for 3–5% of all tumors, and the prognosis is poor [1]. Probably, these tumors acquire the capacity to metastasize before the development of a clinically evident primary lesion [11]. A historical autopsy study showed that the breast was the primary tumor site in CUP syndrome in only 2% of the cases [12, 13].

Immunohistochemistry is fundamental to correctly identify the primary site and, in our case, was essential to decide the therapeutic strategy. Since about 80% of human breast cancer cells express hormone receptors, ER and PR statuses are usually used as reliable markers for breast origin [14]. However, the primary gastric carcinomas can also express sex hormone receptors. According to Tokunaga and colleagues, the rates of positivity are about 26.6% for ER and 20.6% for PR [15]. In a more recent analysis by Matsui et al., the positivity is about 32% and 12% for ER and PR, respectively [16]. For this reason, their use, in association with other supplemental diagnostic markers, can improve the diagnostic accuracy. From an IHC point of view, breast cancer is positive for CK7 and CK18 and negative for CK20, as our patient. CK7 and CK20 are the first steps in the IHC markers' approach used in CUP syndrome. Cytoplasmatic positivity for GCDFP-15 is also highly specific (90%) to identify a malignant breast lesion. GCDFP-15 is a marker of apocrine differentiation and is detected in 62–72% of breast cancers [17, 18].

Probably in the future, the RNA microarray with gene expression tests will play an important role in the diagnosis of CUP. Su et al. defines a predictive algorithm using 110 genes expressed in the 11 most frequent malignancies. In their study, they have been able to predict the anatomical site of the tumor origin for 90% of the 175 carcinomas analyzed, including 9 of the 12 metastatic lesions [19]. The role of RNA profiling is evolving. More studies are ongoing, but the available data are still premature. More studies are needed to understand if gene expression can be different between primary and metastatic lesions.

The management of metastatic linitis plastica of the stomach is totally different from that of primary gastric carcinoma. Surgical resection is the first option for patients with primary gastric cancer without metastasis, but, in our case, gastric lesion was the manifestation of a systemic disease. All international breast cancer guidelines recommend endocrine therapy in luminal metastatic breast cancer without visceral crisis. For this reason, after the resolution of the symptoms with the jejunostomy creation, we decided to start systemic therapy with fulvestrant.

In conclusion, interaction between clinician and pathologist is important to select the correct IHC tests to perform.

Our goal in this case report is twofold: firstly, to improve the knowledge of surgeons and clinicians reminding them the need to rule out the possibility of a breast origin in women with gastric involvement, even in patients without a previous or concurrent history of breast carcinoma; secondly to increase the attention on immunohistochemical analysis.

To our knowledge, our case is the first published paper on CUP syndrome of breast cancer with this peculiar type of presentation. This case could be helpful with other clinicians due to its rarity and its unusual outcome.

Abbreviations

CUP: Carcinoma of unknown primary.

References

[1] K. Fizazi, F. A. Greco, N. Pavlidis, G. Daugaard, K. Oien, and G. Pentheroudakis, "Cancers of unknown primary site: ESMO Clinical Practice Guidelines for diagnosis, treatment and follow-up," *Annals of Oncology*, vol. 26, Supplement 5, pp. v133–v138, 2015.

[2] M. Harris, A. Howell, M. Chrissohou, R. I. Swindell, M. Hudson, and R. A. Sellwood, "A comparison of the metastatic pattern of infiltrating lobular carcinoma and infiltrating duct carcinoma of the breast," *British Journal of Cancer*, vol. 50, no. 1, pp. 23–30, 1984.

[3] G. Corso, M. Intra, C. Trentin, P. Veronesi, and V. Galimberti, "CDH1 germline mutations and hereditary lobular breast cancer," *Familial Cancer*, vol. 15, no. 2, pp. 215–219, 2016.

[4] B. G. Taal, H. Peterse, and H. Boot, "Clinical presentation, endoscopic features and treatment of gastric metastases from breast carcinoma," *Cancer*, vol. 89, no. 11, pp. 2214–2221, 2000.

[5] M. C. Cummings, P. T. Simpson, L. E. Reid et al., "Metastatic progression of breast cancer: insights from 50 years of autopsies," *The Journal of Pathology*, vol. 232, no. 1, pp. 23–31, 2014.

[6] B. G. Taal, F. C. A. den Hartog Jager, R. Steinmetz, and H. Peterse, "The spectrum of gastrointestinal metastases of breast carcinoma: I. Stomach," *Gastrointestinal Endoscopy*, vol. 38, no. 2, pp. 130–135, 1992.

[7] F. Venturini, V. Gambi, S. Di Lernia et al., "Linitis plastica of the rectum as a clinical presentation of metastatic lobular carcinoma of the breast," *Journal of Clinical Oncology*, vol. 34, no. 7, pp. e54–e56, 2016.

[8] K. Yanagisawa, M. Yamamoto, E. Ueno, and N. Ohkouchi, "Synchronous rectal metastasis from invasive lobular carcinoma of the breast," *Journal of Gastroenterology and Hepatology*, vol. 22, no. 4, pp. 601-602, 2007.

[9] A. J. Cano-Maldonado, M. Diaz-Tie, E. Vives-Rodriguez et al., "Rectal metastasis of lobular breast carcinoma," *Revista Española de Enfermedades Digestivas*, vol. 100, no. 7, pp. 440–442, 2008.

[10] R. Arrangoiz, P. Papavasiliou, H. Dushkin, and J. M. Farma, "Case report and literature review: metastatic lobular carcinoma of the breast – an unusual presentation," *International Journal of Surgery Case Reports*, vol. 2, no. 8, pp. 301–305, 2011.

[11] A. Kramer, G. Hubner, A. Schneeweiss, G. Folprecht, and K. Neben, "Carcinoma of unknown primary – an orphan disease?," *Breast Care*, vol. 3, no. 3, pp. 164–170, 2008.

[12] J. L. Abbruzzese, M. C. Abbruzzese, R. Lenzi, K. R. Hess, and M. N. Raber, "Analysis of a diagnostic strategy for patients with suspected tumors of unknown origin," *Journal of Clinical Oncology*, vol. 13, no. 8, pp. 2094–2103, 1995.

[13] T. Le Chevalier, E. Cvitkovic, P. Caille et al., "Early metastatic cancer of unknown primary origin at presentation. A clinical study of 302 consecutive autopsied patients," *Archives of Internal Medicine*, vol. 148, no. 9, pp. 2035–2039, 1988.

[14] L. de Decker, M. Campone, F. Retornaz et al., "Association between oestrogens receptor expressions in breast cancer and

comorbidities: a cross-sectional, population-based study," *PLoS One*, vol. 9, no. 5, article e98127, 2014.

[15] A. Tokunaga, K. Nishi, N. Matsukura et al., "Estrogen and progesterone receptors in gastric cancer," *Cancer*, vol. 57, no. 7, pp. 1376–1379, 1986.

[16] M. Matsui, O. Kojima, S. Kawakami, Y. Uehara, and T. Takahashi, "The prognosis of patients with gastric cancer possessing sex hormone receptors," *Surgery Today*, vol. 22, no. 5, pp. 421–425, 1992.

[17] O. Kaufmann, T. Deidesheimer, M. Muehlenberg, P. Deicke, and M. Dietel, "Immunohistochemical differentiation of metastatic breast carcinomas from metastatic adenocarcinomas of other common primary sites," *Histopathology*, vol. 29, no. 3, pp. 233–240, 1996.

[18] M. R. Wick, T. J. Lillemoe, G. T. Copland, P. E. Swanson, J. C. Manivel, and D. T. Kiang, "Gross cystic disease fluid protein-15 as a marker for breast cancer: immunohistochemical analysis of 690 human neoplasms and comparison with alpha-lactalbumin," *Human Pathology*, vol. 20, no. 3, pp. 281–287, 1989.

[19] A. I. Su, J. B. Welsh, L. M. Sapinoso et al., "Molecular classification of human carcinomas by use of gene expression signatures," *Cancer Research*, vol. 61, no. 20, pp. 7388–7393, 2001.

31

Adult Sporadic Burkitt's Lymphoma Presenting with Rapid Development of Peritoneal Lymphomatosis

Naomi Fei and Nilay Shah

Department of Internal Medicine, West Virginia University Hospital, 1 Medical Center Dr, Morgantown, WV 26505, USA

Correspondence should be addressed to Naomi Fei; naomi.fei@gmail.com

Academic Editor: Josep M. Ribera

Sporadic Burkitt's Lymphoma (BL) is a highly aggressive form of non-Hodgkin's lymphoma which requires prompt diagnosis and treatment. Though usual presentation involves abdominal lymphadenopathy with possible solid organ involvement, sporadic BL can rarely present with peritoneal lymphomatosis. We present a unique case with rapid evolution of BL presenting as peritoneal and omental lymphomatosis with hepatic lesions and pelvic and pericardial adenopathy.

1. Background

Burkitt's lymphoma (BL) is a highly aggressive subtype of B cell non-Hodgkin's lymphoma with a doubling time of 24 hours [1]. Sporadic BL is a clinical variant which comprises <1 percent of adult non-Hodgkin's lymphomas in the US [2]. Typical presentation includes abdominal symptoms of pain and distension secondary to ascites. Mesenteric and retroperitoneal lymph node enlargement is common. Extranodal involvement most commonly involves the GI tract and secondarily includes CNS, liver, spleen, kidneys, testis, and ovaries [1]. Peritoneal lymphomatosis is a rare presentation of extranodal lymphoma, usually associated with diffuse B cell lymphoma [3–5].

2. Case Report

An 18-year-old female, without significant medical history, presented with complaints of progressive abdominal pain and fullness. Additional symptoms included intermittent non-bloody vomiting, shortness of breath, fatigue, and low grade fevers. On physical examination, there was mild abdominal distension with tenderness to palpation in all 4 quadrants. No palpable masses were noted. No extremity edema was noted, and no cervical, axillary, or inguinal lymphadenopathy was present.

On laboratory evaluation, lactate dehydrogenase was markedly elevated (847 U/L) (nL 140–250 U/L) with uric acid (16.3 mg/dL) (nL 3–5.8 mg/dL). CA 125 level was found to be 637 U/mL (nL < 35). Additional labs were within normal limits including CBC/diff, BMP, and LFTs.

CT abdomen and US of abdomen performed one month priorly for similar complaints were without abnormalities. On repeat imaging during admission, computed tomography (CT) of the chest, abdomen, and pelvis was significant for extensive thickening, nodularity, and enhancement of the peritoneum and omentum, read as consistent with carcinomatosis (Figures 1–3). Additional findings included multiple bilobar attenuation hepatic lesions, pelvic and pericardial adenopathy, and moderate size bilateral pleural effusions. PET/CT was significant for hypermetabolic activity throughout peritoneal cavity with omental caking (Figures 4-5). Hypermetabolic liver lesions were noted with retrosternal and bilateral iliac chain nodes also suspicious for malignancy.

Peritoneal fluid cytology was consistent with CD10+ B cell population. Biopsy of omental and peritoneal implants was consistent with Burkitt's Lymphoma. Flow cytometry identified a CD10 positive, kappa-restricted B cell population. Immunohistochemistry found CD20 positive B cells without significant expression of *BCL-2*. Ki-67 was 100%. FISH was positive for *MYC/IGH*. EBV was found to be positive. Final

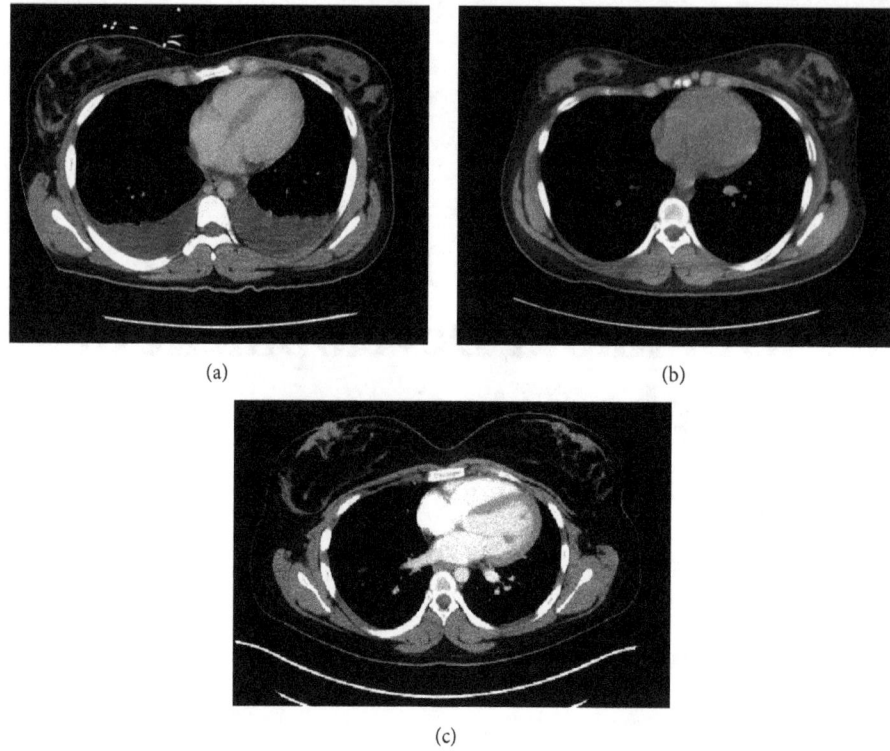

FIGURE 1: Contrast enhanced CT, axial view, upper chest. (a) Completed October 2016 with benign findings. (b) Completed November 2016 with moderate size bilateral pleural effusions. (c) Completed June 2017 with benign findings.

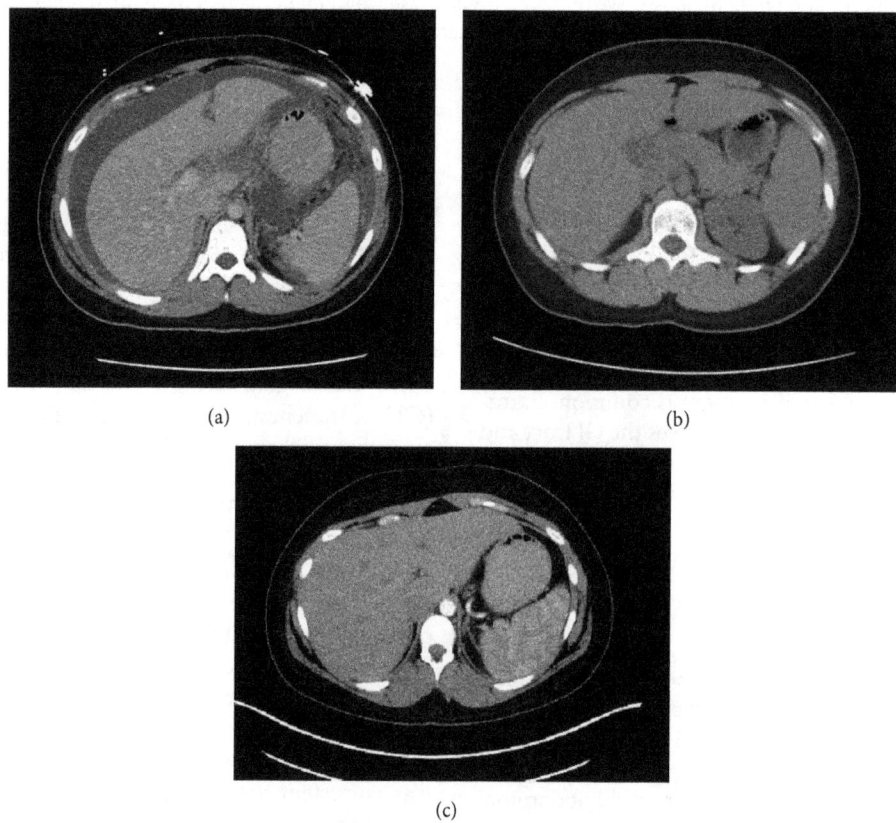

FIGURE 2: Contrast enhanced CT, axial view, upper abdomen. (a) Completed October 2016 with benign findings. (b) Completed November 2016 with multiple bilobar low attenuation indeterminate hepatic lesions. (c) Completed June 2017 with benign findings.

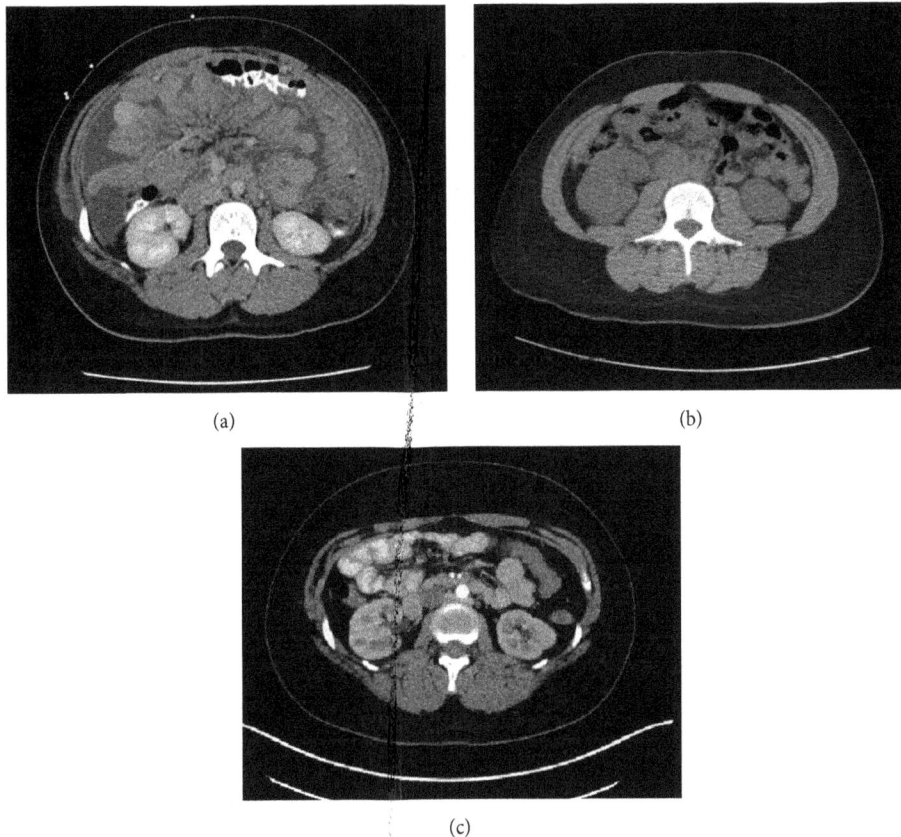

FIGURE 3: Contrast enhanced CT, axial view, mid abdomen. (a) Completed October 2016 with benign findings. (b) Completed November 2016 with extensive thickening, nodularity, and enhancement of the peritoneum and omentum. (c) Completed June 2017 with benign findings.

diagnosis was Ann Arbor stage IV Burkitt's lymphoma, with high-intermediate risk via International Prognostic Index (IPI) scoring.

Five days after presentation, the patient was started on R-Hyper-CVAD alternating with intrathecal MTX/Ara-C. Patient tolerated first 2 cycles well with follow-up PET/CT showing substantial resolution of patient's peritoneal involvement of malignancy and resolved liver lesions. Eight months after initiation of treatment, follow-up PET/CT was consistent with complete response.

3. Discussion

Burkitt's lymphoma (BL) is a highly aggressive subtype of B cell non-Hodgkin's lymphoma with a doubling time of 24 hours [1]. The protooncogene c-MYC on chromosome 8q24 is deregulated in BL allowing for disinhibition of many cell processes including cell growth, division, and death by apoptosis [6]. The World Health Organization (WHO) recognizes three clinical variants according to epidemiology, presentation, and genetic features: endemic, sporadic, and immunodeficiency associated [7].

Sporadic BL comprises <1 percent of adult non-Hodgkin's lymphomas in the US. Median age of diagnosis is 30 years. The majority of patients are male with a 3 or 4 : 1 male : female

ratio. Sporadic BL is more common among Caucasians than African or Asian Americans [2].

In adults, sporadic BL typically presents with abdominal symptoms of pain and distension secondary to ascites. Mesenteric and retroperitoneal lymph node enlargement is common. Extranodal involvement commonly includes the distal ileum, stomach, cecum and/or mesentery, kidney, testis, CNS, and ovaries [1]. Peritoneal lymphomatosis is a rare presentation of extranodal lymphoma, usually associated with diffuse B cell lymphoma [3–5]. On autopsy case series of disseminated lymphoma, 64 (20%) of 322 cases had peritoneal and omental disease [8].

Peritoneal thickening is more commonly caused by peritoneal carcinomatosis secondary to spread of a primary mucinous tumor. Alternative diagnoses of peritoneal thickening include malignant peritoneal mesothelioma and tuberculous peritonitis [9]. Correct interpretation of peritoneal and omental thickening is necessary in the setting of BL given its rapid progression and nonsurgical treatment. When evaluating peritoneal thickening, radiographic signs which favor lymphomatosis rather than carcinomatosis include omental caking with peritoneal and mesenteric soft tissue nodularity and enhancement [5, 10].

It is interesting to note the elevated CA-125 level with which the patient presented. CA-125, a transmembrane glycoprotein, is derived from the epithelia originating

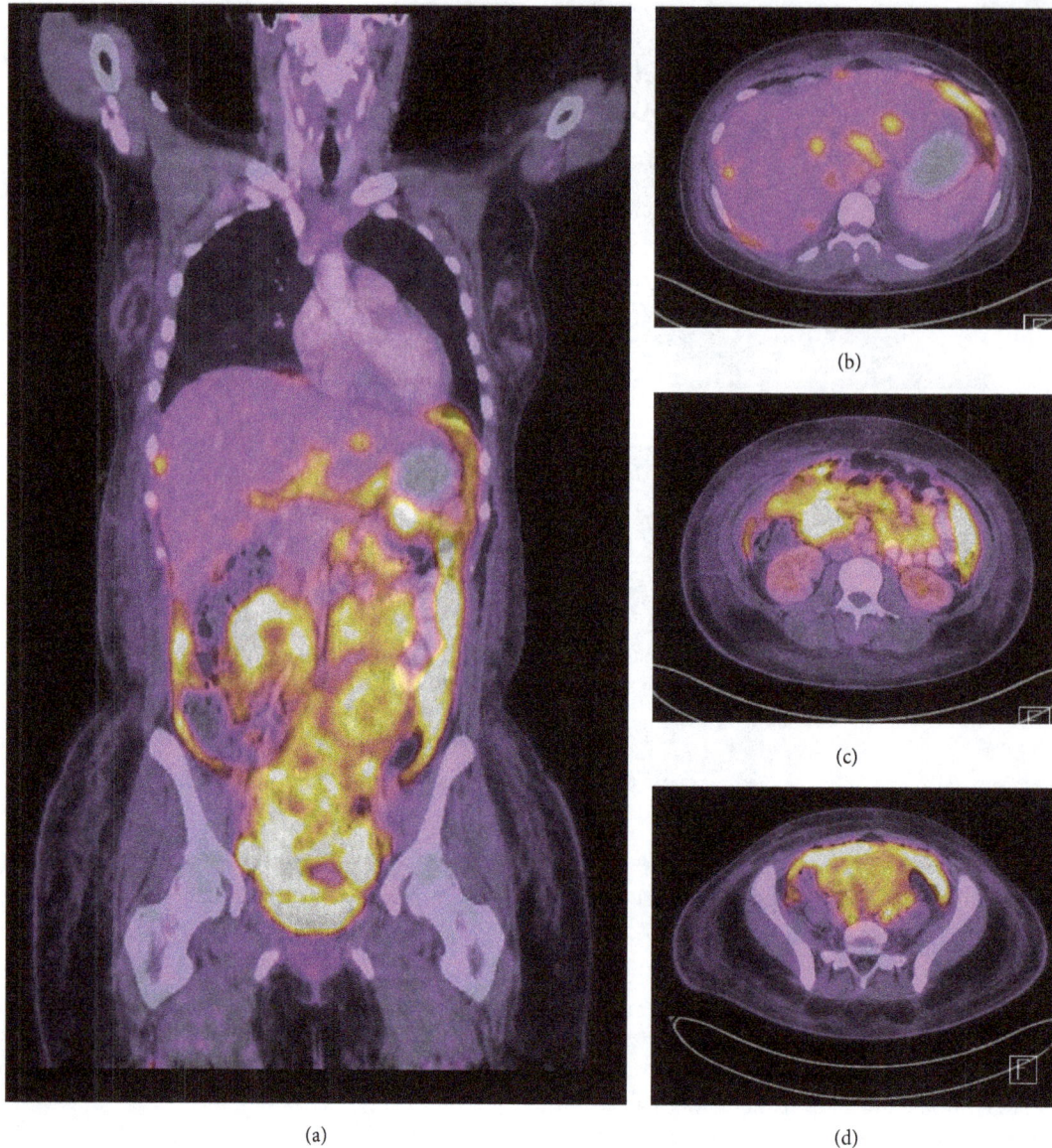

FIGURE 4: PET/CT imaging of the body performed in June 2017. (a) Coronal Body. (b) Axial upper abdomen. (c) Axial mid abdomen. (d) Axial low abdomen. Findings of diffuse and permeative abnormal hypermetabolic activity throughout the cavity corresponding to thickening and caking of the omentum and small pelvic free fluid. Hypermetabolic activity corresponding to multiple low attenuating liver lesions and retrosternal iliac chain nodes suspicious for malignancy.

from coelomic (pericardium, pleura, and peritoneum) and müllerian (fallopian tubal, endometrial, and endocervical) epithelia [11, 12]. Therefore, the elevation in CA-125 in this patient was likely secondary to extensive peritoneal malignancy rather than adnexal malignancy. A similar case report noting elevated CA-125 in a patient with peritoneal lymphoma has been reported by Horger et al. [13]. Inclusion of possible peritoneal sources of CA-125 elevations is crucial when developing a differential diagnosis.

This case report highlights peritoneal lymphomatosis as a rare presentation of BL with an emphasis on the rapidity of progression. Though BL often presents with diffuse abdominal involvement, to our knowledge, this is the first case report which is able to provide comparative imaging to display the rapid growth of tumor. In addition, the case report serves as a reminder of the importance of prompt histological confirmation of etiology of peritoneal thickening.

Abbreviations

BL: Burkitt's lymphoma
WHO: World Health Organization
EBV: Epstein Barr Virus
CVAD: Cyclophosphamide, vincristine, doxorubicin, dexamethasone
MTX: Methotrexate
Ara-C: Cytarabine.

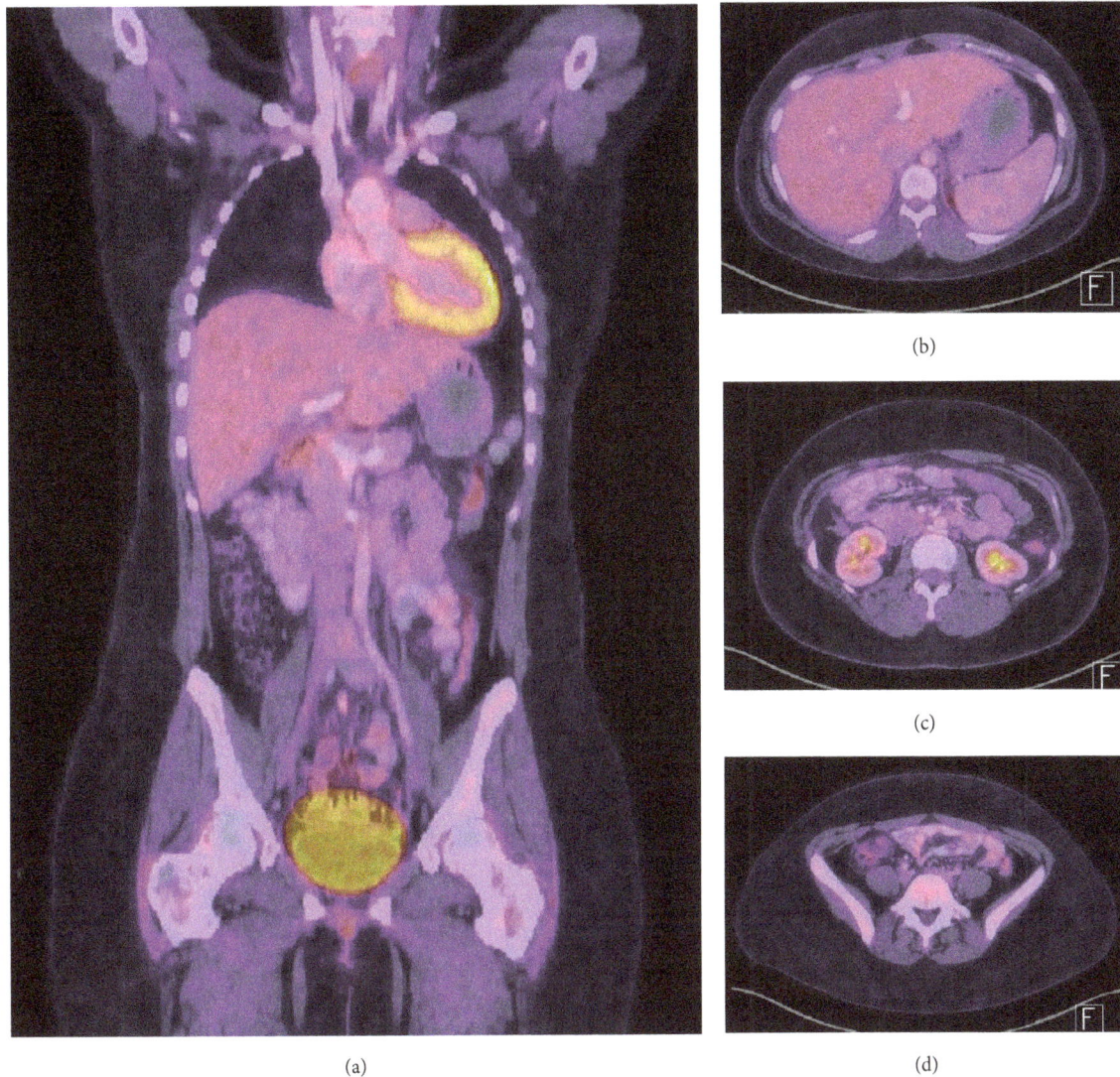

FIGURE 5: PET/CT imaging of the body performed in November 2016. (a) Coronal Body. (b) Axial upper abdomen. (c) Axial mid abdomen. (d) Axial low abdomen. Substantial resolution of patient's peritoneal involvement of malignancy and other changes suggesting malignancy noted. Previously noted liver lesions resolved.

Ethical Approval

Approval from the WVU Ethics Committee regarding the publication of this case report was obtained.

Consent

Approval to submit this case report for publication was obtained from the patient.

Authors' Contributions

Naomi Fei was a major contributor in writing the manuscript. Nilay Shah was a major contributor in editing. All authors read and approved the final manuscript.

Acknowledgments

The authors wish to acknowledge Cara Bryan, M.D., Assistant Professor, Department of Radiology, West Virginia University Hospital, 1 Medical Center Dr, Morgantown, WV 26505, USA.

References

[1] K. A. Blum, G. Lozanski, and J. C. Byrd, "Adult Burkitt leukemia and lymphoma," *Blood*, vol. 104, no. 10, pp. 3009–3020, 2004.

[2] L. M. Morton, S. S. Wang, S. S. Devesa, P. Hartge, D. D. Weisenburger, and M. S. Linet, "Lymphoma incidence patterns by WHO subtype in the United States, 1992–2001," *Blood*, vol. 107, no. 1, pp. 265–276, 2006.

[3] E. Curakova, M. Genadieva-Dimitrova, J. Misevski et al., "NonHodgkin's Lymphoma with Peritoneal Localization," *Case Reports in Gastrointestinal Medicine*, vol. 2014, pp. 1–8, 2014.

[4] M. Horger, M. Müller-Schimpfle, I. Yirkin et al., "Extensive peritoneal and omental lymphomatosis with raised CA 125 mimicking carcinomatosis: CT and intraoperative findings," *British Journal of Radiology*, vol. 77, no. 913, pp. 71–73, 2004.

[5] Y. Kim, O. Cho, S. Song et al., "Peritoneal lymphomatosis: CT findings," *Abdom Imaging*, vol. 23, pp. 87–90, 1998.

[6] R. Dalla-Favera, M. Bregni, J. Erikson et al., "Human c-myc onc gene is located on the region of chromosome 8 that is translocated in Burkitt lymphoma cells," *Proceedings of the National Academy of Sciences of the United States of America*, vol. 79, article 7824, 1982.

[7] World Health Organization, *Classification of TUmours of Hematopoietic and Lymphoid Tissues*, S. H. Swerdlow, E. Campo, and N. L. Harris, Eds., IARC Press, Lyon, France, 2008.

[8] M. A. Lynch, K. C. Cho, R. B. Jeffrey, D. D. Alterman, and M. P. Federle, "CT of peritoneal lymphomatosis," *American Journal of Roentgenology*, vol. 151, pp. 713–716, 1988.

[9] C. Oliveira, H. Matos, P. Serra, R. Catarino, and A. Estevão, "Adult abdominal Burkitt lymphoma with isolated peritoneal involvement," *Journal of Radiology Case Reports*, vol. 8, no. 1, pp. 27–33, 2014.

[10] D. Karaosmanoglu, M. Karcaaltincaba, B. Oguz et al., "Ct findings of lymphoma with peritoneal, omental and mesenteric involvement: peritoneal lymphyomatosis," *European Journal of Radiology*, vol. 71, pp. 313–317, 2009.

[11] I. Jacobs and R. C. Bast, "The CA 125 tumor-associated antigen: a review of the literature," *Human Reprod*, vol. 4, no. 1, article 1, 1989.

[12] O. Dorigo and J. S. Berek, "Personalizing CA125 levels for ovarian cancer screening," *Cancer Prevention Research*, vol. 4, no. 9, pp. 1356–1359, 2011.

[13] M. Horger, M. Müller-Schimpfle, I. Yirkin, M. Wehrmann, and C. D. Claussen, "Extensive peritoneal and omental lymphomatosis and raised CA 125 mimicking carcinomatosis: CT and (913): intraoperative findings," *British Journal of Radiology*, vol. 77, no. 913, pp. 71–73, 2004.

32

Metastatic Sarcomatoid Squamous Cell Carcinoma of the Cervix Presenting with Chest Mass

Lilit Karapetyan,[1] **Manoj Rai,**[1] **Om Dawani,**[1] **and Heather S. Laird-Fick**[2]

[1]*Michigan State University Department of Medicine and EW Sparrow Hospital, 804 Service Rd, Room B301, East Lansing, MI 48824, USA*
[2]*Michigan State University Department of Medicine, 804 Service Rd, Room B316, East Lansing, MI 48824, USA*

Correspondence should be addressed to Lilit Karapetyan; lilit.karapetyan@hc.msu.edu

Academic Editor: Constantine Gennatas

Background. Sarcomatoid squamous cell carcinoma is a rare and aggressive form of cervical cancer. We report a case of metastatic sarcomatoid squamous cell carcinoma (SSCC) of cervix that presented with an anterior chest wall mass. *Case.* A 43-year-old Hispanic female presented with a two-month history of a central chest wall mass. The patient's only past medical history was SSCC of the cervix, stage IIB, diagnosed two years priorly. She underwent neoadjuvant chemoradiation therapy (CRT) with cisplatin followed by radical hysterectomy. Surgical margins were positive which led to adjuvant CRT with carboplatin and paclitaxel. PET scan 4 months after the postoperative treatment was negative for recurrence and metastatic disease. On current presentation, the CT chest revealed anterior mediastinal destructive soft tissue mass involving sternum, and the biopsy showed SSCC. The patient received palliative radiation therapy to her chest with improvement in pain and ability to swallow. After discussing the prognosis she refused further chemotherapy and decided on hospice care. *Conclusion.* Despite good response to first-line therapy, SSCC tends to recur early and does not respond to second-line therapy. Radiation therapy seems to be the most effective modality for treatment, but randomized controlled trials of therapy are impractical.

1. Introduction

Cervical cancer is the fourth most common cancer in women worldwide, causing approximately 270,000 deaths per year. Widespread use of cervical cancer screening has reduced morbidity and mortality in the United States, but in 2017 an estimated 12,900 cases and 4,120 deaths are still expected. Racial and ethnic disparities also persist, with incidence remaining high among Hispanic women [1–3].

The squamous cell histologic subtype accounts for 80% of cervical cancer cases and is classically preceded by precancerous changes detectable by Pap smear. Adenocarcinoma of the cervix behaves similarly, although it develops from the endocervix rather than the transitional zone. Both subtypes of cervical cancer tend to be locally aggressive, with metastases primarily to lymph nodes, lung, and liver [2].

In contrast, sarcomatoid squamous cell carcinoma of the cervix (SSCC) is an extremely rare and aggressive variant, with similar sites of metastasis. There are no well-established guidelines for its treatment; most cases are managed similar to squamous cell carcinoma [3–6].

We report a case of metastatic SSCC of the cervix that presented with an anterior chest wall mass, an unusual site of spread for this rare tumor.

2. Case Presentation

A 43-year-old G6P6 Hispanic female presented with a two-month history of a central chest wall mass (Figure 1). The patient's only past medical history was SSCC of the cervix, stage IIB, diagnosed two years priorly. At that time, she presented with severe vaginal bleeding. Transvaginal and transabdominal ultrasounds showed abnormal enlargement of the uterine cervix. A CT abdomen/pelvis confirmed a heterogenous cervical mass without evidence of metastatic disease. Histopathology revealed SSCC of the cervix, positive

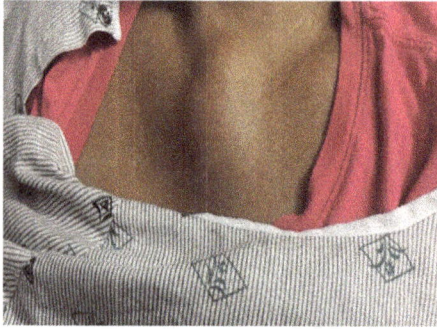

FIGURE 1: Anterior central chest wall mass.

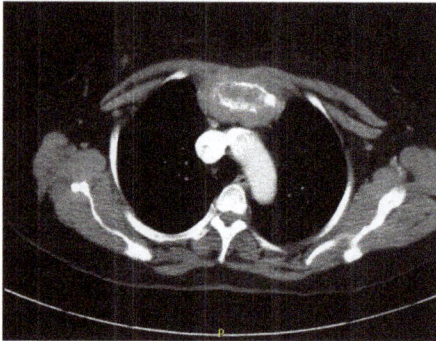

FIGURE 2: 2.1 × 1.5 cm soft tissue infiltrating along the manubrium with underlying destruction of the bone.

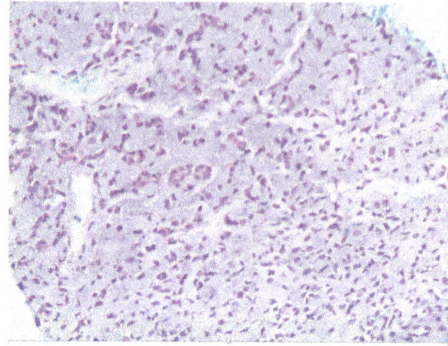

FIGURE 3: HE staining of tumor showing highly cellular epithelial cells with fascicles of short spindle cells.

for human papilloma virus (HPV). The patient was clinically staged as International Federation of Gynecology and Obstetrics (FIGO) stage IIb and subsequently started on chemoradiation therapy with weekly cisplatin and external beam radiation therapy totaling 4140 cGy before undergoing radical hysterectomy. She had microscopically positive margins which led to postoperative adjuvant chemoradiation therapy with carboplatin and paclitaxel. PET scan four months after treatment was negative for recurrent or metastatic disease. She was subsequently lost to follow-up because of lack of insurance and a language barrier.

She again sought medical attention only when she experienced intolerable pain and difficulty in swallowing associated with enlargement of a new mass on her chest (Figure 1). CT chest/abdomen/pelvis and MRI brain/cervical spine showed extensive infiltration by a soft tissue mass, associated bony destruction, and pulmonary nodules (Figure 2). The soft tissue mass extended into the anterior mediastinum, the right upper cervical canal, and neural foramena at the levels of C2–C4 and into the paraspinal muscles at the level of C3. No cord compression was noted. CT-guided core biopsy revealed tumor predominantly composed of spindle cells (Figure 3) with features of SSCC, immunoreactivity for cytokeratin (AE1/AE3), CAM5.2, and vimentin, and weakly positive for muscle actin, S100, and p63. The patient received five palliative radiation treatments to her chest with improvement in pain and swallowing. After discussion of the benefits and risks of palliative chemotherapy, she opted for hospice care.

3. Discussion

Sarcomatoid carcinoma tends to affect the upper aerodigestive tract (i.e., larynx, pharynx, and esophagus) and skin. It comprises only 1-2% of all gynecological malignancies [7]. A comprehensive literature review using the terms "sarcomatoid carcinoma" and "squamous cell carcinoma" identified 20 reported cases, including a case series of nine patients (Brown et al.) [4–6, 8–10]. As with the more common types of cervical cancer, HPV is the primary etiologic factor identified to date; high risk subtypes 16 and 18 have been found in both squamous and sarcomatoid components of the tumor [11].

Two hypotheses exist regarding the development of the sarcomatoid features. In an esophageal model, researchers have described transformation from squamous cell to spindle cell cancer with loss of epithelial cells from the basal layer of the tissue. The spindle cells contain desmosomes and tonofilaments, supporting their squamous cell origin. Alternatively, the carcinoma could be a chimera of squamous and spindle cell components arising from two different stem cell lines [7, 12].

As for the more common subtypes, sarcomatoid tumors are more common with increasing age. The median age at presentation is 67 years. Women are generally symptomatic at the time of diagnosis, with abnormal vaginal bleeding or foul smelling discharge. Cervical lesions are readily visible on physical examination.

Histology demonstrates the pathognomonic squamous and spindle cell components. Immunohistochemistry is usually positive for mesenchymal and epithelial components like cytokeratin and vimentin [7, 12, 13].

The FIGO system is used for staging of the disease. In the absence of evidence for this histologic subtype, most women receive treatments based on the recommendations for squamous cervical carcinoma. Surgery is the preferred choice of treatment for early stage disease. Tumor size, margin status, and tumor biology guide the need for adjuvant radiation therapy after resection for local prevention of recurrence.

Prognosis of SSCC of the cervix, however, is more similar to sarcoma than other types of cervical cancer. It is aggressive, progressive, and generally diagnosed at late stage. The metastases to kidney, peritoneum, and subcutaneous tissue have been described in the literature [7]. Bansal et al. reviewed SEER database for evaluation of outcome of patients with cervical cancer based on different histological types. Five-year survival for stages IB, III, and IV was 80%, 32%, and 17% for squamous cell carcinoma. The patients with adenocarcinoma of stages IB, III, and IV had 83%, 19%, and 9% survival rate. Stage IB, II, and IV sarcomas had survival of 67%, 20%, and 11%, respectively. Similar to sarcomas, SSCC is a highly progressive cancer with low survival rate. Five-year survival plummets with increasing stage, from 90% for stage I to <5% for stage IV. Other prognostic factors include degree of differentiation, extent of the carcinomatous component, size of the tumor, and age at presentation [14–16].

Disease-free survival and response to therapy also vary by stage. Brown et al. reported complete response to first-line therapy in nine patients with SSCC with median disease-free survival of 4.9 months. Two patients, with stage I and II disease, were disease-free for 40 months. After relapse, none of the patients responded to second-line therapies of radiation, surgery, and chemotherapy.

Our patient had a similar course for her stage IIb cancer. She was disease-free for at least four months before being lost to follow-up. Thirteen months later she presented with extensive metastatic disease that had some response to palliative radiotherapy before opting for hospice.

The most common causes of chest mass in adults are inflammatory or infectious conditions and tumors. More than 50% of tumors are malignant. Primary chest wall tumors account for only 5% of thoracic neoplasms. The most common tumors present as local extension of thoracic tumors including breast, lung, pleura, and mediastinum or metastases from thoracic tumors, renal cell carcinoma, thyroid cancer, colon cancer, and melanoma. Lymphomas and chondrosarcoma account for most cases of malignant neoplasms in chest wall [17, 18]. To our knowledge, this is the first case reporting chest mass secondary to metastasis from SSCC of the cervix.

4. Conclusion

In summary, sarcomatoid squamous cell carcinoma of the cervix is a very rare and aggressive cancer. Despite good response to first-line therapy, it tends to recur early and does not respond to second-line therapy. Radiation therapy seems to be the most effective modality for treatment, but randomized controlled trials of therapy are impractical.

References

[1] R. L. Siegel, K. D. Miller, and A. Jemal, "Cancer statistics, 2016," *CA: A Cancer Journal for Clinicians*, vol. 66, no. 1, pp. 7–30, 2016.

[2] J. Barnholtz-Sloan, N. Patel, D. Rollison, K. Kortepeter, J. MacKinnon, and A. Giuliano, "Incidence trends of invasive cervical cancer in the United States by combined race and ethnicity," *Cancer Causes and Control*, vol. 20, no. 7, pp. 1129–1138, 2009.

[3] M. E. Sherman, S. S. Wang, J. Carreon, and S. S. Devesa, "Mortality trends for cervical squamous and adenocarcinoma in the United States: relation to incidence and survival," *Cancer*, vol. 103, no. 6, pp. 1258–1264, 2005.

[4] M. Kumar, A. Bahl, D. Sharma et al., "Sarcomatoid squamous cell carcinoma of uterine cervix: Pathology, imaging, and treatment," *Journal of Cancer Research and Therapeutics*, vol. 4, no. 1, pp. 39–41, 2008.

[5] J. Brown, R. Broaddus, M. Koeller, T. W. Burke, D. M. Gershenson, and D. C. Bodurka, "Sarcomatoid carcinoma of the cervix," *Gynecologic Oncology*, vol. 90, no. 1, pp. 23–28, 2003.

[6] T. H. Nageeti and R. A. Jastania, "Sarcomatoid carcinoma of the cervix," *Annals of Saudi Medicine*, vol. 32, no. 5, pp. 541–543, 2012.

[7] C. C. Anderson, B. H. Le, and B. Robinson-Bennett, "Sarcomatoid Squamous Cell Carcinoma," in *Squamous Cell Carcinoma*, Xiaoming, Ed., InTech, 2012, https://www.intechopen.com/books/squamous-cell-carcinoma/squamous-cell-carcinoma-with-sarcomatoid-features-in-gynecologic-malignancies.

[8] J. G. Batsakis and P. Suarez, "Sarcomatoid carcinomas of the upper aerodigestive tracts," *Advances in Anatomic Pathology*, vol. 7, no. 5, pp. 282–293, 2000.

[9] L. Rodrigues, I. Santana, T. Cunha et al., "Sarcomatoid squamous cell carcinoma of the uterine cervix: case report," *European Journal of Gynaecological Oncology*, vol. 21, no. 3, pp. 287–289, 2000.

[10] L.-C. Pang, "Sarcomatoid squamous cell carcinoma of the uterine cervix with osteoclast-like giant cells: report of two cases," *International Journal of Gynecological Pathology*, vol. 17, no. 2, pp. 174–177, 1998.

[11] C. P. Lin, C. L. Ho, M. R. Shen, L. H. Huang, and C. Y. Chou, "Evidence of human papillomavirus infection, enhanced phosphorylation of retinoblastoma protein, and decreased apoptosis in sarcomatoid squamous cell carcinoma of uterine cervix," *International Journal of Gynecological Cancer*, vol. 16, no. 1, pp. 336–340, 2006.

[12] T. W. Kong, J. H. Kim, S. J. Chang, K. H. Chang, H. S. Ryu, and H. J. Joo, "Sarcomatoid squamous cell carcinoma of the uterine cervix successfully treated by laparoscopic radical hysterectomy: a case report," *The Journal of Reproductive Medicine*, vol. 55, no. 9, pp. 445–448, 2010.

[13] K. Götte, F. Riedel, J. F. Coy, V. Spahn, and K. Hörmann, "Salivary gland carcinosarcoma: Immunohistochemical, molecular genetic and electron microscopic findings," *Oral Oncology*, vol. 36, no. 4, pp. 360–364, 2000.

[14] V. Vinh-Hung, C. Bourgain, G. Vlastos et al., "Prognostic value of histopathology and trends in cervical cancer: a SEER population study," *BMC Cancer*, vol. 7, article 164, 2007.

[15] S. Intaraphet, N. Kasatpibal, S. Siriaunkgul et al., "Prognostic impact of histology in patients with cervical squamous cell carcinoma, adenocarcinoma and small cell neuroendocrine carcinoma," *Asian Pacific Journal of Cancer Prevention*, vol. 14, no. 9, pp. 5355–5360, 2013.

[16] S. Intaraphet, N. Kasatpibal, M. Søgaard et al., "Histological type-specific prognostic factors of cervical small cell neuroendocrine carcinoma, adenocarcinoma, and squamous cell carcinoma," *OncoTargets and Therapy*, vol. 7, pp. 1205–1214, 2014.

[17] J. Warzelhan, E. Stoelben, A. Imdahl, and J. Hasse, "Results in surgery for primary and metastatic chest wall tumors,"

European Journal of Cardio-thoracic Surgery, vol. 19, no. 5, pp. 584–588, 2001.

[18] S. E. Smith and S. Keshavjee, "Primary chest wall tumors," *Thoracic Surgery Clinics*, vol. 20, no. 4, pp. 495–507, 2010.

33

Basal Cell Carcinoma of the Female Breast Masquerading as Invasive Primary Breast Carcinoma: An Uncommon Presentation Site

Mark B. Ulanja (ORCID),[1] **Mohamed E. Taha,**[1] **Arshad A. Al-Mashhadani,**[1]
Marwah Muaad Al-Tekreeti,[2] **Christie Elliot,**[1] **and Santhosh Ambika**[1]

[1]*Department of Internal Medicine, University of Nevada Reno, School of Medicine, 1155 Mill Street, Reno, NV 89502, USA*
[2]*American Public University System, 111 West Congress Street, Charles Town, WV 25414, USA*

Correspondence should be addressed to Mark B. Ulanja; mulanja@unr.edu

Academic Editor: Katsuhiro Tanaka

Skin cancer as a single entity is the most common malignancy in North America, accounting for half of all human cancers. It comprises two types: melanoma and nonmelanoma skin cancers. Of the nonmelanomas, basal cell carcinoma (BCC) constitutes about 80% of the cancers diagnosed every year. BCC usually occurs in sun-exposed areas such as the face and extremities. Occurrence in the nipple areolar complex is very rare. We present a case of a Caucasian woman who presented with what was initially thought to be invasive carcinoma of the breast involving the nipple areolar complex (NAC); however, the diagnosis was revealed to be a basal cell carcinoma after histopathological examination. The tumor was treated with modified radical mastectomy, with negative margins. The importance of this case lies in the rare site of presentation of basal cell carcinoma and the importance of early detection.

1. Introduction

Skin cancer as a single entity is the most common malignancy in North America [1]. They account for half of all human cancers. Generally, they could be divided into two types: melanoma and nonmelanoma skin cancers. The nonmelanoma type, which is the most common form, includes basal cell carcinoma and squamous cell carcinoma. Of the 3.5 million cases of nonmelanoma skin cancer (NMSC) diagnosed each year, 80% are basal cell carcinomas (BCCs), which makes BCCs the most common skin cancer [2]. It is most common among fair-skinned persons, with a lifetime risk of 33% to 39% in white men and 23% to 28% in white women in the United States [1].

The most important environmental risk factor is ultraviolet (UV) light exposure, hence BCC usually occurs in sun-exposed areas [3]. The occurrence of BCC in unexposed areas such as in the nipple areolar complex (NAC) is very rare [4, 5]. We present a case of breast cancer in a Caucasian woman, involving the nipple areolar complex (NAC) which was initially thought to be invasive carcinoma of the breast, but was subsequently diagnosed to be BCC.

2. Case Report

A 64-year-old Caucasian female presented to our emergency department (ED) with a two-day history of bleeding from her left breast. She has had a slowly enlarging growth on her left breast for the past two years, which initially started as a small papular lesion in the nipple areolar complex. Most recently, the mass became ulcerated with active serous discharge; however, due to the lack of health insurance, the patient did not seek any medical attention. For the past two days prior to presentation, she developed significant bleeding and oozing from the ulcerated mass, forcing her to report to the ED. There was associated localized breast pain, but no weight loss, fever, nausea, vomiting, abdominal pain, back pain, abdominal pain, shortness of breath, cough, blurry vision, nor headaches.

She had no prior personal or family history of skin and breast cancers. She had no history of excessive exposure to sunlight, radiation exposure, arsenic ingestion, or a history of immunosuppression.

Physical examination reveals an elderly female in no apparent distress. Vital signs were stable apart from an elevated blood pressure of 164/85 mmHg. Examination of the left breast revealed a large fungating mass of >10 cm in size, occupying most of the mid and outer breast with a distortion of the nipple areolar complex (Figure 1). There were several open wounds with active bleeding and a foul smell. The area of erythema was noted. There were palpable left axillary lymph nodes. The rest of the physical examination was unremarkable.

The provisional diagnosis was breast cancer with possible metastasis. Subsequently, the patient underwent workup to further characterize the mass and assess for metastasis. Computer tomography (CT) scan of the chest, abdomen, and pelvis was positive for a large, partially enhancing heterogeneous mass in the left breast and a calcified granuloma in the right lung field, in addition to mildly enlarged left axillary lymph nodes. No evidence of metastasis was identified in the abdomen and pelvis. Magnetic resonance imaging (MRI) of the brain with and without contrast was negative for brain lesions. There was no evidence of osseous metastatic disease as evident by the negative nuclear medicine bone scintigraphy.

Trucut excisional biopsy of the mass was performed. The initial histopathological exam was suggestive of an epidermal origin of the cancerous cells, raising the possibility of an adnexal primary such as basal cell carcinoma (Figures 2 and 3). Immunohistochemical (IHC) profile also favored a primary skin disorder over a breast primary (Figures 4 and 5). Utilizing NeoGenomics®, the cells were consistent with cutaneous basal cell carcinoma.

Post diagnosis, the patient underwent left modified radical mastectomy with axillary lymph node dissection. After histopathological exam for the dissected tissue and lymph nodes, a final diagnosis of invasive cutaneous basal cell carcinoma was made. The margins were tested negative for carcinoma. All the dissected 16 lymph nodes were negative for cancer. Subsequent treatment and oncological follow-up were scheduled with oncology.

3. Discussion

Basal cell carcinomas (BCCs) are nonmelanoma skin cancers arising from the basal layer of the epidermis and its appendages. They constitute eighty percent of skin cancers. They are slow-growing tumors and very rarely metastasize; however, if left untreated, they tend to grow and invade nearby tissues [6].

Geographically, there is profound variation in the incidence of BCCs due to the effect of ultraviolet light on its development. In the USA for instance, in 1990, the incidence of BCCs in the states which are in close proximity to the

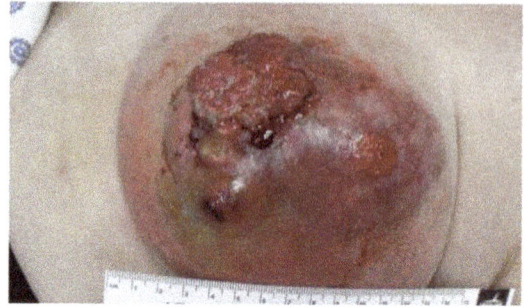

FIGURE 1: Left breast basal cell carcinoma showing ulcerations and bleeding.

equator, like Hawaii, was twice as that of the Midwestern regions [7, 8].

The most important risk factor for BCCs is ultraviolet (UV) light exposure, particularly intermittent, intense UVB light exposure; hence, BCCs most commonly occur in sun-exposed areas [3]. Other risk factors include radiation therapy, chronic arsenic exposure, and long-term immunosuppression. In patients with early-onset or numerous BCCs, a syndromic manifestation of a genetic cause (e.g., basal cell nevus syndrome) should be considered [2].

The occurrence of BCC in the skin of the breast such as the nipple areolar complex (NAC) is very rare [4, 5]. It was first reported in 1893 [9] and as of September 2016, BCCs of the areolar and nipple have been described in 55 individuals of which 35 were males and 20 were females and the onset age ranged from 35 to 86 years [10, 11]. In a study by Betti et al., they found that 74% of the BCCs were located on the head and neck area, 26% were involved in the covered sites of the body, and only two cancers were involved in the nipple and areolar [10]. A histogenic relationship has been noted between pilosebaceous units and the development of BCC [12]. The NAC is deficient in pilosebaceous units and this may explain the paucity of BCCs in this area [13].

In regard to the etiology of BCC in the NAC, some studies have suggested that ultraviolet (UV) irradiation might be the main etiological factor. In one study, a history of extensive sun exposure was evident in three out of six cases with multiple BCC lesions in the NAC [13, 14]. Other potential risk factors include genetic predisposition, immunosuppression, ionizing radiation exposure, arsenic exposure, injuries such as burns or trauma, light-colored skin, previous BCCs at another site, and sunburns [15]. Similar to the majority of the cases of BCC, as well as in our case, no history of risk factors is identified.

Differential diagnosis of a BCC lesion in the NAC includes Paget's disease, eczema, adenoma of the nipple, papilloma of lactiferous ducts, syringomatous adenoma, invasive ductal carcinoma, and melanoma. Therefore, it is crucial to perform histopathological examination to establish the diagnosis [5]. In the NAC, BCC is considered to behave more aggressively than other anatomical sites, but other nonaggressive histological subtypes exist, and tumor recurrence is uncommon after the successful treatment of the primary cancer [15, 16]. In a previous study, a report of 3 out of 31 cases of BCC in the

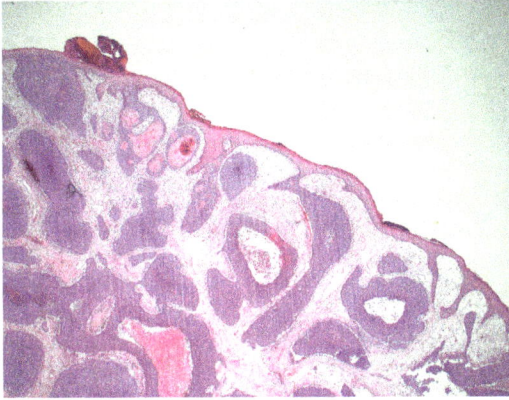

FIGURE 2: Histological findings on excisional biopsy H&E (hematoxylin and eosin stain) 2x, demonstrate nests of tumor cells arising from the surface epidermis.

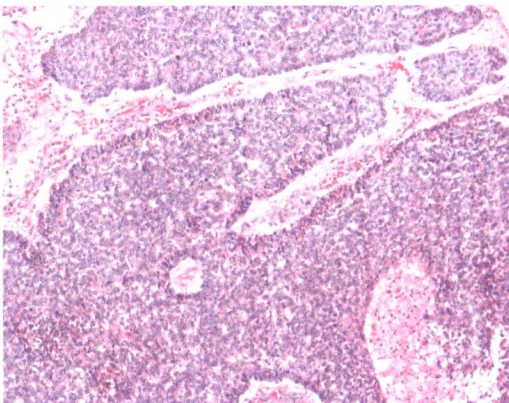

FIGURE 3: Histological findings on excisional biopsy H&E (hematoxylin and eosin stain) 10x show peripheral palisading of the tumor cells at the periphery of the nests.

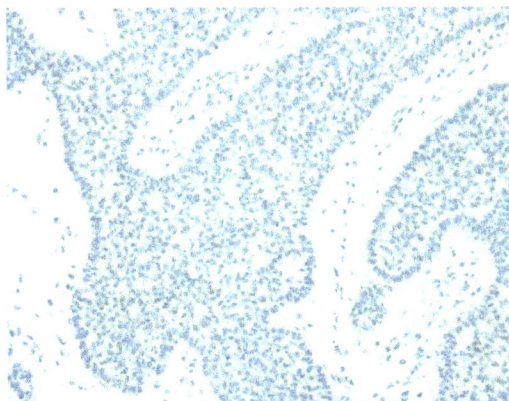

FIGURE 4: Immunohistochemical (IHC) stain 20x shows tumor cells to be negative for GATA3 (note: positive in breast primary).

NAC have developed apparent axillary lymphadenopathy with histologically confirmed cases [15]. Takeno et al. found that axillary lymph node metastasis of basal cell carcinoma was about 11.5% in 26 patients [16], which was apparently

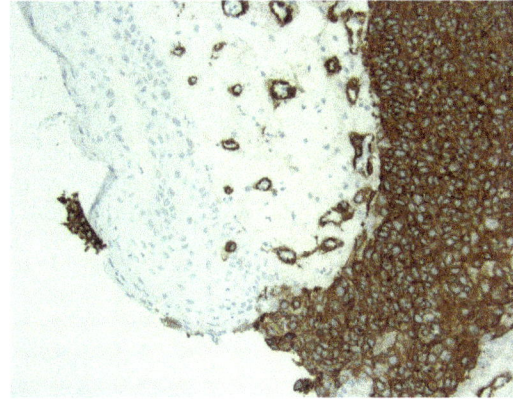

FIGURE 5: IHC stain (SMA—smooth muscle actin) 20x shows the normal epidermis to be negative (which is what is expected), but the tumor cells show strong cytoplasmic positivity. The circles that are also staining is smooth muscle in normal blood vessels (positive internal control).

high compared to the rate of 0.01–0.028% [17] noted by Elder et al. The likely explanation is that the subareolar plexus is rich in a network of lymphatic capillaries and this might provide high potential for metastasis of tumors in this area, hence this relative difference [16, 17].

Varying modalities of treatment are available for BCC in the NAC depending on the characteristics of the lesion. Options include medical treatment, photodynamic therapy, laser therapy, Mohs' microsurgery, and simple surgical excision with or without radiotherapy, as well as partial mastectomy with axillary dissection and surgical reconstruction of the breast [15, 16, 18]. This patient presented late because of the lack of health insurance, and oozing and bleeding were noted from the extensive ulcerated breast lesions. The initial histopathology report was not conclusive and had to be sent for further consultation. It was recommended that given the clinical impression and initial inconclusive histopathology report, mastectomy was most appropriate. It was conceivable that the patient will likely have persistently positive resection margins if reasonable attempts at excision and reexcision was made [19]. Also based on the relatively high incidence of maxillary lymph node metastasis [16], mastectomy was recommended as the best mode of treatment.

Our case presented with a 2-year history of a slowly growing papular lesion in the breast not associated with systemic symptoms except for local breast pain when it began to ulcerate, involving most part of the left breast. It is important to be aware that BCCs can become locally aggressive, without systemic symptoms. Simple mastectomy with left axillary lymph node dissection was performed. Lymph nodes were negative as well as the rest of the metastatic workup. Regular follow-up is very important to assess for recurrence or late manifestation that might develop from micro metastasis. Unfortunately, follow-up was difficult to establish due to health insurance constraints, but the patient was educated thoroughly regarding the examination of her skin and features of recurrence and advised regarding seeking medical help as early as possible.

4. Conclusion

For the past 125 years, only about 62 cases of BCC of the NAC have been reported, which highlights the rarity of this presentation. Clinicians should be aware of the occurrence of BCC in this unexposed region and should consider BCC as a differential diagnosis to other benign and malignant disorders affecting the NAC. Furthermore, given the rich lymphatic nature of the NAC, this cancer has the high potential for distant metastasis, and hence it is of great importance to be recognized early enough to institute appropriate treatment.

Consent

Consent to participate in the study was obtained from the patient. Consent was also obtained from the patient for the publication of materials related to this study.

Authors' Contributions

All authors (Mark B. Ulanja, Mohamed E. Taha, Arshad A. Al-Mashhadani, Marwah Muaad Al-Tekreeti, Christie Elliot, and Santhosh Ambika) contributed equally to the work.

References

[1] D. L. Miller and M. A. Weinstock, "Nonmelanoma skin cancer in the United States: incidence," *Journal of the American Academy of Dermatology*, vol. 30, no. 5, pp. 774–778, 1994.

[2] S. A. Gandhi and J. Kampp, "Skin cancer epidemiology, detection, and management," *The Medical Clinics of North America*, vol. 99, no. 6, pp. 1323–1335, 2015.

[3] A. W. Kopf, "Computer analysis of 3531 basal-cell carcinomas of the skin," *The Journal of Dermatology*, vol. 6, no. 5, pp. 267–281, 1979.

[4] P. Robins, H. S. Rabinovitz, and D. Rigel, "Basal-cell carcinomas on covered or unusual sites of the body," *The Journal of Dermatologic Surgery and Oncology*, vol. 7, no. 10, pp. 803–806, 1981.

[5] H. Yamamoto, Y. Ito, T. Hayashi et al., "A case of basal cell carcinoma of the nipple and areola with intraductal spread," *Breast Cancer*, vol. 8, no. 3, pp. 229–233, 2001.

[6] American Cancer Society, "What are basal and squamous cell skin cancers?," 2016, https://www.cancer.org/cancer/basal-and-squamous-cell-skin-cancer/about/what-is-basal-and-squamous-cell.html.

[7] G. T. Reizner, T. Y. Chuang, D. J. Elpern, J. L. Stone, and E. R. Farmer, "Basal cell carcinoma in Kauai, Hawaii: the highest documented incidence in the United States," *Journal of the American Academy of Dermatology*, vol. 29, no. 2, pp. 184–189, 1993.

[8] T. Y. Chuang, A. Popescu, W. P. D. Su, and C. G. Chute, "Basal cell carcinoma. A population-based incidence study in Rochester, Minnesota," *Journal of the American Academy of Dermatology*, vol. 22, no. 3, pp. 413–417, 1990.

[9] H. Robinson, "Rodent ulcer of the male breast," *Philosophical transactions of the Royal Society of London*, vol. 44, pp. 147–148, 1893.

[10] R. Betti, C. Bruscagin, E. Inselvini, and C. Crosti, "Basal cell carcinomas of covered and unusual sites of the body," *International Journal of Dermatology*, vol. 36, no. 7, pp. 503–505, 1997.

[11] M. Fujii, A. Harimoto, and T. Namiki, "Basalzellkarzinom des Mamillen-Areola-Komplexes mit multiplen Läsionen: Bestrahlung als mögliche Ursache," *Journal der Deutschen Dermatologischen Gesellschaft*, vol. 16, no. 2, pp. 193–195, 2018.

[12] E. Alessi, L. Venegoni, D. Fanoni, and E. Berti, "Cytokeratin profile in basal cell carcinoma," *The American Journal of Dermatopathology*, vol. 30, no. 3, pp. 249–255, 2008.

[13] Y. Oram, C. Demirkesen, A. D. Akkaya, and E. Koyuncu, "Basal cell carcinoma of the nipple: an uncommon but ever-increasing location," *Case Reports in Dermatological Medicine*, vol. 2011, Article ID 818291, 3 pages, 2011.

[14] C. Allemani, T. Matsuda, V. di Carlo et al., "Global surveillance of trends in cancer survival 2000–14 (CONCORD-3): analysis of individual records for 37,513,025 patients diagnosed with one of 18 cancers from 322 population-based registries in 71 countries," *The Lancet*, vol. 391, no. 10125, pp. 1023–1075, 2018.

[15] A. Sinha and J. A. Langtry, "Secondary intention healing following Mohs micrographic surgery for basal cell carcinoma of the nipple and areola," *Acta Dermato-Venereologica*, vol. 91, no. 1, pp. 78-79, 2011.

[16] S. Takeno, N. Kikuchi, T. Miura et al., "Basal cell carcinoma of the nipple in male patients with gastric cancer recurrence: report of a case," *Breast Cancer*, vol. 21, no. 1, pp. 102–107, 2014.

[17] D. E. Elder, R. Elenitsas, B. L. Johnson Jr., G. F. Murphy, and X. Xu, *Lever's Histopathology of the Skin*, Lippincott Williams & Wilkins, Philadelphia, PA, USA, 10th edition, 2008.

[18] A. Sharma, R. M. Tambat, A. Singh, and D. S. Bhaligi, "Basal cell carcinoma of the nipple areola complex," *Journal of Mid-life Health*, vol. 2, no. 2, pp. 89-90, 2011.

[19] H. S. Feigelson, T. A. James, R. M. Single et al., "Factors associated with the frequency of initial total mastectomy: results of a multi-institutional study," *Journal of the American College of Surgeons*, vol. 216, no. 5, pp. 966–975, 2013.

34

Metastatic Cecal Adenocarcinoma to the Gallbladder Presenting with Acute Cholecystitis

Nedal Bukhari[1] **and Marwah Abdulkader**[2]

[1]*Department of Medical Oncology, King Fahad Specialist Hospital, Dammam, Saudi Arabia*
[2]*Department of Pathology, King Fahad Specialist Hospital, Dammam, Saudi Arabia*

Correspondence should be addressed to Nedal Bukhari; nedal.bukhari36@gmail.com

Academic Editor: Jose I. Mayordomo

Colorectal cancer (CRC) is one of the most common cancers and the second highest cause of cancer-related deaths (Jemal et al., 2011). Common presentations of CRC include alterations in bowel habit, weight loss, and lower gastrointestinal bleeding. We report a case of a 74-year-old male who presented with fever and right upper quadrant pain, with positive Murphy's sign on examination. The case was initially managed with a routine cholecystectomy. Histological examination revealed a moderately differentiated adenocarcinoma with a superimposed histologically proven acute acalculous cholecystitis. CT scan done postsurgery showed a cecal mass with retroperitoneal lymphadenopathy. Biopsy result of cecal mass was remarkable for colon adenocarcinoma. We are not aware of any similar prior cases reported in English literature.

1. Introduction

CRC is the third most common cancer in men and the second in women worldwide [1]. Around 20% of patients will have distant metastasis at the time of initial presentation. Regional lymph nodes, liver, lungs, and peritoneum are common metastatic sites for CRC [2].

The intestinal tract venous drainage is through the portal circulation. Therefore, the first site of hematogenous spread of CRC is usually the liver, followed by the lungs, bone, and multiple other sites. However, distal rectal cancers may metastasize initially to the lungs through the inferior rectal vein, which drains into the inferior vena cava rather than into the portal venous system [3].

Throughout the literature search, we came across 2 cases of transverse colon cancers with metastasis to gallbladder masquerading as cholecystitis [4, 5].

2. Case Report

A 74-year-old male with history of stage III sigmoid adenocarcinoma 15 years ago treated with sigmoid colectomy followed by adjuvant 5-fluorouracil (5-FU) chemotherapy presented to his local hospital with acute worsening of epigastric pain associated with nausea and vomiting. On physical examination, the patient was febrile at 38.5°C, tachycardic, and normotensive. Abdominal examination revealed tenderness in the right upper abdomen and rigidity of the abdominal wall with positive Murphy's sign. Laboratory testing revealed a hemoglobin level of 11.5 g/dl and a white cell count of $16/\mu l$ with 80% neutrophils, and other tests were within normal range (which included liver enzymes, bilirubin, LDH, lipase, and amylase).

CA19-9 was elevated at 4945 IU/ml, and the CEA level was measured at $24.11 \, \mu g/l$.

Abdominal ultrasound revealed a sludge and irregular thickness of the gallbladder.

The patient was started on intravenous broad-spectrum antibiotics immediately. Laporascopic cholecystectomy was performed the day after admission. Unfortunately, the postoperative course was complicated by a septic shock and required ICU admission for few days (Figure 1). The initial pathology of the gallbladder showed a moderately differentiated adenocarcinoma of unknown primary possibly due to

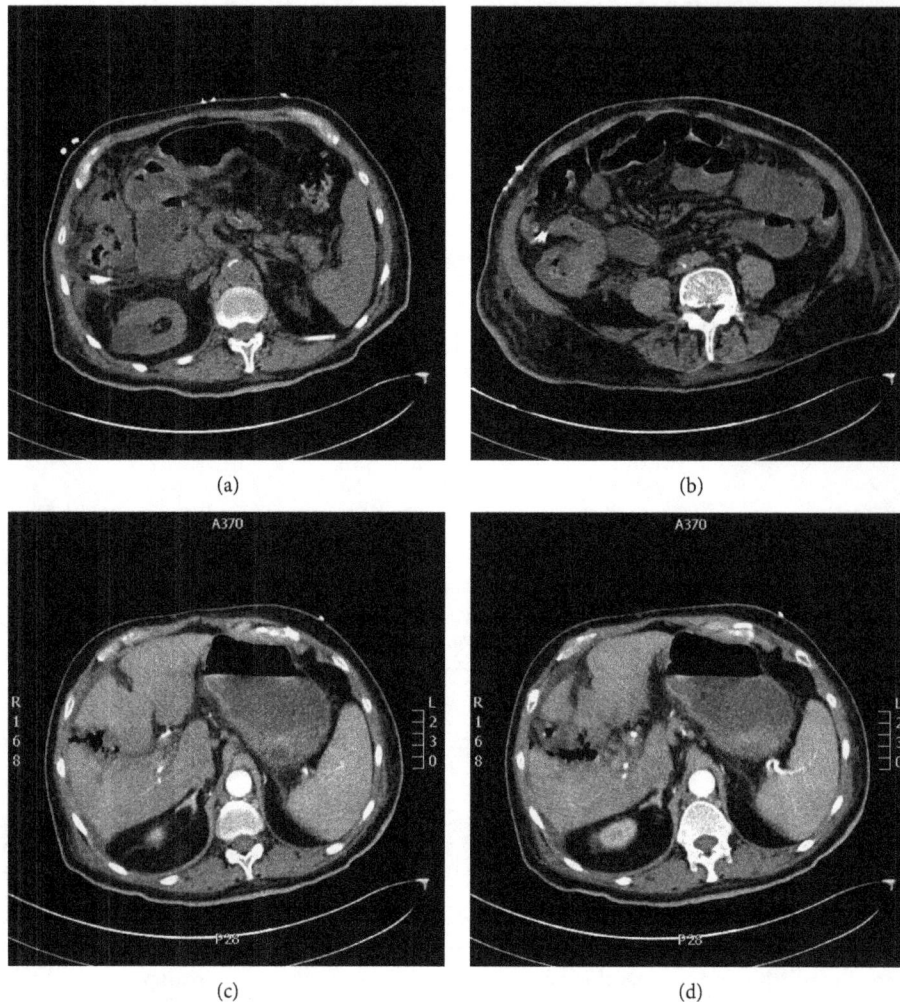

FIGURE 1: (a, b) CT Abdomen showing cecal mass. (c, d) CT abdomen showing post cholecystectomy changes.

gall bladder primary. Further investigations revealed a cecal mass with regional retroperitoneal lymphadenopathy.

The patient was referred to our hospital where he had a biopsy of the latter mass, and the histopathology result was consistent with a moderately differentiated adenocarcinoma of colonic origin. A comprehensive pathological review of the gallbladder specimen was performed, and reexamination and further immunohistochemical analysis including epithelial cytokeratins 7 and 20 (CK7 and CK20) and homeobox protein-2 (CDX-2) were done. Tumor cells isolated from the specimen were positive for CK20 and CDX-2 and negative for CK7.

Our patient was confirmed to have metastatic disease from colon primary; therefore, he was started on palliative capecitabine with significant symptomatic improvement reported after two cycles. He continues to tolerate chemotherapy.

3. Discussion

CRC is one of the most common cancers worldwide. Patients with right-side colon adenocarcinoma usually present with cachexia, weight loss, anemia, and positive fecal occult blood unlike those with left-sided colon cancers, which usually manifest with changes in bowel habit, hematochezia, and symptoms of obstruction.

The gallbladder is an extremely rare site of CRC metastasis, with very few cases reported. However, tumors like melanoma may metastasize to the gallbladder [2]. Other less common primary sites resulting in metastasis include the lung, breast, renal, and cervical malignancies [6, 7]. In a large autopsy series, metastases to the gallbladder were present in 5.8% of patients [8, 9].

Chen et al. reported a case of transverse colon cancer presenting with manifestations of cholecystitis. They suggested that invasion of the gallbladder caused an inflammatory adhesion which resulted in an acute acalculous cholecystitis [4].

Munghate et al. also described a case of transverse colon presenting with cholecystitis [5].

Adenocarcinomas are epithelial cancers arising in glandular tissues. They constitute the largest group of epithelial cancers [10].

CK are keratin proteins found in the cytoskeleton of the epithelium (Figure 2). CK7 and CK20 expression patterns play a major role in the diagnosis of many carcinomas of epithelial etiology [11, 12]. CK7 is found in many ductal and glandular epithelial tissues, including breast, lung, ovary,

(a)

(b)

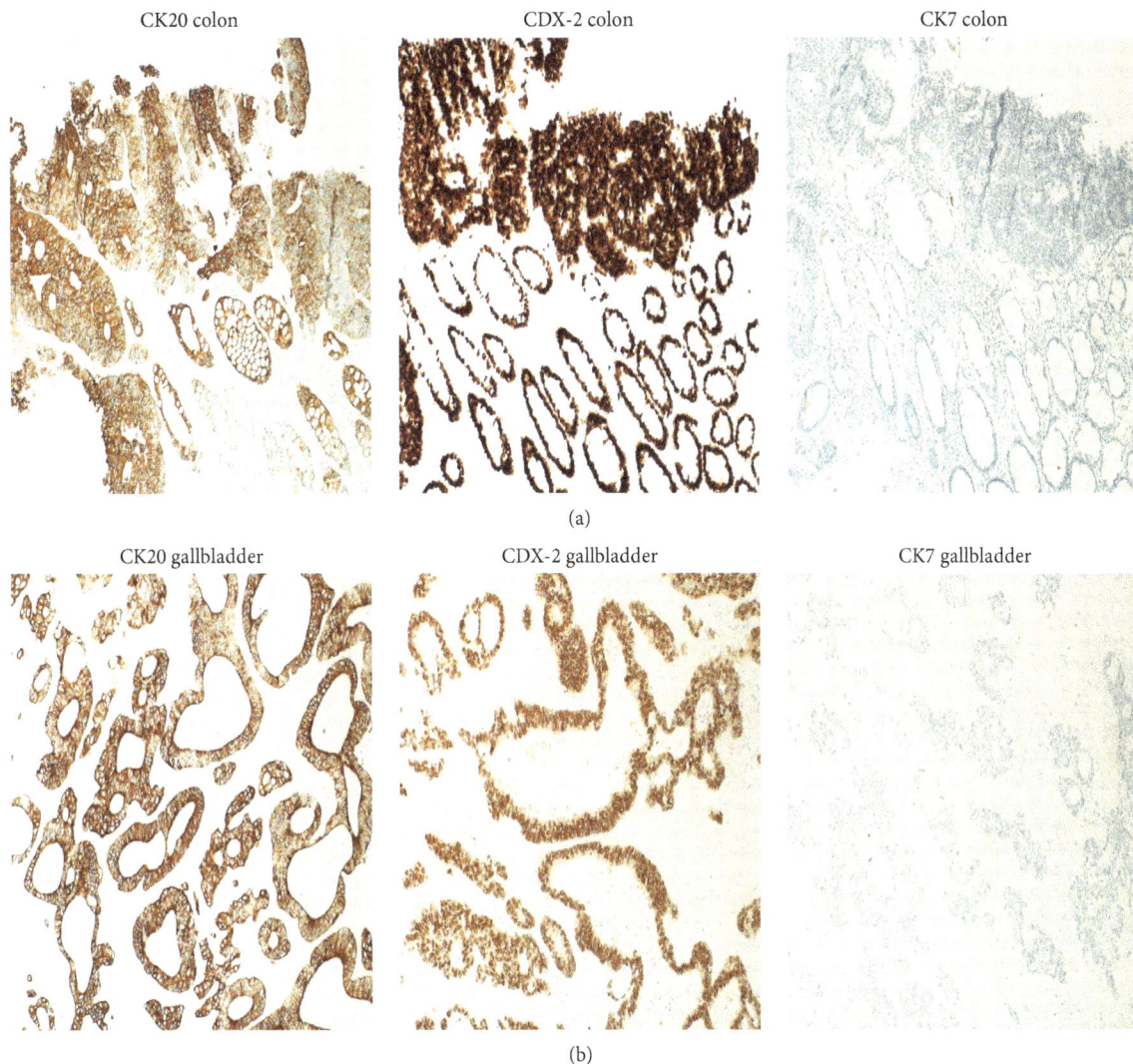

FIGURE 2: (a) Immunohistochemical analysis on the colon specimen. The specimen is CK20 positive, CK7 negative, and CDX-2 positive. (b) Final immunohistochemical analysis on the gallbladder specimen. The specimen is clearly CK20 positive, CK7 negative, and CDX-2 positive.

and endometrium. CK20 is mainly expressed in the gastrointestinal epithelium, Merkel cells, and urothelium [11, 12]. CK20-positive/CK-negative pattern is present in the majority of intestinal adenocarcinoma and also Merkel cell carcinoma whereas the CK7-positive/CK20-negative pattern is found in breast, lung, and ovarian adenocarcinoma. Both CK7 positivity and CK20 positivity are present in gastric, pancreatic, and urothelial carcinoma [11, 12].

The homeobox protein-2 (CDX-2) test result was also helpful in our case to further distinguish colon adenocarcinoma from other gastrointestinal and hepatobiliary tumors.

CDX-2 is normally expressed within the nuclei of the intestinal epithelium, from the duodenum to the rectum, and it is a sensitive and specific marker of adenocarcinomas of intestinal origin [13, 14].

The CK7-negative/CK20-positive expression pattern with CDX2 positivity is consistent with colorectal primary, while gallbladder cancers tend to be both positive for CK7 and CK20 [12–14].

Our case had two distinguishing features; the first one was the primary site being the cecum. The second interesting finding was features of concomitant acute acalculous cholecystitis and metastatic adenocarcinoma. We hypothesize that the local spread resulted in metastasis and subsequently acute cholecystitis mimicking primary gallbladder adenocarcinoma and causing diagnostic confusion.

4. Conclusion

Colon adenocarcinoma metastasizing to the gallbladder is extremely rare. To our knowledge, this is the first case of primary cecal adenocarcinoma with metastasis to the gallbladder presenting with acute acalculous cholecystitis.

References

[1] A. Jemal, F. Bray, M. M. Center, J. Ferlay, E. Ward, and D. Forman, "Global cancer statistics," *CA: a Cancer Journal for Clinicians*, vol. 61, no. 2, pp. 69–90, 2011, Epub 2011 Feb 4.

[2] M. Jung, J. B. Ahn, J. H. Chang et al., "Brain metastases from colorectal carcinoma: prognostic factors and outcome," *Journal of Neuro-Oncology*, vol. 101, no. 1, pp. 49–55, 2011.

[3] J. Fichna, *Introduction to Gastrointestinal Diseases Volume 1*, Springer Nature, 2017, https://www.springer.com/gp/book/9783319490151.

[4] S.-C. Chen, C.-Y. Hsu, S.-M. Wang, and T.-Y. Tai, "Adenocarcinoma of the transverse colon manifested as acute cholecystitis," *American Journal of Emergency Medicine*, vol. 12, no. 3, p. 386, 1994.

[5] A. Munghate, A. Kumar, H. Singh, G. Singh, B. Singh, and M. Chauhan, "Carcinoma transverse colon masquerading as carcinoma gall bladder," *Journal of Gastrointestinal Oncology*, vol. 5, no. 2, pp. E40–E42, 2014.

[6] B. Abdelilah, O. Mohamed, R. Yamoul et al., "Acute cholecystitis as a rare presentation of metastatic breast carcinoma of the Gallbladder: a case report and review of the literature," *Pan African Medical Journal*, vol. 17, p. 216, 2014.

[7] Y. T. N. M. Lee, "Breast carcinoma: pattern of metastasis at autopsy," *Journal of Surgical Oncology*, vol. 23, no. 3, pp. 175–180, 1983.

[8] R. J. Shah, A. Koehler, and J. D. Long, "Bile peritonitis secondary to breast cancer metastatic to the gallbladder," *The American Journal of Gastroenterology*, vol. 95, no. 5, pp. 1379–1381, 2000.

[9] H. L. Abrams, R. Spiro, and N. Goldstein, "Metastases in carcinoma; analysis of 1000 autopsied cases," *Cancer*, vol. 3, no. 1, pp. 74–85, 1950.

[10] H. Herrmann, H. Bär, L. Kreplak, S. V. Strelkov, and U. Aebi, "Intermediate filaments: from cell architecture to nanomechanics," *Nature Reviews Molecular Cell Biology*, vol. 8, no. 7, pp. 562–573, 2007.

[11] R. Bayrak, H. Haltas, and S. Yenidunya, "The value of CDX2 and cytokeratins 7 and 20 expression in differentiating colorectal adenocarcinomas from extraintestinal gastrointestinal adenocarcinomas: cytokeratin 7–/20+ phenotype is more specific than CDX2 antibody," *Diagnostic Pathology*, vol. 7, no. 1, p. 9, 2012.

[12] J. H. Shin, J. H. Bae, A. Lee et al., "CK7, CK20, CDX2 and MUC2 immunohistochemical staining used to distinguish metastatic colorectal carcinoma involving ovary from primary ovarian mucinous adenocarcinoma," *Japanese Journal of Clinical Oncology*, vol. 40, no. 3, pp. 208–213, 2010.

[13] R. W. Werling, H. Yaziji, C. E. Bacchi, and A. M. Gown, "CDX2, a highly sensitive and specific marker of adenocarcinomas of intestinal origin: an immunohistochemical survey of 476 primary and metastatic carcinomas," *American Journal of Surgical Pathology*, vol. 27, no. 3, pp. 303–310, 2003.

[14] http://www.pathologyoutlines.com/topic/stainsck7.html.

35

Pancreatic Adenocarcinoma Producing Parathyroid Hormone-Related Protein

Reiko Yamada,[1] **Kyosuke Tanaka,**[2] **Hiroyuki Inoue,**[1] **Takashi Sakuno,**[1] **Tetsuro Harada,**[1] **Naohiko Yoshizawa,**[1] **Hiroshi Miura,**[1] **Toshihumi Takeuchi,**[1] **Misaki Nakamura,**[1] **Masaki Katsurahara,**[2] **Yasuhiko Hamada,**[2] **Noriyuki Horiki,**[2] **and Yoshiyuki Takei**[1]

[1]Department of Gastroenterology and Hepatology, Mie University Graduate School of Medicine, Tsu, Japan
[2]Department of Endoscopy, Mie University School of Medicine, Tsu, Japan

Correspondence should be addressed to Reiko Yamada; reiko-t@clin.medic.mie-u.ac.jp

Academic Editor: Peter F. Lenehan

A 48-year-old woman presented to our hospital with a 1-year history of a continuous high fever. She was diagnosed with metastatic pancreatic adenocarcinoma accompanied by leukocytosis without infection. Her serum concentration of granulocyte colony-stimulating factor was highly elevated. Forty-five days after initiating chemotherapy, she was readmitted because of a neuropsychiatric disturbance and hypercalcemia. Her serum concentration of parathyroid hormone-related protein (PTH-rP) was elevated. A pretreatment biopsy specimen showed strong cytoplasmic immunoreactivity to anti-PTH-rP antibody, suggesting that overproduction of PTH-rP accounted for the hypercalcemia. Although the patient regained consciousness after treatment, she died of progressive disease 60 days after chemotherapy.

1. Introduction

Paraneoplastic syndromes are sometimes seen in patients with advanced malignancies. Tumors that produce parathyroid hormone-related protein (PTH-rP) can cause a paraneoplastic syndrome characterized by hypercalcemia [1]. The PTH-rP concentration is elevated in more than 90% of patients with squamous cell, renal, ovarian, breast, and endometrial cancer or human T-lymphotropic virus-associated lymphoma [1, 2]; however, it is rarely elevated in patients with pancreatic adenocarcinoma [3–6]. Hence, paraneoplastic production of PTH-rP by pancreatic adenocarcinomas is highly unlikely. We herein report a rare case of a pancreatic adenocarcinoma that produced PTH-rP, resulting in hypercalcemia.

2. Case Report

A 48-year-old woman was referred to our hospital with a 1-year history of a continuous high fever. Significant events in her medical history included Graves' disease at 39 years of age

and the removal of an ovarian cyst at 45 years of age. At the first time when she presented to the referring hospital with a high fever, computed tomography (CT) showed no apparent lesion. After surveillance, her fever was initially thought to be due to tonsillitis. A tonsillectomy was performed at the referring hospital; however, the fever persisted. Follow-up CT revealed a pancreatic body mass and multiple liver masses. Based on these findings, the patient was subsequently referred to our institution for further examination.

Initial laboratory tests showed leukocytosis (white blood cell count, 17,930/mm^3) and an elevated serum C-reactive protein (CRP) concentration (16.79 mg/dL) (Table 1). Blood cultures taken several times showed no signs of infection. Contrast-enhanced CT revealed a pancreatic body tumor with a diameter of 42 mm (Figure 1(a)) and multiple liver masses with marginal enhancement. ^{18}F-Fluorodeoxyglucose (^{18}F-FDG) positron emission tomography combined with CT showed ^{18}F-FDG accumulation in the pancreatic mass [maximum standardized uptake value (SUV max), 7.6], liver masses (SUV max, 9.4), swollen lymph nodes (SUV max, 8.4),

TABLE 1: Laboratory findings on first admission and second admission.

Laboratory data on first admission		Laboratory data on second admission	
WBC	17.930/μL	WBC	58.540/μL
Seg + band	85.7%	Seg + band	96.0%
Lymph.	6.6%	Lymph.	1.5%
Mono.	7.4%	Mono.	2.0%
Eosin.	0.2%	Eosin.	0.5%
Baso.	0.1%	Baso.	0%
RBC	$4.06 \times 10^6/\mu$L	RBC	$2.74 \times 10^6/\mu$L
Hb	10.3 g/dL	Hb	8.8 g/dL
Ht	32.0%	Ht	27.3%
Plt	$352 \times 10^3/\mu$L	Plt	$329 \times 10^3/\mu$L
APTT	38.6 sec	APTT	35.0 sec
PT	13.2 sec	PT	17.2 sec
Alb	3.4 g/dL	Alb	2.0 g/dL
T-bil	0.7 mg/dL	T-bil	2.7 mg/dL
AST	29 U/L	AST	82 U/L
ALT	31 U/L	ALT	47 U/L
LDH	215 U/L	LDH	468 U/L
ALP	669 U/L	ALP	1263 U/L
γ-GTP	127 U/L	γ-GTP	234 U/L
BUN	6 mg/dL	BUN	36 mg/dL
Cre	0.44 mg/dL	Cre	0.85 mg/dL
Glu	117 mg/dL	Glu	117 mg/dL
CRP	16.79 mg/dL	CRP	13.80 mg/dL
Na	130 mmol/L	Na	130 mmol/L
K	3.5 mmol/L	K	4.0 mmol/L
Cl	99 mmol/L	Cl	99 mmol/L
Ca	9.4 mg/dL	Ca	17.1 mg/dL
P	3.5 mg/dL	P	3.9 mg/dL
CEA	5.7 ng/mL	CEA	21.9 ng/mL
CA19-9	1.0 U/mL	CA19-9	1.0 U/mL
CA-125	691.5 U/mL	CA-125	3728.4 U/mL
G-CSF	85.1 pg/mL	PTH-rP	13.7 pmol/L
		PTH	11 pg/mL

WBC, white blood cells; RBC, red blood cells; Hb, hemoglobin; Ht, hematocrit; Plt, platelet count; APTT, activated partial thromboplastin time; PT, prothrombin time; CEA, carcinoembryonic antigen; CA, cancer antigen; G-CSF, granulocyte colony-stimulating factor; TP, total protein; Alb, albumin; T-bil, total bilirubin; AST, aspartate aminotransferase; ALT, alanine aminotransferase; LDH, lactate dehydrogenase; ALP, alkaline phosphatase; ChE, cholinesterase; Glu, glucose; CRP, C-reactive protein; T-chol, total cholesterol; TG, triglycerides; BUN, blood urea nitrogen; Cre, creatine; UA, uric acid; Na, sodium; K, potassium; Cl, chloride; Ca, calcium; P, phosphorus; PTH-rP, parathyroid hormone-related peptide; PTH, parathyroid hormone.

and several lung masses (SUV max, 1.0); however, there were no signs of bone metastasis (Figure 1(b)).

To obtain a definitive diagnosis, endoscopic ultrasound-guided fine-needle aspiration biopsy (EUS-FNAB) was performed using a 22-gauge FNA needle (EchoTip; Cook Medical, Bloomington, IN) (Figure 2). EUS revealed a dumbbell-shaped mass in the body of the pancreas. Histopathologic examination of the biopsy specimen showed necrotic tissue and tumor cells with highly atypical nuclei (Figure 3(a)), indicating a diagnosis of pancreatic adenocarcinoma. Tumor fever was the most likely cause of fever, because several blood cultures showed no signs of infection. The serum granulocyte colony-stimulating factor (G-CSF) concentration was 85.1 pg/mL (normal range, <39 pg/mL); however,

immunohistochemical (IHC) staining of the EUS-FNAB specimen for G-CSF showed demonstrated negative findings.

Oral administration chemotherapy of S-1, which is an oral fluoropyrimidine preparation, at 30 mg/m^2 twice daily on days 1 to 28 of each 42-day cycle was initiated. Although the treatment had been progressing without side effect, the patient was urgently admitted to the hospital 45 days after the commencement of chemotherapy because of neuropsychiatric symptoms during a scheduled follow-up visit; she had hallucinations and was wandering in her house at the day before admission. On admission, she was confused but able to localize pain and open her eyes in response to call.

Hematologic examination showed marked leukocytosis (white blood cell count, 58,540/mm^3), an elevated CRP

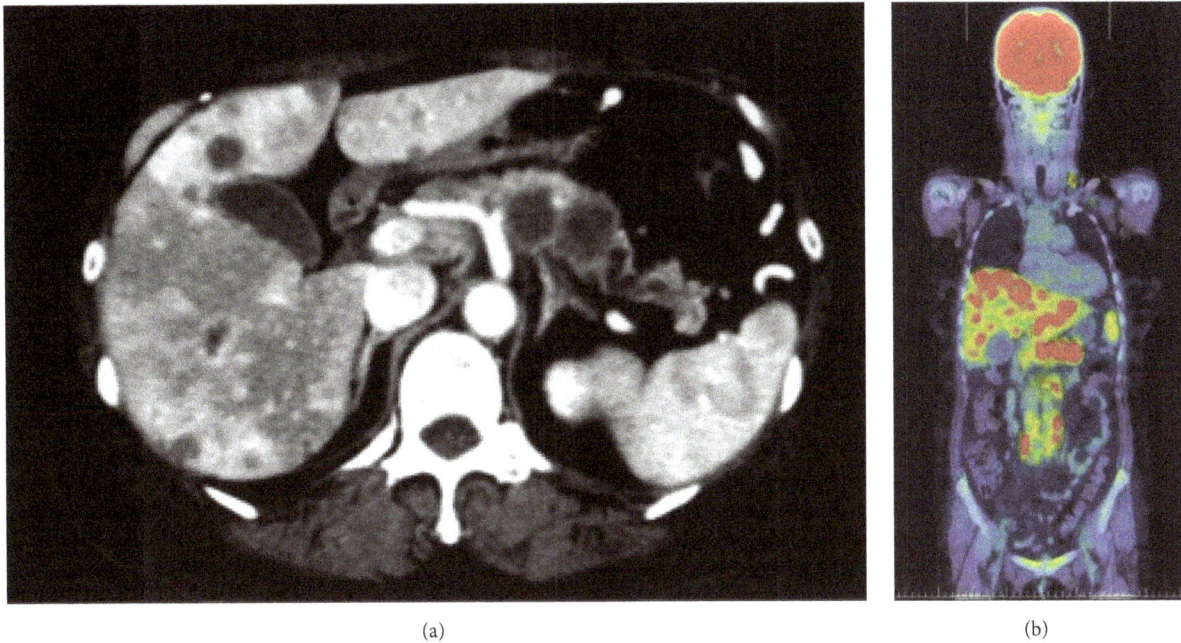

(a)   (b)

FIGURE 1: Computed tomography findings. (a) Contrast-enhanced computed tomography showed a hypovascular tumor in the pancreatic body and multiple liver masses with marginal enhancement. (b) Positron emission tomography-computed tomography showed accumulation of ^{18}F-fluorodeoxyglucose in the pancreatic body mass [maximum standardized uptake value (SUV max), 7.6], liver masses (SUV max, 9.4), swollen lymph nodes (SUV max, 8.4), and lung masses (SUV max, 1.0).

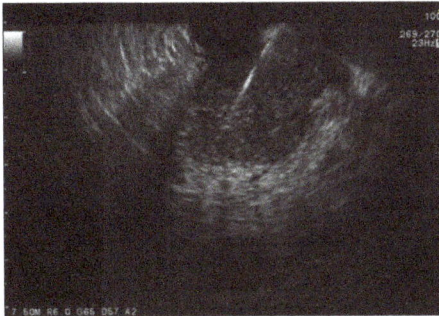

FIGURE 2: Endoscopic ultrasound findings. A dumbbell-shaped mass was present in the body of the pancreas.

concentration (13.80 mg/dL), and severe hypercalcemia (calcium concentration, 18.7 mg/dL, corrected for the albumin of 2 mg/dL) (Table 1). In addition, the serum PTH-rP concentration was 13.7 pmol/mL, which well exceeded the normal range (<1.1 pmol/mL). Production of PTH-rP by the tumor was confirmed via IHC staining of the pretreatment EUS-FNAB specimen previously obtained; strong expression of PTH-rP in the tissue of pancreatic adenocarcinoma was observed (Figure 3(b)). Hence, the hypercalcemia was likely caused by tumor-derived PTH-rP.

Parenteral hydration combined with furosemide was performed, followed by administration of synthetic calcitonin and bisphosphonate. The patient regained consciousness, and her serum calcium level normalized to 9.0 mg/dL. She was communicative and in good spirits for several days thereafter.

However, she ultimately died of progressive disease 60 days after the commencement of chemotherapy.

3. Discussion

In the present case, the serum PTH-rP and G-CSF concentrations were markedly elevated in a patient with a pancreatic adenocarcinoma. The strong expression of PTH-rP in the tissue of pancreatic adenocarcinoma was observed; thus production of PTH-rP by the tumor was confirmed, whereas IHC staining for G-CSF was negative in spite of markedly elevated serum G-CSF concentration. Hence, G-CSF elevation might occur secondary to inflammation.

PTH-rP is a single-chain peptide with an amino terminal domain that is very similar to that of PTH. PTH-rP is also known as an oncofetal protein expressed in both normal tissues and many malignancies, including squamous cell, renal, ovarian, breast, and endometrial cancers; however, it is rarely elevated in patients with pancreatic adenocarcinoma [2–6]. PTH-rP seems to play a role in cell growth, proliferation, and angiogenesis [7]. By interacting with its classic bone and kidney receptors, excess PTH-rP triggers an endocrine response that results in hypercalcemia.

Our patient exhibited an attenuated inflammatory reaction along with a continuous high fever and high serum CRP concentration. These findings suggest that inflammatory cytokines played a key role in the production of PTH-rP by cancer cells and the high serum G-CSF concentration. An association between hypercalcemia and inflammatory cytokines has been reported [8–10]. Our findings suggest that

(a)

(b)

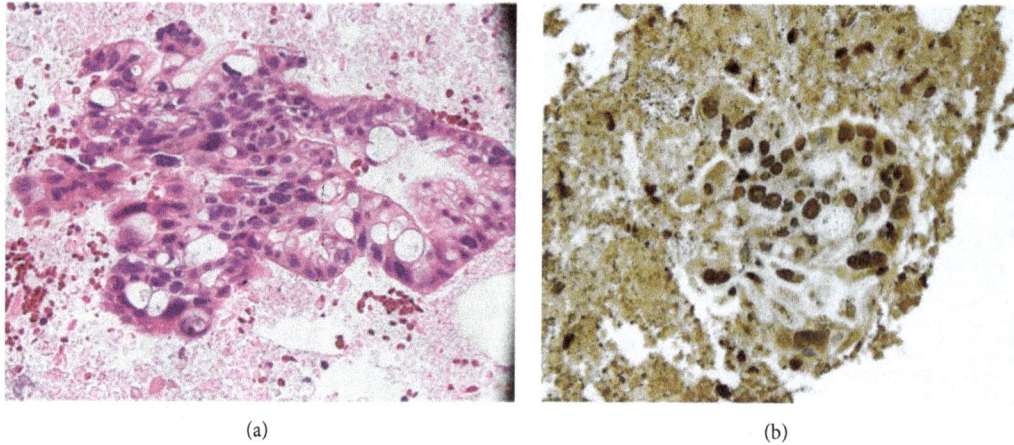

FIGURE 3: Pathologic examination findings. (a) Examination of an endoscopic ultrasound-guided fine-needle aspiration specimen showed necrotic tissue and tumor cells with highly atypical nuclei. Based on the histological findings, the final diagnosis was pancreatic adenocarcinoma. (b) Immunohistochemical staining of an endoscopic ultrasound-guided fine-needle aspiration specimen showed strong expression of parathyroid hormone-related protein.

continuous inflammation in association with rapid tumor growth may exacerbate the severe hypercalcemia caused by excess PTH-rP, ultimately resulting in the poor prognosis of pancreatic adenocarcinomas. However, further in vitro and in vivo studies are needed to confirm this theory in patients with pancreatic adenocarcinomas.

In conclusion, if a patient with pancreatic adenocarcinoma becomes an abnormal neuropsychiatric condition, hypercalcemia due to PTH-rP production by cancer cells should also be considered.

Ethical Approval

The study design was exempt from ethics review board approval.

Consent

The patient provided informed consent.

Acknowledgments

The authors thank Dr. Kazuo Fukutome from the Department of Pathology and Matrix Biology, Mie University, for his kind support.

References

[1] A. F. Stewart, "Clinical practice. Hypercalcemia associated with cancer," *The New England Journal of Medicine*, vol. 352, no. 4, pp. 373–379, 2005.

[2] T. Inoue, S. Nagao, H. Tajima et al., "Adenosquamous pancreatic cancer producing parathyroid hormone-related protein," *Journal of Gastroenterology*, vol. 39, no. 2, pp. 176–180, 2004.

[3] I. Tachibana, S. Nakano, T. Akiyama et al., "Parathyroid hormone-related protein mediates hypercalcemia in an exocrine pancreatic cancer," *American Journal of Gastroenterology*, vol. 89, pp. 1580-1581, 1994.

[4] M. Yamamoto, S. Nakano, M. Mugikura, I. Tachibana, Y. Ogami, and M. Otsuki, "Pancreatic cancer and hypercalcemia associated with von Recklinghausen's disease," *Journal of Gastroenterology*, vol. 31, no. 5, pp. 728–731, 1996.

[5] M. S. Rasnake, C. Glanton, D. Ornstein, M. Osswald, and M. Garrison, "Hypercalcemia mediated by parathyroid hormone-related protein as an early manifestation of pancreatic adenocarcinoma metastasis: A case report," *American Journal of Clinical Oncology: Cancer Clinical Trials*, vol. 24, no. 4, pp. 416-417, 2001.

[6] M. Bouvet, S. R. Nardin, D. W. Burton et al., "Human pancreatic adenocarcinomas express parathyroid hormone-related protein," *Journal of Clinical Endocrinology and Metabolism*, vol. 86, no. 1, pp. 310–316, 2001.

[7] J. J. Grzesiak, K. C. Smith, D. W. Burton, L. J. Deftos, and M. Bouvet, "GSK3 and PKB/Akt are associated with integrin-mediated regulation of PTHrP, IL-6 and IL-8 expression in FG pancreatic cancer cells," *International Journal of Cancer*, vol. 114, no. 4, pp. 522–530, 2005.

[8] N. Asanuma, K. Hagiwara, I. Matsumoto et al., "PTHrP-producing tumor: Squamous cell carcinoma of the liver accompanied by humoral hypercalcemia of malignancy, increased IL-6 and leukocytosis," *Internal Medicine*, vol. 41, no. 5, pp. 371–376, 2002.

[9] C. W. G. M. Löwik, G. van der Pluijm, H. Bloys et al., "Parathyroid hormone (PTH) and PTH-like protein (PLP) stimulate interleukin-6 production by osteogenic cells: A possible role of interleukin-6 in osteoclastogenesis," *Biochemical and Biophysical Research Communications*, vol. 162, no. 3, pp. 1546–1552, 1989.

[10] M. Weissglas, D. Schamhart, C. Lowik, S. Papapoulos, P. Vos, and K.-H. Kurth, "Investigative Urology: Hypercalcemia and Cosecretion of Interleukin-6 and Parathyroid Hormone Related Peptide by a Human Renal Cell Carcinoma Implanted Into Nude Mice," *The Journal of Urology*, vol. 153, no. 3, pp. 854–857, 1995.

36

Primary CNS Burkitt Lymphoma: A Case Report of a 55-Year-Old Cerebral Palsy Patient

Kathryn Bower ⓘ[1] **and Nilay Shah**[2]

[1]Section of Hematology/Oncology, West Virginia University, Morgantown, WV, USA
[2]Alexander B. Osborn Hematopoietic Malignancy and Transplantation Program, West Virginia University, Morgantown, WV, USA

Correspondence should be addressed to Kathryn Bower; kathryn.bower@hsc.wvu.edu

Academic Editor: Jeanine M. Buchanich

With primary central nervous system lymphoma (PCNSL) being a rare disease, the subtype of Burkitt lymphoma (BL) presenting as a sole CNS lesion is an even more exceptional diagnosis. A case of coexistent primary CNS Burkitt lymphoma (PCNSBL) with cerebral palsy (CP) is presented. A 55-year-old Caucasian male presented with increasing bilateral lower extremity weakness above his baseline in addition to signs of increased intracranial pressure. Four abnormal enhancing masses were detected on MRI with biopsy results consistent with Burkitt lymphoma. Complete staging workup was completed with no evidence of extra-CNS disease noted on PET/CT, bone marrow biopsy, or cerebral spinal fluid analysis. The patient was treated with intravenous as well as intrathecal chemotherapy and found to be in a complete remission at six months. Recurrence in the CNS was observed four months later with treatment consisting of whole brain radiation as well as intrathecal chemotherapy. Thirty months after diagnosis, the patient remains disease-free. To our knowledge, this is the first case of PCNSBL in the setting of CP. A review of literature regarding treatment options in this controversial setting is provided.

1. Introduction

Primary central nervous system lymphoma (PCNSL) has historically been an uncommon disease entity since it was first discovered. Recent reviews, however, indicate that cases continue to arise at increasing numbers [1–3]. Incidence rose three-fold between the years of 1973 and 1984; however, the rate of increase is currently trending toward stabilization [4]. This is perhaps due to the invention of highly active antiretroviral therapy (HAART) for acquired immunodeficiency syndrome (AIDS) as immunocompromised individuals remain at 300% increased risk for PCNSL [3], and the average age of diagnosis is 40 in the immunosuppressed population versus 55–61 years of age in those who are immunocompetent [3]. Even as the incidence of PCNSL rises, it remains a rare disease with a mere 7% incidence rate. The subset of those individuals with primary CNS Burkitt lymphoma (PCNSBL) constitutes an even scarcer population comprising just 3–5% of the PCNSL cases [1–3]. Only 36

cases of PCNSBL were found worldwide after a thorough literature review (Table 1).

With such diminutive evidence on the most effective way to treat these patients, no standard of care exists, and the chosen therapy has been anything but uniform. Many have elected various combinations of intravenous (IV) chemotherapy, intrathecal (IT) chemotherapy, and radiation therapy. A backbone of IV high-dose methotrexate (HD-MTX) proves to be the most significant prognostic variable with regard to treatment [3]. However, the optimal role for IT MTX as well as radiation has yet to be defined.

Recently, there has been doubt amongst professionals whether whole brain radiation therapy (WBRT) should be implored for these patients. In those who receive WBRT, approximately 61% relapse within the radiation field, and the risk of significant neurotoxicity, is 25–35% at 5 years with death occurring in one-third of those patients [4–6]. This toxicity proves especially detrimental in individuals greater than 60 years of age [4], with recent assertions that using

TABLE 1: Reported PCNSBL cases. Cy: cyclophosphamide; OS: overall survival; WBRT: whole brain radiation therapy; CHOP: cyclophosphamide, doxorubicin, vincristine, and prednisone; Dex: dexamethasone; IVIG: intravenous immunoglobulin; MTX: methotrexate.

Author	Year	Age/sex	How it is diagnosed (LP versus mass)	Treatment and OS
Gawish [18]	1976	8/M	Left frontoparietal mass extending across midline and through the skull	Complete resection with recurrence. Subtotal resection with Cy. OS of 3 years
Valsamis et al. [19]	1976	6 m/M	Left parietal, bilateral temporal, and post pituitary mass with abdominal and periaortic nodal involvement	Resection, steroids, WBRT, and spinal irradiation with recurrence, IT MTX. OS of 23 months
Tanaka et al. [20]	1977	49/M	Right thalamus to midbrain mass	Subtotal resection. OS of 4.5 years
Tanaka et al. [20]	1977	58/M	Right temporal mass	Subtotal resection. Recurrence. OS 3 months
Tanaka et al. [20]	1977	42/M	Left deep parietal to occipital mass	Pred with partial resection. Recurrence. Vincristine and Cy with radiation. Vincristine, bleomycin, Cy, steroids. OS of 2.5 years
Giromini et al. [11]	1981	11/M	Left temporooccipital mass	Complete resection
Hegedüs [21]	1984	50/F	Right lower parietal lobe mass	Post mortem finding
Kobayashi [22]	1984	55/F	Right temporoparietal mass	Complete resection. Recurrence with reresection. OS of 2 months
Pui et al. [23]	1985	6/M	T2-5 mass	Laminectomy and CHOP (without prednisone). OS > 2 years
Pui et al. [23]	1985	7/M	C7-T4 mass	Laminectomy, radiation, dex, and Cy. Recurrence. OS of 5 months
Pui et al. [23]	1985	12/M	T7-10 mass	Laminectomy, CHOP (substituting dex for prednisone). OS of 4 months
Mizugami et al. [24]	1987	6/M	T10 mass	Near complete resection, radiation, and chemotherapy. Leukemic transformation then CSF recurrence. IT MTX and cranial irradiation. OS of 20 months
Mizugami et al. [24]	1987	5/M	Epidural T12-L4 mass	Near complete resection, radiation, and chemotherapy with recurrence. OS of 7 months
Mizugami et al. [24]	1987	7/F	T11 mass	Near complete resection. Spinal radiation and chemotherapy with progression of disease. OS of 3 months
Shigemori et al. [25]	1991	49/F	Left frontal lobe mass	Resection, radiation, CHOP, and IT MTX. OS of >6 months
Tekkök et al. [12]	1991	5/M	Parasellar mass, extending to bilateral sphenoids and sella turcica	Partial resection, craniospinal radiation, CHOP, and IT MTX/cytarabine/prednisone. OS > 18 months
Toren et al. [26]	1994	6/F	CSF	Steroids, IVIG, doxorubicin, vincristine, HD MTX, with IT MTX, cytarabine, and hydrocortisone. Changed to CHOP with MTX and IT MTX, cytarabine, hydrocortisone. OS of >2 years
Mora and Wollner [7]	1999	18/M	T11 mass	Laminectomy with CHOP substitute daunorubicin for doxorubicin and radiation. Relapse and refused further treatment. OS > 8 months
Mora and Wollner [7]	1999	9/M	Epidural T9-11 mass	Laminectomy, dex, radiation, and CHOP (substituting daunorubicin for doxorubicin). Recurrence and given chemotherapy via LSA3 protocol. Second recurrence, received palliative radiation. OS > 1 year
Spath-Schwalbe et al. [27]	1999	40/M	Cerebellum and pons masses	MTX and WBRT. OS > 1 year
Wilkening et al. [28]	2001	43/F	L2-3 epidural tumor involving the dura and cauda equina	Complete resection, radiation, IT MTX, and MTX with ifosfamide and CHOP (with dex substituted for prednisone). OS of >2 years
Monabati et al. [29]	2002	49/F	Right parietal mass	Complete resection, CHOP, and craniospinal radiation. Refused further treatment. OS of >6 months
Daley et al. [30]	2003	13/F	L1-2 epidural mass	Complete excision, CHOP with MTX, and IT MTX and cytarabine and steroids. OS of >5 years

TABLE 1: Continued.

Author	Year	Age/sex	How it is diagnosed (LP versus mass)	Treatment and OS
Shehu [31]	2003	8/M	Left temporal and right orbit masses	Cy, vincristine, and MTX with IT cytosine arabinoside. OS of 11 months
Abel et al. [32]	2006	50/M	Central and right thalamus mass	Unknown
Gobbato et al. [15]	2006	38/M	Right frontotemporoparietal subdural mass	Craniotomy. OS of 11 days
Kozáková et al. [33]	2008	60/F	Sellar/pituitary mass	Complete resection
Gu et al. [34]	2010	75/F	Third and left lateral ventricle masses	WBRT. OS of >9 months
Takasu et al. [35]	2010	71/M	Hypothalamus and third ventricle mass	Partial resection and WBRT
Jiang et al. [36]	2011	14/M	Right lateral ventricle mass	Complete resection, radiation, and MTX, vincristine, predisone, and leucovorin. OS of >18 months
Lim et al. [10]	2011	43/F	Medulla oblongata mass, CSF involvement	MTX, vincristine, and procarbazine with IT MTX and WBRT. OS of 7 months
Akhaddar et al. [37]	2012	13/F	Right infratemporal and cavernous/maxillary/sphenoethmoidal sinus mass	Chemotherapy
Jiang et al. [38]	2012	69/M	Right temporal and occipital lobe, cervical spine, and cauda equina masses; CSF involvement	DLBCL/BL subtype. WBRT, spinal radiation with recurrence. HD MTX and cytarabine with rituximab
Yoon et al. [39]	2012	10/M	Suprasellar, cerebellum, and 3rd ventricle masses; CSF involvement	HD MTX and cytarabine with IT cytarabine, MTX, and hydrocortisone. OS of >7 years
Yoon et al. [39]	2012	32 m/M	Sellar mass extending to orbit/sphenoid, CSF involvement	HD MTX and cytarabine with IT cytarabine, MTX, and hydrocortisone. Relapse, treated with IT cytarabine, MTX, and hydrocortisone with WBRT and spinal radiation. Then received prednisone, vincristine, and cyclophosphamide with IT. OS of 9 months
Alabdulsalam et al. [40]	2014	18/M	4th ventricle mass	Craniotomy with HD MTX with rituximab-CHOP and IT MTX, cytarabine, and hydrocortisone. OS of >18 months

WBRT in children is no longer necessary or acceptable due to significant risk of long-term neurotoxicity [7]. The German PCNSL Study Group is the largest and only phase III randomized trial comparing IV chemotherapy ± WBRT which revealed no significant difference in overall survival (OS) (44.2 versus 59.0 months, $p = 0.78$) when WBRT was added to HD-MTX-based chemotherapy in those patients with a complete response (CR) [8]. In a subset of patients who did not reach a CR, however, the addition of WBRT did show prolonged progression-free survival (PFS) (5.0 versus 2.9 months, $p = 0.002$) but did reveal a difference in OS (27.4 versus 18.2 months, $p = 0.119$) [8].

Several different therapeutic options, including IT chemotherapy and complete surgical resection, have also been questioned. As IV HD-MTX crosses the blood-brain barrier, many believe IT only increases toxicity with little to no additional benefit. Complete resection of the tumor has also been challenged in the past as it potentially increases neurologic deficits without any survival benefit [5]. Recently, the German PCNSL Study Group-1 (GPSG-1) trial has refuted this, stating there may be significant PFS [2]. Discrepancies may be attributed to the advances that have been made in neurosurgical techniques over the last decade [2].

Patients with PCNSL have an extremely poor prognosis, with an OS of approximately 12–18 months [1, 3, 9]. Without treatment, this number dwindles to 1.5–3.3 months [10]. Therefore, it is imperative that this disease be treated with the best available option to improve the expected survival of these individuals. Here, we present a case of an adult HIV-negative male with PCNSBL in the setting of cerebral palsy (CP) and our approach to treatment with long-term follow-up.

2. Case

A 55-year-old Caucasian male with past medical history of cerebral palsy (CP) presented with nausea, vomiting, thirty-pound weight loss, and worsening bilateral lower extremity weakness for one month. A computerized tomography (CT) angiogram of the brain revealed a suprasellar mass facilitating transfer to our institution for further management. Magnetic resonance imaging (MRI) of the brain indicated abnormal enhancement along the ependymal margin of the frontal horns of the bilateral lateral ventricles with four distinct abnormal enhancing mass lesions in the hypothalamus ($11 \times 12 \times 13$ mm), pineal gland ($8 \times 8 \times 9$ mm), the trigon of the right lateral ventricle ($5 \times 5 \times 4$ mm), and the

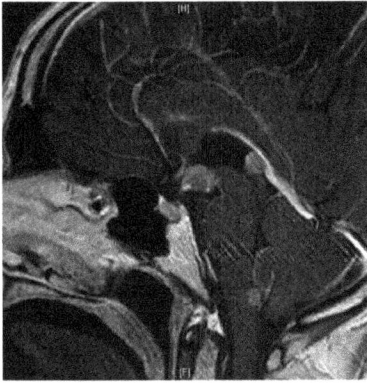

FIGURE 1: MRI brain, T1 sagittal + gadolinium, demonstrated lesions within hypothalamus, pineal gland, trigon of the right lateral ventricle, and foramen of Magendie at diagnosis.

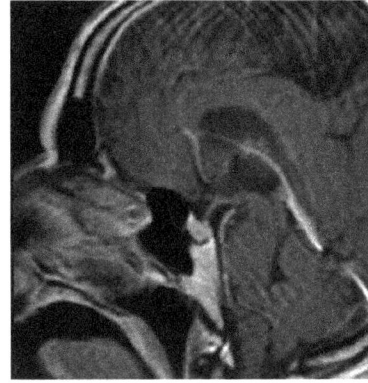

FIGURE 2: MRI brain, T1 sagittal + gadolinium, revealing complete resolution of all four mass lesions after receiving IV and IT chemotherapy.

foramen of Magendie ($7 \times 6 \times 9$ mm) which demonstrated restriction diffusion indicating hypercellularity (Figure 1).

An endoscopic biopsy of the third ventricle floor lesion was performed with pathology revealing sheets of intermediate size monotonous lymphoid cells displaying high nuclear-to-cytoplasmic ratio with dispersed chromatin and indistinct nucleoli. Numerous apoptotic cells and mitotic figures with foci of necrosis were observed. The tumor cells displayed CD 20 with coexpression of CD 10 and were negative for BCL 2, BCL 6, CD 3, and CD 5. EBER in situ hybridization was also negative. Fluorescent in situ hybridization was positive for [11, 12] (MYC/IHG) fusion in 97% of the cells and loss of BCL2 in 96%. These results appeared to be consistent with Burkitt lymphoma.

Staging workup was obtained which only revealed concern for extra cranial disease present at T12-L1 and L2-L3 consistent with subarachnoid nodular pial metastases on MRI of the lumbosacral spine. PET/CT disclosed no evidence of extra-CNS disease. A lumbar puncture and bone marrow biopsy were performed and found to be negative for disease. In the absence of extra-CNS disease, the patient was diagnosed with PCNSBL.

Patient was started on IV HD-MTX (3.5 grams per meter squared) and cytarabine (2 grams per meter squared) per Ferreri regimen [13] with the addition of IT MTX/cytarabine every 21 days for four cycles. Dose was reduced by 25% for cycle three due to persistent cytopenias and toxicity including renal dysfunction with delayed MTX clearance. A repeat brain MRI was obtained after 6 months which indicated complete remission with no evidence of disease (Figure 2).

Four months later, the patient began having generalized weakness with visual disturbances and headaches. A repeat brain MRI at that time revealed interval development of markedly abnormal signal in the pons extending to the midbrain and dorsal medulla. Repeat cerebral spinal fluid (CSF) analysis showed rare atypical lymphocytes consistent with relapse of lymphoma. He underwent WBRT, receiving 30 Gray (Gy) over 17 fractions with an additional boost to the midbrain lesion with 9 Gy in 8 fractions. Currently, he is disease-free at 30 months s/p diagnosis.

3. Discussion

To our knowledge, our patient is the only PCNSBL case with a past medical history of CP. No literature was discovered that revealed a connection between these two diseases, and further research may be warranted if similar cases develop in the future. It would have been easy to dismiss the presenting symptoms as part of his CP; therefore, caution must be taken to not be blinded by a patient's past medical history in attempting to decipher the etiology of new symptoms. Primary CNS lymphoma should remain a consideration for those presenting with neurological symptoms regardless of their history.

The optimal treatment for PCNSBL continues to elude us, and no standard of care exists at this time. The paucity of cases provides little opportunity for randomized controlled trials; therefore, clinicians have been forced to extrapolate based upon recommendations for Burkitt lymphoma residing outside as well as PCNSL regimens. Many of the reported cases of PCNSBL used HD-MTX +/−, some variation of cyclophosphamide, doxorubicin, vincristine, and prednisone (CHOP) therapy. A few studies attempted additional agents such as ifosfamide and procarbazine, but had little success. Several used IT MTX alone or in combination with cytarabine and steroids.

Our treatment decision was based upon the Ferreri regimen, which is the only randomized trial for PCNSL [13]. Since our patient suffered from the added rarity of Burkitt lymphoma subtype, the addition of IT chemotherapy was made based on standard practice for extra-CNS Burkitt lymphoma as it has a high incidence of CNS penetration. While there has been some debate regarding the need for IT chemotherapy in addition to IV HD-MTX, these patients were mostly non-Burkitt type (diffuse large B cell) PCNSL. Even with the baseline cognitive deficits of our patient, he was able to tolerate an aggressive chemotherapy regimen that included IT and eventually WBRT without any permanent neurological complications to date. Although he did develop some mild delirium while hospitalized for WBRT and IT MTX after relapse, this promptly resolved prior to discharge. The decision at that time was made to withhold any further

IT therapy as no further evidence of disease was present and the risk of toxicities outweighed the current benefits. He remains disease-free at 30 months.

The role of IT therapy has been challenged in the face of HD-MTX therapy being able to cross the BBB. Ferreri et al. have shown that there is no survival benefit when using IT in addition to HD-MTX with regard to PCNSL of all types, with 2-year OS rates of 51 ± 5% with IT versus 50 ± 6% without IT [14]. There are also reports of increased neurotoxicity when adding concurrent IT to HD-MTX with no survival benefit [8]. Neither of these studies separated those with Burkitt subtype, however. Therefore, our decision for IT administration was based upon extrapolation from accepted therapy for extra-CNS Burkitt lymphoma being IT MTX/Ara-C in addition to systemic chemotherapy.

We present a case of relapsed lymphoma that responded to WBRT of 30 Gray in 17 fractions with boost of 9 Gray in 8 fractions which was tolerated well with a complete response (CR), and no evidence of disease at 18 months after radiation was completed. Many studies have attempted to investigate the benefits and toxicities associated with the use of WBRT, which challenges the prior approach to this entity. There seems to be a trend away from WBRT, especially in those individuals > 60 years of age and children with no evidence of residual disease after IV chemotherapy, as long-term neurocognitive consequences have been found to outweigh the benefit gained by these patients with neurotoxicity being fatal even without evidence of recurrent disease [4].

Recent studies have shown no OS benefit when adding upfront WBRT to HD-MTX-containing regimens. Ferreri et al. have shown an OS of 25 ± 4% at 2 years with WBRT alone which was significantly inferior to both MTX-containing chemotherapy as well as MTX combined with WBRT, revealing a 2-year OS of 34 ± 10% and 45 ± 3%, respectively [14]. This OS difference between WBRT with MTX versus MTX alone was not significant; therefore, it is suggested that those individuals at a high risk of neurotoxicity forego WBRT unless relapse or refractory disease is apparent. We therefore chose to forego WBRT in the initial setting, reserving it for relapsed disease in our patient. Debate also exists regarding the optimal dose of WBRT, as each study utilized different fractions and dosages. Hyperfractionation has also been noted to have increase toxicity as compared to standard dosage with neurotoxicity rates of 23% and 3.7%, respectively [5]. This has been shown to be most prevalent in those receiving > 50 Gray [9].

The concept of complete surgical resection has fallen under scrutiny in recent years as well. Previously, many subscribed to complete resection of the mass with recent reports challenging this citing an increase in postoperative neurological deficits with no OS benefit [2, 3, 15]. Currently, the decision for excision when CNS lesions are the only areas of disease is made on a case by case basis with regard to tumor location and expected postsurgical deficits.

Despite adequate initial treatment with chemotherapy with or without WBRT, approximately 40–50% of PCNSL patients relapse within the first 5 years [3]. This obviates the need for obtaining better treatment modalities, not only first line but also for relapsed or refractory disease. The

median post relapse survival rate approximates 2 months with a 2-year OS of 8% [3]. Our patient is now 18 months status post a second CR. A few small studies have evaluated the role of bone marrow transplant as a potential treatment for PCNSL in the relapsed and refractory setting as these individuals have a significantly increased risk of death [2, 16, 17]. Randomized phase II trials must be undertaken to thoroughly evaluate this option with regard to such a specific disease population.

Our patient subscribed to the current statistics of recurrence of disease within the first five years despite a complete response to initial treatment. He is currently disease-free for 18 months after reinduction with WBRT, which is longer than the average survival of such individuals, and remains without any significant neurotoxicity. Using our approach of IV and IT chemotherapy in PCNSBL upfront and reserving WBRT for the relapsed setting, our patient has far exceeded the median post relapse survival rate. This suggests a potential benefit to our approach. Regardless of the relatively favorable outcome of our patient, it remains that clear optimal treatment continues to be elusive. Substantial advances are required with regard to PCNSBL, as it remains a significant challenge to patients and physicians alike.

References

[1] D. C. Miller, F. H. Hochberg, N. L. Harris, M. L. Gruber, D. N. Louis, and H. Cohen, "Pathology with clinical correlations of primary central nervous system non-Hodgkin's lymphoma. The Massachusetts general hospital experience 1958-1989," *Cancer*, vol. 74, no. 4, pp. 1383–1397, 1994.

[2] J. L. Rubenstein, N. K. Gupta, G. N. Mannis, A. K. LaMarre, and P. Treseler, "How I treat CNS lymphomas," *Blood*, vol. 122, no. 14, pp. 2318–2330, 2013.

[3] J. Y. Blay, P. Ongolo-Zogo, C. Sebban et al., "Primary cerebral lymphomas: unsolved issues regarding first-line treatment, follow-up, late neurological toxicity and treatment of relapses," *Annals of Oncology*, vol. 11, Supplement_1, pp. S39–S44, 2000.

[4] T. Batchelor and J. S. Loeffler, "Primary CNS lymphoma," *Journal of Clinical Oncology*, vol. 24, no. 8, pp. 1281–1288, 2006.

[5] L. M. DeAngelis, W. Seiferheld, S. C. Schold, B. Fisher, C. J. Schultz, and Radiation Therapy Oncology Group Study 93-10, "Combination chemotherapy and radiotherapy for primary central nervous system lymphoma: radiation therapy oncology group study 93-10," *Journal of Clinical Oncology*, vol. 20, no. 24, pp. 4643–4648, 2002.

[6] M. Reni, A. J. M. Ferreri, N. Guha-Thakurta et al., "Clinical relevance of consolidation radiotherapy and other main therapeutic issues in primary central nervous system lymphomas treated with upfront high-dose methotrexate," *International Journal of Radiation Oncology*Biology*Physics*, vol. 51, no. 2, pp. 419–425, 2001.

[7] J. Mora and N. Wollner, "Primary epidural non-Hodgkin lymphoma: spinal cord compression syndrome as the initial

form of presentation in childhood non-Hodgkin lymphoma," *Medical and Pediatric Oncology*, vol. 32, no. 2, pp. 102–105, 1999.

[8] A. Korfel, E. Thiel, P. Martus et al., "Randomized phase III study of whole-brain radiotherapy for primary CNS lymphoma," *Neurology*, vol. 84, no. 12, pp. 1242–1248, 2015.

[9] B. Bataille, V. Delwail, E. Menet et al., "Primary intracerebral malignant lymphoma: report of 248 cases," *Journal of Neurosurgery*, vol. 92, no. 2, pp. 261–266, 2000.

[10] T. Lim, S. J. Kim, K. Kim et al., "Primary CNS lymphoma other than DLBCL: a descriptive analysis of clinical features and treatment outcomes," *Annals of Hematology*, vol. 90, no. 12, pp. 1391–1398, 2011.

[11] D. Giromini, J. Peiffer, and T. Tzonos, "Occurrence of a primary Burkitt-type lymphoma of the central nervous system in an astrocytoma patient," *Acta Neuropathologica*, vol. 54, no. 2, pp. 165–167, 1981.

[12] İ. H. Tekkök, K. Tahta, A. Erbengi, M. Büyükpamukçu, Ş. Ruacan, and M. Topçu, "Primary intracranial extradural Burkitt-type lymphoma," *Child's Nervous System*, vol. 7, no. 3, pp. 172–174, 1991.

[13] A. J. M. Ferreri, M. Reni, M. Foppoli et al., "High-dose cytarabine plus high-dose methotrexate versus high-dose methotrexate alone in patients with primary CNS lymphoma: a randomised phase 2 trial," *The Lancet*, vol. 374, no. 9700, pp. 1512–1520, 2009.

[14] A. J. M. Ferreri, M. Reni, F. Pasini et al., "A multicenter study of treatment of primary CNS lymphoma," *Neurology*, vol. 58, no. 10, pp. 1513–1520, 2002.

[15] P. L. Gobbato, A. A. Pereira Filho, G. David et al., "Primary meningeal Burkitt-type lymphoma presenting as the first clinical manifestation of acquired immunodeficiency syndrome," *Arquivos de Neuro-Psiquiatria*, vol. 64, no. 2b, pp. 511–515, 2006.

[16] A. J. M. Ferreri, L. E. Abrey, J. Y. Blay et al., "Summary statement on primary central nervous system lymphomas from the eighth international conference on malignant lymphoma, Lugano, Switzerland, June 12 to 15, 2002," *Journal of Clinical Oncology*, vol. 21, no. 12, pp. 2407–2414, 2003.

[17] A. J. M. Ferreri, R. Crocchiolo, A. Assanelli, S. Govi, and M. Reni, "High-dose chemotherapy supported by autologous stem cell transplantation in patients with primary central nervous system lymphoma: facts and opinions," *Leukemia & Lymphoma*, vol. 49, no. 11, pp. 2042–2047, 2008.

[18] H. H. A. Gawish, "Primary Burkitt's lymphoma of the frontal bone," *Journal of Neurosurgery*, vol. 45, no. 6, pp. 712–715, 1976.

[19] M. P. Valsamis, P. H. Levine, I. Rapin, M. Santorineou, and K. Shulman, "Primary intracranial Burkitt's lymphoma in an infant," *Cancer*, vol. 37, no. 3, pp. 1500–1507, 1976.

[20] T. Tanaka, A. Nishimoto, A. Doi et al., "Primary intracranial malignant lymphomas with particular reference to their pathogenesis," *Acta Pathologica Japonica*, vol. 27, no. 6, pp. 927–940, 1977.

[21] K. Hegedüs, "Burkitt-type lymphoma and reticulum-cell sarcoma. An unusual mixed form of two intracranial primary malignant lymphomas," *Surgical Neurology*, vol. 21, no. 1, pp. 23–29, 1984.

[22] H. Kobayashi, T. Sano, K. Li, and K. Hizawa, "Primary Burkitt-type lymphoma of the central nervous system," *Acta Neuropathologica*, vol. 64, no. 1, pp. 12–14, 1984.

[23] C. H. Pui, G. V. Dahl, H. O. Hustu, and S. B. Murphy, "Epidural spinal cord compression as the initial finding in childhood acute leukemia and non-Hodgkin lymphoma," *The Journal of Pediatrics*, vol. 106, no. 5, pp. 788–792, 1985.

[24] T. Mizugami, A. Mikata, H. Hajikano, K. Asanuma, H. Ishida, and C. Nakamura, "Primary spinal epidural Burkitt's lymphoma," *Surgical Neurology*, vol. 28, no. 2, pp. 158–162, 1987.

[25] M. Shigemori, T. Tokunaga, J. Miyagi et al., "Multiple brain tumors of different cell types with an unruptured cerebral aneurysm," *Neurologia Medico-Chirurgica*, vol. 31, no. 2, pp. 96–99, 1991.

[26] A. Toren, M. Mandel, E. Shahar et al., "Primary central nervous system Burkitt's lymphoma presenting as Guillain-Barré syndrome," *Medical and Pediatric Oncology*, vol. 23, no. 4, pp. 372–375, 1994.

[27] E. Spath-Schwalbe, I. Genvresse, H. Stein et al., "Primary cerebral highly-malignant B-cell lymphoma of the Burkitt type," *Deutsche Medizinische Wochenschrift*, vol. 124, no. 15, pp. 451–455, 1999.

[28] A. Wilkening, M. Brack, A. Brandis, F. Heidenreich, R. Dengler, and K. Weibetaenborn, "Unusual presentation of a primary spinal Burkitt's lymphoma," *Journal of Neurology, Neurosurgery, & Psychiatry*, vol. 70, no. 6, pp. 794–797, 2001.

[29] A. Monabati, S. M. Rakei, P. V. Kumar, M. Taghipoor, and A. Rahimi, "Primary Burkitt lymphoma of the brain in an immunocompetent patient," *Journal of Neurosurgery*, vol. 96, no. 6, pp. 1127–1129, 2002.

[30] M. F. Daley, M. D. Partington, N. Kadan-Lottick, and L. F. Odom, "Primary epidural Burkitt lymphoma in a child: case presentation and literature review," *Pediatric Hematology and Oncology*, vol. 20, no. 4, pp. 333–338, 2003.

[31] B. B. Shehu, "Primary central nervous system Burkitt's lymphoma presenting with proptosis," *Annals of Tropical Paediatrics*, vol. 23, no. 4, pp. 319–320, 2003.

[32] T. W. Abel, M. A. Thompson, J. Kim, A. Yenamandra, and M. W. Becher, "Primary central nervous system Burkitt lymphoma: report of a case confirmed with identification of t(8;14) by FISH," *Brain Pathology*, vol. 16, Supplement 1, pp. 96-97, 2006.

[33] D. Kozáková, K. Macháleková, P. Brtko, P. Szépe, P. Vanuga, and M. Pura, "Primary B-cell pituitary lymphoma of the Burkitt type: case report of the rare clinic entity with typical clinical presentation," *Casopis lekaru ceskych*, vol. 147, no. 11, pp. 569–573, 2008.

[34] Y. Gu, Y. Hou, X. Zhang, and F. Hu, "Primary central nervous system Burkitt lymphoma as concomitant lesions in the third and the left ventricles: a case study and literature review," *Journal of Neuro-Oncology*, vol. 99, no. 2, pp. 277–281, 2010.

[35] M. Takasu, S. Takeshita, N. Tanitame et al., "Primary hypothalamic third ventriclular Burkitt's lymphoma: a case report with emphasis on differential diagnosis," *The British Journal of Radiology*, vol. 83, no. 986, pp. e43–e47, 2010.

[36] M. Jiang, J. Zhu, Y. Guan, and L. Zou, "Primary central nervous system Burkitt lymphoma with non-immunoglobulin heavy chain translocation in right ventricle: case report," *Pediatric Hematology and Oncology*, vol. 28, no. 5, pp. 454–458, 2011.

[37] A. Akhaddar, M. Zalagh, H. Belfquih, and M. Boucetta, "Burkitt's lymphoma: a rare cause of isolated trigeminal neuralgia in a child," *Child's Nervous System*, vol. 28, no. 7, pp. 1125-1126, 2012.

[38] L. Jiang, Z. Li, L. E. Finn et al., "Primary central nervous system B cell lymphoma with features intermediate between diffuse large B cell lymphoma and Burkitt lymphoma," *International Journal of Clinical and Experimental Pathology*, vol. 5, no. 1, pp. 72–76, 2012.

[39] J. H. Yoon, H. J. Kang, H. Kim et al., "Successful treatment of primary central nervous system lymphoma without irradiation in children: single center experience," *Journal of Korean Medical Science*, vol. 27, no. 11, pp. 1378–1384, 2012.

[40] A. Alabdulsalam, S. Z. A. Zaidi, I. Tailor, Y. Orz, and S. Al-Dandan, "Primary Burkitt lymphoma of the fourth ventricle in an immunocompetent young patient," *Case Reports in Pathology*, vol. 2014, Article ID 630954, 6 pages, 2014.

37

A Definitive IMRT-SIB with Concomitant Chemotherapy for Synchronous Locally Advanced Anal Canal Cancer and Prostate Cancer

Tubin Slavisa(D) **and Raunik Wolfgang**

Institut für Strahlentherapie/Radioonkologie, Feschnigstraße 11, 9020 Klagenfurt am Wörthersee, Austria

Correspondence should be addressed to Tubin Slavisa; slavisa.tubin@kabeg.at

Academic Editor: Jose I. Mayordomo

Currently, there are no specific recommendations regarding the management of the synchronous tumours due to the lack of either specific guidelines or individuals' clinical experiences relative to these clinical situations. In the presence of a locally advanced double primary tumour and with the lymph node metastases in addition, from the radiotherapeutical point of view, it must be challenging to manage this complicated situation that requires a more delicate treatment planning, due to higher doses prescribed to greater volumes concomitantly with the chemotherapy. A 68-year-old Caucasian male with a synchronous intermediate-risk prostate adenocarcinoma and locally advanced anal canal carcinoma underwent IMRT-SIB with concomitant chemotherapy at our institute. Two years after the treatment, the restaging CT and MRI scan showed no evidence of the disease and the patient reported no significant gastrointestinal or genitourinary toxicity. Our experience is unique, since it is the first report on using the IMRT-SIB technique simultaneously with chemotherapy in the management of the synchronous prostate and anal canal carcinomas. Therefore, we find it important to provide the current literature with the results from our experience which show good feasibility, efficacy, and tolerability of the definitive concomitant IMRT-SIB-chemotherapy for the synchronous anal canal cancer and prostate cancer.

1. Background

Generally speaking, synchronous tumours are very rare clinical entities, and for that reason, the recommendations for their treatment, as well as the epidemiological data, are still lacking in the available papers. However, for some categories, like those found among the synchronous colorectal neoplasms, there are few details that are available in papers that best show how rare these clinical entities are, with the incidence between 0.17% and 0.69%, in the case of 2-3 synchronous lesions [1]. But, for the eventual prostate and anal canal synchronous cancers, the epidemiological data does not exist at all, due to an extremely rare clinical situation. By considering those tumours separately, it has already been well established that the prostate cancer is the most common cancer in Europe for males [2], while the anal canal carcinoma is much less common. The American Cancer Society estimated

that, in 2016, approximately 2.6% of the new cases of anal canal, anorectum, or anus cancers, among the digestive system cancers, will be diagnosed [3]. Even though its incidence rate has increased in the recent years, the squamous cell anal carcinoma is still considered a rare malignancy, and in Europe, its annual incidence ranges from 3 per 100,000 (men; Geneva, Switzerland) to less than 1 per 100,000 (both sexes; England and the Netherlands) [4]. Usually, small carcinomas of the anal margin are well treated with local excision, while the concomitant radio-chemotherapy, using 5-fluorouracil and mitomycin C, is a standard first-line treatment for all other cases; salvage surgery is reserved for the local relapses [5]. Based on the tumour stage, a patient's performance status and life expectancy treatment options for the prostate cancer include radical prostatectomy, radiotherapy (external beam radiotherapy and/or brachytherapy), and hormonal therapy [6]. While the existing National

Comprehensive Cancer Committee (NCCN) guidelines consider and contain the specific recommendations on the treatment for single tumours, among those mentioned above, there are no recommendations regarding the management of the same tumours when they are synchronous. Considering the fact that, in certain clinical situations, the definitive radiotherapy and/or radio-chemotherapy for those tumours could induce significant toxicity, even when treated individually, we find it important to report on managing an even more complicated situation than this, with synchronous locally advanced tumours that require a more delicate treatment planning, due to higher doses prescribed to greater volumes concomitantly with chemotherapy.

Therefore, we thought that reporting the results of our experience shall be interesting, due to the lack of either specific guidelines or individuals' clinical experiences relative to these kinds of clinical situations, and it can provide the currently available papers with the results on feasibility, efficacy, and tolerability of the definitive concomitant IMRT-SIB-chemotherapy for the synchronous locally advanced anal canal cancer and intermediate-risk prostate cancer.

2. Case Description

The current disease story of our 68-year-old Caucasian male started two years ago, when this patient observed a hard lesion in the anal canal, which, in the first months since he observed it, was neither officially diagnosed nor treated. Ten months after that, he underwent cholecystectomy due to cholelithiasis, and the perioperative diagnostic examination revealed some suspicious lesions in the anal canal and some enlarged pelvic lymph nodes. His comorbidities included only gout, and his Karnofsky performance status was 90. He has never been treated with radiotherapy, and he had a second-degree family history for malignancies. At that time, a digital rectal examination identified mild prostatomegaly, with a palpable suspicious nodule in the left prostate lobe, without any signs of the extracapsular extension. Also, a large ulcerated mass was palpable at the dorsal anal canal wall, without lymphadenopathies in the inguinal region. Subsequent colonoscopy confirmed the presence of a suspicious lesion on the posterior anal canal, extending above up to the anorectal junction. A magnetic resonance imaging (MRI) for the regional staging confirmed an infiltrative lesion of the anal canal with a maximum diameter of 3.2 cm, with a high-grade suspicion of sphincter infiltration, and two enlarged lymphadenopathies in the mesorectum and in the right internal iliac region, respectively, both with a maximal diameter of 2 cm, which is suspicious of tumour metastases. Further, an area with a maximal diameter of 2 cm within the left prostate basis having a restricted diffusion with a lower apparent diffusion coefficient (ADC) than that in the surrounding healthy prostate tissue, which appeared hypointense on ADC maps but hyperintense on the diffusion-weighted maps, was also described. Afterwards, biopsies confirmed a poorly differentiated squamous cell carcinoma of the anal canal, as well as a moderately differentiated prostate adenocarcinoma, with a Gleason score of 7 (3 + 4) in both lobes. He resulted human immunodeficiency

virus- (HIV-) negative, and his carcinoembryonic antigen (CEA) and prostate-specific antigen (PSA) were 2.09 U/L (reference range = 0–5.0 U/L) and 0.74 ng/mL (reference range = 0–4.0 ng/mL), respectively. Additional staging with the whole-body computed tomography (CT) scans excluded the presence of any distant metastases. Therefore, our patient had a synchronous intermediate-risk stage IIB cT2cN0M0 prostate adenocarcinoma and stage IIIB cT2N2M0 anal canal squamous cell carcinoma.

A multidisciplinary team which included surgical, medical, and radiation oncologists evaluated this case and passed a decision to submit the patient to the definitive concurrent radio-chemotherapy.

Regarding this clinical entity, the current papers are "blind," and at this moment, they can provide us only with one case report on early-stage I metachronous small anal canal squamous cell carcinoma (cT1N0) and intermediate-risk prostate cancer (cT1cN0) that was published in 2011 [7]. Due to the relative lack of experience in the intensity-modulated radiation therapy (IMRT) at the time, which should be a more appropriate radiotherapy technique for managing this kind of conditions, the authors planned a conventional 3D conformal radiotherapy by using a wide anterior-posterior/posterior-anterior field arrangement with concurrent mitomycin C (12 mg/m^2 i.v. bolus on day 1) and 5-fluorouracil (1000 mg/m^2 on days 1–4 (week 1) and 29–32 (week 5) by continuous 24 h i.v. infusion). Due to the use of this technique, the prescribed doses for the anal canal carcinoma and the prostate carcinoma were 50.4 Gy and 73.8 Gy, respectively. That treatment has been well tolerated, without any significant gastrointestinal or genitourinary toxicity, except for one-week treatment break, due to the moist desquamation in the bilateral inguinal and intergluteal areas. The last restaging eighteen months later showed no evidence of the disease or of the cancer whatsoever.

3. Treatment Planning

The presence of the two synchronous cancers, as in our abovementioned case, which should be treated at the same time, is a difficult circumstance in itself, and our case was even further complicated with the four nearby volumes that should have been covered with a high-dose radiotherapy, due to the presence of the locally advanced cT2N2 anal canal carcinoma. Therefore, our choice was the IMRT-SIB technique targeted at improving the therapeutic ratio. The simulation of the treatment was performed in the supine position, with a comfortably full bladder, after which the planned CT (performed with 2 mm slice thickness) was then fused with the diagnostic MRI for the subsequent treatment planning. FeetSTEP and KneeSTEP were used in combination, to achieve the maximum accuracy in positioning and repositioning the hip and lower limbs. In order to ensure the best possible localization and contouring of the small bowel, the patient got three deciliters of the oral contrast 60 minutes prior to the simulation. The anal marker was used to mark the anal verge. Also, the patient was instructed on what diet to maintain during the treatment to ensure the regular bowel

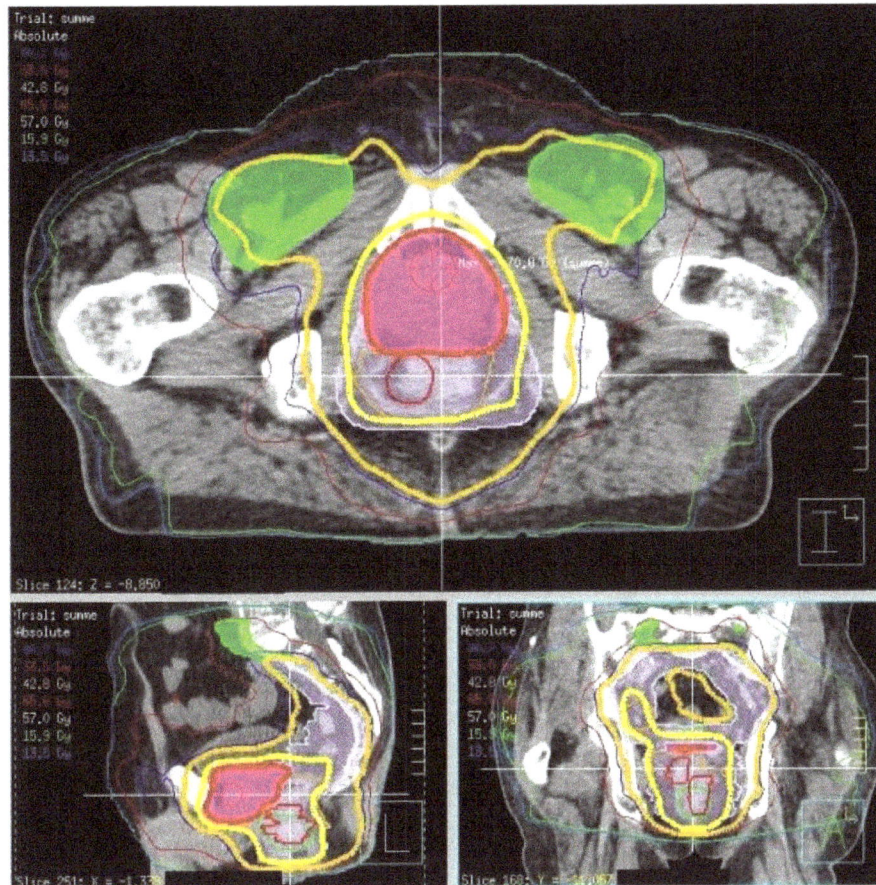

FIGURE 1: Dose distribution in the sum plan at the level of both primary tumours.

function. The IMRT-SIB plan was designed by using Pinnacle[3] Treatment Planning (Philips) (Figures 1 and 2).

Elective clinical target volume (CTV) included the anal canal with the perineum, the entire mesorectum (perirectal nodal region) to the pelvic floor, the inguinal and pelvic nodal regions (internal iliac, external iliac, and presacral). For the contouring of the elective nodal CTV, the 8 mm margin in soft tissue (excluding uninvolved bone and muscle but including small lymph nodes) around the iliac blood vessels has been added. The inferior extent of the inguinal nodal region was 2 cm caudal to the saphenous/femoral junction. CTV included 2 cm of the apparently normal perianal skin around the anal verge, 1 cm of the posterior bladder to account for day-to-day variation in the bladder position, and just a 5 mm beyond the levator muscles in the lower pelvis. The posterior and lateral margins of CTV extended to pelvic sidewall musculature or, where absent, bone. The superior extent of CTV was where the common iliac vessels bifurcate into external/internal ilia (approximate boney landmark: sacral promontory) including the rectosigmoid junction. At midline, CTV extended 1 cm anterior to the sacrum, to cover properly the presacral nodal region. Boost CTV was created by adding a 5 mm margin to the involved pelvic lymph nodes and a 2 cm margin on the gross tumour within the anal canal. An additional margin of 8 mm was added to CTV to create the planning target volume (PTV). For a definition of the target volumes, the anorectal contouring atlas published by RTOG [8] was used. CTV prostate included a whole prostate gland together with a neurovascular bundle and 1 cm of the proximal seminal vesicles to which an additional 7 mm margin was then added to create prostate PTV.

As regards the tumour extension, the four different PTV dose volumes were defined:

(1) PTV1: the uninvolved inguinal lymph nodes (cN0) have been irradiated with a single dose of 1.8 Gy up to 36 Gy.

(2) PTV2: the uninvolved pelvic lymph nodes (cN0) have been irradiated with a single dose of 1.8 Gy up to 45 Gy.

(3) PTV3: the involved pelvic lymph nodes (cN2) and primary tumour of the anal canal have been irradiated with a single dose of 1.8 Gy up to 59.4 Gy.

(4) PTV4: the prostate has been irradiated with a single dose of 2.1 Gy up to 69.3 Gy.

The dose that was prescribed to the prostate (PTV4) was slightly hypofractionated and has biologically corresponded to the 72 Gy equivalent dose in 2 Gy fractions (EQD2) considering the α/β ratio of 1.2/1.5 Gy for the prostate cancer. Before being delivered with 11 fields by 15 MV

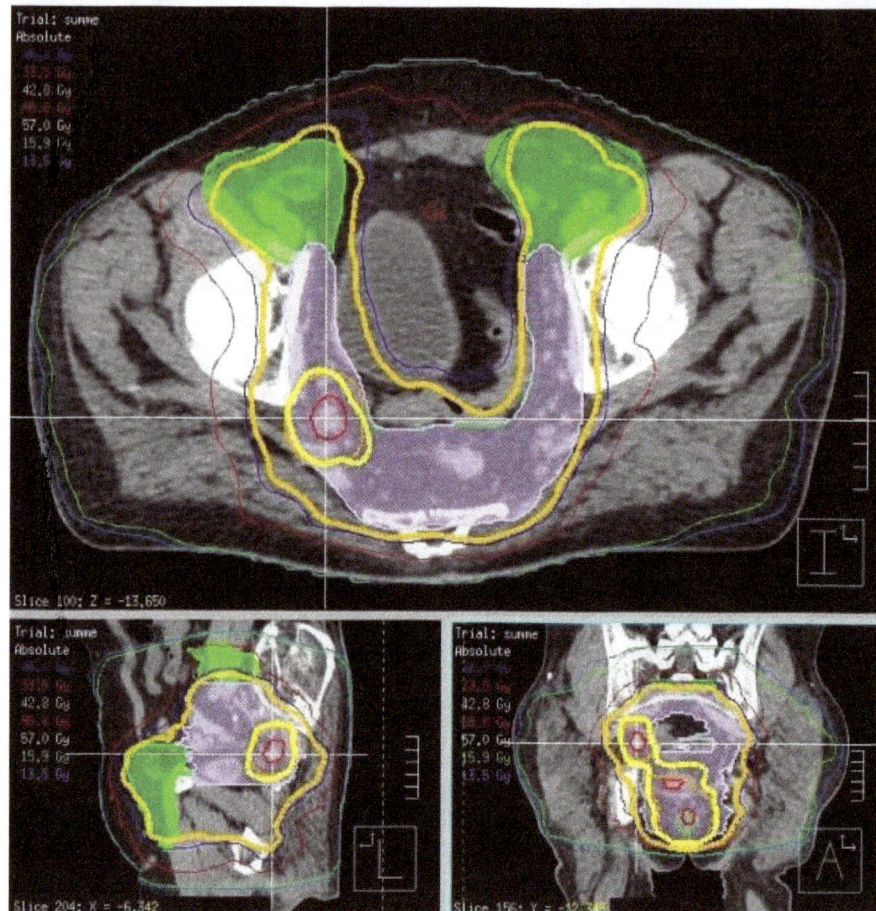

FIGURE 2: Dose distribution in the sum plan at the level of the right internal iliac lymph node metastasis.

LINAC, the radiotherapy plan has been submitted for the quality assurance, to be approved for the delivery accuracy. To ensure good tolerability of the treatment that was performed, the constraints published by RTOG have been met [9]. The toxicity was assessed with the CTCAE score. The patient was regularly followed up weekly during the treatment and then every 4 months after the completion of treatment.

4. Results

The patient has tolerated chemoradiotherapy very well presenting only with an acute toxicity grade 2 erythema in the perianal region, which did not require the suspension of his treatment, and grade 1 anemia. During the follow-up, few months after his treatment, he reported very mild late radiation proctitis and fecal incontinence which regressed spontaneously without requiring any medical treatment. At his last follow-up two years after the treatment, the restaging CT and MRI scan showed no evidence of the disease and he reported no gastrointestinal or genitourinary toxicity.

5. Conclusions

As already mentioned, the current papers present only one case report on the metachronous early-stage anal canal cancer and prostate cancer, so this is the first report on using the IMRT-SIB technique simultaneously with chemotherapy in the management of the synchronous prostate and anal canal carcinomas. By using this treatment option and by achieving a complete remission among all four evident tumour sites, with the acceptable low toxicity profile, we conclude that this therapeutic option is feasible, effective, and well tolerable.

References

[1] A. Lasser, "Synchronous primary adenocarcinomas of the colon and rectum," *Diseases of the Colon and Rectum*, vol. 21, no. 1, pp. 20–22, 1978.

[2] J. Ferlay, E. Steliarova-Foucher, J. Lortet-Tieulent et al., "Cancer incidence and mortality patterns in Europe: estimates for 40 countries in 2012," *European Journal of Cancer*, vol. 49, no. 6, pp. 1374–1403, 2013.

[3] R. L. Siegel, K. D. Miller, and A. Jemal, "Cancer statistics, 2016," *CA: a Cancer Journal for Clinicians*, vol. 66, no. 1, pp. 7–30, 2016.

[4] D. M. Parkin, S. L. Whelan, J. Ferlay, L. Teppo, and D. B. Thomas, *Cancer Incidence in Five Continents. Vol. VIII IARC Scientific Publications No. 155*, IARC Press, Lyon, 2002.

[5] R. Glynne-Jones, J. M. A. Northover, A. Cervantes, and On behalf of the ESMO Guidelines Working Group, "Anal cancer: ESMO Clinical Practice Guidelines for diagnosis, treatment and follow-up," *Annals of Oncology*, vol. 21, Supplement 5, pp. v87–v92, 2010.

[6] N. Mottet, J. Bellmunt, M. Bolla et al., "EAU-ESTRO-SIOG Guidelines on prostate cancer. Part 1: screening, diagnosis, and local treatment with curative intent," *European Urology*, vol. 71, no. 4, pp. 618–629, 2016.

[7] E. F. Miles, L. L. Jacimore, and J. W. Nelson, "Metachronous anal canal and prostate cancers with simultaneous definitive therapy: a case report and review of the literature," *Case Reports in Oncological Medicine*, vol. 2011, Article ID 864371, 4 pages, 2011.

[8] R. J. Myerson, M. C. Garofalo, I. El Naqa et al., "Elective clinical target volumes for conformal therapy in anorectal cancer: a radiation therapy oncology group consensus panel contouring atlas," *International Journal of Radiation Oncology, Biology, Physics*, vol. 74, no. 3, pp. 824–830, 2009.

[9] L. A. Kachnic, K. Winter, R. J. Myerson et al., "RTOG 0529: a phase 2 evaluation of dose-painted intensity modulated radiation therapy in combination with 5-fluorouracil and mitomycin-C for the reduction of acute morbidity in carcinoma of the anal canal," *International Journal of Radiation Oncology, Biology, Physics*, vol. 86, no. 1, pp. 27–33, 2013.

38

T Cell Histiocyte Rich Large B Cell Lymphoma Presenting as Hemophagocytic Lymphohistiocytosis: An Uncommon Presentation of a Rare Disease

Uroosa Ibrahim,[1] Gwenalyn Garcia,[1] Amina Saqib,[2] Shafinaz Hussein,[3] and Qun Dai[1]

[1]Department of Hematology/Oncology, Staten Island University Hospital, 475 Seaview Avenue, Staten Island, NY 10305, USA
[2]Department of Pulmonary/Critical Care, Staten Island University Hospital, 475 Seaview Avenue, Staten Island, NY 10305, USA
[3]Department of Pathology, Staten Island University Hospital, 475 Seaview Avenue, Staten Island, NY 10305, USA

Correspondence should be addressed to Uroosa Ibrahim; uroosaibrahim@gmail.com

Academic Editor: Jeanine M. Buchanich

T cell histiocyte rich large B cell lymphoma (THRLBCL) is a rare subtype of non-Hodgkin's lymphoma characterized by malignant B cells with reactive T lymphocytes. The pathophysiology is thought to involve cytokine-mediated evasion of T cell immune response by malignant B cells. It usually presents at an advanced stage with extranodal involvement. An extremely unusual manifestation of the disease is hemophagocytic lymphohistiocytosis (HLH) which is a hyperinflammatory disorder. We present a case of a 43-year-old male who presented with recurrent fever and recent radiologic imaging showing splenomegaly and right inguinal lymphadenopathy. On presentation, he had a fever of 105°F. Laboratory work-up was consistent with pancytopenia, elevated lactate dehydrogenase, elevated D-dimer, and a ferritin of 24,247 ng/mL. The patient was started on steroid therapy. An excisional biopsy of the right inguinal lymph node was consistent with a diagnosis of THRLBCL and the patient subsequently received six cycles of chemotherapy with R-CHOP (Rituximab, Cyclophosphamide, Doxorubicin, Vincristine, and Prednisone) after which a PET-CT scan showed no evidence of biologically active disease and ferritin was down to 822 ng/mL. We discuss the clinical manifestations and diagnostic and therapeutic considerations of this rare disease along with a review of reported cases in the literature.

1. Introduction

T cell histiocyte rich large B cell lymphoma (THRLBCL) is a rare subtype of diffuse large B cell lymphoma (DLBCL) characterized by malignant B cells with an infiltrate of reactive T lymphocytes. It is often an aggressive malignancy requiring prompt recognition and treatment. Hemophagocytic lymphohistiocytosis (HLH) is an uncommon hyperinflammatory disorder with an acute and potentially fatal presentation. It can be familial or acquired as a result of an underlying disorder such as an infection, malignancy, or an autoimmune phenomenon. Hematologic malignancies account for majority of the cases of secondary HLH. We describe a rare case of HLH secondary to THRLBCL presenting with persistent high fever. We discuss the unfolding of the diagnosis which can be challenging in these clinical scenarios, as well as management considerations with reference to five other cases reported to date.

2. Case

A 43-year-old male presented to our hospital with complaints of recurrent high fever for a few weeks. On an Urgent Care visit eight weeks prior to presentation, the patient was found to be positive for influenza. He was thereafter treated with Levaquin for persistent febrile episodes, later requiring hospitalization during which work-up revealed pancytopenia and hyperferritinemia. On computed tomography (CT) scan of the abdomen, multiple hypodense dense lesions were seen within the spleen with the largest one in the medial posterior part measuring 4.5×3.8 cm, and right inguinal lymphadenopathy. A bone marrow aspirate smear was adequately cellular with left shifted myeloid and erythroid maturation. A histiocyte with hemophagocytosis was seen. There was no evidence of malignancy. The patient was subsequently discharged from the facility and was scheduled for a CT-guided lymph node biopsy.

Four days later, the patient presented to our emergency department with a fever of 105°F. CBC revealed pancytopenia with a total white count of 1×10^9 cells/L, hemoglobin of 7 g/dL, and a platelet count of 60×10^9/L. Renal function and electrolytes were normal. Total bilirubin was 1.4 mg/dL, aspartate aminotransferase, alanine aminotransferase, and alkaline phosphatase were normal. Uric acid was 1.7 mg/dL, LDH 913 U/L, triglycerides 302 mg/dL, PT 14.7 seconds, and PTT 39 seconds. CT of the abdomen and pelvis with contrast revealed multiple enlarged abdominal lymph nodes including perigastric and pancreatic lymph nodes measuring up to 2.2 cm and retroperitoneal lymphadenopathy including a large retrocaval lymph node measuring up to 3.6 cm. There was a right inguinal conglomerate of lymph nodes measuring up to 6.6 × 4.1 cm. The spleen was enlarged with diffuse enhancement. There was no focal hepatic lesion identified. Further work-up revealed an elevated D-dimer at 7123 ng/mL and ferritin 24,247 ng/mL. Haptoglobin was less than 20 mg/dL. Rheumatologic work-up including anti-CCP antibody, SSA and B, ANA, ANCA, anti-myeloperoxidase antibody, and rheumatoid factor was negative. Viral serology including HIV and hepatitis B and C was negative. Soluble IL-2 receptor alpha was elevated at 9726 U/mL (Normal 406–100 U/mL).

The differential diagnosis at this point included a lymphoproliferative disorder, hemophagocytic lymphohistiocytosis, or other inflammatory disorder. The patient had an excisional biopsy of the right inguinal lymph node that showed effacement of normal nodal architecture. The cellular elements comprised predominantly of small lymphoid cells and histiocytes with scattered large atypical cells. These atypical cells showed irregular nuclei with distinct nucleoli. Immunophenotypically, they were positive for CD20, PAX5, OCT2, BCL6, and MUM1 while they were negative for CD10, CD15, and CD30. In situ hybridization for EBV encoded RNA (EBER) was negative. The background small lymphocytes consisted mostly of T cells and histiocytes. While numerous small and some large B cells were seen in the abnormal follicles surrounding the atypical infiltrate, they were absent in the diffuse histiocyte rich areas. Small T cells positive for CD3, CD2, CD5, CD7, and CD43 were present both in the abnormal follicles and the histiocyte infiltrate. Ki 67 staining was approximately 30% with preferential staining of the larger cells [Figure 1]. The slides were sent for a second opinion and the overall findings were supportive of a diagnosis of T cell histiocyte rich large B cell lymphoma.

The patient was started on dexamethasone 20 mg given intravenously daily. He responded well and subsequently the dose of intravenous steroids was reduced and he was switched to oral Prednisone. A Positron Emission Tomography (PET) scan was performed that showed splenomegaly (15.7 cm) with multiple mass-like areas of increased uptake with a maximum SUV of 10.2. Patchy uptake was seen in the liver with a maximum SUV of 8.9 in the posterior right lobe. Multiple FDG-avid subdiaphragmatic, perigastric, peripancreatic, periportal, mesenteric, retroperitoneal, right iliac chain, and right external iliac lymph nodes were identified.

Following the diagnosis of THRLBCL, the patient was treated with R-CHOP (Rituximab, Cyclophosphamide,

Doxorubicin, Vincristine, and Prednisone) given the lack of data to support use of a more aggressive regimen such as DA-R-EPOCH (dose-adjusted Rituximab, Etoposide, Prednisone, Vincristine (Oncovin), Cyclophosphamide, and Doxorubicin). A PET scan performed after three cycles of chemotherapy showed a decrease in the size of the spleen (now 13.4 cm) with conversion to non-FDG-avid status. The multiple enlarged retroperitoneal lymph nodes also decreased in size and were no longer FDG-avid. The ferritin level decreased to 3304 ng/mL. The patient completed a total of six cycles of chemotherapy without complications at the end of which his ferritin was 822 ng/mL, LDH 170 U/L, and PET-CT scan showed no evidence of biologically active disease. The patient remains in remission after six months of completion of therapy.

3. Discussion

T cell histiocyte rich large B cell lymphoma (THRLBCL) is a rare subtype of lymphoma accounting for 1-2% of diffuse large B cell lymphoma (DLBCL). It is histologically characterized by few scattered large malignant B cells (typically <10% of the cell population) in a background of reactive T cells and histiocytes. The pathophysiology of this disease is thought to involve cytokine-mediated evasion of the T cell immune response by the malignant B cells. It is an aggressive lymphoma, presenting at an advanced stage and with extranodal involvement in over 60% of cases. Five-year overall survival with R-CHOP is reported at 46% [1, 2].

Hemophagocytic lymphohistiocytosis (HLH) is an immune-mediated disorder characterized by fever, splenomegaly, and cytopenias. Laboratory features include hypertriglyceridemia, hypofibrinogenemia, hemophagocytosis, low or absent NK-cell activity, hyperferritinemia, and an elevated soluble CD 25. The diagnosis is made with either the presence of molecular aberrations consistent with HLH, for example, pathologic mutations in PRF1, UNC13D, or STX11, or with fulfilment of five of eight clinical criteria outlined above. The pathophysiology of HLH involves the uncontrolled activation of T cells, histiocytes, and macrophages, resulting in an overproduction of inflammatory cytokines and consequent multiorgan damage [3, 4].

Serum levels of soluble interleukin-2 receptor alpha (sIL-2R alpha) and soluble CD163 (sCD163) reflect the degree of activation and expansion of T cells and phagocytic macrophages, respectively. The IL-2 receptor complex is a trimer, consisting of alpha, beta, and gamma chains, that interact with IL-2. A soluble form of IL-2R appears in serum and plasma, concomitantly with increased cell surface expression. Serum-soluble interleukin-2 receptor (sIL-2r) level is considered an important diagnostic test and disease marker in HLH [5].

HLH may occur as a primary or familial disorder, or it may be secondary to a triggering event. Infections and malignancies are the most commonly identified triggers. Lymphoma is the most common malignancy known to trigger HLH. Primary HLH is treated with a regimen of dexamethasone and etoposide, with intrathecal methotrexate and hydrocortisone in patients with central nervous system

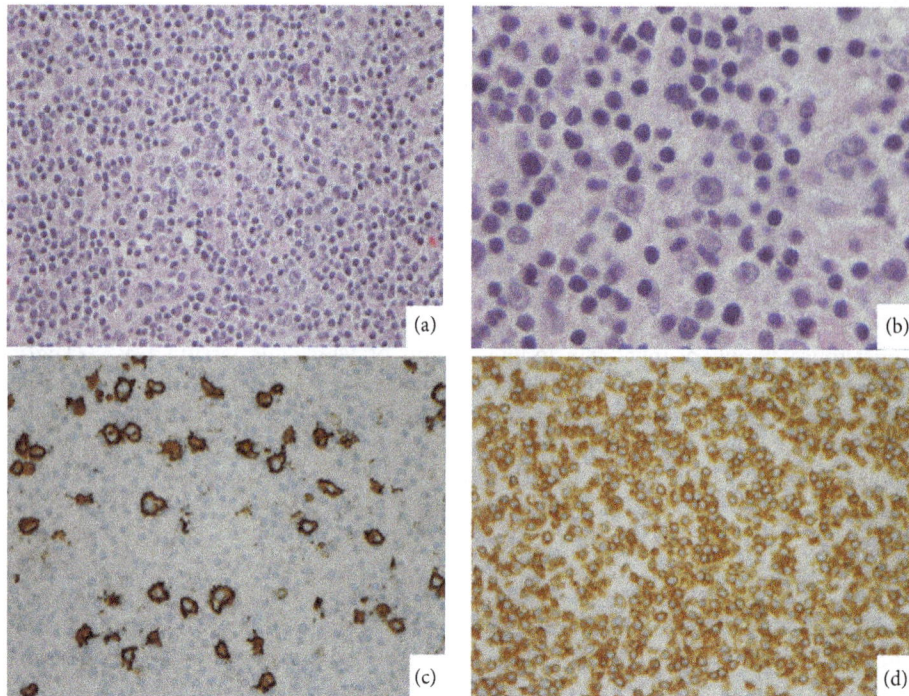

FIGURE 1: The lymph node showed effacement of normal architecture comprised predominantly of small lymphocytes and histiocytes ((a), H&E, ×200). Scattered large atypical cells with irregular nuclei and nucleoli were observed ((b), H&E, ×1000). CD20 highlights the large cells while CD3 stains numerous small T cells in the background ((c) and (d), ×400).

involvement. The optimal management of malignancy-associated HLH is uncertain; HLH-directed therapy, malignancy-directed therapy, or a combination of both may be offered depending on the clinical scenario [3, 6].

Treatment of THRLBCL is on the lines of DLBCL treatment. To date, only five cases of HLH occurring in the setting of THRLBCL have been described in the English literature [7–11]. Of the prior documented cases [Table 1], two achieved complete remission (CR) with R-CHOP, with one of the patients relapsing ten months later [6, 8]. A third patient achieved CR with DA-R-EPOCH; and a fourth patient achieved CR with high-dose chemotherapy followed by autologous stem cell transplantation [9, 10]. The last patient achieved remission with salvage therapy but developed a fatal relapse several months later [11].

An intriguing fact is that THRLBCL has been shown to express cytokines such as tumor necrosis factor-α, interferon-Υ, and interleukin 6; and the same cytokines have also been implicated in the pathogenesis of HLH [2, 4, 12]. It is interesting to note that a predominantly B cell malignancy evokes a cytotoxic T cell response which is thought to be largely ineffective [13]. Genetic profiling studies have demonstrated tolerogenic immune response signatures in THRLBCL and may explain the aggressive nature of the disease. What may not be entirely coincidental is also the finding of programmed death ligand 1 (PD-L1) expression by both tumor cells and the histiocytes in the microenvironment, which may be responsible for rendering the T cells ineffective as mentioned

above [14]. The question then arises is if this can be a potential target of immune therapy in the disease. Given the rarity of this condition, its acuity, and aggressiveness, chemotherapy and steroids remain the standard treatment. The role of immune modulation, apart from glucocorticoids, is yet to be explored.

Treatment options for refractory or recurrent disease include alemtuzumab, a monoclonal antibody to the CD52 protein expressed on the surface of mature T cells and possibly NK cells. This acts as a bridge towards hematopoietic stem cell transplant. Patients with hematologic malignancies may have recurrent episodes of HLH given that the malignancy persists as a trigger. These patients must be referred for transplant which can be allogeneic or autologous depending on the primary disease. Avenues of ongoing research include an anti-interferon-gamma monoclonal antibody and the study of pegaspargase together with liposomal Doxorubicin, etoposide, and high-dose methylprednisolone (L-DEP) as an initial treatment for Epstein Barr virus-induced hemophagocytic lymphohistiocytosis [15].

4. Conclusion

HLH is a potentially fatal condition and when it is secondary to an aggressive malignancy, prompt diagnosis and initiation of treatment can be life-saving for the patient. While awaiting pathology results, treating the HLH is important for symptom control; however, treating the primary disease remains a priority in the long-term management of patients.

TABLE 1: Reported cases of hemophagocytic lymphohistiocytosis secondary to T cell histiocyte rich large B cell lymphoma.

Serial #	Age/sex [ref]	Presentation	Site of involvement	Immunophenotype	Treatment	Outcome
1	20/M [7]	Jaundice, malaise, abdominal pain, fever	LN, liver	CD3+ CD5+ CD7+ CD45+ T cell infiltrate Scattered large CD20+ PAX5+ CD15– CD30– Alk-1– B-cells	R-CHOP × 6 IT-MTX	Alive
2	52/M [8]	Fever, DOE, weight loss	LN	Scattered large CD20+ cells CD3+ T cells CD30– CD15– EBV–	R-CHOP × 8, IT-MTX, cytarabine, MP	Recurrence at 10 m, salvage therapy
3	30/M [9]	Fever, jaundice, weight loss, ARF	LN, lung	Large CD20+ CD15– CD30– B cells CD3+ CD5+ CD7+ CD8+ TIA-1+ T cells CD68+ histiocytes	DA-R-EPOCH	Alive
4	30/F [10]	Pruritus, night sweats, fever, weight loss	LN, liver	CD79a+ Mib-1+ large cells	MOPP-ABV then high dose MTX, vincristine and etoposide, then AHSCT	Alive at 24 m
5	34/M [11]	Fever, abdominal pain, jaundice	BM	ND	ND	DOD
6	43/M [current case]	Fever	LN	Large atypical cell CD20+, PAX5+, BCL-6+, MUM1+, EMA (weak), Kappa (weak) CD3+, CD2+, CD5+, CD7+, CD43+ T cells	R-CHOP × 6	Alive

AHSCT: autologous hematopoietic stem cell transplant; BM: bone marrow; DA-R-EPOCH: dose adjusted Rituximab, Etoposide, Prednisone, Vincristine (Oncovin), Cyclophosphamide, and Doxorubicin; DOE: dyspnea on exertion; DOD: died of disease; IT-MTX: intrathecal methotrexate; LN: lymph node; M: months; MOPP-ABV: mechlorethamine, vincristine, procarbazine, prednisone/doxorubicin bleomycin, and vincristine; MP: methylprednisolone; ND: not described; R-CHOP: Rituximab, Cyclophosphamide, Doxorubicin, Vincristine, and Prednisone.

References

[1] A. El Weshi, S. Akhtar, W. A. Mourad et al., "T-cell/histiocyte-rich B-cell lymphoma: clinical presentation, management and prognostic factors: report on 61 patients and review of literature," *Leukemia and Lymphoma*, vol. 48, no. 9, pp. 1764–1773, 2007.

[2] T. Tousseyn and C. De Wolf-Peeters, "T cell/histiocyte-rich large B-cell lymphoma: an update on its biology and classification," *Virchows Archiv*, vol. 459, no. 6, pp. 557–563, 2011.

[3] M. B. Jordan, C. E. Allen, S. Weitzman, A. H. Filipovich, and K. L. McClain, "How I treat hemophagocytic lymphohistiocytosis," *Blood*, vol. 118, no. 15, pp. 4041–4052, 2011.

[4] M. Ramos-Casals, P. Brito-Zerón, A. López-Guillermo, M. A. Khamashta, and X. Bosch, "Adult haemophagocytic syndrome," *The Lancet*, vol. 383, no. 9927, pp. 1503–1516, 2014.

[5] J. Bleesing, A. Prada, D. M. Siegel et al., "The diagnostic significance of soluble CD163 and soluble interleukin-2 receptor α-chain in macrophage activation syndrome and untreated new-onset systemic juvenile idiopathic arthritis," *Arthritis and Rheumatism*, vol. 56, no. 3, pp. 965–971, 2007.

[6] K. Lehmberg, K. E. Nichols, J.-I. Henter et al., "Consensus recommendations for the diagnosis and management of hemophagocytic lymphohistiocytosis associated with malignancies," *Haematologica*, vol. 100, no. 8, pp. 997–1004, 2015.

[7] M. Mehta, J. Wang, R. McHenry, and S. Zucker, "T-cell/histiocyte-rich large B-cell lymphoma masquerading as autoimmune hepatitis with clinical features of hemophagocytic lymphohistiocytosis," *Journal of Gastrointestinal & Digestive System*, vol. 5, article 3, 2015.

[8] E. M. Mahtat, M. Zine, M. Allaoui et al., "Hemophagocytic lymphohistiocytosis complicating a T-cell rich B-cell lymphoma," *BMC Hematology*, vol. 16, no. 1, article 28, 2016.

[9] K. Devitt, J. Cerny, B. Switzer et al., "Hemophagocytic lymphohistiocytosis secondary to T-cell/histiocyte-rich large B-cell lymphoma," *Leukemia Research Reports*, vol. 3, no. 2, pp. 42–45, 2015.

[10] M. Mitterer, N. Pescosta, C. Mc Quain et al., "Epstein-Barr virus related hemophagocytic syndrome in a T-cell rich B-cell lymphoma," *Annals of Oncology*, vol. 10, no. 2, pp. 231–234, 1999.

[11] O. S. Aljitawi and J. M. Boone, "Lymphoma-associated hemophagocytic lymphohistiocytosis," *Blood*, vol. 120, no. 5, article 932, 2012.

[12] S. Nakayama, T. Yokote, Y. Hirata, K. Iwaki, M. Tsuji, and T. Hanafusa, "Multiple cytokine- and chemokine-producing T-cell/histiocyte-rich large B-cell lymphoma," *British Journal of Haematology*, vol. 160, no. 6, article 734, 2013.

[13] P. Van Loo, T. Tousseyn, V. Vanhentenrijk et al., "T-cell/histiocyte-rich large B-cell lymphoma shows transcriptional features suggestive of a tolerogenic host immune response," *Haematologica*, vol. 95, no. 3, pp. 440–448, 2010.

[14] B. J. Chen, B. Chapuy, J. Ouyang et al., "PD-L1 expression is characteristic of a subset of aggressive B-cell lymphomas and virus-associated malignancies," *Clinical Cancer Research*, vol. 19, no. 13, pp. 3462–3473, 2013.

[15] S. Weitzman, "Approach to hemophagocytic syndromes," *Hematology/The Education Program of the American Society of Hematology*, vol. 2011, no. 1, pp. 178–183, 2011.

39

Rapid Onset of B12 Deficiency in the Setting of Worsening Multiple Myeloma: Correlations between B12 Deficiency and Multiple Myeloma

Karan Seegobin, Satish Maharaj, Grant Nelson, Jeremy Carlson, Cherisse Baldeo, and Rafik Jacob

Department of Internal Medicine, University of Florida College of Medicine, Jacksonville, FL 32209, USA

Correspondence should be addressed to Karan Seegobin; karanseegobin@hotmail.com

Academic Editor: Kaiser Jamil

A 67-year-old female with a relapse of multiple myeloma after being in remission for approximately 2 years following autologous stem cell transplant presented with worsening pancytopenia, over a three-month period. There were an increase in her monoclonal spike at 3.13 g/dL on serum protein electrophoresis, low serum B12 levels, and positive intrinsic factor antibodies. Three months before, she had normal B12 levels and a significantly lower monoclonal spike of 1.07 g/dL. She was diagnosed with B12 deficiency with pernicious anaemia in the setting of her worsening myeloma. Multiple myeloma (MM) has been linked with B12 deficiency and pernicious anaemia. Several mechanisms have been described regarding the pathogenesis of B12 deficiency in such patients. Increased tumour activity can further perpetuate the development of B12 deficiency in such patients. With regard to our case, the increase in tumour activity and onset of pernicious anaemia could have contributed to the rapid development of B12 deficiency. In contrast to this, rapid development of B12 deficiency could also signify relapse or worsening of the myeloma as seen in our case. Physicians ought to consider B12 deficiency in patients with worsening pancytopenia and myeloma.

1. Background

Multiple myeloma is a clonal malignancy of plasma cells characterized by an overproduction of monoclonal antibodies [1]. The IgG and IgM paraproteinemia of the kappa type as well as IgA myeloma have been linked with pernicious anaemia [1–3]. Generation of specific autoreactive antibodies, anti-intrinsic-factor-like activity of the IgM paraprotein, increased tumour burden, immunomodulatory properties of lenalidomide, and disruption of renal mechanisms of B12 absorption are some of the described mechanisms by which B12 deficiency can occur in these patients [1, 4, 5]. Physicians ought to be aware of the association between B12 deficiency and multiple myeloma as its onset can signify worsening of the disease. Further research is needed into the usefulness of B12 levels as a marker of worsening myeloma. We described a case of myeloma that presented with worsening pancytopenia and was found to have B12 deficiency, pernicious anaemia, and worsening of the disease activity, signified by

increase in monoclonal paraprotein levels. As paraprotein levels increased, the B12 levels decreased in our case. Further research is needed to show the usefulness of B12 levels in multiple myeloma with regard to disease activity. We further review the mechanisms of B12 deficiency in these patients and discuss the utility of monitoring vitamin B12 levels in these patients.

2. Case Presentation

We report a case of a 67-year-old female with multiple myeloma and hypertension who was previously treated with chemotherapy and autologous stem cell transplant with good response, having no evidence of monoclonal gammopathy on serum immunofixation. The patient subsequently had a relapse of the disease two years after the transplant, with reoccurrence of the IgG lambda monoclonal paraprotein on serum immunofixation. The patient did not wish for another stem cell transplant; she was then managed with

TABLE 1: Displaying the trend of B12 levels, CBC, and paraprotein levels.

Laboratory test	Time of presentation	Three months before	24 months before
B12 levels (211–946 pg/mL)	94	631.5 pg/ml	751 pg/ml
WCC (4.5–11 × 103/uL)	2.5	4.67	4.5
Hb (12–16 g/dL)	6	11.7	11.1
Platelet (140–440 thou/cu mm)	7	142	143
Intrinsic factor antibody (0–1.1 AU/mL)	11.9		
Monoclonal spike (0.7–1.60 g/dL)	3.13	1.07	0.4

TABLE 2: Complete blood count on admission and prior to discharge.

Hematologic parameter	On admission	Prior to discharge
White cell count (4.5–11 × 103/uL)	2.5	4.75
Hemoglobin 12–16 g/dL	6	8
Platelet 140–440 thou/cu mm	7	14

lenalidomide and dexamethasone which were stopped when she experienced worsening pancytopenia over a three-month period. Despite stopping the medications, the pancytopenia still progressed. She also complained of intermittent rash on both upper extremities over this time which would resolve on its own. On examination, she was not in respiratory distress, with vital signs within normal limits. She had petechial bruising on bilateral upper extremities, as well as the thorax. Other aspects of the clinical examination were noncontributory.

Her white cell count was 2.5 (4.5–11 × 103/uL); absolute neutrophil count 449; haemoglobin (Hb) 6 (12–16 g/dL); MCV 100 (82–101 fl); platelet 7 (140–440 thou/cu mm); reticulocyte count 0.9% (0.5–1.5%); reticulated haemoglobin 44.7 (28.8–37.7 pg); reticulocyte index 0.8%; vitamin B12 94 (211–946 pg/mL); intrinsic factor antibody 11.9 (0–1.1 AU/mL); creatinine 1.07 (0.5–0.95 mg/dL), and serum protein electrophoresis showed a monoclonal spike 3.13 g/dL in the gamma region corresponding to IgG lambda paraprotein. Three months before, she had a monoclonal spike of 1.07 g/dL in the gamma region. Furthermore, her B12 levels were 631.5 pg/ml and 751 pg/ml, respectively, 3 and 24 months before. These results are further outlined in Table 1.

She was diagnosed with B12 deficiency and pernicious anaemia in the setting of relapsed myeloma and started on B12 replacements, together with other supportive treatments including blood and platelet transfusions. The patient did not wish to pursue further chemotherapy and preferred palliative and hospice care. She was discharged after improvement in her cytopenias (Table 2); however she was lost to follow-up thereafter.

3. Discussion

Multiple myeloma (MM) is a clonal malignancy of plasma cells characterized by an overproduction of monoclonal antibodies [1]. Clinically, this entity is characterized by skeletal lesions, anaemia, hypercalcemia, and renal failure [1]. The incidence of MM is 6.1/100,000 people per year and increases to 30.4/100,000 people per year in those older than 65 years [1]. The median age of diagnosis of MM is 71 years in Caucasians and 67 years in African-Americans [1].

Multiple myeloma (MM) has been linked with several autoimmune conditions in the medical literature [1]. Yet, the significance of these associations is not well understood [1]. In this case the patient was being managed for a relapse of multiple myeloma when she presented with worsening pancytopenia and was found to have B12 deficiency, pernicious anaemia with worsening disease activity.

There are several case reports of pernicious anaemia developing in patients with multiple myeloma [6]. Some studies established that the incidence of cobalamin deficiency in patients with IgA multiple myeloma and MGUS is approximately 13.6% [1]. Another estimated that the prevalence of pernicious anaemia in patients with MM ranged from 4.3% to 5.8% in 1962 [4]. The research has advocated screening for vitamin B12 deficiency in this population [6]. From our case, screening for B12 deficiency may have had three benefits in first detecting the onset of B12 deficiency, early diagnosis of pernicious anaemia, and earlier detection of worsening of the disease activity.

Our patient had elevated IgG lambda paraprotein. Pernicious anaemia has been reported in a case of IgG and IgM paraproteinemia of the kappa type as well as IgA multiple myeloma. [3]. There are several reported mechanisms for the development of B12 deficiency in patients with myeloma which include the following:

[a] Myeloma triggers intrinsic immune alterations and promotes generation of specific autoreactive antibodies, as reported in cases of ITP developing after myeloma [1]. We postulate that worsening of myeloma demonstrated by the increase in the monoclonal spike in our case may have been an underlying trigger for autoantibody production and subsequent development of pernicious anaemia.

[b] The M protein could have anti-intrinsic-factor-like activity or may in some other way interfere with the normal vitamin B12 absorptive process [4].

[c] Malignant plasma cells may more rapidly consume the body's store of vitamin B12 and, hence, increase the likelihood that a patient develops vitamin B12 deficiency [4]. Bone marrow-derived MM cells were shown to have increased uptake and accumulation of vitamin B12 in culture [4]. Concluded from this report is that one would expect a higher prevalence of vitamin B12 deficiency among patients who have MM and among patients who have larger myeloma

burden [4]. In our case the B12 levels had a downward trend over the 24-month period, and the monoclonal paraprotein levels had an upward trend as seen in Table 1. This further supports the theory above that plasma cells contribute to development of B12 deficiency.

[d] Excess free light chains (FLCs), readily measurable by the serum FLC assay, could disrupt the renal proximal tubule receptors megalin and cubilin where B12 is reabsorbed [5]. The authors went on to suggest that the prevalence of B12 deficiency would be higher in plasma cell dyscrasias patients with higher free light chain burden [5].

[e] Immunomodulatory properties of lenalidomide are linked with the development of autoimmune diseases [7]. In one report, there was a 4.3% absolute risk of autoimmune disorders in MM patients treated with lenalidomide especially if they had prior autologous transplant [7] Though autoimmune haemolytic anaemia, idiopathic thrombocytopenic purpura, Evans syndrome, autoimmune thyroiditis, optic neuritis, cutaneous vasculitis, and polymyositis have been reported, to the best of our knowledge, we have not seen any cases of pernicious anaemia with lenalidomide [1]. It is possible that lenalidomide contributed to the development of our patient's pernicious anaemia; however this association would have to be validated in larger studies.

An interplay of all these mechanisms above could have contributed to the development of B12 deficiency in our patient. Furthermore, the increased tumour activity in our case could have contributed to her rapid development of B12 deficiency over three months. Our patient had normal B12 levels 24 months prior to presentation and developed low B12 levels during the three-month period when she had worsening pancytopenia with elevation in the monoclonal spike in the gamma region from 1.07 to 3.03. The likelihood that she was B12 deficient prior to the worsening of her myeloma was unlikely since < 5% of patients with serum vitamin B12 levels > 300 pg/mL have biochemical evidence of vitamin B12 deficiency [4]. Furthermore, a serum vitamin B12 level < 200 pg/mL has a high specificity for vitamin B12 deficiency [4].

Vitamin B12 deficiency is a known cause of pancytopenia [8]. We suspect this would have contributed to the patient's pancytopenia. However, the relapse of myeloma and history of lenalidomide use could have also contributed to this hematologic finding. Failure of the pancytopenia to recover after stopping the lenalidomide and dexamethasone made this agent as the underlying cause unlikely. As discussed above, lenalidomide is known to cause pancytopenia; however the hematological indices would be expected to improve after discontinuation of the drug [9].

MM remains incurable with an important life-expectancy shortening [10]. Although the incorporation of the novel agents thalidomide, bortezomib, and lenalidomide in the front-line therapy has resulted in significant improvement, many patients do not have a sustained response making the treatment of relapsed/refractory MM a real challenge [10]. The duration of responses is limited and all patients will develop progressive disease [10]. In light of its nature to relapse and progress, awareness about the association of multiple myeloma with B12 deficiency and pernicious anaemia is important as these can mimic a relapse of myeloma or even signify the onset of worsening disease activity.

4. Conclusion

B12 deficiency and pernicious anaemia can develop in patients with relapsed multiple myeloma. Furthermore, its onset can signify worsening disease activity. The development of B12 deficiency can be rapid; additionally, serum B12 levels may be of use in monitoring disease activity. The pathophysiology of B12 deficiency in these patients is not well understood and there is a need for further research in this area.

Consent

Written consent was obtained from the patient for publication of this manuscript.

Disclosure

The authors of this manuscript certify that they have no affiliations with or involvement in any organization or entity with any financial interest (such as honoraria; educational grants; participation in speakers' bureaus; membership, employment, consultancies, stock ownership, or other equity interest; and expert testimony or patent-licensing arrangements) or nonfinancial interest (such as personal or professional relationships, affiliations, knowledge, or beliefs) in the subject matter or materials discussed in this manuscript.

Authors' Contributions

The idea for reporting this case was that of Karan Seegobin. Further intellectual content and editing were done by all the authors. All the authors reviewed, edited, and approved the final version. Karan Seegobin assumes responsibility for the integrity of the content.

References

[1] A. Shimanovsky, J. A. Argote, S. Murali, and C. A. Dasanu, "Autoimmune manifestations in patients with multiple myeloma and monoclonal gammopathy of undetermined significance," *BBA Clinical*, vol. 6, pp. 12–18, 2016.

[2] C. M. McShane, L. J. Murray, O. Landgren et al., "Prior autoimmune disease and risk of monoclonal gammopathy of undetermined significance and multiple myeloma: a systematic review," *Cancer Epidemiology Biomarkers and Prevention*, vol. 23, no. 2, pp. 332–342, 2014.

[3] K. Kjeldsen, J. Clausen, and A. Froland, "Pernicious anaemia, paraproteinaemia with unusual features, and chromosome aberrations," *Acta Medica Scandinavica*, vol. 186, no. 1-6, pp. 209–215, 1969.

[4] R. Baz, C. Alemany, R. Green, and M. A. Hussein, "Prevalence of vitamin B12 deficiency in patients with plasma cell dyscrasias: a retrospective review," *Cancer*, vol. 101, no. 4, pp. 790–795, 2004.

[5] C. Braschi, J. Doucette, and A. Chari, "Characterization of B12 deficiency in patients with plasma cell disorders," *Blood*, vol. 126, p. 5330, 2015.

[6] P. E. Perillie, "Myeloma and pernicious anemia," *The American Journal Of The Medical Sciences*, vol. 275, no. 1, pp. 93–98, 1978.

[7] V. Montefusco, M. Galli, and F. Spina, "Autoimmune diseases during treatment with immunomodulatory drugs in multiple myeloma: selective occurrence after lenalidomide," *Leuk Lymphoma*, vol. 55, pp. 2032–2037, 2014.

[8] T. R. Halfdanarson, J. A. Walker, M. R. Litzow, and C. A. Hanson, "Severe vitamin B12 deficiency resulting in pancytopenia, splenomegaly and leukoerythroblastosis," *European Journal of Haematology*, vol. 80, no. 5, pp. 448–451, 2008.

[9] C. A. Dasanu and D. T. Alexandrescu, "A case of severe aplastic anemia secondary to treatment with lenalidomide for multiple myeloma," *European Journal of Haematology*, vol. 82, no. 3, pp. 231–234, 2009.

[10] J. Bladé, L. Rosiñol, and C. Fernández de Larrea, "How I treat relapsed myeloma," *Blood*, vol. 125, no. 10, pp. 1532–1540, 2015.

40

Spontaneous Rupture of Hepatic Metastasis from Pancreatic Adenocarcinoma

Anil Rahul, Fernandes Robin, and Hiremath Adarsh

Internal Medicine, MD Anderson Cancer Center, 1400 Pressler Street, Houston, TX 77030, USA

Correspondence should be addressed to Anil Rahul; drrahulanil@gmail.com

Academic Editor: Jorg Kleeff

A 58-year-old man with advanced-stage pancreatic adenocarcinoma presented with fatigue and dyspnea. Examination revealed tachycardia (102 b/min) with mild tenderness in right upper quadrant. His hemoglobin (Hb) was 7.9 g/dL (10 days prior to presentation 12.2 g/dL), International normalized ratio (INR), platelet count was normal, and the stool guaiac test was negative. On admission, abdominal computed tomography (CT) scan showed hepatic metastatic lesion with a rupture and hemoperitoneum communicating to the subdiaphragmatic space. This rapid progression of anemia along with presenting symptoms and CT imaging were attributed to diagnosis of spontaneous rupture of liver metastasis from pancreatic adenocarcinoma. Patient received blood transfusion and hemoglobin was monitored in successive intervals. His general condition and anemia improved with conservative management and he was discharged in 3 days. Repeated CT after 4 months showed resolving hemoperitoneum and stable hemoglobin levels. The patient deceased 9 months after being diagnosed. A literature search revealed limited data regarding the incidence and management of spontaneous rupture of metastatic lesion secondary to pancreatic adenocarcinoma which has been managed conservatively and thus we are reporting our experience.

1. Introduction

Spontaneous ruptures secondary to malignant liver metastasis are uncommon occurrences that clinically present with similar symptoms/signs as the more common spontaneous rupture of liver secondary to hepatocellular carcinoma (HCC). HCC is consistently reported to have a poor prognosis and, due to its prevalence, continues to be the most lethal and life-threatening hallmark of advanced disease, attributing to 25–75% mortality in the acute phase HCC [1]. Hepatic metastatic rupture, on the other hand, has a comparably poorer prognosis owing to confounding clinical presentation and delayed diagnosis. Several invasive interventional methods have been developed to prevent fatal sequelae of intraperitoneal hemorrhage. Thus, these invasive interventions have become the most prevalent methods of treatment, far surpassing conservative therapies. However, the interventional strategies do not significantly improve median survival and result in recurrent complications and interruptions to chemotherapy. Herein, we present a rare case of successful conservative management of spontaneous rupture of liver metastasis secondary to advanced pancreatic adenocarcinoma with no delay in resuming immunotherapy for cancer.

2. Case Report

A 58-year-old man presented with a 2-week history of fatigue and dyspnea. Two years prior to the presentation, he was diagnosed with pancreatic adenocarcinoma in the body and tail which subsequently metastasized to the liver, left lung, 6th cervical vertebra (c-6), splenic artery, ascitic fluid, and diaphragm which was confirmed by biopsies at aforementioned sites. In the interim, he underwent several lines of chemotherapy, radiation, and molecularly targeted therapy. Surgical procedures included wedge resection of the left lung lesions, cervical corpectomy and fusion, abdominal paracentesis, and gastrostomy tube placement. Past medical history includes type 2 diabetes mellitus and tubulovillous adenoma for which he underwent polypectomy. On admission, the patient was in minimal distress with tachycardia (102 beats/min), blood pressure of 99/62 mmHg, and mild

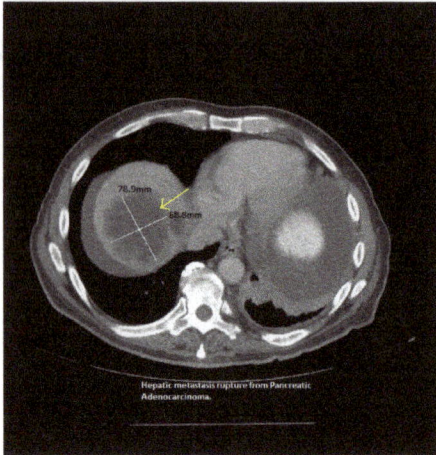

FIGURE 1: Axial contrast enhanced CT image showing metastasis in liver dome (large yellow arrow) had grown since earlier study (Figure 2).

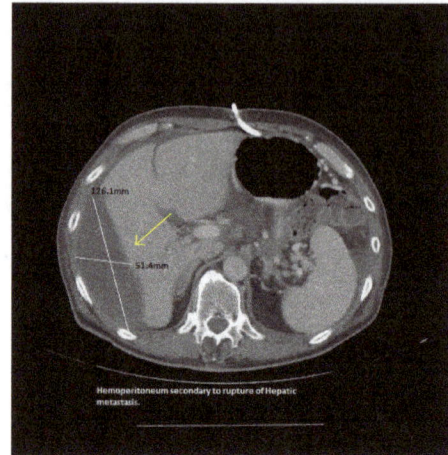

FIGURE 2: Previous CT (contrast enhanced) showing liver metastases (yellow arrow) smaller at that time and no perihepatic fluid.

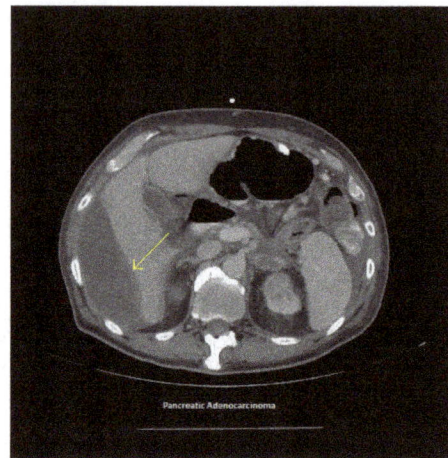

FIGURE 3: Axial contrast enhanced CT image (same study as in Figure 1) showing (yellow arrow) subcapsular liver collection.

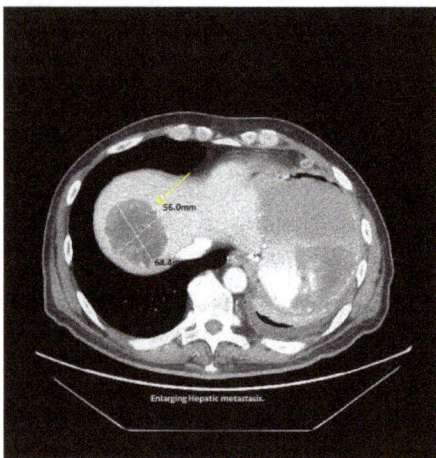

FIGURE 4: Axial contrast enhanced CT obtained 4 months after study in Figures 1 and 3 showing decreasing size of subcapsular liver collection.

tenderness in the right upper quadrant of abdomen. Laboratory data revealed hemoglobin (Hb): 7.9 g/dL; hematocrit (Hct): 24.9%; platelet count: 210,000/mm^3; prothrombin time (PT): 14 s; INR: 1.08; activated partial thromboplastin time: 27.7 s; stool guaiac test that was negative; LFT's and RFT's that were within normal limits. 10 days prior to this presentation, his Hb and Hct levels were 12.2 g/dL and 37.7%, respectively, suggesting rapid progression of anemia. Abdominal contrast enhanced CT was immediately performed and revealed an enlarging hepatic metastatic lesion (78.9 × 68.8 mm) with a rupture (Figure 1) and hemoperitoneum (126.1 × 51.4 mm) with communication to the subdiaphragmatic space (Figure 3). Previous CT imaging showed a hepatic metastatic lesion measuring (56.0 × 64.4 mm) (Figure 2). Follow-up imaging revealed resolving hemoperitoneum (Figure 4).

Considering the guarded condition and vitals being the lower limits of normalcy, the medical team consisting of a hospitalist, interventional radiologist, and oncologist decided upon managing the patient's treatment conservatively. The patient was given a blood transfusion; Hb and Hct were monitored serially in successive intervals during hospitalization. Subsequently, his general condition and anemia improved (Hb to 9.9 g/dL and Hct to 30.9%). Throughout his hospitalization, the patient's condition was stable and improved solely with conservative management. Since this approach was undertaken, there was no undue delay in resuming the patient's immunotherapy for pancreatic cancer. Repeated CT after 4 months showed resolving hemoperitoneum and stable Hb. The patient deceased 9 months after being diagnosed with hemoperitoneum secondary to metastatic hepatic rupture.

3. Discussion

Pancreatic cancer is one of the deadliest cancers, evidenced by the fact that its mortality equals its incidence [2]. Early diagnosis and treatment are limited for this condition because of the tumor's aggressively invasive nature and early metastatic properties. Pancreatic cancer metastasizes early in its course and liver is the most common site for distant metastasis, followed by the peritoneal cavity [3]. Massive hemorrhage related to ruptured liver metastases is quite exceptional and less than 50 cases are reported in the literature. Spontaneous rupture of a metastatic liver tumor is rare and uncommon when compared to hepatic rupture of primary lesion (HCC) leading to hemoperitoneum, which is a devastating complication of both primary and metastatic hepatic tumors [4, 5].

Pivotal clinical features of hemoperitoneum indicating hepatic metastatic rupture include history of malignancy, abdominal pain, hypotension, severe anemia, elevated liver enzymes, and, in extreme cases, surgical abdomen. Choi et al. reported that peripheral location of the tumor, protruding, contour, discontinuity of hepatic surface, and surrounding hemoperitoneum are helpful diagnostic indicators of ruptured HCC [6]. The aforementioned clinical and imaging (CT) findings helped us to yield to a diagnosis of metastatic hepatic rupture in our patient.

Treatment of hemoperitoneum secondary to spontaneous rupture of metastatic liver tumor depends on several factors, including tumor size, location, and severity of exsanguination. The major objective of treatment is to control the hemorrhage quickly and effectively; this can be accomplished by hepatic wedge resection/lobectomy or suture ligation of the bleeding source/hepatic artery. Recent studies suggested that a two-staged therapeutic approach in managing ruptured hepatic lesion consists of initial management with conservative approach, hemostasis achieved via transarterial embolization or surgery, followed by staged hepatic resection [7]. Transcatheter hepatic arterial embolization (TAE) may seem to be ideal for these patients, due to its various merits. Greatest benefit of TAE would be being done under local anesthesia and less invasive nature of the procedure [8]. That said, it also has some demerits, like recurrent bleeding and liver failure [8, 9], peritoneal abscess [10], implanted metastases, and patients who need to have preserved liver functions (not beyond Child-Pugh B) [11]. In addition, long-term results are poor if it is used as a solitary treatment approach without being followed by surgery [12]. On the other hand, even though surgery showed better mortality benefit [13], it has numerous risk like infections, and secondary bleeding, high morbidity [14], and last but not the least it puts a far greater toll on inevitable interruptions in chemo/immunotherapies, increase in hospital stay and cost.

However, conservative treatment focuses on achieving hemostatsis by correcting coagulopathy, close monitoring, and follow-up medical imaging to confirm hemostasis after initial resuscitation [9]. A study by Hsueh et al. showed patients who received hepatectomy, either immediate or staged after posttransarterial embolization, and reported higher survival rates of 85.2% at 30 days and 62.2% at 1 year. By comparison, similar populations treated conservatively exhibited a reduction in liver function, prolonged INR, and increased 30-day mortality [15]. Contrary to the above study Leung et al. in their retrospective study on 112 patients with ruptured HCC, comparing the in-hospital mortality and median survival in patients treated with conservative and surgical approach, concluded that the conservative approach

gave similar results to that of surgical approach [(62% versus 51%) and (7 days' versus 12 days) resp.] [16]. Having arrived at the diagnosis, with consideration of the risk factors in this patient, we agreed on managing the patient's treatment conservatively despite the odds of poor prognosis, and he responded very well and was discharged home in stable condition to resume immunotherapy for pancreatic cancer without any interruptions.

4. Conclusion

In conclusion, we convey that spontaneous metastatic liver rupture secondary to advanced pancreatic adenocarcinoma is rare and has a poor prognosis. Clinical findings and CT are of great help in making a quick diagnosis of hemoperitoneum due to metastatic liver rupture. Although the literature supports invasive intervention (extrapolating from data for HCC) in advanced-stage pancreatic cancer, conservative treatment alone (if medically stable) can be employed to combat the sequelae of intraperitoneal hemorrhage and improve survival with fewer complications and minimal interruption or delays in necessary chemotherapy or cancer-directed treatments.

References

[1] T. Aoki, N. Kokudo, Y. Matsuyama et al., "Prognostic impact of spontaneous tumor rupture in patients with hepatocellular carcinoma: an analysis of 1160 cases from a nationwide survey," *Annals of Surgery*, vol. 259, no. 3, pp. 532–542, 2014.

[2] R. Siegel, J. Ma, Z. Zou, and A. Jemal, "Cancer statistics, 2014," *CA Cancer Journal for Clinicians*, vol. 64, no. 1, pp. 9–29, 2014.

[3] S. Yachida, S. Jones, I. Bozic et al., "Distant metastasis occurs late during the genetic evolution of pancreatic cancer," *Nature*, vol. 467, no. 7319, pp. 1114–1117, 2010.

[4] C.-F. Tung, C.-S. Chang, W.-K. Chow, Y.-C. Peng, J.-I. Hwang, and M.-C. Wen, "Hemoperitoneum secondary to spontaneous rupture of metastatic epidermoid carcinoma of liver: case report and review of the literature," *Hepato-Gastroenterology*, vol. 49, no. 47, pp. 1415–1417, 2002.

[5] Z.-Y. Chen, Q.-H. Qi, and Z.-L. Dong, "Etiology and management of hemmorrhage in spontaneous liver rupture: a report of 70 cases," *World Journal of Gastroenterology*, vol. 8, no. 6, pp. 1063–1066, 2002.

[6] B. G. Choi, S. H. Park, J. Y. Byun, S. E. Jung, K. H. Choi, and J.-Y. Han, "The findings of ruptured hepatocellular carcinoma on helical CT," *The British Journal of Radiology*, vol. 74, no. 878, pp. 142–146, 2001.

[7] L. M. Veltchev, "Spontaneous rupture of hepatocellular carcinoma and hemoperitoneum-management and long term survival," *Journal of IMAB*, vol. 1, no. 2009, pp. 3–102, 2009.

[8] C. S. Leung, C. N. Tang, K. H. Fung, and M. K. W. Li, "A retrospective review of transcatheter hepatic arterial embolisation for ruptured hepatocellular carcinoma," *Journal of the Royal College of Surgeons of Edinburgh*, vol. 47, no. 5, pp. 685–688, 2002.

[9] A. Tanaka, R. Takeda, S. Mukaihara et al., "Treatment of ruptured hepatocellular carcinoma," *International Journal of Clinical Oncology*, vol. 6, no. 6, pp. 291–295, 2001.

[10] Y. Yokoi, S. Suzuki, T. Sakaguchi et al., "Subphrenic abscess formation following superselective transcatheter chemoembolization for hepatocellular carcinoma," *Radiation Medicine*, vol. 20, no. 1, pp. 45–49, 2002.

[11] C.-N. Yeh, H.-M. Chen, M.-F. Chen, and T.-C. Chao, "Peritoneal implanted hepatocellular carcinoma with rupture after TACE presented as acute appendicitis," *Hepato-Gastroenterology*, vol. 49, no. 46, pp. 938–940, 2002.

[12] A. Rossetto, G. L. Adani, A. Risaliti et al., "Combined approach for spontaneous rupture of hepatocellular carcinoma," *World Journal of Hepatology*, vol. 2, no. 1, pp. 49–51, 2010.

[13] Y.-J. Jin, J.-W. Lee, S.-W. Park et al., "Survival outcome of patients with spontaneously ruptured hepatocellular carcinoma treated surgically or by transarterial embolization," *World Journal of Gastroenterology*, vol. 19, no. 28, pp. 4537–4544, 2013.

[14] W.-K. Chen, Y.-T. Chang, Y.-T. Chung, and H.-R. Yang, "Outcomes of emergency treatment in ruptured hepatocellular carcinoma in the ED," *The American Journal of Emergency Medicine*, vol. 23, no. 6, pp. 730–736, 2005.

[15] K.-C. Hsueh, H.-L. Fan, T.-W. Chen et al., "Management of spontaneously ruptured hepatocellular carcinoma and hemoperitoneum manifested as acute abdomen in the emergency room," *World Journal of Surgery*, vol. 36, no. 11, pp. 2670–2676, 2012.

[16] K. L. Leung, W. Y. Lau, P. B. S. Lai, R. Y. C. Yiu, W. C. S. Meng, and C. K. Leow, "Spontaneous rupture of hepatocellular carcinoma: conservative management and selective intervention," *Archives of Surgery*, vol. 134, no. 10, pp. 1103–1107, 1999.

41

Testicular Signet-Ring Cell Metastasis from a Carcinoma of Unknown Primary Site: A Case Report and Literature Review

Aristomenes Kollas,[1] George Zarkavelis,[1] Anna Goussia,[2] Aikaterini Kafantari,[1] Anna Batistatou,[2] Zoi Evangelou,[2] Eva Sintou,[3] and Nicholas Pavlidis[1]

[1]*Department of Medical Oncology, University Hospital of Ioannina, 45500 Ioannina, Greece*
[2]*Department of Pathology, University Hospital of Ioannina, 45500 Ioannina, Greece*
[3]*Department of Cytology, University Hospital of Ioannina, 45500 Ioannina, Greece*

Correspondence should be addressed to Nicholas Pavlidis; npavlid@uoi.gr

Academic Editor: Constantine Gennatas

Signet-ring cell carcinoma is a highly malignant adenocarcinoma consisting of cells characterized as cytoplasmic vacuoles filled with mucin. The most common primary location of this type of cancer is the stomach, but it may also be found in other organs such as prostate, testis, bladder, ovaries, or colon. To date, metastatic signet-ring cell carcinoma of unknown primary (CUP) site to the testis is an extremely rare entity in daily practice. Reviewing the literature, we have been able to detect only three cases of testicular metastases from CUP, two with histological diagnosis of a signet-ring cell carcinoma and one with an adenocarcinoma. In this short paper, we report a case of a 56-year-old man who presented to our Department with testicular mass and ascites. Following a standard diagnostic approach no primary tumor could be identified. CUP was the final clinical diagnosis, histologically characterized as poorly differentiated adenocarcinoma with signet-ring cells involving the peritoneum and the testicular structures.

1. Introduction

CUP is a clinical syndrome, which is defined by the presence of metastatic disease without establishment of the primary site. Throughout the literature, the term occult is also used when referring to a type of malignancy with uncertain site of uncertain origin outcome, without definitive IHC findings and clinical manifestations. Its frequency is estimated about 3% to 5% of all malignancies and it is represented with various clinical and histologic characteristics. The natural history of the disease is characterized by a short time of symptoms and rapid dissemination of the disease. The diagnostic algorithm is based on patient's symptoms, clinical examination, laboratory findings, and imaging studies. A more favorable prognosis has been associated with lymph nodal disease, female sex, good performance status, normal LDH levels, and small number of metastatic sites [1, 2].

In order to identify the primary site, a thorough physical examination, a complete medical history, and basic laboratory tests such as complete blood count, serum biochemistry, chest X-ray, CT scans, mammography, and tumor markers should be performed [2, 3]. Accumulating data emphasize the limited role of PET/CT in diagnosing a probable primary site, mainly if head and neck cancer is suspected [4–6]. Basic IHC stains are used to increase the ability to identify the primary organ sites, such as CK7, CK20, chromogranin, synaptophysin, NSE, TTF-1, thyroglobulin, CDX-2, PSA, AFP, b-hCG, vimentin, S100, HMB 45, ER, or PR [7]. At the same time, more accurate methods such as Molecular Tumor Profiling technics (MTP) are available to help oncologists define the primary site [8]. The primary goal of medical oncologists is to rule out the presence of a potentially treatable or curable malignancy (i.e., germ-cell tumors, lymphomas, and breast cancer) [2].

Association of CUP with signet-ring histology is very rare, especially with the presence of testicular metastasis. We, therefore, introduce a case of a 56-year-old man, who presented to our Department with a testicular mass and ascites, without the presence of a primary site following

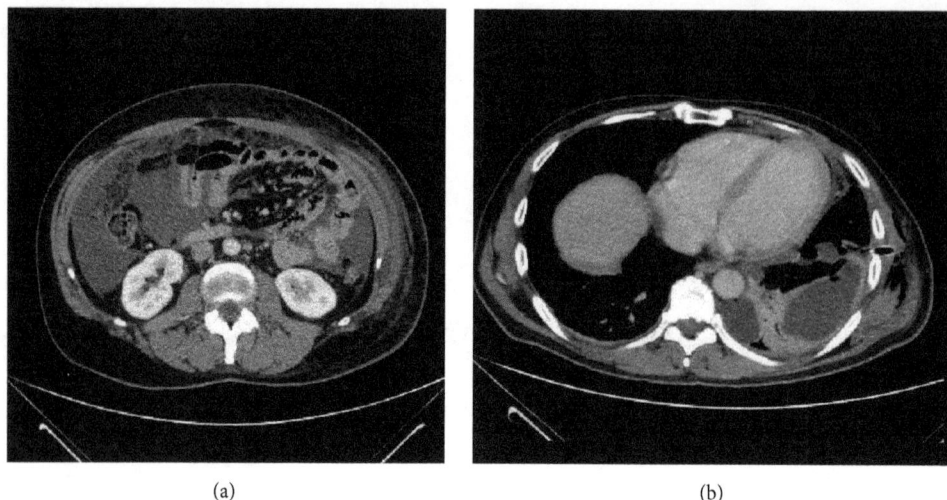

(a)

(b)

FIGURE 1: (a) At the time of diagnosis diffuse peritoneal fluid in the abdomen and peritoneal implants are presented through the CT scan. (b) Pleural effusion on the left (progressive disease) presented after the third cycle of Capecitabine/Oxaliplatin chemotherapy.

extensive diagnostic work-up. Our final diagnosis was cancer of unknown primary.

2. Case Presentation

A 56-year-old male Caucasian, 60-pack-year smoker with a past medical history of sleep apnea presented as an outpatient with gradual abdominal distention. During the last 2 months he reported painless swelling of the right testis. Physical examination revealed ascites and right scrotal hard mass with enlarged testis. Complete blood count and biochemistry were normal, while serum CA 125 was increased (319 μ/mL). In November of 2015 he was admitted to the Oncology Department for further investigation.

Computed tomography of the thorax and abdomen revealed a minimal pleural effusion of the left hemithorax, diffuse peritoneal fluid in the abdomen, and peritoneal implants (Figure 1(a)). Since no solid literature data exist (apart from the sensitivity of PET/CT scan in hidden primaries mainly of head neck) no PET/CT scan was requested in our case. Upper and lower GI endoscopy revealed no abnormalities. Patient had a scrotal ultrasound imaging that revealed an enlarged right epididymis with small amount of fluid in the right side of the scrotum. Abdominal paracentesis revealed exudative fluid with neoplastic signet-ring cells indicative of metastatic adenocarcinoma. Gross evaluation of the tissue specimen revealed several poorly defined, whitish, and hard in consistency foci throughout the testicular parenchyma, the epididymis, and the spermatic cord. The tunicae surrounding the testis were thickened. Microscopical examination of multiple tissue sections taken from the grossly described foci showed the presence of a poorly differentiated carcinoma composed of signet-ring cells (Figure 2(a)). Perineural and neural invasion as well as vascular invasion were observed.

By histochemical stains (PAS, Alcian Blue) a large amount of mucin was demonstrated in the cytoplasm of tumor cells

(Figure 2(b)). Immunohistochemically, the neoplastic cells were diffusely positive for cytokeratin 20 and EMA, focally positive for cytokeratin 7, CEA, and c-kit (CD117), and negative for PLAP, a-fetoprotein, CD30, inhibin, calretinin, PSA, p504S (AMACR), TTF-1, and Melan A (Figure 2(c)). The pathological diagnosis was in favor of a metastatic adenocarcinoma, probably of gastrointestinal origin. Tissue HER2 was negative.

Taking into consideration the aforementioned findings, the primary site could not be established and the case was classified as CUP. In November 2015 he started on systemic therapy consisting of Capecitabine and Oxaliplatin. Up till January 2015, he has received three cycles of the above regimen with good partial remission of his ascites and excellent drug toleration. However, just before the fourth cycle he developed right pleural effusion with accompanying moderate dyspnea (Figure 1(b)). Pleural fluid cytology was positive for metastatic adenocarcinoma with signet-ring cells.

A second-line regimen consisting of Doxorubicin, Cyclophosphamide, and Fluorouracil (DCF) was administered. Up till now, the patient has received six cycles of DCF with complete response of the disease on abdominal and thoracic CT scans as well as normalisation of serum CA 125 (6 μ/mL).

3. Discussion

Cancer of unknown primary remains a neoplastic entity usually with an aggressive natural history and poor outcome. At the time of patient presentation an extensive investigation is needed in order to identify the primary site. Failure to identify the primary site leads to the establishment of CUP diagnosis. Cisplatin based chemotherapy in combination with a taxane is the main recommended empirical regimen.

Histologically, CUP includes well and moderately differentiated adenocarcinomas, squamous cell carcinomas,

(a)

(b)

(c)

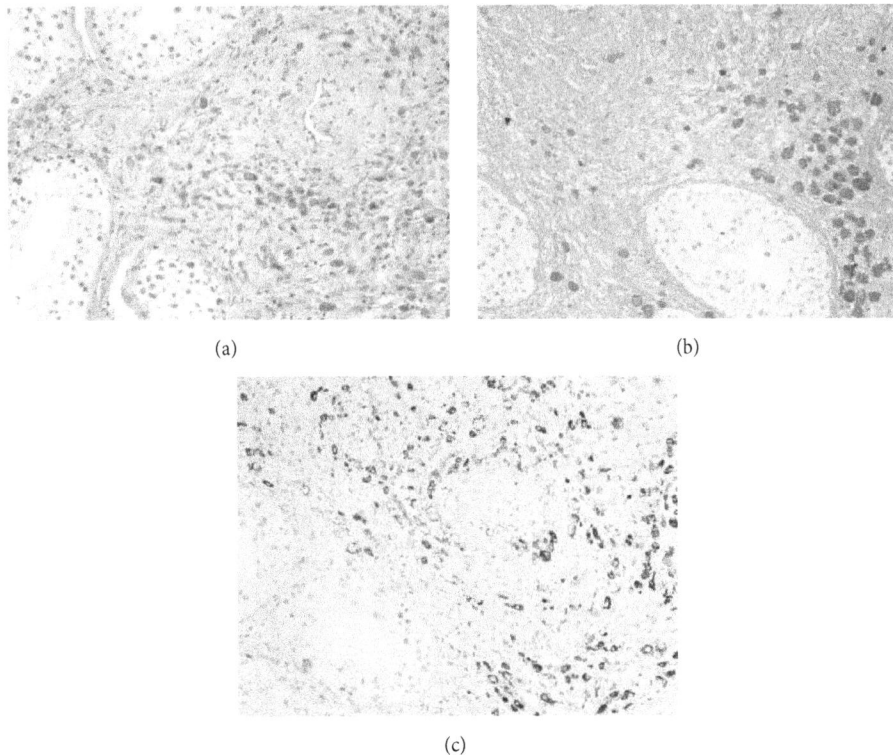

FIGURE 2: (a) The testicular parenchyma is infiltrated by neoplastic signet-ring cells (hematoxylin-eosin ×200). (b) Tumor cells exhibit positivity for mucin stains (arrows). (c) Immunohistochemically the tumor cells were positive for cytokeratin 20 (arrows).

neuroendocrine carcinomas, poorly differentiated carcinomas, and undifferentiated carcinomas. CUP is distinguished between favourable (nodal disease and neuroendocrine tumors) and unfavourable (splanchnic metastases) subsets [2]. CUP can also be presented as isolated effusion or peritoneal carcinomatosis [12, 13]. To date, few cases of signet-ring carcinomas of occult primary site with metastases in the testicles have been reported. In particular, there are two similar cases through the literature with poor prognosis despite the therapeutic efforts that have been made.

Although the testicles are considered to be an inhospitable environment for cancer cells due to the low temperature, rarely neoplastic cells are able to invade them through the systematic venous, lymphatic circulation, or direct tumor invasion [14]. Although testicular metastases from other solid tumors have been rarely described, it is known that prostate cancer is the commonest primary tumor with such a predilection [15, 16]. In this paper, we presented the fourth case of a CUP patient diagnosed with a metastatic scrotal lesion (see Table 1).

In 2004 Salesi et al. reported a case of a 62-year-old man who presented with dyspnea, while a testicular mass and lung metastases with pleural effusion were noted. The final diagnosis according to the IHC studies was occult gastrointestinal adenocarcinoma [16].

In 2008 Chimakurthi and Lalit reported a case of a 37-year-old man with a history of alcoholism and alcoholic liver disease, who presented with ascites and right scrotal swelling. Testicular biopsy revealed metastatic adenocarcinoma with

signet-ring cell features of an unknown primary site [10]. It was in 2011 when Saredi et al. reported a case of a 77-year-old man complaining of right testicular swelling. Orchiectomy revealed metastasis from poorly differentiated neoplasm with signet-ring cells, while prostatic biopsy revealed a unilateral acinar prostatic adenocarcinoma. Despite detailed diagnostic investigations, no primary site was detected and the final diagnosis was CUP with testicular signet-ring metastasis [11].

As a take home message, it should always be kept in mind that the clinical differential diagnosis of testicular mass—apart from primary cancers such as germ-cell tumors or non-Hodgkin's lymphomas—metastatic lesions from various solid tumors must be ruled out.

4. Conclusion

To date, several cases of metastatic adenocarcinomas to the testicles with primary tumors in prostate, lung, stomach, colon, or kidney have been reported. However, the diagnosis of signet-ring cell metastases to the testis from an unknown primary carcinoma is very uncommon. Conclusively, oncologists have to take into account the case of occult primary testicular metastasis with signet-ring cells as an extremely rare but existing possibility.

TABLE 1: Reported cases of CUP with testicular metastases.

Author	Patient	Presenting symptom	Disease extent	Histological findings
Salesi et al. 2004 [9]	62-year-old male	Dyspnea and left testicular mass	Multiple lung metastases, pleural effusion, mediastinal node involvement, brain metastasis, and testicular metastasis	Metastatic adenocarcinoma (testicular biopsy and VATS)
Chimakurthi and Lalit 2008 [10]	37-year-old male	Ascites and right scrotal swelling	Diffuse carcinomatosis involving most of the abdominal organs, bowel obstruction, and frozen retroperitoneum	Metastatic adenocarcinoma with signet ring cells (testicular biopsy and omental biopsy)
Saredi et al. 2011 [11]	77-year-old male	Right testicular swelling	Pulmonary metastases and peritoneal carcinomatosis	Signet ring adenocarcinoma (testicular biopsy) Acinar prostatic adenocarcinoma (prostatic biopsy)
Kollas et al. 2006 (present case)	56-year-old male	Ascites and right testicular swelling	Peritoneal, testicular, and pleural metastases	Poorly differentiated carcinoma composed of signet ring cells

References

[1] N. Pavlidis and K. Fizazi, "Carcinoma of unknown primary (CUP)," *Critical Reviews in Oncology/Hematology*, vol. 69, no. 3, pp. 271–278, 2009.

[2] N. Pavlidis and G. Pentheroudakis, "Cancer of unknown primary site," *The Lancet*, vol. 379, no. 9824, pp. 1428–1435, 2012.

[3] G. Pentheroudakis and N. Pavlidis, "Serum tumor markers," in *Metastatic Carcinomas of Unknown Origin*, M. R. Wick, Ed., pp. 165–175, Demos Medical Publishing, New York, NY, USA, 2008.

[4] R. C. Delgado-Bolton, C. Fernández-Pérez, A. González-Maté, and J. L. Carreras, "Meta-analysis of the performance of 18F-FDG PET in primary tumor detection in unknown primary tumors," *Journal of Nuclear Medicine*, vol. 44, no. 8, pp. 1301–1314, 2003.

[5] P. Sève, C. Billotey, C. Broussolle, C. Dumontet, and J. R. Mackey, "The role of 2-deoxy-2-[F-18]fluoro-D-glucose positron emission tomography in disseminated carcinoma of unknown primary site," *Cancer*, vol. 109, no. 2, pp. 292–299, 2007.

[6] F. Keller, G. Psychogios, R. Linke et al., "Carcinoma of unknown primary in the head and neck: comparison between positron emission tomography (PET) and PET/CT," *Head and Neck*, vol. 33, no. 11, pp. 1569–1575, 2011.

[7] K. A. Oien, "Pathologic evaluation of unknown primary cancer," *Seminars in Oncology*, vol. 36, no. 1, pp. 8–37, 2009.

[8] P. Economopoulou, G. Mountzios, N. Pavlidis, and G. Pentheroudakis, "Cancer of Unknown Primary origin in the genomic era: elucidating the dark box of cancer," *Cancer Treatment Reviews*, vol. 41, no. 7, pp. 598–604, 2015.

[9] N. Salesi, A. Fabi, B. Di Cocco et al., "Testis metastasis as an initial manifestation of an occult gastrointestinal cancer," *Anticancer Research*, vol. 24, no. 2, pp. 1093–1096, 2004.

[10] R. Chimakurthi and K. Lalit, "Signet-ring cell metastasis with unknown primary," *Gastrointestinal Cancer Research*, vol. 2, no. 5, supplement 3, pp. S17–S21, 2008.

[11] G. Saredi, M. Rivalta, M. C. Sighinolfi et al., "Testicular metastasis of signet ring cell tumour of unknown origin: diagnostic features of a tricky case," *Andrologia*, vol. 43, no. 3, pp. 222–223, 2011.

[12] G. Pentheroudakis and N. Pavlidis, "Serous papillary peritoneal carcinoma: unknown primary tumour, ovarian cancer counterpart or a distinct entity? A systematic review," *Critical Reviews in Oncology/Hematology*, vol. 75, no. 1, pp. 27–42, 2010.

[13] N. Pavlidis, E. Briasoulis, J. Hainsworth, and F. A. Greco, "Diagnostic and therapeutic management of cancer of an unknown primary," *European Journal of Cancer*, vol. 39, no. 14, pp. 1990–2005, 2003.

[14] F. Blefari and O. Risi, "Rare secondary carcinoma from colon to testis. Review of literature and report of a new case," *Archivio Italiano di Urologia, Nefrologia, Andrologia*, vol. 61, no. 3, pp. 275–278, 1989.

[15] S. R. Patel, R. L. Richardson, and L. Kvols, "Metastatic cancer to the testes: a report of 20 cases and review of the literature," *The Journal of Urology*, vol. 142, no. 4, pp. 1003–1005, 1989.

[16] A. Schneider, A. Kollias, J. Woziwodzki, and G. Stauch, "Testicular metastasis of a metachronous small cell neuroendocrinic prostate cancer after anti-hormonal therapy of a prostatic adenocarcinoma. Case report and literature review," *Urologe A*, vol. 45, no. 1, pp. 75–80, 2006.

42

Metastatic Melanoma of Uncertain Primary with 5-Year Durable Response after Conventional Therapy: A Case Report with Literature Review

Jomjit Chantharasamee ⓘ[1] and Jitsupa Treetipsatit[2]

[1]Division of Medical Oncology, Department of Medicine, Faculty of Medicine, Siriraj Hospital, Mahidol University, Bangkok, Thailand
[2]Department of Pathology, Faculty of Medicine, Siriraj Hospital, Mahidol University, Bangkok, Thailand

Correspondence should be addressed to Jomjit Chantharasamee; jomjit025@hotmail.com

Academic Editor: Jose I. Mayordomo

A 51-year-old Thai woman presented with bilateral leg edema and painful left inguinal mass for 6 months. Physical examination revealed matted bilateral inguinal lymph nodes up to 9 cm in size. Otherwise, physical examinations including skin were unremarkable. The result of the lymph node incisional biopsy is consistent with that of metastatic melanoma. The extensive investigation demonstrated multiple intra-abdominal and inguinal lymph nodes without detectable primary tumor. Palliative radiation and conventional chemotherapy were prescribed. The CT scan between treatments showed that the response was stable disease, but the following CT scan demonstrated a gradual decrease in size from August 2012 to November 2017 including the lesions outside radiation fields. Moreover, she developed vitiligo during a follow-up visit. The previous data reported the median overall survival among the patients who were treated with conventional chemotherapy ranging from 9.1 to 9.3 months and whose 5-year survival was less than 10%. This case represented a metastatic melanoma of unknown primary who achieved a durable response by conventional treatment. The clinical features including nodal-only disease, vitiligo, and abscopal effect of radiation were considered to be the favorable factors.

1. Introduction

Malignant melanoma is an uncommon skin malignancy accounting for about 4% of skin cancer [1, 2]. An incidence rate of melanoma is increasing worldwide but varies between different studies ranging from 0.3 to 3.6% [1] depending on the predominant skin type and geographical location. The *prevalence* for men and women varies with the *highest prevalence* at the *fifth decade* of age [2, 3]. Malignant melanoma of unknown primary (MUP) was reported to be 2–2.4% of melanoma [2, 4]. Compared to the other areas, Asian populations have a significantly lower incidence rate that was estimated about 0.2 to 0.5 per 100,000 patient-years; this incidence rate is mostly of melanoma of known primary (MKP), so that makes MKP in Asian population extremely rare [1, 2]. Most of the literatures in the different geographic regions demonstrated better overall survival of MUP than of MKP [2, 5, 6].

A 5-year overall survival of MUP before the era of the immune checkpoint inhibitor was reported to range from 8 to 18% [3, 4, 7]. The most common metastatic site is the lymph node and GI tract [2, 3]. Many hypotheses were documented in relation to the etiology of MUP including spontaneous regression of primary melanoma, undiagnosed excised melanoma, small primary in the visceral site, and primary melanoma in the lymph node [2, 8, 9]. This study was aimed at reporting a patient with metastatic melanoma of uncertain primary who achieved durable response longer than expected after being treated with conventional treatments.

2. Case Report

A 51-year-old Thai woman was hospitalized in July 2012 with edema at the left lower extremities and painful left inguinal mass for 6 months.

Physical examination revealed matted bilateral inguinal lymph nodes up to 9 cm in size with hard consistency, erythema, and tenderness without fluctuation or ulcer. Marked swelling at both lower extremities was observed. There was no other superficial lymphadenopathy. Otherwise, physical examinations were normal.

Incisional biopsy of the left inguinal lymph node revealed metastatic round cell tumor which is immunohistochemistry positive for vimentin, S100, and HMB-45. The immunophenotype is consistent with malignant melanoma (Figure 1).

Therefore, primary tumors in the lower extremities, abdominal cavity, and anogenital organ were suspected. By complete skin examination, no cutaneous lesion was identified. Ophthalmoscopy, gastroscopy, colonoscopy, and cystoscopy were completely normal. Genital and pelvic examinations did not show any evidence of lesion. She denied previous abnormal or removal of cutaneous lesion. Computer tomography of the whole abdomen showed multiple enlarged lymph nodes throughout the abdominal and pelvic cavity up to 9.5 cm, along with compression of both iliac veins without an organ-specific lesion (Figure 2). CT chest was unremarkable. The patient was diagnosed with metastatic melanoma of unknown primary. The molecular testing had not been done due to the patient's reimbursement issue, and the specimen was poor in quality for further testing. During the investigation, she developed severe pain requiring high-dose opioid, so she has undergone 20 Gy of palliative radiotherapy for bilateral inguinal lymph nodes. Despite radiotherapy, the remaining tumors were up to 7.4 cm based on the CT scan. For the subsequent systemic therapy, according to a national reimbursement policy, she could not access an immune checkpoint inhibitor or targeted drug. Chemotherapy was prescribed with carboplatin (AUC5) and paclitaxel 175 mg/m^2 for 6 cycles. After completion of the planned chemotherapy, the symptom was slightly improved. The CT scan at the first 3 months showed that the response was stable disease, but the following CT scan demonstrated a gradual decrease in size over time from August 2012 to November 2017 (Figure 3). During the follow-up period, the patient developed multiple depigmented patches around the lips, trunk, and periorbital and inguinal area, which are typical of vitiligo.

3. Discussion

Systemic treatments of metastatic melanoma were developed for many decades since conventional chemotherapy has been considered a standard approach until the emergence of new drugs such as targeted therapy and immunotherapy over the last 10 years. The dramatic and durable response occurred by taking targeted therapy or immunotherapy but not by taking chemotherapy. In the patients who did not have access to those drugs, chemotherapy is a mainstay treatment. Previous data reported the median overall survival among the patients who were treated with conventional chemotherapy ranging from 7.7 to 16 months and whose 5-year survival was 8–18% [4, 6, 7, 10, 11].

This case report represents a patient with metastatic melanoma of unknown primary with durable response by conventional chemotherapy and palliative radiation. When comparing prognosis, MUP tends to have a better prognosis than MKP as reported in previous studies [2, 4–6, 8, 12]. The aforementioned hypotheses of unknown primary including an immunological response that leads to spontaneous regression of primary tumor, unrecognized primary tumor, and the occurrence of malignant ectopic nevus cells in the lymph node itself can be considered the etiology of MUP in this patient, who denied previous removal of cutaneous lesion [2, 8, 9]. The data from Dana-Farber Institute reported that the nodal-only metastasis was an independent favorable prognostic factor of MUP compared to metastasis at other sites [3]. This patient had nodal-only metastasis, which explains that this is a favorable clinical feature. The survival outcome of metastatic melanoma according to the molecular alteration was reported in many literatures. For Asian population, the study reported by Kong et al. [13] showed that KIT mutation was an independent prognostic factor for a shorter survival compared to KIT wild type (30 versus 58 months). Another study by Si et al. [14] reported that BRAF and NRAS mutation was associated with worse overall survival compared to wild-type melanoma (33 versus 53 months). Regarding the effect of palliative chemotherapy, the recent studies showed that the response rate was 10–30% [10, 11, 15] consistent with the response rate of this patient. After completion of chemotherapy, the tumors still had a detectable size as same as previous, but after regular visits, the tumors gradually decreased in size based on the interval CT scan. The possibility of clinical response from the conventional chemotherapy can be explained by the genomic profile. The correlation of somatic mutations with the clinical outcome of melanoma patients treated with carboplatin/paclitaxel either with or without sorafenib was reported by Melissa et al. The patients harboring BRAF mutation and wild type seemed to have longer survival than those harboring NRAS mutation (15.6 versus 5.6 months) in a chemotherapy arm [16]. Another study from Jilaveanu et al. [17] reported the association between marker expression and response to sorafenib plus chemotherapy. This study revealed that the patients with high VEGFR-R2/low ERK1/2 expression correlated with a higher response rate compared to those with low VEGFR-R2/high ERK1/2. However, we could not demonstrate the molecular alteration in our patient due to the unaffordable cost of testing at the time of diagnosis and the poor quality of the 5-year archival specimen. In addition to the chemotherapy treatment, the tumors outside the radiation field also decreased in size which could be either the effect of chemotherapy or the abscopal effect of radiation [18]. This late-response phenomenon could be the effect of the immune response rather than of the chemotherapy itself. According to the effect of radiotherapy, irradiation can induce the host antitumor immune response resulting in the late response after treatment as presented in this case [19]. The hypotheses of presentation of vitiligo concomitant with melanoma by the process of autoimmune-related vitiligo were published in many literatures. The several data-reported specific antigens of melanoma such as TRP1 and TRP2 that were shared by normal melanocytes caused immune response to both melanoma and normal

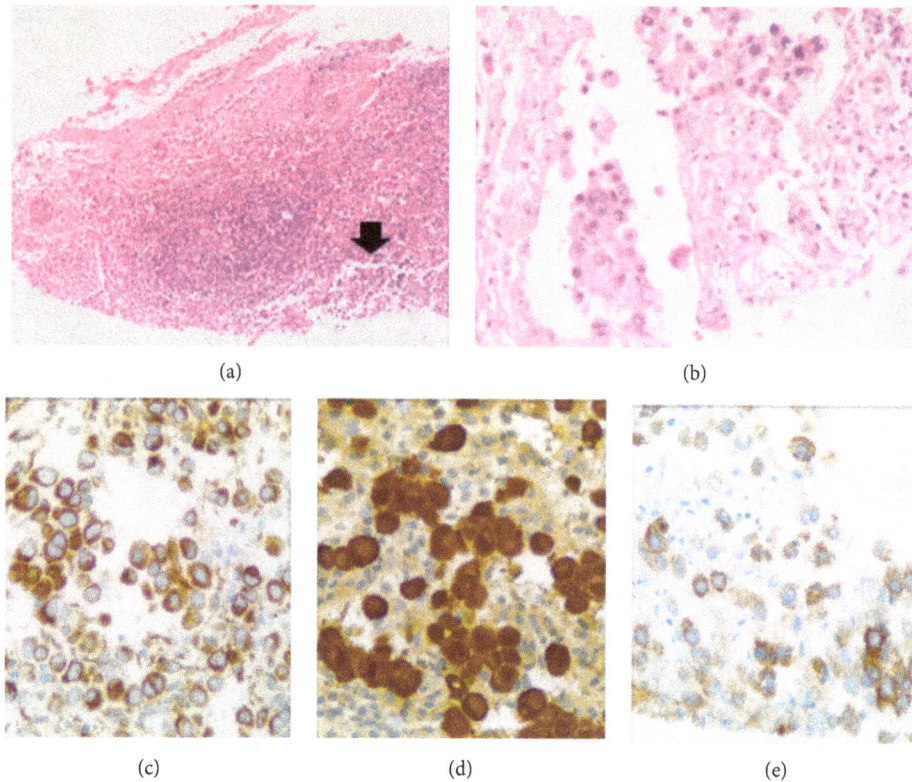

FIGURE 1: Metastatic malignant melanoma in the left inguinal lymph node: (a) H&E at ×40 and (b) H&E at ×400. The tumor cells are positive for vimentin (c), S100 (d), and HMB-45 (e).

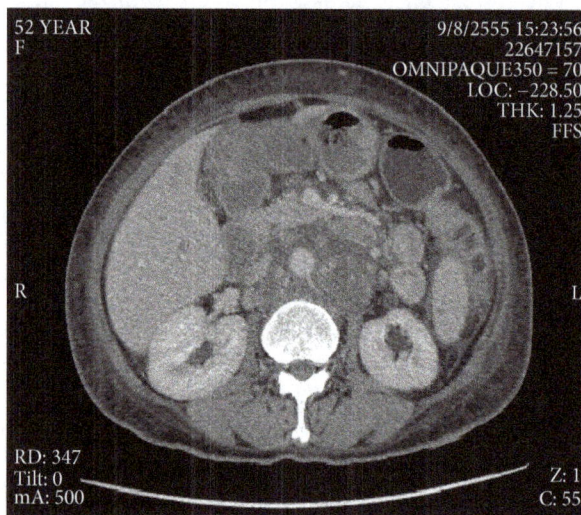

FIGURE 2: Abdominal CT scan at the time of diagnosis demonstrated matted paraaortic nodes.

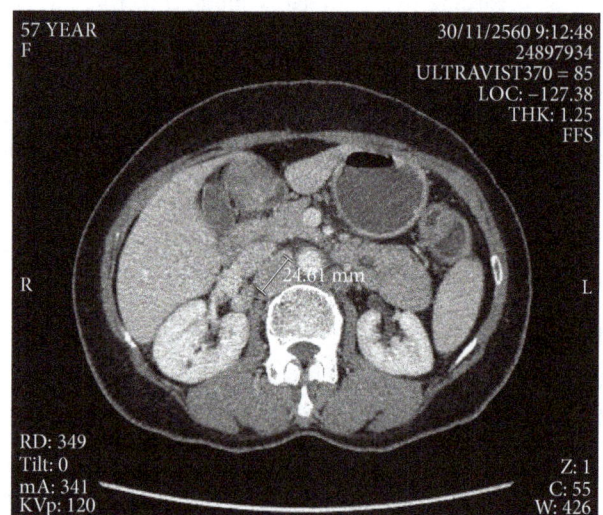

FIGURE 3: The following CT scan revealed a marked decrease in size of intra-abdominal lymph nodes.

melanocytes [20–22]. In addition, some preclinical evidence supported the role of CD8 T-cell-mediated melanoma in vitiligo. The result from an ex vivo study demonstrated that melanoma cells can be killed by CD8 T-cells taken from a vitiligo lesion and T-cells taken from melanoma that caused apoptosis of melanocytes [21, 23, 24]. Moreover, the report from Becker et al. [25] showed the clonotypically identical

T-cell infiltration within the melanoma and vitiligo lesion. All those theories can explain the correlation between melanoma and vitiligo. The evidence supports that the presence of vitiligo may be a favorable prognostic factor for survival theoretically due to the immune mechanism responsible for melanocytic proliferation causing depigmentation of skin and spontaneous regression of primary melanoma which were reported [26–28]. One of the studies reported by Nordlund et al. [28] showed that a 10-year survival rate among patients with nonmetastatic melanoma with vitiligo was 49%. This patient who has vitiligo may benefit from this mechanism in terms of disease control. This patient had a tumor response along with vitiligo later after the complete treatment which was probably from the effect of the immune process. The molecular basis in this patient was not yet known to be a prognostic marker for survival.

4. Conclusion

Metastatic melanoma can achieve durable response by conventional chemotherapy and radiotherapy in patients with some clinical characteristics. The presence of the nodal-only disease, vitiligo, and effect of radiation seemed to be the favorable factors for better survival.

References

[1] F. Erdmann, J. Lortet-Tieulent, J. Schüz et al., "International trends in the incidence of malignant melanoma 1953–2008—are recent generations at higher or lower risk?," *International Journal of Cancer*, vol. 132, no. 2, pp. 385–400, 2013.

[2] J. F. Scott, R. Z. Conic, C. L. Thompson, M. R. Gerstenblith, and J. S. Bordeaux, "Stage IV melanoma of unknown primary: a population-based study in the United States from 1973 to 2014," *Journal of the American Academy of Dermatology*, vol. 18, pp. 30472–30479, 2018.

[3] K. A. Katz, E. Jonasch, F. S. Hodi et al., "Melanoma of unknown primary: experience at Massachusetts general hospital and Dana-Farber Cancer Institute," *Melanoma Research*, vol. 15, no. 1, pp. 77–82, 2005.

[4] A. E. Chang, L. H. Karnell, and H. R. Menck, "The National Cancer Data Base report on cutaneous and noncutaneous melanoma," *Cancer*, vol. 83, no. 8, pp. 1664–1678, 1998.

[5] J. M. Bae, Y. Y. Choi, D. S. Kim et al., "Metastatic melanomas of unknown primary show better prognosis than those of known primary: a systematic review and meta-analysis of observational studies," *Journal of the American Academy of Dermatology*, vol. 72, no. 1, pp. 59–70, 2015.

[6] C. C. Lee, M. B. Faries, L. A. Wanek, and D. L. Morton, "Improved survival for stage IV melanoma from an unknown primary site," *Journal of Clinical Oncology*, vol. 27, no. 21, pp. 3489–3495, 2009.

[7] G. Vijuk and A. S. Coates, "Survival of patients with visceral metastatic melanoma from an occult primary lesion: a retrospective matched cohort study," *Annals of Oncology*, vol. 9, no. 4, pp. 419–422, 1998.

[8] P. Savoia, P. Fava, S. Osella-Abate et al., "Melanoma of unknown primary site: a 33-year experience at the Turin Melanoma Centre," *Melanoma Research*, vol. 20, no. 3, pp. 227–232, 2010.

[9] G. Tchernev, A. Chokoeva, and L. V. Popova, "Primary solitary melanoma of the lymphatic nodes or a single metastasis of unknown melanoma: do we need a new staging system?,"

Open Access Macedonian Journal of Medical Sciences, vol. 5, no. 7, pp. 970–973, 2017.

[10] S. Aamdal, I. Wolff, S. Kaplan et al., "Docetaxel (Taxotere) in advanced malignant melanoma: a phase II study of the EORTC early clinical trials group," *European Journal of Cancer*, vol. 30, no. 8, pp. 1061–1064, 1994.

[11] M. B. Atkins, J. Hsu, S. Lee et al., "Phase III trial comparing concurrent biochemotherapy with cisplatin, vinblastine, dacarbazine, interleukin-2, and interferon alfa-2b with cisplatin, vinblastine, and dacarbazine alone in patients with metastatic malignant melanoma (E3695): a trial coordinated by the eastern cooperative oncology group," *Journal of Clinical Oncology*, vol. 26, no. 35, pp. 5748–5754, 2008.

[12] F. Egberts, I. Bergner, S. Krüger et al., "Metastatic melanoma of unknown primary resembles the genotype of cutaneous melanomas," *Annals of Oncology*, vol. 25, no. 1, pp. 246–250, 2014.

[13] Y. Kong, L. Si, Y. Zhu et al., "Large-scale analysis of *KIT* aberrations in Chinese patients with melanoma," *Clinical Cancer Research*, vol. 17, no. 7, pp. 1684–1691, 2011.

[14] L. Si, Y. Kong, X. Xu et al., "Prevalence of BRAF V600E mutation in Chinese melanoma patients: large scale analysis of BRAF and NRAS mutations in a 432-case cohort," *European Journal of Cancer*, vol. 48, no. 1, pp. 94–100, 2012.

[15] E. Bajetta, M. del Vecchio, P. Nova et al., "Multicenter phase III randomized trial of polychemotherapy (CVD regimen) versus the same chemotherapy (CT) plus subcutaneous interleukin-2 and interferon-α2b in metastatic melanoma," *Annals of Oncology*, vol. 17, no. 4, pp. 571–577, 2006.

[16] M. A. Wilson, F. Zhao, R. Letrero et al., "Correlation of somatic mutations and clinical outcome in melanoma patients treated with carboplatin, paclitaxel, and sorafenib," *Clinical Cancer Research*, vol. 20, no. 12, pp. 3328–3337, 2014.

[17] L. Jilaveanu, C. Zito, S. J. Lee et al., "Expression of sorafenib targets in melanoma patients treated with carboplatin, paclitaxel and sorafenib," *Clinical Cancer Research*, vol. 15, no. 3, pp. 1076–1085, 2009.

[18] M. A. Postow, M. K. Callahan, C. A. Barker et al., "Immunologic correlates of the abscopal effect in a patient with melanoma," *The New England Journal of Medicine*, vol. 366, no. 10, pp. 925–931, 2012.

[19] C. A. Perez, A. Fu, H. Onishko, D. E. Hallahan, and L. Geng, "Radiation induces an antitumour immune response to mouse melanoma," *International Journal of Radiation Biology*, vol. 85, no. 12, pp. 1126–1136, 2010.

[20] A. Houghton, M. Eisinger, A. P. Albino, J. Cairncross, and L. Old, "Surface antigens of melanocytes and melanomas. Markers of melanocyte differentiation and melanoma subsets," *Journal of Experimental Medicine*, vol. 156, no. 6, pp. 1755–1766, 1982.

[21] M. J. Turk, J. D. Wolchok, J. A. Guevara-Patino, S. M. Goldberg, and A. N. Houghton, "Multiple pathways to tumor immunity and concomitant autoimmunity," *Immunological Reviews*, vol. 188, no. 1, pp. 122–135, 2002.

[22] H. Uchi, R. Stan, M. J. Turk et al., "Unraveling the complex relationship between cancer immunity and autoimmunity: lessons from melanoma and vitiligo," *Advances in Immunology*, vol. 90, pp. 215–241, 2006.

[23] A. Anichini, C. Maccalli, R. Mortarini et al., "Melanoma cells and normal melanocytes share antigens recognized by HLA-A2-restricted cytotoxic T cell clones from melanoma patients,"

Journal of Experimental Medicine, vol. 177, no. 4, pp. 989–998, 1993.

[24] K. Oyarbide-Valencia, J. G. van den Boorn, C. J. Denman et al., "Therapeutic implications of autoimmune vitiligo T cells," *Autoimmunity Reviews*, vol. 5, no. 7, pp. 486–492, 2006.

[25] J. C. Becker, P. Guldberg, J. Zeuthen, E.-B. Bröcker, and P. t. Straten, "Accumulation of identical T cells in melanoma and vitiligo-like leukoderma," *Journal of Investigative Dermatology*, vol. 113, no. 6, pp. 1033–1038, 1999.

[26] E. A. Cho, M. A. Lee, H. Kang, S. D. Lee, H. O. Kim, and Y. M. Park, "Vitiligo-like depigmentation associated with metastatic melanoma of an unknown origin," *Annals of Dermatology*, vol. 21, no. 2, pp. 178–181, 2009.

[27] P. Quaglino, F. Marenco, S. Osella-Abate et al., "Vitiligo is an independent favourable prognostic factor in stage III and IV metastatic melanoma patients: results from a single-institution hospital-based observational cohort study," *Annals of Oncology*, vol. 21, no. 2, pp. 409–414, 2010.

[28] J. J. Nordlund, J. M. Kirkwood, B. M. Forget, G. Milton, D. M. Albert, and A. B. Lerner, "Vitiligo in patients with metastatic melanoma: a good prognostic sign," *Journal of the American Academy of Dermatology*, vol. 9, no. 5, pp. 689–696, 1983.

43

Atypical Proliferating Trichilemmal Cyst with Malignant Breast Skin Transformation: A Case Report and Review of the Literature

Marino Antonio Capurso-García,[1,2] **Verónica Bautista-Piña,**[3]
Alan Pomerantz,[2] **Javier Andrés Galnares-Olalde,**[2] **Ruben Blachman-Braun,**[2]
Sergio Rodríguez-Rodríguez,[2] **and Monica Goldberg-Murow**[2]

[1]*Departamento de Oncología Mamaria Quirúrgica, Instituto de Enfermedades de la Mama (IEM),*
 La Fundación del Cáncer de Mama (FUCAM), 40980 Mexico City, Mexico
[2]*Facultad de Ciencias de la Salud, Universidad Anáhuac México Norte, 52786 Huixquilucan, MEX, Mexico*
[3]*Departamento de Patología, Instituto de Enfermedades de la Mama (IEM), La Fundación del Cáncer de Mama (FUCAM),*
 40980 Mexico City, Mexico

Correspondence should be addressed to Alan Pomerantz; cancercancer0@gmail.com

Academic Editor: Jose I. Mayordomo

Proliferating trichilemmal tumors (PTTs) are benign adnexal skin neoplasms that arise from the outer root sheath of the hair follicle. These tumors are most commonly observed on the scalp and occur, most of the time, in elderly women. Malignant transformation of these neoplasms is a rare event; less than 50 cases have been reported in the English medical literature. We present the case of a 39-year-old Hispanic woman with a tumor located on the skin of one of her breasts that in her third surgical procedure the histologic examination revealed the presence of a malignant proliferating trichilemmal tumor (MPTT). Furthermore, a review of the medical literature and a discussion of the clinical and pathologic features of this rare entity are provided.

1. Introduction

Proliferating trichilemmal tumors (PTTs) are benign adnexal skin neoplasms that arise from the outer root sheath of the hair follicle. Most of these tumors arise within the wall of a preexisting trichilemmal cyst [1]. Moreover, these tumors, from a histopathological standpoint, are very similar to a squamous cell carcinoma (SCC) [2]. PTTs were first described in 1966 by Wilson-Jones as epidermoid proliferating cysts [3]. However, it was not until 1995 that epidermoid proliferating cysts and PTTs were distinguished as different lesions [2].

PTTs encompass only 0.1% of all skin tumors. Additionally, most of the patients that present these lesions are elderly women, and in 90% of the cases these tumors occur on the scalp [4]. PTTs rarely exhibit malignant transformation (characterized by invading neighboring tissues and the presence of anaplasia and necrosis) into malignant proliferating

trichilemmal tumors (MPTTs) [5–7], a fact substantiated by the presence of less than 50 cases of MPTTs reported in the English medical literature.

In this paper, the first case reported in Latin America regarding the malignant transformation of a PTT, we present the case of a woman with a tumor located on the skin of one of her breasts that in her third surgical procedure the histologic examination revealed the presence of a MPTT. In addition, a literature review and a discussion of the clinical and pathologic features of this rare entity are provided.

2. Case Report

A 39-year-old Hispanic woman was referred to our hospital due to the sudden appearance of a painful, mobile, fixed mass of about 5 cm in diameter in the internal upper quadrant of her right breast. The lesion was classified as a breast cyst, and

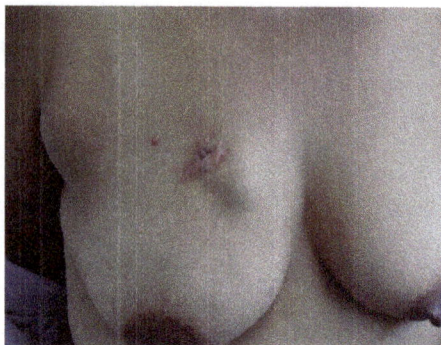

FIGURE 1: Photography of recurrent tumor in the right breast beneath the previous site of resection. Note the nodule under the scar deforming the overlying skin.

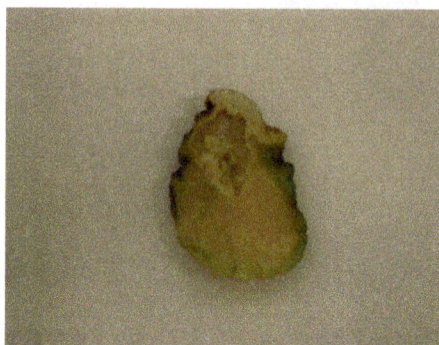

FIGURE 2: Pale yellow, firm, solid, lobulated, poorly defined mass, of 2.8 cm in length and 2.5 in width, covered by mature adipose tissue.

a puncture of it was performed. Hyaline fluid was aspirated from the mass, with a subsequent decrease in its size. After two months, in the next follow-up, the growth reappeared. Therefore, the mass was surgically resected. The resected lesion was sent to the pathology department and a diagnosis of chronic granulomatous mastitis and fat necrosis was made.

Three months after the surgery, the patient presented again for an evaluation due to the presence of a keloid scar of about 5 cm. When the breast was examined a 2 cm nodule located under the scar was palpated. The mass had well-defined borders and was not fixed to superficial or deep tissue (Figure 1). A breast ultrasound was performed, and it showed a cystic tumor of 2.33 cm, with well-defined borders and mixed echodensity. Due to the result of the ultrasound, the growth was described as a recurrent, complicated right breast skin cyst.

The patient underwent surgery in order to remove the tumorous growth. The lump was excised with amplified margins of 2 cm. The macroscopic appearance of the tumor was of a pale yellow, firm, solid, lobulated, poorly defined mass, of 2.8 cm in length and 2.5 in width, covered by mature adipose tissue (Figure 2). Microscopically, the tumor was described as a mixed tissue tumor, consisting of solid and cystic areas. The solid part of the neoplastic lesion was formed by squamous cells disposed as cordons, exhibiting peripheral palisades, with the presence of abrupt keratinization of the outer layers and focal calcifications. The cystic part presented a wall showing stratified squamous epithelium, multiple pleomorphic mitotic cells, and intraluminal keratin deposits (Figures 3 and 4). In some areas of the adjacent stroma, the pathologist observed squamous epithelial cell nests, with desmoplastic reaction and lymphocytic proliferation (Figure 5). The immunohistochemistry report was as follows: CD34 negative in the neoplastic cells, positive cytokeratin AE1/AE3, and positive p53 in 40% of the tumor. Finally, the diagnosis of MPTT was made, and the patient has been followed up since the diagnosis without any signs that the neoplasia has relapsed.

3. Discussion

PTTs are rare, and the malignant transformation of these tumors is a rarer pathological finding. Moreover, only two

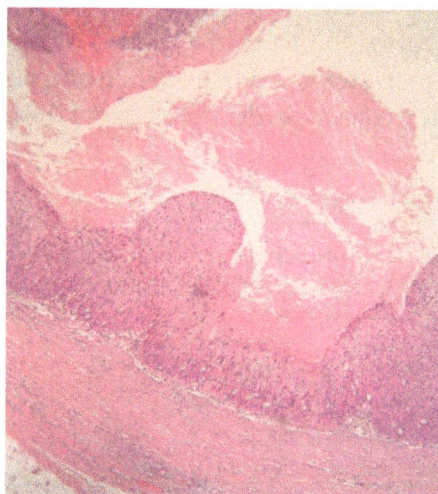

FIGURE 3: Cystic tumor portion where keratin amorphous deposits are observed (H and E, ×10).

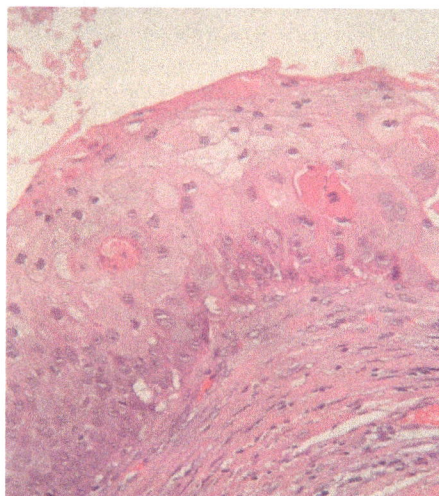

FIGURE 4: High magnification micrograph showing squamous epithelium keratinization (H and E, ×20).

cases in the literature have reported the presence of a MPTT over the skin of the breast [8, 9]. PTTs usually appear in

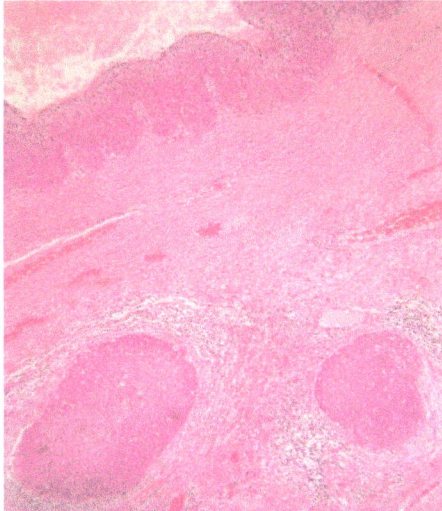

FIGURE 5: Photomicrograph showing epithelial cell nests in the stroma with desmoplastic reaction (H and E, ×10).

women, 80–87% of the cases, between 27 and 83 years of age, with a peak in the sixth and seventh decades of life [4, 10]. They typically appear in sun-exposed areas and regions with abundant hair growth, thus explaining why these tumors appear most frequently on the scalp [5].

Histologically, PTTs are characterized by an abrupt transition of the nucleated epithelium to anucleated keratinized cells without a granular layer, a phenomenon known as trichilemmal keratinization. MPTTs can occur de novo but most often occur due to the malignant transformation of a PTT. A stepwise transformation of MPTTs has been described from an adenomatous to an epitheliomatous and then to a carcinomatous stage [11]. Additionally, in a study in which 76 patients were evaluated, the clinicopathological categorization of PTTs into three groups was proposed [4, 7].

(i) Group 1 Tumors. They are considered completely benign and present minimal nuclear atypia, trichilemmal keratinization, and stromal invasion with mononuclear cells, plasma cells, lymphocytes, and giant cells.

(ii) Group 2 Tumors. They are considered locally aggressive and present irregular and local invasive contours, with moderate cytological atypia, foci of single cell necrosis, and abrupt keratinization with desmoplastic stromal response.

(iii) Group 3 Tumors. They are considered malignant and present marked nuclear polymorphism, atypical mitosis, foci of single cell necrosis, abrupt keratinization, and lymphovascular invasion.

Even though the diagnosis of MPTTs is mostly done in a histopathological fashion, the use of immunohistochemistry can help to distinguish MPTTs from PTTs and SCCs. CD34 is a marker that is closely associated with trichilemmal keratinization, and because it is absent in SCCs and present

in MPTTs it can help in differentiating one condition from the other (an important distinction because MPTTs have a greater chance of recurring and metastasizing) [7, 12]. As with this case, there have been reports of MPTTs where a negative staining with CD34 is observed. Moreover, some authors have postulated that a loss of CD34 staining is related to a decrease in the differentiation of the tumor. Ki-67 and p53 can help in the distinction of MPTTs from PTTs, as both markers are usually absent or dimly expressed in PTTs [7].

In order to evaluate possible local and distant metastases, imaging studies are warranted. It has been reported that on imaging studies MPTTs can manifest as either a cystic or a solid mass. Computed tomography scan is useful for the evaluation of focal bone involvement and erosion, and assessment of possible metastases; meanwhile, magnetic resonance imaging is reserved to evaluate soft tissue infiltration and signs of malignancy. Malignancy findings include poorly defined margins, penetration of tissue planes, and local invasion [1, 4].

As with other skin lesions, surgical excision remains the treatment of choice. Wide excision with margins of at least 1 cm is recommended [1, 4]. With a local recurrence rate of 3.7%, even for benign PTTs, Mohs micrographic surgery has been suggested as a better technique for the excision of MPTTs due to its superior margin control [13].

Due to the rarity of MPTTs, the efficacy of alternative treatments cannot be evaluated. In cases with distant metastases the use of CAV (cisplatin, adriamycin, and vindesine) chemotherapy, a regimen that has been used for advanced squamous cell carcinoma, has been attempted. Nonetheless, the results have not been promising [13]. Therefore, patients suspected of having this condition should be diagnosed and treated in an expedite manner, with a close follow-up after the excision of the tumor.

4. Conclusion

We report a case of a MPTT that occurred in an atypical location, which represented a clinical challenge in both the diagnosis and definitive treatment, due to the nonspecific clinical presentation and rarity of this condition. The recurrences that the patient presented may have occurred due to the fact that excision margins of less than 1 cm were used in the previous resection. Furthermore, it is important to state that the clinician should be alert to this diagnosis, especially in the presence of a cyst with recent rapid growth after remaining unchanged for a long time and tendency to recur after the tumor has been excised.

Acknowledgments

The authors acknowledge the Universidad Anáhuac México Norte for the support provided in the publication of this paper.

References

[1] A. K. Satyaprakash, D. J. Sheehan, and O. P. Sangüeza, "Proliferating trichilemmal tumors: a review of the literature," *Dermatologic Surgery*, vol. 33, no. 9, pp. 1102–1108, 2007.

[2] N. Uchida, Y. Tsuzuki, T. Ando et al., "Malignant proliferating trichilemmal tumor in the skin over the breast: a case report," *Breast Cancer*, vol. 7, no. 1, pp. 79–82, 2000.

[3] E. W. Jones, "Proliferating epidermoid cysts," *Archives of Dermatology*, vol. 94, no. 1, pp. 11–19, 1966.

[4] B. D. Deshmukh, M. P. Kulkarni, Y. A. Momin, and K. R. Sulhyan, "Malignant proliferating trichilemmal tumor: a case report and review of literature," *Journal of Cancer Research and Therapeutics*, vol. 10, no. 3, pp. 767–769, 2014.

[5] P. K. Shetty, S. Jagirdar, K. Balaiah, and D. Shetty, "Malignant proliferating trichilemmal tumor in young male," *Indian Journal of Surgical Oncology*, vol. 5, no. 1, pp. 43–45, 2014.

[6] S. Goyal, B. B. Jain, S. Jana, and S. K. Bhattacharya, "Malignant proliferating trichilemmal tumor," *Indian Journal of Dermatology*, vol. 57, no. 1, pp. 50–52, 2012.

[7] O. Alici, M. K. Keles, and A. Kurt, "A rare cutaneous adnexal tumor: malignant proliferating trichilemmal tumor," *Case Reports in Medicine*, vol. 2015, Article ID 742920, 4 pages, 2015.

[8] M. Aydin and A. Aslaner, "Proliferating trichilemmal tumors on breast and scalp: report of a case," *International Journal of Surgery*, vol. 7, no. 2, pp. 1–4, 2005.

[9] T. Saida, K. Oohara, Y. Hori, and S. Tsuchiya, "Development of a malignant proliferating trichilemmal cyst in a patient with multiple trichilemmal cysts," *Dermatologica*, vol. 166, no. 4, pp. 203–208, 1983.

[10] S. Rao, R. Ramakrishnan, D. Kamakshi, S. Chakravarthi, S. Sundaram, and D. Prathiba, "Malignant proliferating trichilemmal tumour presenting early in life: an uncommon feature," *Journal of Cutaneous and Aesthetic Surgery*, vol. 4, no. 1, pp. 51–55, 2011.

[11] J. Ye, O. Nappi, P. E. Swanson, J. W. Patterson, and M. R. Wick, "Proliferating pilar tumors: a clinicopathologic study of 76 cases with a proposal for definition of benign and malignant variants," *American Journal of Clinical Pathology*, vol. 122, no. 4, pp. 566–574, 2004.

[12] E. D. Mathis, J. B. Honningford, H. E. Rodriguez, K. P. Wind, M. M. Connolly, and F. J. Podbielski, "Malignant proliferating trichilemmal tumor," *American Journal of Clinical Oncology: Cancer Clinical Trials*, vol. 24, no. 4, pp. 351–353, 2001.

[13] D. R. Fieleke and G. D. Goldstein, "Malignant proliferating trichilemmal tumor treated with Mohs surgery: proposed protocol for diagnostic work-up and treatment," *Dermatologic Surgery*, vol. 41, no. 2, pp. 292–294, 2015.

44

Pulmonary Metastases from an Undifferentiated Embryonal Sarcoma of the Liver: A Case Report and Review

Mingxia Shi⊙,[1] Hongzhi Xu,[1] Guillermo P. Sangster,[2] and Xin Gu[1]

[1]*Department of Pathology and Translational Pathobiology, Louisiana State University Health Science Center-Shreveport, 1501 Kings Highway, Shreveport, LA 71130, USA*
[2]*Department of Radiology, Louisiana State University Health Science Center-Shreveport, 1501 Kings Highway, Shreveport, LA 71130, USA*

Correspondence should be addressed to Mingxia Shi; mshi@lsuhsc.edu

Academic Editor: Ossama W. Tawfik

Undifferentiated embryonal sarcoma of the liver (UESL) is a rare malignant hepatic tumor that occurs primarily in children. Only a limited number of cases have been reported in the literature due to low incidence of one per million, and reports of metastatic lesion of UESL are even rarer. We hereby describe the case of a 13-year-old male who presented with a palpable mass with imaging findings suggestive of a large complex tumor in the right lobe of the liver. He underwent extended right hepatectomy followed by adjuvant chemotherapy. The tumor was confirmed to be UESL by postoperative pathology and immunohistochemical staining analysis. Four years later, surveillance imaging revealed a small lung nodule in the left lower lobe. Complete removal of the lung tumor by wedge resection was performed, and a histological diagnosis of metastatic UESL was made. The patient also received postoperative adjuvant chemotherapy and is currently in a good general condition and tumor-free in the present eight-month period. This case is presented with emphasis on clinicopathological and immunohistochemical findings of the primary UESL and lung metastases with the aim of collecting more data and expanding our understanding of this rare malignancy.

1. Introduction

Malignant liver tumors represent approximately for 1% to 4% of all solid tumors in children [1]. Undifferentiated embryonal sarcoma of the liver (UESL), first described by Stocker and Ishak in 1978 as a rare aggressive mesenchymal tumor of the liver [2], accounts for approximately 9–13% of all childhood malignant hepatic tumors [3] and is the third most common hepatic malignancy in children after hepato-blastoma and hepatocellular carcinoma. It occurs predominantly in children, with a peak incidence between 6 and 10 years of age [2]. It has also infrequently been reported in adults. Due to its low incidence of one per million [4], only a limited number of cases have been reported in the literature.

Diagnosis of UESL relies on postoperative pathological examination and immunohistochemical results. It is based on the tumor morphology, patient's age, and tumor location (primary hepatic mass) together with a panel of undifferentiated pathologic markers including vimentin, desmin, CD10, CD68, alpha1-antitrypsin, and ruling out of other pathologies. In the past, prognosis of UESL had been poor due to local recurrence, tumor rupture, and metastatic disease [2, 5]. More recently, aggressive treatment regimens that combine complete surgical resection of the hepatic tumor and effective multiagent chemotherapy have improved survival substantially [6, 7]. Although metastases of UESL have been reported to occur in 5–13% of children [8, 9], only very rare cases of metastatic UESL, which mostly are present at time of diagnosis, have been reported in the literature [4, 10, 11]. The optimal treatment for metastatic UESL has not been defined, likely due to the rarity of the disease and a paucity of data.

Herein, we report a case of UESL found in a 13-year-old male who developed a lung metastasis four years after hepatectomy and adjuvant chemotherapy and highlight the clinicopathological and immunohistochemical features of the primary and metastatic lesion.

2. Case Presentation

A 13-year-old male was transferred to our Pediatric Hematology/Oncology Clinic for evaluation of a large liver mass detected by an abdominal computed tomography (CT) scan in an outside hospital. He presented with increasing abdominal distension of several months' duration and denied fever, abdominal pain, nausea, vomiting, or loss of appetite. During his admission, a physical examination revealed that the liver edge was palpable 6 cm below the right costal margin and no abdominal tenderness or guarding was present. Laboratory investigations demonstrated slightly elevated lactate dehydrogenase (263 U/L, normal range: 74–250 U/L). His blood count, liver function tests, and other liver enzymes as well as serum alpha-fetoprotein (AFP) were within normal range. Ultrasonography revealed a partially defined hepatic mass with multiple internal cystic foci, and an increased intralesional vascularization is identified (Figure 1(a)). Magnetic resonance imaging (MRI) of the abdomen revealed a $17 \times 18 \times 20$ cm heterogeneous predominantly cystic mass with thick internal septations, residual solid tissue, and peripheral neovascular formation in the right hepatic lobe (Figures 1(b)–1(d)). Extended right hepatectomy was performed. Intraoperative frozen section was submitted with interpretation of malignant neoplasm. Grossly, the resected specimen consisted of a $19.5 \times 14 \times 16$ cm well-circumscribed mass with a fibrous pseudocapsule. Cut surface of the tumor showed a variegated appearance of gray, solid glistening tumor alternating with soft gelatinous areas with dark-brown and yellow-green areas of hemorrhage and necrosis (Figure 2(a)). On microscopic examination, the tumor contains alternating hypocellular myxoid areas and hypercellular areas. It was comprised predominantly of pleomorphic cells that are spindle, oval, or stellate shaped and distributed in a fibrous or myxoid stroma (Figures 2(b)–2(d)). Some areas showed fibroblast-like fascicles and bundles. Focally, tumor cells were highly bizarre, with occasional large anaplastic multinucleated giant cells. Atypical mitotic figures were easily identified. Few sharply defined eosinophilic hyaline globules in the tumor cell cytoplasm were observed (Figure 2(e)). Entrapped bile ducts and hepatic cords were present in areas at the periphery of the tumor (Figure 2(f)). By immunohistochemistry, tumor cells stained positively for vimentin and alpha1-antitrypsin, partially positive for desmin, and negative for myogenin, smooth muscle actin (SMA), and pancytokeratin (AE1/AE3) (Figures 3(a)–3(f)). The AE1/AE3 stain highlighted the entrapped bile ducts (Figure 3(f)). The surgical margin was free. On the basis of these findings, a pathological diagnosis of UESL was made. Postoperative positron emission tomography (PET) scan did not reveal residual or metastatic disease. A five-month course of chemotherapy (VAdrC/VIE) including vincristine, doxorubicin, cyclophosphamide, ifosfamide, and etoposide was received, starting at 4 weeks after the operation, and he tolerated the chemotherapy well. The patient has been followed with imaging studies, including a whole-body PET scan.

At 48 months of follow-up, surveillance MRI showed a hyperintense, 7 mm lung lesion on T2-weighted images but

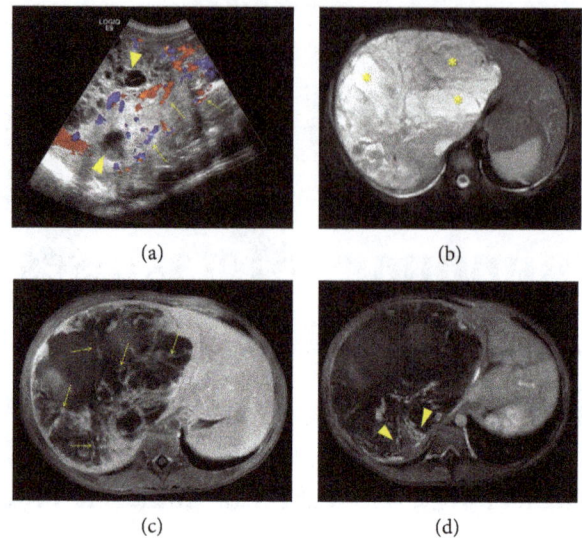

(a)　　　　　　　　　　(b)

(c)　　　　　　　　　　(d)

FIGURE 1: (a) Ultrasonography of the liver. Grayscale with Doppler image demonstrates a partially defined hepatic mass with multiple internal cystic foci (arrowheads) and increased intralesional vascularization (arrows). MRI of the abdomen with axial T2 fat saturation (b) and LAVA (liver acquisition with volume acceleration sequence) after intravenous contrast administration at 5 min (c) and 20 min (d) show a large heterogeneous mass within the right hepatic lobe. A predominant intralesional cystic/necrotic component (*), multiple internal septations (arrows), and residual solid tissue (arrowheads) are seen.

PET scan was negative. Chest CT imaging at 50 months following the hepatectomy revealed a 1.7×1.4 cm lung nodule in the left lower lobe (Figure 4(a)) with no pleural or pericardial effusions. There was left hepatic lobe hypertrophy with no evidence of local tumor recurrence. The patient underwent lateral thoracotomy with wedge resection of the left lower lobe nodule. Macroscopically, the resected specimen consisted of a well-demarcated mass measuring $1.5 \times 1.2 \times 0.9$ cm with soft and gelatinous cut surface. Histopathological studies revealed that the tumor was composed of pleomorphic stellate and spindled neoplastic cells in a predominantly myxoid matrix; scattered bizarre multinucleated giant cells and atypical mitotic figures were frequently seen (Figures 4(b)–4(d)). No evident intracellular or extracellular eosinophilic hyaline globules were observed. There were bronchioles entrapped within and at the periphery of the tumor (Figures 4(e) and 4(f)). Few isolated bronchioles were focally destroyed by the infiltrating tumor. Background lung parenchyma revealed atelectasis and marked vascular congestion. By immunohistochemistry, the tumor cells were strongly and diffusely positive for vimentin, α1-antitrypsin, and CD10, patchy positive for desmin, CD56, and BCL2, rare staining for CD68, and negative for myogenin and AE1/AE3 (Figures 5(a)–5(i)). The entrapped bronchiolar epithelium was highlighted by AE1/AE3 (Figure 5(i)). The pathological findings are consistent with metastases of the UESL. A chemotherapy regimen with olaratumab plus doxorubicin was received. At the time of this report, he is 9 months after wedge resection and remains well with no evidence of tumor recurrence.

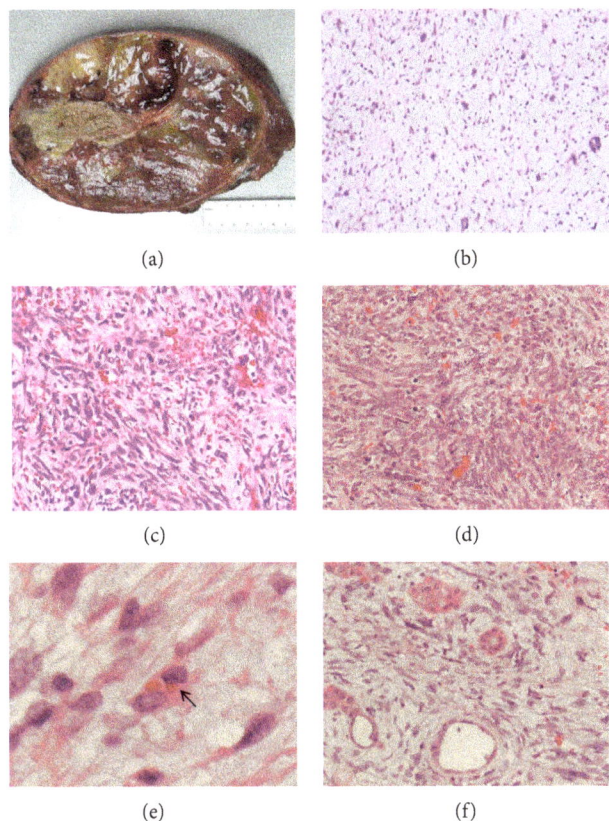

FIGURE 2: Pathological findings of the UESL. (a) Macroscopic appearance of the tumor. Histological examination showed (b, c, and d) hypocellular myxoid and hypercellular areas containing stellate and spindle-shaped malignant cells with scattered bizarre multinucleated giant cells, (e) the presence of cytoplasmic eosinophilic hyaline globules (arrow), and (f) cords of hepatocytes and bile ducts entrapped within the tumor (hematoxylin and eosin stain; original magnification: (b) ×100; (c, d, and f) ×200; (e) ×400).

3. Discussion

Undifferentiated embryonal sarcoma of the liver (UESL) is a relatively new distinct clinicopathologic entity that describes a rare malignancy arising from the primitive mesenchymal tissue of the liver [2]. It is mainly seen in young children and adolescents without gender predilection. UESL is rare among adults, with a female preponderance [12]. It represents fewer than 1% of all primary liver neoplasms in adults [13].

Patients with UESL usually have variable and nonspecific symptoms, with abdominal pain and abdominal mass reported to be the most common presenting complaints [14]. Other complaints, such as fever, nausea, vomiting, weight loss, fatigue, anorexia, and jaundice, may be presented. Spontaneous rupture resulting in intraperitoneal hemorrhage due to rapid tumor growth has also been reported [15]. There are no distinctive laboratory findings for UESL. Mild leukocytosis or leukopenia, low albumin, anemia, and slightly elevated transaminase levels and erythrocyte sedimentation rates may be seen. Evaluation of some tumor markers including AFP, cancer antigen 19-9, and

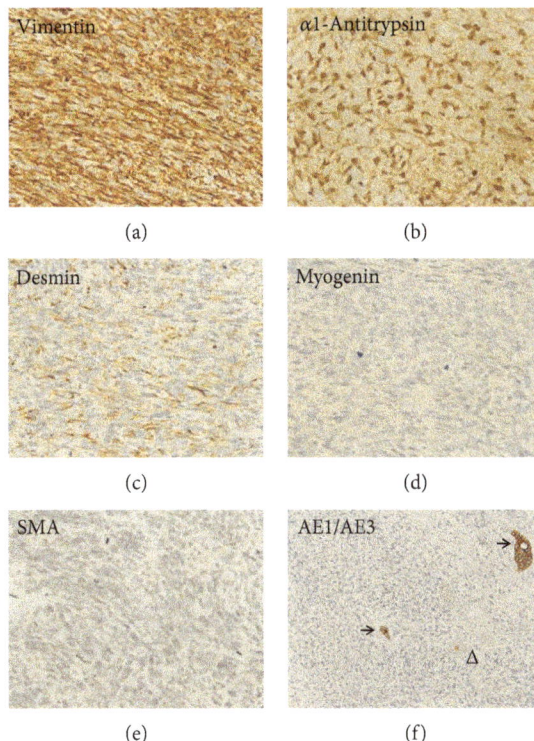

FIGURE 3: Immunohistochemical staining of the tumor cells in the UESL showed strong positivity for vimentin (a) and α1-antitrypsin (b), patchy positivity for desmin (c), and negative for myogenin (d), smooth muscle actin (SMA) (e), and pancytokeratin AE1/AE3 (f). The entrapped hepatic cords were negative for AE1/AE3 (f) (arrowhead), but AE1/AE3 highlighted the entrapped bile ducts (f) (arrow) (immunoperoxidase; original magnification: ×200).

carcinoembryonic antigen often yields normal results, but rare cases with increased levels of AFP and cancer antigen 125 have been reported [16]. There is one reported case of UESL that secretes erythropoietin, which was used as a marker of the tumor recurrence [17]. Our patient presented with asymptomatic abdominal mass and unremarkable laboratory findings, which is similar to what have been reported previously in most cases of childhood UESL.

The results of imaging studies of UESL are often nonspecific and inconclusive. On ultrasound (US) imaging, UESL usually appears as a hypoechoic solid mass. CT and MRI scans typically demonstrate a large mass with cystic attenuation. UESL is occasionally misdiagnosed as a benign hepatic lesion based on the cystic appearance seen on CT and MRI. This diagnostic pitfall may cause delayed management. There have been several case reports of UESL being mistaken for hydatid disease [18, 19]. Discrepancy of internal architecture on US and CT was considered one of the important characteristics of UESL. Such discordant or inconsistent imaging findings of a large hepatic lesion that has a seemingly cystic appearance on CT or MRI and a predominantly solid appearance on ultrasound should raise suspicion for this tumor [20, 21]. On angiography, UESL is most often hypovascular; however, avascular and hypervascular appearances have been reported [22]. Our case showed consistent images of the multicystic hepatic mass on US and CT. These

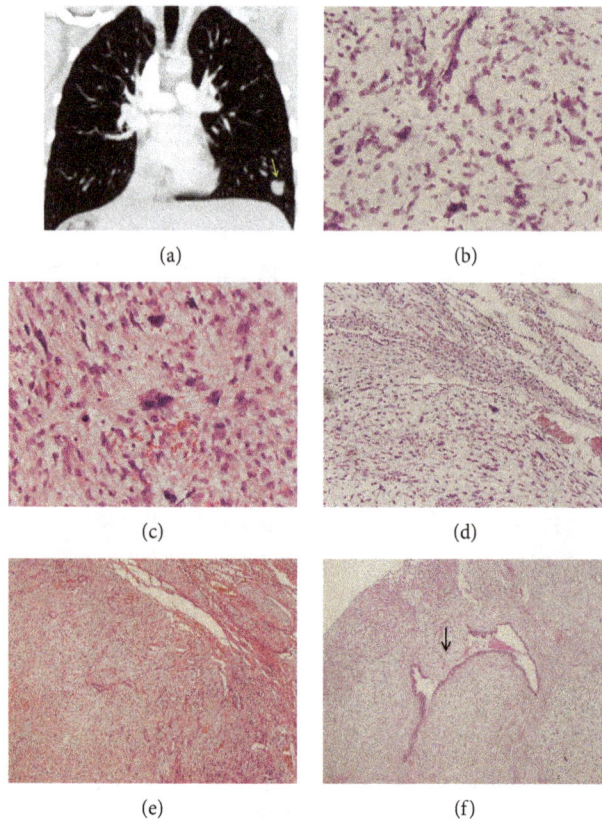

(a)   (b)

(c)   (d)

(e)   (f)

FIGURE 4: Pulmonary metastatic lesion of UESL. (a) CT of the thorax showed a well-defined solid nodular lesion (arrow) in the left lower lobe. (b, c) Histological examination of the lung lesion. (d) The uninvolved pulmonary parenchyma (to upper right of the center) is compressed. (e, f) Bronchioles entrapped within and at the periphery of the tumor. An isolated bronchiole is surrounded and focally destroyed by the infiltrating tumor (f) (arrow) (hematoxylin and eosin stain; original magnification: (f) ×40; (d) and (e) ×100; (b) and (c) ×200).

characteristic imaging patterns account for the increased water content within the abundant myxoid stroma of UESL.

Preoperative diagnosis of UESL is challenging due to the lack of characteristic clinical manifestations and tumor markers, nonspecific radiological imaging, and the rarity of the disease. Definitive diagnosis relies on postoperative pathological examination and immunohistochemical results. UESL usually occurs as a large (10–30 cm), solitary well-circumscribed mass that is mostly localized in the right lobe of the liver, while it rarely develops in the hepatic left lobe or the bilateral lobes. The mass often has a fibrous pseudo-capsule with compressed liver parenchyma. Cut surface reveals a heterogeneous appearance that is predominately solid but often has foci of cystic or gelatinous degeneration. Hemorrhagic and necrotic areas are common [19, 22–24]. Microscopically, UESL consists of medium to large sized spindle, oval, or stellate shaped pleomorphic cells that may be arranged either compactly or loosely in abundant myxoid matrix or fibrous stroma. Multinucleated giant cells, bizarre cells, and atypical mitosis are often seen. Trapped hepatocytes and bile duct cells can be observed at peripheral area of the tumor. Variable sized eosinophilic globules can be seen

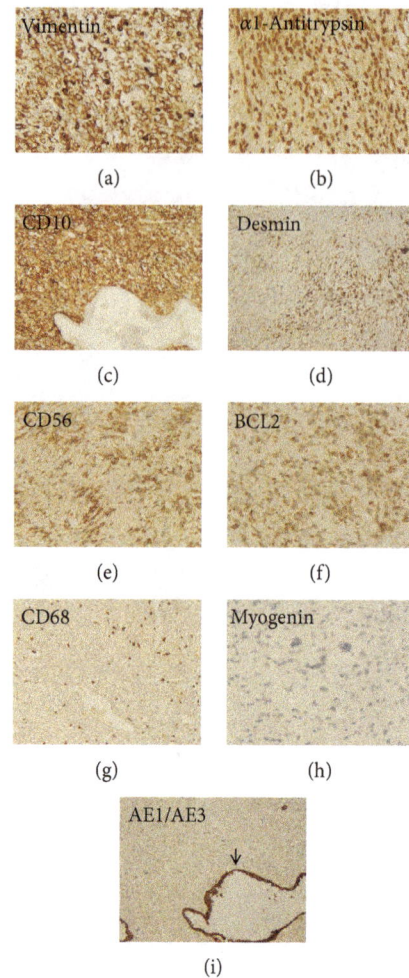

(a)   (b)

(c)   (d)

(e)   (f)

(g)   (h)

(i)

FIGURE 5: Immunohistochemical staining of the pulmonary metastatic lesion showed strong and diffuse positivity for vimentin, α1-antitrypsin, and CD10 (a–c), patchy positivity for desmin, CD56, and BCL2 (d–f), rare staining for CD68 (g), and negative for myogenin and AE1/AE3 (h and i). The entrapped bronchiolar epithelium was highlighted by AE1/AE3 (i) (arrow) (immunoperoxidase; original magnification: (c, d, g, and i) ×100; (a, b, e, f, and h) ×200).

in the tumor cell cytoplasm and extracellular matrix [19, 22–26]. These hyaline globules are diastase-resistant and periodic acid-Schiff- (PAS-) positive and correspond with the prominent electron-dense complexes under an electron microscope [22]. The histopathologic characteristics of UESL in our case are similar to those described in the previous reports. Also in the literature, focal osteoid picture was reported in one adult case [26]. Extramedullary hematopoiesis has been noted in some of the cases [2, 27].

Immunohistochemically, the staining pattern of UESL is variable and nonspecific. The divergent staining or combined expression of fat, muscle, histiocytic, and epithelial markers suggests the origin of primitive mesenchymal stem cell, which may display partial differentiation. Usually, multiple immunostains are performed to help with the diagnosis as they also facilitate the exclusion of other tumors in the differential diagnosis, which includes poorly differentiated or sarcomatoid hepatocellular carcinoma, embryonal rhabdomyosarcoma, and other sarcomas. Tumor cells of UESL are consistently positive for vimentin and α1-antitrypsin. There is variable staining for desmin, smooth-muscle actin, CD68, CD56, BCL2, and CD10. No immunoreactivity has been described for HepPar-1, myogenin, CD34, CD117, S-100, Alk-1, or AFP [22–25]. Glypican 3 (GPC3) and paranuclear dot-like staining for cytokeratin has been reported [14, 27]. The immunohistochemical profiles in our case are consistent with a diagnosis of UESL.

In the past, prognosis of UESL had been poor; initial reports described mortality within 12 months of diagnosis, and the long-term disease-free survival rate was less than 37% [2, 5]. Poor prognosis of UESL is associated with local recurrence, tumor rupture, and its metastasis to other parts of the body. Since the widespread use of multimodal therapy, including primary resection, neoadjuvant or adjuvant chemotherapy, and radiation, the long-term survival rate of UESL patients has improved significantly and is currently reported to be >70% [4, 6, 7]. Currently, complete resection of hepatic tumor, combined with adjuvant chemotherapy, appears to be the mainstay of treatment. The chemotherapy regimens reported in the literature are varied as no standard regimens designed specifically for UESL. In addition, liver transplantation has been reported to improve survival for refractory, unresectable, or recurrent tumors [4, 6, 7].

Pulmonary metastases are a common manifestation of sarcoma. The pulmonary arteries are the most common route for metastases. Tumors most likely to metastasize to the lungs include those with a rich vascular supply draining directly into the systemic venous system. Metastases of UESL have been reported to occur in 5–13% of children [8, 9], and metastatic sites such as the lung, adrenal gland, peritoneum, and pleura have been reported [4, 10, 11, 28]. The tumor cells might spread hematogenously, via lymphatics or by direct extension. Tumor may also show direct involvement of the heart, with inferior vena cava tumor extension to the right atria [27]. The cases of metastatic UESL that reported in the literature are mostly present at the time of primary diagnosis. Plant et al. reported one patient with UESL recurred 2 years from diagnosis with bilateral paraspinal masses [28]. Our case reported an interval of 4 years between primary tumor treatment and development of lung metastasis. The mechanism of lung metastases occurring years after curative resection remains to be elucidated.

The optimal treatment of patients with metastases remains controversial. Some cases have shown that surgical resection combined with chemotherapy appears to be the most beneficial treatment strategy [8]. Xie et al. reported a case of UESL with lung metastasis in which they have achieved a good result using immunotherapy [10]. However, only rare cases of metastatic UESL have been reported in the literature, and knowledge of the metastatic lesions and its optimal treatment is tempered by the few cases available and large amounts of missing data.

4. Conclusions

Although current aggressive multimodal therapy is associated with favorable outcomes in children with UESL,

intensive surveillance and follow-up for early detection of metastases is crucial to increase the chances of long-term survival. The patient reported herein developed a lung metastasis four years after hepatectomy and adjuvant chemotherapy. This case is presented with emphasis on clinicopathological and immunohistochemical findings of the primary UESL and lung metastases with the aim of collecting more data and expanding our understanding of this rare malignancy. Pulmonary metastasectomy for the isolated lung metastases of UESL with adjuvant chemotherapy may provide a reasonable long period of survival.

References

[1] N. Howlader, A. B. Mariotto, S. Woloshin, and L. M. Schwartz, "Providing clinicians and patients with actual prognosis: cancer in the context of competing causes of death," *Journal of the National Cancer Institute. Monographs*, vol. 2014, no. 49, pp. 255–264, 2014.

[2] J. T. Stocker and K. G. Ishak, "Undifferentiated (embryonal) sarcoma of the liver. Report of 31 cases," *Cancer*, vol. 42, no. 1, pp. 336–348, 1978.

[3] Z. G. Wei, L. F. Tang, Z. M. Chen, H. F. Tang, and M. J. Li, "Childhood undifferentiated embryonal liver sarcoma: clinical features and immunohistochemistry analysis," *Journal of Pediatric Surgery*, vol. 43, no. 10, pp. 1912–1919, 2008.

[4] Y. Shi, Y. Rojas, W. Zhang et al., "Characteristics and outcomes in children with undifferentiated embryonal sarcoma of the liver: a report from the National Cancer Database," *Pediatric Blood & Cancer*, vol. 64, no. 4, article e26272, 2017.

[5] E. E. Lack, B. L. Schloo, N. Azumi, W. D. Travis, H. E. Grier, and H. P. W. Kozakewich, "Undifferentiated (embryonal) sarcoma of the liver. Clinical and pathologic study of 16 cases with emphasis on immunohistochemical features," *The American Journal of Surgical Pathology*, vol. 15, no. 1, pp. 1–16, 1991.

[6] P. Techavichit, P. M. Masand, R. W. Himes et al., "Undifferentiated embryonal sarcoma of the liver (UESL): a single-center experience and review of the literature," *Journal of Pediatric Hematology/Oncology*, vol. 38, no. 4, pp. 261–268, 2016.

[7] H. Ismail, B. Dembowska-Bagińska, D. Broniszczak et al., "Treatment of undifferentiated embryonal sarcoma of the liver in children—single center experience," *Journal of Pediatric Surgery*, vol. 48, no. 11, pp. 2202–2206, 2013.

[8] M. E. Horowitz, E. Etcubanas, B. L. Webber et al., "Hepatic undifferentiated (embryonal) sarcoma and rhabdomyosarcoma in children. Results of therapy," *Cancer*, vol. 59, no. 3, pp. 396–402, 1987.

[9] G. Bisogno, T. Pilz, G. Perilongo et al., "Undifferentiated sarcoma of the liver in childhood: a curable disease," *Cancer*, vol. 94, no. 1, pp. 252–257, 2002.

[10] S. Xie, X. Wu, G. Zhang et al., "Remarkable regression of a lung recurrence from an undifferentiated embryonal sarcoma of the liver treated with a DC vaccine combined with immune cells: a case report," *Cellular Immunology*, vol. 290, no. 2, pp. 185–189, 2014.

[11] M. K. Lee, C. G. Kwon, K. H. Hwang et al., "F-18 FDG PET/CT findings in a case of undifferentiated embryonal sarcoma of the liver with lung and adrenal gland metastasis in a child," *Clinical Nuclear Medicine*, vol. 34, no. 2, pp. 107–108, 2009.

[12] F. Lenze, T. Birkfellner, P. Lenz et al., "Undifferentiated embryonal sarcoma of the liver in adults," *Cancer*, vol. 112, no. 10, pp. 2274–2282, 2008.

[13] K. Noghuchi, H. Yokoo, K. Nakanishi et al., "A long-term survival case of adult undifferentiated embryonal sarcoma of liver," *World Journal of Surgical Oncology*, vol. 10, no. 1, p. 65, 2012.

[14] X. W. Li, S. J. Gong, W. H. Song et al., "Undifferentiated liver embryonal sarcoma in adults: a report of four cases and literature review," *World Journal of Gastroenterology*, vol. 16, no. 37, pp. 4725–4732, 2010.

[15] T. Y. Hung, D. Lu, and M. C. Liu, "Undifferentiated (embryonal) sarcoma of the liver complicated with rupture in a child," *Journal of Pediatric Hematology/Oncology*, vol. 29, no. 1, pp. 63–65, 2007.

[16] T. Sakellaridis, I. Panagiotou, T. Georgantas, G. Micros, D. Rontogianni, and C. Antiochos, "Undifferentiated embryonal sarcoma of the liver mimicking acute appendicitis. Case report and review of the literature," *World Journal of Surgical Oncology*, vol. 4, no. 1, p. 9, 2006.

[17] J. M. Lin, J. E. Heath, W. S. Twaddell, and R. J. Castellani, "Undifferentiated sarcoma of the liver: a case study of an erythropoietin-secreting tumor," *International Journal of Surgical Pathology*, vol. 22, no. 6, pp. 555–558, 2014.

[18] A. M. Halefoglu and A. Oz, "Primary undifferentiated embryonal sarcoma of the liver misdiagnosed as hydatid cyst in a child: a case report and review of the literature," *Journal of the Belgian Society of Radiology*, vol. 97, no. 4, pp. 248–250, 2014.

[19] H. Zhang, L. Lei, C. W. Zuppan, and A. S. Raza, "Undifferentiated embryonal sarcoma of the liver with an unusual presentation: case report and review of the literature," *Journal of Gastrointestinal Oncology*, vol. 7, Supplement 1, pp. S100–S106, 2016.

[20] W. K. Moon, W. S. Kim, I. O. Kim et al., "Undifferentiated embryonal sarcoma of the liver: US and CT findings," *Pediatric Radiology*, vol. 24, no. 7, pp. 500–503, 1994.

[21] K. S. Sodhi, E. Bekhitt, and C. Rickert, "Paradoxical hepatic tumor: undifferentiated embryonal sarcoma of the liver," *Indian Journal of Radiology and Imaging*, vol. 20, no. 1, pp. 69–71, 2010.

[22] J. Putra and K. Ornvold, "Undifferentiated embryonal sarcoma of the liver: a concise review," *Archives of Pathology & Laboratory Medicine*, vol. 139, no. 2, pp. 269–273, 2015.

[23] Q. Cao, Z. Ye, S. Chen, N. Liu, S. Li, and F. Liu, "Undifferentiated embryonal sarcoma of liver: a multi-institutional experience with 9 cases," *International Journal of Clinical and Experimental Pathology*, vol. 7, no. 12, pp. 8647–8656, 2014.

[24] A. Mori, K. Fukase, K. Masuda et al., "A case of adult undifferentiated embryonal sarcoma of the liver successfully treated with right trisectionectomy: a case report," *Surgical Case Reports*, vol. 3, no. 1, p. 19, 2017.

[25] D. Treitl, A. Roudenko, S. El Hussein, M. Rizer, and P. Bao, "Adult embryonal sarcoma of the liver: management of a massive liver tumor," *Case Reports in Surgery*, vol. 2016, Article ID 5625762, 6 pages, 2016.

[26] J. H. Chen, C. H. Lee, C. K. Wei, S. M. Chang, and W. Y. Yin, "Undifferentiated embryonal sarcoma of the liver with focal osteoid picture-a case report," *Asian Journal of Surgery*, vol. 36, no. 4, pp. 174–178, 2013.

[27] N. Lightfoot and M. Nikfarjam, "Embryonal sarcoma of the liver in an adult patient," *Case Reports in Surgery*, vol. 2012, Article ID 382723, 4 pages, 2012.

[28] A. S. Plant, R. W. Busuttil, A. Rana, S. D. Nelson, M. Auerbach, and N. C. Federman, "A single-institution retrospective cases series of childhood undifferentiated embryonal liver sarcoma (UELS): success of combined therapy and the use of orthotopic liver transplant," *Journal of Pediatric Hematology/Oncology*, vol. 35, no. 6, pp. 451–455, 2013.

45

Combination of Superselective Arterial Embolization and Radiofrequency Ablation for the Treatment of a Giant Renal Angiomyolipoma Complicated with Caval Thrombus

Konstantinos N. Stamatiou,[1] Hippocrates Moschouris,[2] Kiriaki Marmaridou,[2] Michail Kiltenis,[2] Konstantinos Kladis-Kalentzis,[2] and Katerina Malagari[3]

[1]Department of Urology, Tzaneio General Hospital, 18536 Piraeus, Greece
[2]Department of Diagnostic and Interventional Radiology, Tzaneio General Hospital, 18536 Piraeus, Greece
[3]2nd Department of Radiology, University of Athens, Attikon Hospital, Chaidari, 12462 Athens, Greece

Correspondence should be addressed to Kiriaki Marmaridou; kiriaki.marmaridou@gmail.com

Academic Editor: Cesar V. Reyes

This is a case of a 78-year-old male patient with multiple angiomyolipomas of a solitary right kidney. The largest of these tumors (maximum diameter: 13.4 cm) caused significant extrinsic compression of the inferior vena cava complicated by thrombosis of this vessel. Treatment of thrombosis with anticoagulants had been ineffective and the patient had experienced a bleeding episode from the largest right renal angiomyolipoma, which had been treated by transarterial embolization in another institution, 4 months prior to our intervention. Our approach included superselective transarterial embolization of the dominant, right kidney angiomyolipoma with hydrogel microspheres, which was combined, 20 days later, with ultrasonographically guided radiofrequency ablation. Both interventions were uneventful. Computed tomography 2 months after ablation showed a 53% reduction in tumor volume, reduced space-occupying effect on inferior vena cava, and resolution of caval thrombus. Nine months after intervention the patient has had no recurrence of thrombosis or hemorrhage and no tumor regrowth has been observed. The combination of superselective transarterial embolization and radiofrequency ablation seems to be a feasible, safe, and efficient treatment of large renal angiomyolipomas.

1. Introduction

Angiomyolipomas (AMLs) have been classified among the perivascular epithelioid cells tumor group (PEComas). They are composed of variable amounts of three components: blood vessels (angioid), smooth muscle (myoid), and mature fat (lipoid) components. AMLs represent the most common benign, noncystic renal lesion [1]. Two types have been described: sporadic and multiple. The first occurs as a single tumor in one kidney. It accounts for 80% of renal AMLs and it is typically identified in adults, with a strong female predilection. The second occurs as larger tumor and/or multiple tumors in both kidneys and accounts for 20% of renal AMLs. It affects both sexes at a younger age than sporadic AML. It is seen in association with tuberous sclerosis

and lymphangioleiomyomatosis. AMLs are benign and usually asymptomatic. Although most AMLs are incidentally diagnosed on cross-sectional imaging, they do have the risk of rupture with bleeding or secondary damage of surrounding structures, as they grow. The risk of bleeding and surrounding tissue damage is proportional to the size of the lesion (diameter > 4 centimeters). AMLs may also be associated with palpable mass, flank pain, urinary tract infections, haematuria, renal failure, hypertension, and, rarely, renal vein and/or inferior vena cava thrombosis. AMLs found incidentally are usually small and so require no therapy. Lesions that present with retroperitoneal hemorrhage often require emergency transarterial embolization as a life-saving measure [2]. Although embolization is effective for this purpose, some authors report a significant percentage of

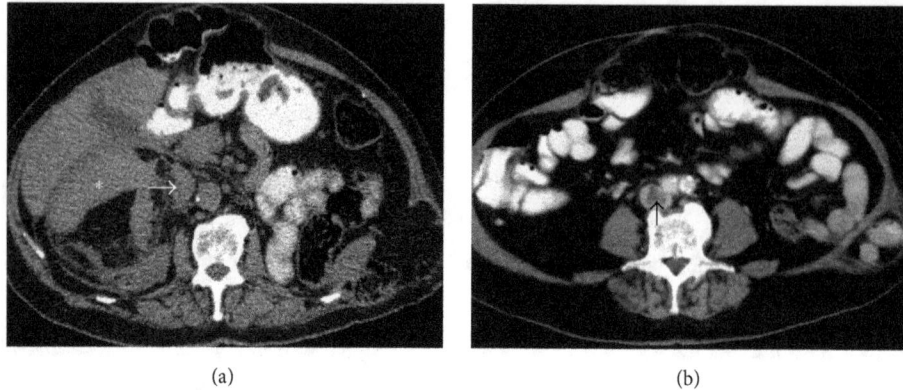

(a)   (b)

FIGURE 1: Axial CT images prior to intervention. (a) Unenhanced image shows the typical appearance of a large angiomyolipoma with fat and soft-tissue (∗) densities. The mass compresses the inferior vena cava (arrow). (b) Contrast-enhanced image (venous phase) shows a thrombus causing an enhancement defect (arrow) at the lowest part of the inferior vena cava.

recurrent hemorrhage, recurrent symptoms, or inadequate tumor shrinkage after embolization [3].

We herein describe a complicated case of a giant renal AML, which was successfully managed by a combined interventional radiologic approach.

2. Case Presentation

A 78-year-old male patient presented to our institution with a history of complicated renal AMLs. One year earlier, the patient had undergone a left nephrectomy for the management of massive spontaneous hemorrhage from a giant AML of the ipsilateral kidney. The right kidney was affected by several small (<2 cm) AMLs and by a dominant tumor measuring 13.4 × 10.5 × 7.5 cm. The composition of this tumor was primarily fat, with a soft-tissue component at the upper pole of the tumor. This component caused significant extrinsic compression of the inferior vena cava, and a thrombus was observed at the lower part of this vein (Figure 1). Treatment of the caval thrombus with anticoagulants (acenocoumarol per os, with target International Normalized Ratio of 2.5) for 5 months had proven ineffective. During that period, the patient had experienced an episode of severe hemorrhage from the dominant tumor of the right kidney, which was managed with transarterial embolization in another institution. The patient also complained of moderate right flank pain. The rest of his medical history was unremarkable and there were no clinical or imaging findings indicative of a congenital disorder.

The patient was evaluated by a multidisciplinary team consisting of urologist, interventional radiologist, nephrologist, vascular surgeon, and pathologist. It was decided to utilize a combined interventional treatment, in order to reduce the risk of future hemorrhage, achieve a degree of tumor shrinkage, and minimize the adverse effects on the integrity and function of the solitary right kidney. Superselective arterial embolization (SAE) was performed first. Vascular access was gained via the right common femoral artery, with Seldinger technique, and, after a flush aortogram, the right renal artery was selectively catheterized with a 5-French, Cobra-1 angiographic catheter. The

large upper pole AML was fed by a few, relatively thin arteries arising from the right renal capsular artery. No aneurysms or arteriovenous shunts were observed. Superselective approach was achieved by means of 2.2-French Microcatheter (Stridesmooth, Asahi Intecc Co. Ltd., Aichi, Japan) and embolization was performed with tightly calibrated, hydrogel microspheres (Embozene, Celonova Bio-Sciences, San Antonio, Texas, USA) with diameters of 250 and 400 micrometers (μm). Postembolization angiogram showed devascularization of the AML and no signs of renal infarction. With the exception of right flank pain, the procedure was well tolerated and the patient was discharged the following day. A radiofrequency ablation (RFA) of the dominant angiomyolipoma of the left kidney was performed 20 days later (Figure 2). With the patient in left lateral decubitus position, an oblique coronal sonogram of the tumor was acquired and the upper portion of the tumor (which compressed the IVC) was targeted. A 17-gauge, water cooled, radiofrequency electrode with a 3 cm active tip was utilized (Jet-Tip, RF Medical Co., Seoul, Korea). The electrode was successively inserted at two sites at the upper portion of the tumor and a 12-minute ablation cycle was applied to each site. The RF power output was automatically adjusted by the generator and ranged from 60 to 140 Watts. During ablation, a slow infusion of 20 mL of normal saline was performed by means of a dedicated pump, through the electrode into the tumoral tissue, to improve coagulation and to prevent carbonization. Medication for pain control included ropivacaine hydrochloride (15 mL of Naropeine 0.2%, as local injection) and pethidine (100 mg/2 mL, as slow intravenous infusion). The ablation was monitored ultrasonographically. At the end of the procedure, scanning at multiple planes showed that the largest part of the upper pole of the tumor had been covered by high-level echoes (ablation-related gas formation). Finally, the electrode tract was ablated to decrease the risk of bleeding. The patient received intravenous hydration and antibiotics and was discharged the following day.

A computed tomography (CT) scan performed 8 weeks after RFA revealed shrinkage of the dominant AML of the right kidney, with 17% reduction in maximum tumor diameter and 53% reduction in tumor volume. There was a

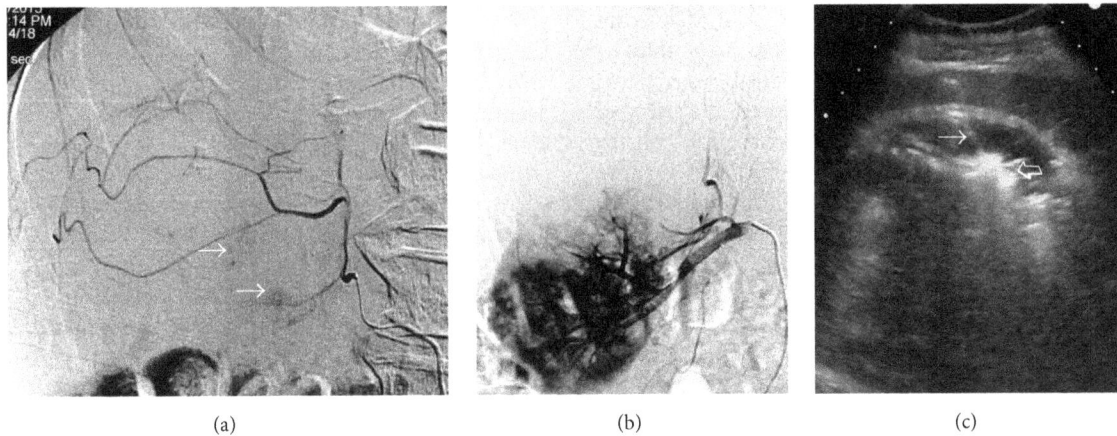

FIGURE 2: Representative images from the interventions. (a) Digital subtraction angiography (DSA) image after superselective catheterization of the tumor feeders shows relatively few and thin tumoral arteries and a limited tumor blush (arrows). (b) DSA image after embolization shows devascularization of the tumor with preservation of the renal enhancement. (c) Coronal oblique sonographic image during ablation shows the electrode (arrow), which has been advanced into the soft-tissue part of the tumor. Strong echoes (open arrow) caused by tissue vaporization are noted around the electrode tip.

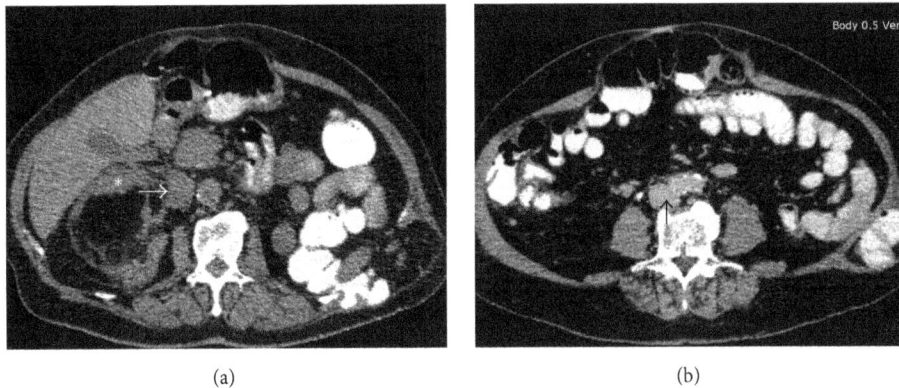

FIGURE 3: Axial CT images after embolization and ablation. (a) Unenhanced image shows that the angiomyolipoma is smaller, with relative shrinkage of the soft-tissue component (∗) in favor of the fat. The compression of the IVC (arrow) is now less striking. (b) Contrast-enhanced image (venous phase) shows disappearance of the caval thrombus (arrow).

significant (75%) reduction in the volume of the soft-tissue component. The extrinsic compression of the IVC was also relieved and complete resolution of the caval thrombus was noted (Figure 3). Three months after intervention, acenocoumarol treatment was terminated. Nine months posttreatment the patient reported partial resolution of the right flank pain and sonography showed a minimal further decrease in maximum tumor diameter and no evidence of IVC thrombus. Serum creatinine values were near the upper normal limits prior to treatment and throughout the follow-up period.

3. Discussion

To manage both the hemorrhagic potential and the space-occupying effect of the large AML of our case, we adopted a combined interventional radiologic approach.

SAE was performed first, in order to devascularize the tumor and to reduce the risk of hemorrhage (either spontaneous or iatrogenic). SAE is a widely accepted intervention for the treatment of symptomatic AMLs and for prophylactic treatment of asymptomatic AMLs larger than 4 cm [2]. A variety of embolic agents have been used for SAE of AML and no widely accepted guidelines exist. In our institution we treat non-aneurysm bearing AMLs exclusively with the aforementioned type of microspheres. The properties of these microspheres (spherical shape, smooth surface, tight diameter calibration, and insignificant inflammatory reaction of surrounding tissues) allow for predictable, complete, and well tolerated vessel occlusion. Regarding the selected size of the microspheres, we, like others [2], have concerns about the safety of SAE with smaller microspheres (<150–200 μm). On the other hand, taking into account the size of the tumor feeders of our case, we thought that microspheres of larger diameters ($\geq$500 μm) would probably cause a very early and very proximal occlusion, with inadequate filling of the tumor's vascular bead and with increased risk of backflow.

We decided to combine our endovascular treatment with RFA, because our experience, as well as published data [3, 4], suggests that SAE alone may not always cause significant tumor shrinkage. This is particularly true for larger and fat-rich (at least 50% fat content) AMLs [4]. We also speculated that the ischemic effect of SAE might increase the safety of the subsequent ablative procedure, by limiting the risk for iatrogenic hemorrhage. It is also known that RFA is more effective when applied on devascularized tissue; otherwise, tissue cooling (caused by circulating blood) limits the heating effect of the ablation. Moreover, with RFA, we were able to target the upper and medial part of the tumor, which primarily caused compression of the IVC. The result of our combined treatment was a small reduction in the maximum tumor diameter, but a significant reduction in tumor volume and in the volume of the soft-tissue component. There was also a clinical benefit, since the patient symptoms improved and the reduction of tumor bulk was followed by resolution of the IVC thrombus. We acknowledge that our hypothesis regarding the relationship between the IVC thrombus and the mass effect of the AML is based only on imaging, and not on histopathology. Nevertheless, there was no other underlying cause of IVC thrombosis, and its resolution occurred only after tumor debulking. Contrary to our experience, almost all of the published cases of AML-related thrombus are caused by direct extension of aggressive AMLs (of epithelioid histology) into the renal vein and/or IVC [5]. Effective treatment of such cases is based on surgical (nephron-sparing surgery or nephrectomy plus thrombectomy) and not on interventional radiologic procedures.

RFA has emerged as a valuable treatment option of renal AML. RFA can be considered a nephron-sparing technique, since it can target the solid and vascular elements of the tumor, without damaging any normal renal tissue. The efficacy of RFA against AML has been assessed in relatively small series and mainly for small AMLs [6–8]: Castle et al. treated successfully 15 small renal AMLs with a low complication rate (13.3%) and complete disappearance of tumoral enhancement on CT, at a mean follow-up of 21 months [6]. However, changes in tumor size were not reported. Prevoo et al. reported a decrease in tumor size from 4.5 cm to 2.9 cm at 12 months after RFA of a sporadic AML in a patient with a solitary kidney. No complications occurred and no AML recurrence was observed during the 12-month follow-up [7]. Gregory et al. treated four large AMLs (maximal axis 6.1–32.4 cm). They reported no complications, no hemorrhagic events, and significant decrease in mean soft-tissue-to-total tumor ratio during a follow-up of 48 months. Nevertheless, the total tumor volume did not change significantly [8]. The same authors experienced problems of impedance when applying RF energy to the lipomatous parts of tumors and attributed the high impedance to the natural insulating properties of fat. We did not encounter similar problems, perhaps because we utilized different equipment and different ablation protocol and we primarily targeted the nonlipomatous parts of the tumor. Contrary to other authors, we used ultrasound instead of CT for guidance and monitoring of RFA. Since the CT-scanner in our institution is busy with diagnostic imaging, we usually reserve CT for tumors which cannot be safely and easily targeted by ultrasound. Moreover, insertion and manipulation of RF probes are often troublesome when the patient is in the CT-gantry. We recognize that sonographic monitoring of ablation is impaired by the echogenic "cloud" that appears around the RF electrode. Accurate depiction of untreated areas during ablation is crucial in the case of renal carcinoma (which should be, ideally, completely ablated); however the clinical context of our case was different and a detailed delineation of residual tumor was unnecessary. We believe that careful planning of the electrode trajectory, successful initial targeting of the lesion, and correct interpretation of intraprocedural sonographic findings can reduce the impact of the limitations of sonography.

Although experience regarding the combination of SAE and RFA is limited to a few cases, it appears that this combination is safe, feasible, and efficient. RFA may be applied after clinical failure of SAE, which may manifest as inadequate tumor shrinkage, tumor regrowth, or persistence of symptoms after SAE. Sooriakumaran et al. ablated 3 large sporadic AMLs (9–19 cm) previously treated with SAE and found a reduction in tumor mass of 20% and significantly reduced enhancement of the treated areas on CT or MRI after a median follow-up of 7.5 months [9]. Two of the patients of the aforementioned study of Gregory et al. also had a history of unsuccessful SAE [8].

Another remarkable feature of the presented case is that the multiple (and initially bilateral) AMLs of our patient were not associated with a congenital disorder, as shown by the clinical and imaging evaluation. No genetic testing was available. Multiple and bilateral AMLs may also be encountered (albeit rarely) on a sporadic basis [10].

We conclude that the combination of SAE and RFA may be a safe and effective option for the treatment of challenging cases of renal AMLs. This combination is worth being assessed in the context of a large study with adequate follow-up.

References

[1] M. Jinzaki, S. G. Silverman, H. Akita, Y. Nagashima, S. Mikami, and M. Oya, "Renal angiomyolipoma: a radiological classification and update on recent developments in diagnosis and management," *Abdominal Imaging*, vol. 39, no. 3, pp. 588–604, 2014.

[2] D. Li, B. B. Pua, and D. C. Madoff, "Role of embolization in the treatment of renal masses," *Seminars in Interventional Radiology*, vol. 31, no. 1, pp. 70–81, 2014.

[3] T. E. Murray, F. Doyle, and M. Lee, "Transarterial embolization of angiomyolipoma: a systematic review," *Journal of Urology*, vol. 194, no. 3, pp. 635–639, 2015.

[4] A. Hocquelet, F. Cornelis, Y. Le Bras et al., "Long-term results of preventive embolization of renal angiomyolipomas: evaluation of predictive factors of volume decrease," *European Radiology*, vol. 24, no. 8, pp. 1785–1793, 2014.

[5] G. Shen, Q. Mao, H. Yang, and C. Wang, "Aggressive renal angiomyolipoma with vena cava extension: a case report and

literature review," *Oncology Letters*, vol. 8, no. 5, pp. 1980–1982, 2014.

[6] S. M. Castle, V. Gorbatiy, O. Ekwenna, E. Young, and R. J. Leveillee, "Radiofrequency ablation (RFA) therapy for renal angiomyolipoma (AML): an alternative to angio-embolization and nephron-sparing surgery," *BJU International*, vol. 109, no. 3, pp. 384–387, 2012.

[7] W. Prevoo, M. A. A. J. van den Bosch, and S. Horenblas, "Radiofrequency ablation for treatment of sporadic angiomyolipoma," *Urology*, vol. 72, no. 1, pp. 188–191, 2008.

[8] S. M. Gregory, C. J. Anderson, and U. Patel, "Radiofrequency ablation of large renal angiomyolipoma: median-term follow-up," *CardioVascular and Interventional Radiology*, vol. 36, no. 3, pp. 682–689, 2013.

[9] P. Sooriakumaran, P. Gibbs, G. Coughlin et al., "Angiomyolipomata: challenges, solutions, and future prospects based on over 100 cases treated," *BJU International*, vol. 105, no. 1, pp. 101–106, 2010.

[10] A. Fittschen, I. Wendlik, S. Oeztuerk et al., "Prevalence of sporadic renal angiomyolipoma: a retrospective analysis of 61,389 in- and out-patients," *Abdominal imaging*, vol. 39, no. 5, pp. 1009–1013, 2014.

46

Uncommon BRAF Mutations Associated with Durable Response to Immunotherapy in Patients with Metastatic Melanoma

Brenen P. Swofford[1] and Jade Homsi[2]

[1]*University of Arizona College of Medicine-Phoenix, Phoenix, AZ, USA*
[2]*University of Texas Southwestern, Dallas, TX, USA*

Correspondence should be addressed to Brenen P. Swofford; brenen.swofford@bannerhealth.com and
Jade Homsi; jade.homsi@utsouthwestern.edu

Academic Editor: Kaiser Jamil

Melanoma is a disease process which has been increasing in incidence over the past three decades and metastatic melanoma carries a poor prognosis. Through genetic studies of this disease, it has been determined that the BRAF V600 mutation plays a major role in the pathophysiology of the disease and this has led to the utilization of targeted therapy (BRAF and MEK inhibitors) in its treatment. Other BRAF mutations (non-V600 mutations) are rare in melanoma and targeted therapy is not indicated for patients with these mutations due to reduced response rates. An emerging option for metastatic melanoma with uncommon BRAF mutations is immunotherapy using checkpoint inhibitors such as PD-1 inhibitors or CTLA-4 inhibitors. Currently, it is unknown how patients with BRAF non-V600 mutations respond to immunotherapy. This report will examine the effect of immunotherapy on two distinct metastatic melanoma patients, each with uncommon BRAF mutations, occurring outside the V600 locus (E586K and G469E). These patients were noted to have a durable, complete response when treated with immunotherapy and continue to exhibit a response 9 and 15 months after discontinuing therapy. Further research and clinical trials are needed to study patients with uncommon BRAF mutations and the potential therapeutic benefit of immunotherapy.

1. Introduction

Melanoma is currently the fifth most common cancer in American men and seventh most common in American women [1]. Additionally, the incidence of this disease process is increasing dramatically [1, 2]. Patients with localized disease often only require surgical resection [2]. For those who have metastatic melanoma, it was originally a diagnosis with a poor prognosis (roughly 10% 5-year survival rate) and very limited, effective treatment options; however, with the utilization of targeted and immune therapies, the median survival time is now approaching 2-3 years [2, 3].

An expanded evaluation of molecular biology and pathogenesis of melanoma cells has led to the discovery of a new category of therapy often called targeted therapy. Available targeted therapies are directed at the mitogen-activated protein kinase (MAPK) pathway, a key signaling pathway that is activated in melanomas [4]. The serine/threonine kinases BRAF and CRAF are perhaps the most important downstream mediators of this pathway and mutations lead to clonal expansion and tumor progression [5, 6]. When activated, these kinases interact with the extracellular sign-regulated kinase (ERK), which initiates MEK phosphorylation, leading to phosphorylation of ERK and subsequent promotion of cellular growth of the tumor cells [5, 6]. BRAF mutations commonly affect exons 11 and 15 [7]. Currently, ~100 mutations of the BRAF gene have been determined to be associated with cancers, with the majority occurring at the glycine P loop (involved in stabilizing the phosphate groups of ATP during enzyme binding) and the activation segment (stabilizing the inactive form of the kinase) [8].

In patients with BRAF mutations, 80–90% contain an activating mutation occurring at the V600 locus (with the most common mutations being V600E and V600K) [3]. Vemurafenib and Dabrafenib are two targeted BRAF inhibitors that have demonstrated the ability to induce tumor regression and prolong overall survival in patients with metastatic melanoma possessing the V600 mutation [3, 6, 9]. In the BRIM-3 trial, patients with the V600 mutation experienced a significantly longer median overall survival when treated with Vemurafenib [9]. However, one associated negative finding from targeted therapies is the development of resistance to treatment by the tumor cells [9]. There are multiple factors that may be involved in the development of resistance by these tumor cells. One factor being studied is the association between resistant melanoma tumor cells and the CRAF protein [10].

Immunotherapy attempts to stimulate the immune system to destroy cells by inducing, enhancing, or suppressing the immune response to the cancer cells. In regard to melanoma, current immunotherapy options include checkpoint inhibitors (Ipilimumab, Pembrolizumab, and Nivolumab) [11]. Ipilimumab is a monoclonal antibody to CTLA-4 which augments cellular proliferation by binding to the cytotoxic T-lymphocyte associated antigen 4 (CTLA-4) [12, 13]. CTLA-4, in melanoma, is bound by tumor antigen leading to down-regulation of T-cell activation pathways [12, 13]. Ipilimumab blocks the CTLA-4 receptor allowing for enhanced T-cell activation/proliferation [12, 13]. Pembrolizumab and Nivolumab are monoclonal antibodies which inhibit programmed cell death by binding to the PD-1 receptor on T-cells [11, 14]. This binding inhibits the negative immune regulation caused by the tumor and antigen presenting cells [11, 14]. Anti-PD-1 antibodies reverse the T-cell suppression allowing an antitumor response [11, 14]. Clinical trials of immunotherapy in melanoma are still relatively new and the outcome with immunotherapy in patients with uncommon BRAF mutations is unknown. This report will examine the effect of immunotherapy on two distinct metastatic melanoma patients, each with uncommon BRAF mutations, occurring outside the V600 locus (E586K and G469E).

2. Cases

The first patient is a 55-year-old male with metastatic melanoma of unknown primary source diagnosed in March of 2015 after presenting with right hip pain of several weeks duration. The radiographs of the right hip revealed a 5.5 cm lytic lesion of the proximal femoral shaft and MRI further characterized the lesion as having aggressive features. Bone biopsy and pathologic evaluation demonstrated metastatic melanoma. Molecular testing revealed a BRAF E586K mutation; NRAS and C-Kit mutations were not detected. The patient underwent palliative surgery for tumor burden removal with negative margins and was started on Ipilimumab 3 mg/kg ×4 doses and palliative radiation to the affected area. The patient tolerated therapy and completed it in July 2015. He was asymptomatic and repeat imaging indicated no evidence of disease. In June of 2016 the patient presented with a left cervical mass and cervical lymphadenopathy; recurrent metastatic melanoma was confirmed by biopsy (Figure 1(a)). Given the previous response to Ipilimumab, the patient was reinitiated on this therapy ×4 cycles using the same dosage. The patient tolerated the treatment and imaging post treatment has indicated complete response to therapy (Figure 1(a)). The patient continues to demonstrate a complete response more than 9 months later.

The second patient is a 79-year-old male who was initially diagnosed with melanoma after a biopsy of the left nasal ala in April of 2014. A CT of the neck was concerning for necrotic lymph nodes on the left. Wide, local excision of the primary melanoma and left cervical lymph node dissection demonstrated a 9 mm nonulcerated melanoma and 4/25 positive lymph nodes for metastatic melanoma. He underwent adjuvant radiation therapy to the neck. Nine months later, he had a biopsy proven recurrent disease in the left and right cervical lymph nodes (Figure 1(b)). BRAF mutation testing indicated a G469E mutation and NRAS mutation was not detected. CT scans also demonstrated multiple bilateral lung nodules. The patient was initiated on Pembrolizumab 2 mg/kg every three weeks intravenously in May 2015 and staging scans in September 2015 (after 4 doses) revealed complete response to therapy in the lymph nodes and lungs (Figure 1(b)). He was continued on Pembrolizumab with the last dose occurring in May of 2016 and is being followed with close observation. The patient tolerated the treatment well and scans continue to show complete response lasting more than 15 months.

3. Discussion

Metastatic melanoma is a disease of increasing incidence and one of poor prognosis [2]. The BRAF V600 mutation is an important factor to direct proper treatment through targeted therapy [6]. However, for those patients with uncommon BRAF mutations (non-V600), as exhibited by the two patients presented in this case report, immunotherapy may offer a potential treatment option. Studies indicate that Ipilimumab can induce long-lasting disease control, that is not influenced by BRAF status [12, 13]. Additionally, anti-PD-1 agents such as Pembrolizumab have shown higher response rates, with most response rates lasting greater than 12 months [11, 14]. The first patient possessed a BRAF E586K mutation and was treated with Ipilimumab twice with significant disease regression and complete response radiographically noted now for 9 months. The second patient possessed a BRAF G469E mutation and was started on Pembrolizumab, with a complete response for more than 15 months, and remains off therapy. The durable response rates noted with these patients, combined with the benefits in tolerance, may represent the future of metastatic melanoma with uncommon BRAF mutation therapy.

While V600 is the most common mutation detected in patients with melanoma, more than 100 mutations on exons 11 and 15 have been reported by the Catalog of Somatic Mutations in Cancer database [7]. In regard to melanoma, data is limited but it is estimated that ~10% to as high as 30% of patients with melanoma have a non-V600 mutation [10, 15]. Current research regarding patients with non-V600 mutations is incomplete but patients with non-V600 mutations generally have a more aggressive clinical course and are not usually responsive to the selective BRAF therapy options [10, 15]. Data on the outcome of immunotherapy in patients with metastatic melanoma and uncommon BRAF mutations is unstudied.

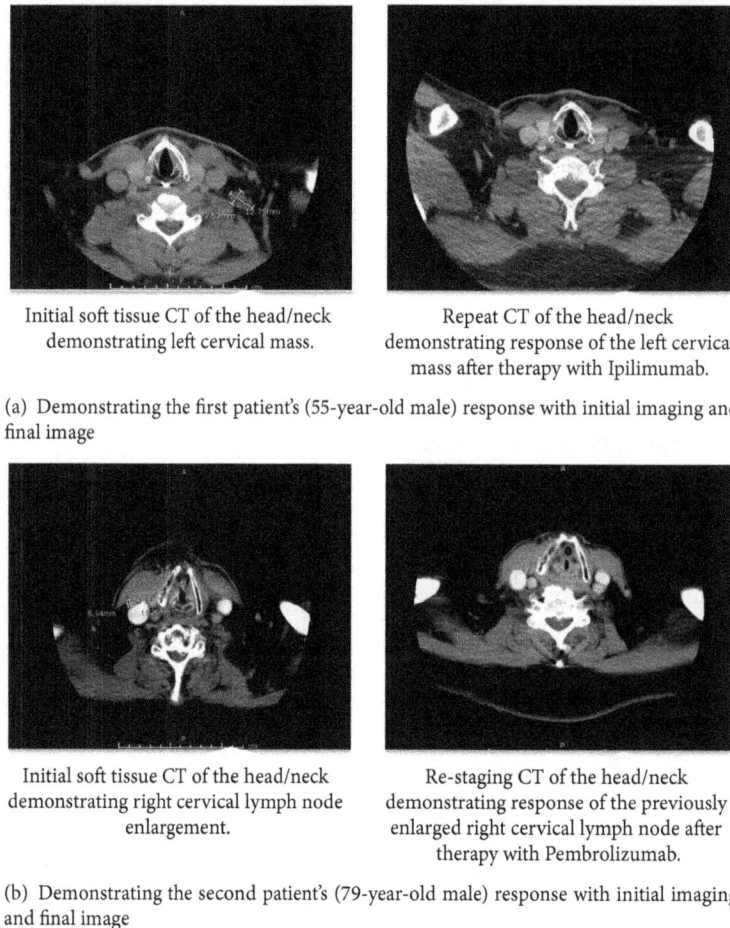

Initial soft tissue CT of the head/neck demonstrating left cervical mass.

Repeat CT of the head/neck demonstrating response of the left cervical mass after therapy with Ipilimumab.

(a) Demonstrating the first patient's (55-year-old male) response with initial imaging and final image

Initial soft tissue CT of the head/neck demonstrating right cervical lymph node enlargement.

Re-staging CT of the head/neck demonstrating response of the previously enlarged right cervical lymph node after therapy with Pembrolizumab.

(b) Demonstrating the second patient's (79-year-old male) response with initial imaging and final image

FIGURE 1

The exact mechanism of action and tumor pathogenesis regarding immunotherapy and the durable treatment response is still being investigated. One hypothesis relates to the CRAF serine kinase. CRAF is related to the plasma membrane and can activate MAPK signaling [10]. CRAF has other functions independent of the MAPK pathway such as an association with mitochondria where it regulates apoptosis and cellular death [10]. Preliminary research of CRAF and non-V600 mutations demonstrates that, with CRAF knockdown, induced apoptosis in melanoma cells occurs [10]. It is possible that immunotherapy inhibits or down-regulates the CRAF kinase leading to apoptosis of the melanoma tumor cells. Additionally, an association between resistant melanoma tumor cells and elevated CRAF proteins is being studied [16]. It is believed that the CRAF protein decreases the bioavailability of therapeutic agents in tumor cells [16]. It is possible that immunotherapy may modulate or affect the CRAF protein levels, thereby decreasing the development of resistance as both of these patients have experienced a durable response with repeated use of their respective immunotherapy agents. Further hypotheses and clinical studies could examine uncommon BRAF mutations and tumor cells, to evaluate if these mutations yield greater

production of PDL-1 ligands or decreased tumor antigen leading to a greater activity of CTLA-4 antibodies, which confers a greater response to their respective immunotherapy agents as indicated by these two cases.

Based upon the significant, durable responses experienced by the two patients presented in this case report, perhaps immunotherapy could be considered first-line therapy for patients with uncommon BRAF mutations. Further research is needed to assess the mechanism of action, evaluate for differences in outcomes with various immunotherapy options, and determine the long-term response rates/potential side effects of immunotherapy in this population.

References

[1] B. A. Kohler, R. L. Sherman, N. Howlader et al., "Annual Report to the Nation on the Status of Cancer, 1975-2011, Featuring Incidence of Breast Cancer Subtypes by Race/Ethnicity, Poverty,

and State," *Journal of the National Cancer Institute*, vol. 107, no. 6, p. djv048, 2015.

[2] B. F. Cole, R. D. Gelber, J. M. Kirkwood, A. Goldhirsch, E. Barylak, and E. Borden, "Quality-of-life-adjusted survival analysis of interferon alfa-2b adjuvant treatment of high-risk resected cutaneous melanoma: An Eastern Cooperative Oncology Group Study," *Journal of Clinical Oncology*, vol. 14, no. 10, pp. 2666–2673, 1996.

[3] G. V. Long, A. M. Menzies, A. M. Nagrial et al., "Prognostic and clinicopathologic associations of oncogenic BRAF in metastatic melanoma," *Journal of Clinical Oncology*, vol. 29, no. 10, pp. 1239–1246, 2011.

[4] K. Omholt, A. Platz, L. Kanter, U. Ringborg, and J. Hansson, "NRAS and BRAF mutations arise early during melanoma pathogenesis and are preserved throughout tumor progression," *Clinical Cancer Research*, vol. 9, no. 17, pp. 6483–6488, 2003.

[5] H. Chong and K.-L. Guan, "Regulation of Raf through phosphorylation and N terminus-C terminus interaction," *Journal of Biological Chemistry*, vol. 278, no. 38, pp. 36269–36276, 2003.

[6] C. Wellbrock and A. Hurlstone, "BRAF as therapeutic target in melanoma," *Biochemical Pharmacology*, vol. 80, no. 5, pp. 561–567, 2010.

[7] W. O. Greaves, S. Verma, K. P. Patel et al., "Frequency and spectrum of BRAF mutations in a retrospective, single-institution study of 1112 cases of melanoma," *Journal of Molecular Diagnostics*, vol. 15, no. 2, pp. 220–226, 2013.

[8] S. K. Hanks and T. Hunter, "Protein kinases 6. The eukaryotic protein kinase superfamily: Kinase (catalytic) domain structure and classification," *The FASEB Journal*, vol. 9, no. 8, pp. 576–596, 1995.

[9] P. B. Chapman, A. Hauschild, C. Robert et al., "Improved survival with vemurafenib in melanoma with BRAF V600E mutation," *New England Journal of Medicine*, vol. 364, no. 26, pp. 2507–2516, 2011.

[10] K. S. M. Smalley, M. Xiao, J. Villanueva et al., "CRAF inhibition induces apoptosis in melanoma cells with non-V600E BRAF mutations," *Oncogene*, vol. 28, no. 1, pp. 85–94, 2009.

[11] D. B. Johnson, C. M. Lovly, R. J. Sullivan, R. D. Carvajal, and J. A. Sosman, "Melanoma driver mutations and immune therapy," *OncoImmunology*, vol. 5, no. 5, Article ID e1051299, 2016.

[12] P. A. Ascierto, E. Simeone, V. C. Sileni et al., "Clinical experience with ipilimumab 3 mg/kg: Real-world efficacy and safety data from an expanded access programme cohort," *Journal of Translational Medicine*, vol. 12, no. 1, article no. 116, 2014.

[13] A. Snyder, V. Makarov, and T. Merghoub, "Genetic basis for clinical response to CTLA-4 blockade in melanoma," *The New England Journal of Medicine*, vol. 371, pp. 2189–2199, 2014.

[14] S. L. Topalian, F. S. Hodi, J. R. Brahmer et al., "Safety, activity, and immune correlates of anti-PD-1 antibody in cancer," *New England Journal of Medicine*, vol. 366, no. 26, pp. 2443–2454, 2012.

[15] G. Zheng, L.-H. Tseng, G. Chen et al., "Clinical detection and categorization of uncommon and concomitant mutations involving BRAF," *BMC Cancer*, vol. 15, article 779, 2015.

[16] C. Montagut, S. V. Sharma, T. Shioda et al., "Elevated CRAF as a potential mechanism of acquired resistance to BRAF inhibition in melanoma," *Cancer Research*, vol. 68, no. 12, pp. 4853–4861, 2008.

47

Recurrent Gastrointestinal Stromal Tumors in the Imatinib Mesylate Era: Treatment Strategies for an Incurable Disease

Rebecca M. Platoff,[1] William F. Morano,[1] Luiz Marconcini,[2] Nicholas DeLeo,[1] Beth L. Mapow,[3] Michael Styler,[2] and Wilbur B. Bowne[1]

[1]Department of Surgery, Drexel University College of Medicine, Philadelphia, PA, USA
[2]Department of Medicine, Division of Hematology/Oncology, Drexel University College of Medicine, Philadelphia, PA, USA
[3]Department of Pathology and Laboratory Medicine, Drexel University College of Medicine, Philadelphia, PA, USA

Correspondence should be addressed to Wilbur B. Bowne; wilbur.bowne@drexelmed.edu

Academic Editor: Jaime De la Garza

Introduction. Recurrence of gastrointestinal stromal tumors (GISTs) after surgical resection and imatinib mesylate (IM) adjuvant therapy poses a significant treatment challenge. We present the case of a patient who underwent surgical resection after recurrence and review the current literature regarding treatment. *Case Presentation.* A 58-year-old man with a large intra-abdominal jejunal GIST was treated with complete surgical resection followed by IM. The patient experienced disease recurrence 3.5 years later and underwent IM dose escalation and reresection. *Conclusion.* Current strategies to treat recurrent GIST include dose escalation, modifying adjuvant tyrosine kinase inhibitor therapy, and surgery. High-level evidence will be required to better define the combinatory roles of tyrosine kinase inhibitor therapy, guided by molecular profiling, and surgery in the management of recurrent GIST.

1. Introduction

Although rare, with an estimated incidence of 1.5 cases per 100,000 person years, gastrointestinal stromal tumors (GISTs) are the most common mesenchymal neoplasm of the gastrointestinal tract [1–5]. They arise from the interstitial cells of Cajal and most commonly occur in the stomach (50–60%), duodenum and small bowel (20–35%), rectum (5%), esophagus (2%), and rarely in the omentum, mesentery, and retroperitoneum [1, 6, 7].

A breakthrough in the management of GISTs was the development of tyrosine kinase inhibitors (TKIs), most notably imatinib mesylate (IM), which targets a mutation in *c-Kit*, a gene encoding a tyrosine kinase receptor and found in 80-90% of patients with GIST [1, 6, 8–12]. Before the development of targeted therapy, greater than 50% recurred within two years of surgery [1, 6, 10, 13]. IM is recommended by the FDA in the adjuvant setting for intermediate/high-risk disease as a result of the Z9001 trial and has been used in the neoadjuvant setting for potentially resectable disease

[9, 14, 15]. DeMatteo et al. demonstrated in this randomized controlled trial that one year of IM improved recurrence-free survival as compared to placebo, regardless of tumor size [9]. In 2012, Joensuu et al. further showed that three years of adjuvant imatinib conferred an overall survival advantage compared with one year of treatment [16]. This therapy has become the mainstay of adjuvant treatment for intermediate/high-risk GISTs [6, 17].

Despite remarkable improvements, management of recurrent disease remains largely undefined, in particular the role of surgical resection in recurrent disease. We present a case of recurrent GIST managed surgically after progression on adjuvant TKI therapy and review the current literature regarding management strategies for recurrent GIST.

2. Case Report

A 58-year-old man presented to his primary care physician with vague abdominal pain, constipation, and one year of urinary hesitancy. Abdominopelvic CT scan revealed

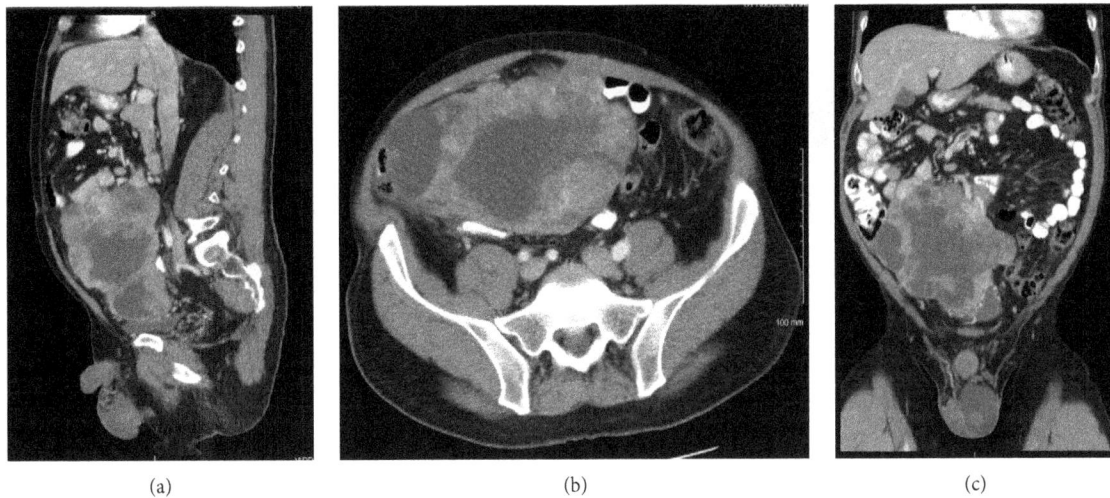

(a)   (b)   (c)

FIGURE 1: Sagittal (a), axial (b), and coronal (c) images of CT with IV contrast showing the large, lobulated primary mass that was discovered in January 2013.

a complex, lobulated, enhancing, intraperitoneal mass measuring $18 \times 19 \times 10$ cm, extending from the umbilicus to the level of the superior acetabulum (Figure 1). He underwent resection of the mass, including small bowel and partial bladder resection in January 2013. Pathology confirmed complete resection (R0) of high-grade GIST originating from the proximal jejunum, stage IIIB (pT4a, pNx). The tumor was spindle-cell subtype, with the mitotic rate of 8/10 HPF, and necrosis. Immunohistochemistry (IHC) showed membrane positivity for CD117, beta-catenin, vimentin, and smooth muscle actin (SMA). Mutational analysis demonstrated no mutations in the *c-Kit* proto-oncogene or platelet-derived growth factor receptor alpha (*PDGFRA*). Risk of recurrence was determined to be 90% [18–23]. He began imatinib mesylate 400 mg daily postoperatively. No evidence of tumor recurrence was detected over three years postoperatively. The patient tolerated imatinib well, except for mild diarrhea (grade 1 CTCAE) [24].

In May 2016, surveillance CT revealed a 3.5×2.8 cm left lower quadrant mass abutting the sigmoid colon (Figure 2). IM dosage was empirically increased from 400 mg to 800 mg daily, but repeat imaging in July 2016 showed disease progression. The left lower quadrant lesion had grown in size to $4.0 \times 3.3 \times 3.2$ cm, with extrinsic compression on the sigmoid colon, with a $2.4 \times 2.1 \times 2.5$ cm periumbilical lesion. Additionally, a new right upper quadrant lesion was noted, approximately $5.3 \times 3.7 \times 2.1$ cm. In late July 2016, diagnostic laparoscopy was performed (detecting a right lower quadrant peritoneal nodule), followed by laparotomy, small bowel resection, resection of right upper quadrant lesion, sigmoidectomy, and resection of right lower quadrant peritoneal nodule (Figure 3). The pathology revealed high-grade GIST with negative margins and absence of *c-Kit* mutation. Molecular profiling and next-generation sequencing (NGS) of the recurrent disease indicated susceptibility to sunitinib based on the presence of wild-type (WT) *c-Kit*. Accordingly, the patient was switched from imatinib to sunitinib. Follow-up CT in May 2017 showed no

signs of tumor recurrence, with patient follow-up at three-month intervals [14].

3. Discussion

In the case of primary GIST, surgery remains the definitive therapy for patients with low- and intermediate-risk disease [25]. For patients with high-risk disease (defined by the NIH Consensus Criteria as [1] size >10 cm, [2] mitotic rate > 10/50 hpf field or [3] mitotic rate > 5/50 hpf and tumor size > 5 cm, or [4] tumor rupture spontaneously or at surgery), adjuvant TKI therapy has been shown to add significant survival benefit [9, 26].

The Z9001 Trial revolutionized the treatment of GIST, demonstrating improvement in 1-year recurrence-free survival of 98% versus 83% in treatment and placebo groups, respectively [9]. Thereafter, the Scandinavian Sarcoma Group (SSG) trial, comparing 1 and 3 years of imatinib therapy, showed improved 5-year recurrence-free survival of 47.9% and 65.6%, respectively [16]. Of note, approximately 15% of GISTs have no detectable *c-Kit* or *PDGFRA* mutation [27]. The benefit from adjuvant imatinib is minimal in *c-Kit/PDGFRA*-WT patients. Specifically, in the study by Corless et al., imatinib was associated with higher recurrence-free survival versus placebo in patients with *c-Kit* exon 11 deletions but was not significantly associated with *PDGFRA* mutation or wild-type tumors [28]. Thus, risk of recurrence is higher, and treatment with imatinib is debated [29]. Nevertheless, NCCN recommendations suggest continued use of adjuvant imatinib therapy for these patients.

GIST recurrence in the IM era is largely considered incurable, and treatment strategies are aimed at delaying progression [6, 16]. Despite response to TKI therapy, many patients with high-risk GIST eventually develop recurrent disease [6]. In the SSG study, 65.6% of those who completed 3 years of adjuvant imatinib were alive without recurrence 5 years after study entry. However, 34.4% of those treated experienced recurrence requiring further management [16].

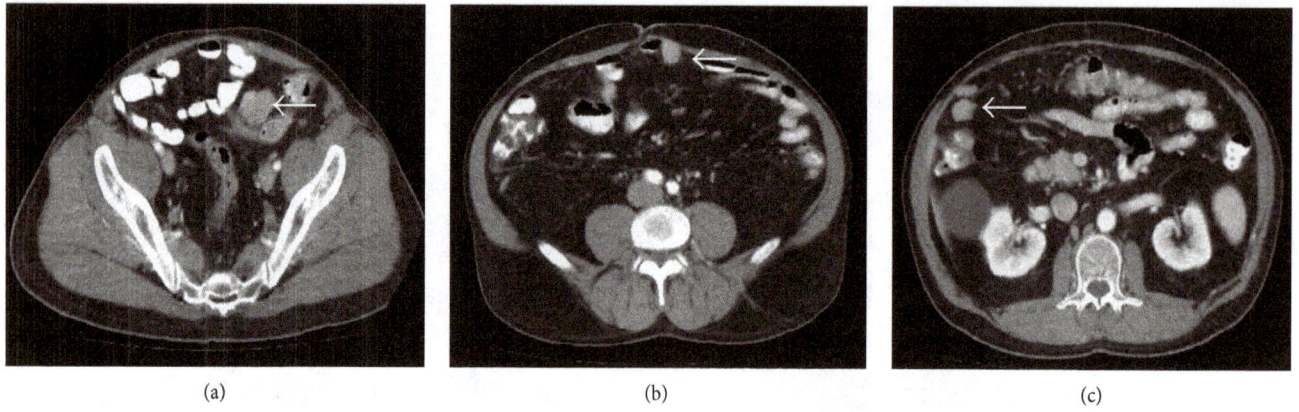

FIGURE 2: Axial CT images demonstrating recurrent lesions (white arrows) in the left lower quadrant (a), adherent to the anterior abdominal wall (b), and in the right upper quadrant (c).

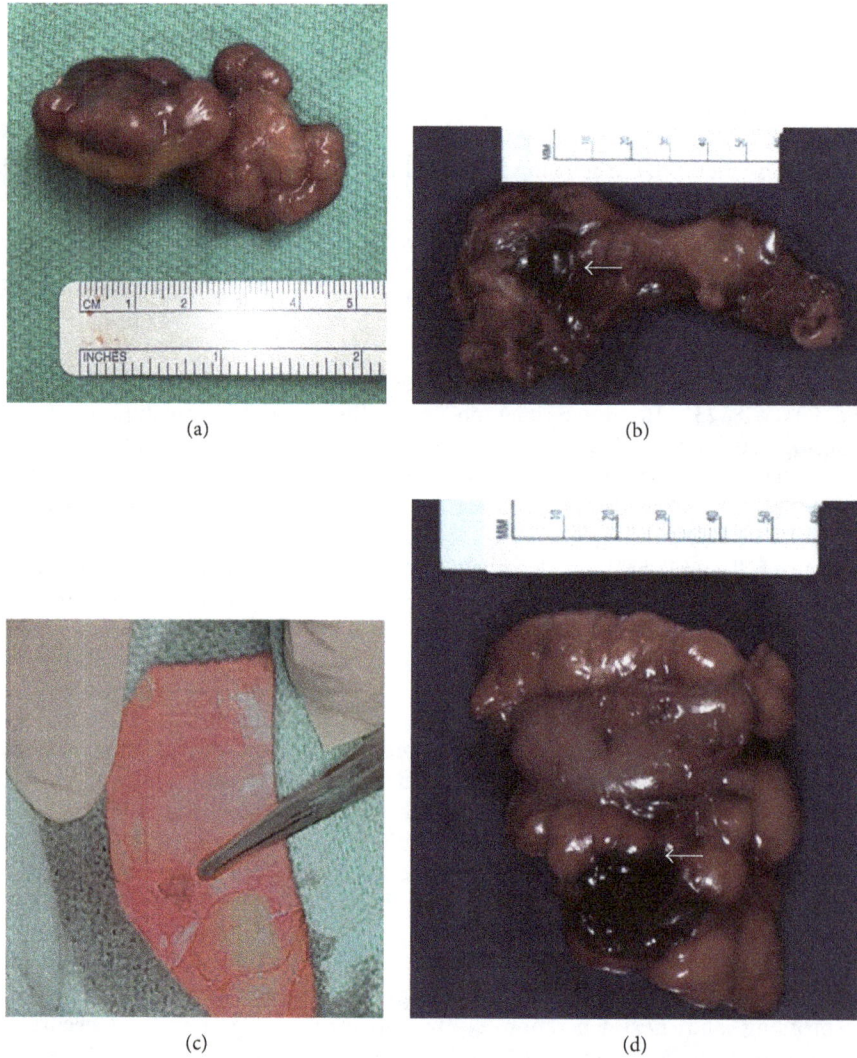

FIGURE 3: (a) Gross specimen of right upper quadrant recurrent GIST lesion. (b) Anterior abdominal wall mass (white arrow) adherent to the resected loop of the small intestine. (c) Small nodule within the mesentery discovered on diagnostic laparoscopy and resected. (d) Gross specimen demonstrating necrotic sigmoid lesion (white arrow) adherent to resected sigmoid.

TABLE 1: Institutional studies demonstrating benefit of TKI therapy for recurrent GIST.

	Study design	Number of patients	Primary endpoint	Main findings
Demetri et al. [30]	Randomized, double-blind, placebo-controlled, multicenter, international trial comparing sunitinib versus placebo after imatinib failure	321 (207 sunitinib versus 105 placebo patients)	Tumor progression	Median time to tumor progression: 27.3 weeks in patients receiving sunitinib versus 6.4 weeks with placebo
MetaGIST [31]	Analysis of two large, randomized, cooperative group studies comparing two doses of IM (400 mg daily versus twice daily) in 1640 patients with advanced GISTs	1640 (data analysis after 344 and 321 cases of progression or death in each study)	PFS and OS	High-dose imatinib 800 mg daily improved PFS but not OS compared to imatinib 400 mg daily
Reichardt et al. [32]	Randomized phase III open-label trial comparing nilotinib versus best supportive care with advanced GIST following prior imatinib/sunitinib failure	248 (2 : 1 randomization nilotinib or best supportive care)	PFS, OS	Subset analysis of patients with one prior regimen each of imatinib and sunitinib showed significant increase in median OS in favor of nilotinib versus best supportive care
Demetri et al. [33]	Randomized, double-blinded, placebo-controlled, multicenter, international trial comparing regorafenib versus placebo after imatinib/sunitinib failure	199 (133 regorafenib versus 66 placebo patients)	PFS	Median PFS 4.8 months for regorafenib versus 0.9 months for placebo
Seifert et al. [34]	Analysis of 85 patients with GISTs to determine expression of immune checkpoint molecules and effects of combination IM + PD-1/PD-L1 blockade in murine GISTs	85 (blood samples from patients with GISTs)	PD-1 receptor expression in T-cells of human GISTs T-cell function in mice with GISTs treated with IM and PD-1/PD-L1 inhibitor	The PD-1 inhibitory receptors were upregulated on tumor-infiltrating T-cells compared with T-cells from matched blood PD-1 expression on T-cells was highest in IM-treated human GISTs PD-1/PD-L1 blockade in vivo had no efficacy alone but enhanced antitumor effects of IM by increasing T-cell effector function

IM = imatinib mesylate, PFS = progression-free survival, OS = overall survival.

Table 1 highlights current institutional studies demonstrating benefit of TKI therapy for recurrent GIST. Treatment options are to initially escalate TKI dose or switch to a second-line drug, typically sunitinib malate [6, 13]. Imatinib can be increased from 400 mg to 800 mg daily, with an approximate 30% response rate in patients with KIT exon 9 mutations and acceptable toxicity profile [6, 31]. While c-Kit exon 11 mutations tend to have a higher response to imatinib, primary resistance in the first 6 months of treatment can occur with c-Kit exon 9, exon 18, and PDGFRA mutations [35–37]. Secondary resistance after six months can be observed with acquisition of new KIT kinase mutations such as in c-Kit exon 17 or c-Kit kinase domain 1 [38–40].

Sunitinib targets c-Kit and PDGFR-alpha and -beta receptors, among others [6]. In our patient, after resection of recurrence, NGS demonstrated a WT c-Kit, signaling potential benefit with sunitinib. Clinical benefit (partial response or stable disease for greater than or equal to 6 months) with sunitinib was observed with progression-free and overall survival in imatinib-resistant GIST [41]. In patients with WT c-Kit, Heinrich et al. showed a median progression-free survival of 19 months for patients treated with sunitinib after progression on imatinib versus 5.1 months for those with exon 11 mutations ($p = 0.03$) [41]. Similarly, a study by Demetri et al. showed improved median time to tumor progression for sunitinib versus placebo of approximately

27 weeks versus 6 weeks [30]. Subsequent progression from second-line therapy can then be treated with regorafenib, an oral multikinase inhibitor with increased progression-free survival but not overall survival compared to placebo [33].

A key principle in treatment of recurrent and/or metastatic GIST is to continue imatinib or second-line therapy indefinitely, as it has been shown that patients who discontinue therapy have higher rates of disease progression [6]. Moreover, recent studies have found strong linear correlations between survival time and duration of TKI therapy after diagnosis of recurrence/metastasis [1, 13, 26, 42]. NGS of the 592 genes most commonly associated with cancer, should expand our understanding of clonal evolution and pathogenesis of disease (high-risk primary and recurrence).

Another avenue in the early phase of exploration is treatment with immunotherapy. Seifert et al. analyzed 85 patients with GIST to determine expression of immune checkpoint molecules and the effects of combination imatinib and PD-1/PD-L1 blockade in KitV558Δ/+ mice that develop GIST. The PD-1 inhibitory receptors were upregulated on tumor-infiltrating T-cells as compared to T-cells from matched blood. PD-1 and PD-L1 blockade in vivo had no efficacy alone but enhanced the antitumor effects of imatinib by increasing T-cell effector function [34].

In addition to TKIs, surgery remains an important consideration in the management of recurrent GIST (Table 2).

TABLE 2: Institutional studies demonstrating benefit of surgery for recurrent GIST.

	Study design	Number of patients	Primary endpoint	R0 resection	Main findings
Bischof et al. [1]	Multi-institutional retrospective cohort	158 (87 locally advanced, 71 recurrent/metastatic)	RFS, OS	69% (recurrent/ metastatic) versus 87.4% (locally advanced)	TKI-sensitive recurrent/metastatic disease—improved RFS, OS after surgery
Du et al. [43]	Phase III multicenter trial for recurrent/metastatic on IM +/− surgery for residual disease	41 (19 IM + surgery, 22 IM alone)	PFS	73.6%	Trend towards improved PFS in surgery group
Tan et al. [13]	Retrospective cohort—upfront surgery versus TKI for recurrence	186 (56 recurrent—30 resectable, 24 underwent surgery for recurrence)	DFS, OS	75% (18 of 24) in upfront surgery group	Improved OS and DFS with surgery
Chang et al. [17]	Prospectively collected retrospective review—imatinib + surgery (early versus late groups) versus IM only	182 (89 metastatic, 93 recurrent, 76 underwent surgery)	Clinical response, PFS, OS	31.5% (early surgery) versus 59.1% (late surgery)	Improved CR, PR, PFS, OS in early surgery group; improved CR, PR, OS in late surgery group
Sato et al. [25]	Retrospective cohort comparing IM + surgery to surgery only	737 (93 recurrent/ metastatic—50 surgery + TKI therapy, 43 TKI therapy alone)	DFI, OS	58% (29 of 50)	Improved survival from surgery + TKI after complete resection, response to TKI, < 4 metastatic lesions, lesions < 100 mm total

TKI = tyrosine kinase inhibitor, IM = imatinib mesylate, OS = overall survival, DFS = disease-free survival, PFS = progression-free survival, CR = complete response, PR = partial response, RFS = recurrence-free survival, DFI = disease-free interval.

GISTs may follow disease-specific patterns that make recurrence amenable to resection [10, 42]. To demonstrate the benefit of surgery itself, studies have focused on its role in GIST recurrence regardless of patients' TKI use. A 2015 retrospective review of 186 patients showed that surgery for resectable, recurrent GIST was associated with increased overall survival compared to patients with resectable disease on TKI therapy alone [13]. In this study, 56 patients experienced recurrence, 30 with resectable disease. Twenty-four of those patients underwent upfront surgery (of which 18 received imatinib postoperatively) and 6 opted for nonoperative management. Their results showed a 1-year survival of 100% for those who underwent surgery compared to 50% with medical management alone, with 3-year survival rates of 80% versus 50% ($p = 0.04$), respectively. While surgery alone improved survival over TKI therapy only, their data also demonstrated a median disease-free survival of 2.9 years for patients who underwent surgery while on imatinib, as compared to 1.4 years after surgery alone. This study established the benefit of upfront surgery for GIST recurrence regardless of response to adjuvant TKI therapy, while also highlighting the combinatory effect of these two treatment strategies. The authors suggest that in patients with resectable, recurrent disease, complete resection of recurrent GIST may eliminate possible mutant strains, avoiding the need for escalation of TKI dosage [13, 15].

Further studies into surgical management of recurrent GIST have shown optimal recurrence-free and overall survival if patients are responding to TKI therapy at the time of surgery. Winer and Raut recommend that imatinib therapy commence prior to surgery, and surgeons should wait a minimum of six months before proceeding with resection [6]. Furthermore, retrospective reviews from the

Istituto Nazionale dei Tumori, Memorial Sloan Kettering Cancer Center, and Brigham and Women's Hospital/Dana-Farber Cancer Center demonstrated that these patients benefit most when disease progression has stabilized on imatinib, or less commonly on sunitinib [44–46]. Similarly, Chang et al. showed that timing of surgery relative to TKI therapy may contribute to outcome in a review of 182 patients with advanced/recurrent GIST [17]. In this study, 76 patients undergoing cytoreductive surgery were divided into an "early" group (prior to imatinib use, $n = 54$) and a "late" group (after imatinib use, $n = 22$). Those in the late surgery group had a higher rate of R0 resection (59.1% versus 31.6%, $p = 0.02$), higher complete and partial response rates (100% versus 79.6%, $p = 0.02$), and improved trend in overall survival. The authors imply that as surgery reduces tumor burden, this may delay time to development of secondary resistance, and offers a survival benefit when imatinib therapy is initiated prior to surgery [17].

The quality of resection for GIST recurrence has been found to play a pivotal role in survival [6, 25]. A 2016 study by Sato et al., analyzing data from forty Japanese institutions, showed that overall survival is significantly improved with R0/R1 resection [25]. Of the 93 included patients who experienced recurrence, 50 underwent surgery. Those with R0/R1 resection ($n = 34$) had significantly higher 5-year overall survival as compared to R2 resection ($n = 13$) (82.2% versus 47.0%, $p = 0.018$). Notably, the authors found a survival benefit from curative resection but reduced 5-year overall survival for R2 resection as compared to TKI therapy only (47% versus 60.2%). Their study concluded that surgical intervention should be reserved only for patients with possibility of achieving R0/R1 resection, 6–12 months after initiation of imatinib therapy. Importantly, R0/R1 resection of residual disease had a benefit when the number of metastatic lesions was less than 4, total tumor size was less than 100 cm, and disease remained stable or responsive to TKI therapy [25].

Laparoscopy has become an important consideration in the management of primary GISTs, both for diagnostic and therapeutic purposes, yet literature is sparse regarding its contribution for recurrence. Currently, NCCN guidelines support the use of a laparoscopic approach for resection of GIST in anatomically favorable locations (anterior wall of the stomach, ileum, and jejunum), while also noting that its use may expand after further studies due to the decreased short-term morbidity of this approach [14]. Likewise, diagnostic laparoscopy may be a valuable adjunct when approaching these patients with recurrent or metastatic disease to determine resectability or detect lesions not visualized on imaging.

CT remains the imaging modality of choice for surveillance and selection of patients with recurrence that may be candidates for surgical resection. This allows for monitoring disease progression via a change in size, development of new lesions, or alteration in density on CT demonstrating a response to TKI therapy. Tumor treatment-response, or lack thereof, will help guide whether surgical resection of recurrent disease is appropriate [47]. However, in our patient, laparoscopy allowed for detection of a subradiographic lesion not previously visualized on CT, facilitating complete resection in this patient with high-grade, recurrent GIST.

Paucity of high-level evidence investigating the management of recurrent GIST calls for prospective, randomized controlled studies to evaluate the benefit of surgery compared with TKI therapy alone. The difficulty with conducting such trials is elaborated by Du et al. who explain that in their experience, both patients and surgeons are resistant to the idea that a computer algorithm is the decision maker for randomizing an intervention as major as surgery. Their prospective, randomized trial comparing surgery and IM therapy for recurrent/metastatic GIST enrolled 41 patients, far short of the planned 210. This study investigated only patients with recurrence and continued response to IM and showed that median overall survival was prolonged in patients who underwent surgery. While their findings were encouraging, they lacked statistical significance due to poor patient accrual [43].

4. Conclusion

Recent literature demonstrates a survival benefit with surgical intervention in patients with recurrent GISTs. Factors that may improve survival after surgical management of recurrent GIST include quality of resection, limited burden of disease, and response to TKI therapy. If recurrence develops while on TKI therapy, progression-free survival may be improved with dose escalation or next-generation TKIs. Further studies are now needed to elucidate the relative importance of these factors, particularly their impact on patient survival, such as ours, who progressed on TKI therapy, but otherwise had resectable disease

with few metastases and optimal performance status. Current literature offers insight into the role of surgery for improving survival in patients with recurrent GIST, with the most significant deficit being whether surgery can provide survival benefit to patients no longer responding to TKI therapy. Clearly, the roles of TKIs and surgery for improving survival in patients with recurrent GIST are not mutually exclusive. Prospective, randomized trials will be required to develop treatment algorithms to delineate combinatory roles of TKIs, guided by molecular profiling, and surgery in the management of recurrent GIST.

Consent

Written informed consent was obtained from the patient for publication of this case report and any accompanying image.

Authors' Contributions

Rebecca M. Platoff and William F. Morano contributed equally to the production of this manuscript.

References

[1] D. A. Bischof, Y. Kim, I. Blazer et al., "Surgical management of advanced gastrointestinal stromal tumors: an international multi-institutional analysis of 158 patients," *Journal of the American College of Surgeons*, vol. 219, no. 3, pp. 439–449, 2014.

[2] P. G. Casali, L. Jost, P. Reichardt, M. Schlemmer, J.-Y. Blay, and ESMO Guidelines Working Group, "Gastrointestinal stromal tumors: ESMO clinical recommendations for diagnosis, treatment and follow-up," *Annals of Oncology*, vol. 19, no. 2, pp. ii35–ii38, 2008.

[3] M. Miettinen and J. Lasota, "Gastrointestinal stromal tumors—definition, clinical, histological, immunohistochemical, and molecular genetic features and differential diagnosis," *Virchows Archiv*, vol. 438, no. 1, pp. 1–12, 2001.

[4] B. Nilsson, P. Bümming, J. M. Meis-Kindblom et al., "Gastrointestinal stromal tumors: the incidence, prevalence, clinical course, and prognostication in the preimatinib mesylate era," *Cancer*, vol. 103, no. 4, pp. 821–829, 2005.

[5] G. Tryggvason, H. G. Gíslason, M. K. Magnússon, and J. G. Jónasson, "Gastrointestinal stromal tumors in Iceland, 1990-2003: the Icelandic GIST study, a population-based incidence and pathologic risk stratification study," *International Journal of Cancer*, vol. 117, no. 2, pp. 289–293, 2005.

[6] J. H. Winer and C. P. Raut, "Management of recurrent gastrointestinal stromal tumors," *Journal of Surgical Oncology*, vol. 104, no. 8, pp. 915–920, 2011.

[7] C. E. Woodall III, G. N. Brock, J. Fan et al., "An evaluation of 2537 gastrointestinal stromal tumors for a proposed clinical staging system," *Archives of Surgery*, vol. 144, no. 7, pp. 670–678, 2009.

[8] C. L. Corless, C. M. Barnett, and M. C. Heinrich, "Gastrointestinal stromal tumours: origin and molecular oncology," *Nature Reviews Cancer*, vol. 11, no. 12, pp. 865–878, 2011.

[9]   R. P. DeMatteo, K. V. Ballman, C. R. Antonescu et al., "Adjuvant imatinib mesylate after resection of localised, primary gastrointestinal stromal tumour: a randomised, double-blind, placebo-controlled trial," *The Lancet*, vol. 373, no. 9669, pp. 1097–1104, 2009.

[10] R. P. DeMatteo, J. J. Lewis, D. Leung, S. S. Mudan, J. M. Woodruff, and M. F. Brennan, "Two hundred gastrointestinal stromal tumors: recurrence patterns and prognostic factors for survival," *Annals of Surgery*, vol. 231, no. 1, pp. 51–58, 2000.

[11] G. D. Demetri, M. von Mehren, C. D. Blanke et al., "Efficacy and safety of imatinib mesylate in advanced gastrointestinal stromal tumors," *New England Journal of Medicine*, vol. 347, no. 7, pp. 472–480, 2002.

[12] H. Joensuu, P. J. Roberts, M. Sarlomo-Rikala et al., "Effect of the tyrosine kinase inhibitor STI571 in a patient with a metastatic gastrointestinal stromal tumor," *New England Journal of Medicine*, vol. 344, no. 14, pp. 1052–1056, 2001.

[13] G. H. C. Tan, J. S. M. Wong, R. Quek et al., "Role of upfront surgery for recurrent gastrointestinal stromal tumours," *ANZ Journal of Surgery*, vol. 86, no. 11, pp. 910–915, 2015.

[14] M. von Mehren, R. L. Randall, R. S. Benjamin et al., "Soft tissue sarcoma, version 2.2016, NCCN clinical practice guidelines in oncology," *Journal of the National Comprehensive Cancer Network*, vol. 14, no. 6, pp. 758–786, 2016.

[15] B. L. Eisenberg, J. Harris, C. Blanke et al., "Phase II trial of neoadjuvant/adjuvant imatinib mesylate (IM) for advanced primary and metastatic/recurrent operable gastrointestinal stromal tumor (GIST): early results of RTOG 0132/ACRIN 6665," *Journal of Surgical Oncology*, vol. 99, no. 1, pp. 42–47, 2009.

[16] H. Joensuu, M. Eriksson, K. Sundby Hall et al., "One vs three years of adjuvant imatinib for operable gastrointestinal stromal tumor: a randomized trial," *Journal of the American Medical Association*, vol. 307, no. 12, pp. 1265–1272, 2012.

[17] S.-C. Chang, C.-H. Liao, S.-Y. Wang et al., "Feasibility and timing of cytoreduction surgery in advanced (metastatic or recurrent) gastrointestinal stromal tumors during the era of imatinib," *Medicine*, vol. 94, no. 24, p. e1014, 2015.

[18] E. Downs-Kelly, B. P. Rubin, and J. R. Goldblum, "Mesenchymal tumors of the gastrointestinal tract," in *Odze and Goldblum's Surgical Pathology of the GI Tract, Liver, Biliary Tract, and Pancreas*, R. D. Odze and J. R. Goldblum, Eds., Elsevier: Saunders, Philadelphia, PA, USA, 3rd edition, 2015.

[19] M. Miettinen, M. Furlong, M. Sarlomo-Rikala, A. Burke, L. H. Sobin, and J. Lasota, "Gastrointestinal stromal tumors, intramural leiomyomas, and leiomyosarcomas in the rectum and anus: a clinicopathologic, immunohistochemical, and molecular genetic study of 144 cases," *American Journal of Surgical Pathology*, vol. 25, no. 9, pp. 1121–1133, 2001.

[20] M. Miettinen, J. Kopczynski, H. R. Makhlouf et al., "Gastrointestinal stromal tumors, intramural leiomyomas, and leiomyosarcomas in the duodenum: a clinicopathologic, immunohistochemical, and molecular genetic study of 167 cases," *American Journal of Surgical Pathology*, vol. 27, no. 5, pp. 625–641, 2003.

[21] M. Miettinen and J. Lasota, "Gastrointestinal stromal tumors: pathology and prognosis at different sites," *Seminars in Diagnostic Pathology*, vol. 23, no. 2, pp. 70–83, 2006.

[22] M. Miettinen, H. Makhlouf, L. H. Sobin, and J. Lasota, "Gastrointestinal stromal tumors of the jejunum and ileum: a clinicopathologic, immunohistochemical, and molecular genetic study of 906 cases before imatinib with long-term follow-up," *American Journal of Surgical Pathology*, vol. 30, no. 4, pp. 477–489, 2006.

[23] M. Miettinen, L. H. Sobin, and J. Lasota, "Gastrointestinal stromal tumors of the stomach: a clinicopathologic, immunohistochemical, and molecular genetic study of 1765 cases with long-term follow-up," *American Journal of Surgical Pathology*, vol. 29, no. 1, pp. 52–68, 2005.

[24] U.S Dept. of Health and Human Services, "Common Terminology Criteria for Adverse Events (CTCAE) Version 4.0, 2010," April 2017, https://evs.nci.nih.gov/ftp1/CTCAE/CTCAE_4.03_2010-06-14_QuickReference_8.5x11.pdf.

[25] S. Sato, T. Tsujinaka, T. Masuzawa et al., "Role of metastasectomy for recurrent/metastatic gastrointestinal stromal tumors based on an analysis of the Kinki GIST registry," *Surgery Today*, vol. 47, no. 1, pp. 58–64, 2017.

[26] H. Joensuu, "Risk stratification of patients diagnosed with gastrointestinal stromal tumor," *Human Pathology*, vol. 39, no. 10, pp. 1411–1419, 2008.

[27] D. Gasparotto, S. Rossi, M. Polano et al., "Quadruple-negative GIST is a sentinel for unrecognized neurofibromatosis type 1 syndrome," *Clinical Cancer Research*, vol. 23, no. 1, pp. 273–282, 2017.

[28] C. L. Corless, K. V. Ballman, C. R. Antonescu et al., "Pathologic and molecular features correlate with long-term outcome after adjuvant therapy of resected primary GI stromal tumor: the ACOSOG Z9001 trial," *Journal of Clinical Oncology*, vol. 32, no. 15, pp. 1563–1570, 2014.

[29] H. Joensuu, P. Hohenberger, and C. L. Corless, "Gastrointestinal stromal tumour," *The Lancet*, vol. 382, no. 9896, pp. 973–983, 2013.

[30] G. D. Demetri, A. T. van Oosterom, C. R. Garrett et al., "Efficacy and safety of sunitinib in patients with advanced gastrointestinal stromal tumour after failure of imatinib: a randomised controlled trial," *The Lancet*, vol. 368, no. 9544, pp. 1329–1338, 2006.

[31] Gastrointestinal Stromal Tumor Meta-Analysis Group (MetaGIST), "Comparison of two doses of imatinib for the treatment of unresectable or metastatic gastrointestinal stromal tumors: a meta-analysis of 1,640 patients," *Journal of Clinical Oncology*, vol. 28, no. 7, pp. 1247–1253, 2010.

[32] P. Reichardt, J. Y. Blay, H. Gelderblom et al., "Phase III study of nilotinib versus best supportive care with or without a TKI in patients with gastrointestinal stromal tumors resistant to or intolerant of imatinib and sunitinib," *Annals of Oncology*, vol. 23, no. 7, pp. 1680–1687, 2012.

[33] G. D. Demetri, P. Reichardt, Y. K. Kang et al., "Efficacy and safety of regorafenib for advanced gastrointestinal stromal tumours after failure of imatinib and sunitinib (GRID): an international, multicentre, randomised, placebo-controlled, phase 3 trial," *The Lancet*, vol. 381, no. 9863, pp. 295–302, 2013.

[34] A. M. Seifert, S. Zeng, J. Q. Zhang et al., "PD-1/PD-L1 blockade enhances T-cell activity and antitumor efficacy of imatinib in gastrointestinal stromal tumors," *Clinical Cancer Research*, vol. 23, no. 2, pp. 454–465, 2017.

[35] M. C. Heinrich, C. L. Corless, G. D. Demetri et al., "Kinase mutations and imatinib response in patients with metastatic gastrointestinal stromal tumor," *Journal of Clinical Oncology*, vol. 21, no. 23, pp. 4342–4349, 2003.

[36] M. C. Heinrich, K. Owzar, C. L. Corless et al., "Correlation of kinase genotype and clinical outcome in the North American Intergroup Phase III Trial of imatinib mesylate for treatment of advanced gastrointestinal stromal tumor: CALGB 150105 study by Cancer and Leukemia Group B and Southwest

Oncology Group," *Journal of Clinical Oncology*, vol. 26, no. 33, pp. 5360–5367, 2008.

[37] S. Farag, N. Somaiah, H. Choi et al., "Clinical characteristics and treatment outcome in a large multicenter observational cohort of pdgfra exon 18 mutated gastrointestinal stromal tumor (GIST) patients," *European Journal of Cancer*, vol. 76, no. 5, pp. 76–83, 2017.

[38] C. R. Antonescu, P. Besmer, T. Guo et al., "Acquired resistance to imatinib in gastrointestinal stromal tumor occurs through secondary gene mutation," *Clinical Cancer Research*, vol. 11, no. 11, pp. 4182–4190, 2005.

[39] L. L. Chen, J. C. Trent, E. F. Wu et al., "A missense mutation in KIT kinase domain 1 correlates with imatinib resistance in gastrointestinal stromal tumors," *Cancer Research*, vol. 64, no. 17, pp. 5913–5919, 2004.

[40] M. C. Heinrich, C. L. Corless, C. D. Blanke et al., "Molecular correlates of imatinib resistance in gastrointestinal stromal tumors," *Journal of Clinical Oncology*, vol. 24, no. 29, pp. 4764–4774, 2006.

[41] M. C. Heinrich, R. G. Maki, C. L. Corless et al., "Primary and secondary kinase genotypes correlate with the biological and clinical activity of sunitinib in imatinib-resistant gastrointestinal stromal tumor," *Journal of Clinical Oncology*, vol. 26, no. 33, pp. 5352–5359, 2008.

[42] A. P. Conley, A. Guerin, M. Sasane et al., "Treatment patterns, prescribing decision drivers, and predictors of complete response following disease recurrence in gastrointestinal stromal tumor patients: a chart extract-based approach," *Journal of Gastrointestinal Cancer*, vol. 45, no. 4, pp. 431–440, 2014.

[43] C.-Y. Du, Y. Zhou, C. Song et al., "Is there a role of surgery in patients with recurrent or metastatic gastrointestinal stromal tumours responding to imatinib: a prospective randomised trial in China," *European Journal of Cancer*, vol. 50, no. 10, pp. 1772–1778, 2014.

[44] C. P. Raut, M. Posner, J. Desai et al., "Surgical management of advanced gastrointestinal stromal tumors after treatment with targeted systemic therapy using kinase inhibitors," *Journal of Clinical Oncology*, vol. 24, no. 15, pp. 2325–2331, 2006.

[45] R. P. DeMatteo, R. G. Maki, S. Singer, M. Gonen, M. F. Brennan, and C. R. Antonescu, "Results of tyrosine kinase inhibitor therapy followed by surgical resection for metastatic gastrointestinal stromal tumor," *Annals of Surgery*, vol. 245, no. 3, pp. 347–352, 2007.

[46] A. Gronchi, M. Fiore, F. Miselli et al., "Surgery of residual disease following molecular-targeted therapy with imatinib mesylate in advanced/metastatic GIST," *Annals of Surgery*, vol. 245, no. 3, pp. 341–346, 2007.

[47] W. B. Bowne, "Imaging strategies to detect recurrent GIST after surgery: controversies, consensus and guidelines," *GIST Cancer Journal*, vol. 3, no. 1, pp. 10–15, 2016.

48

A Case of Undiagnosed HIV Infection in a 57-Year-Old Woman with Multiple Myeloma: Consequences on Chemotherapy Efficiency and Safety

I. Poizot-Martin,[1,2] S. Brégigeon,[1] C. Tamalet,[3] R. Bouabdallah,[4] O. Zaegel-Faucher,[1] V. Obry-Roguet,[1] A. Ivanova,[1] C.E. Cano,[1] and C. Solas[5]

[1] Aix Marseille Université, APHM Hôpital Sainte-Marguerite, Service d'Immuno-Hématologie Clinique, 270 boulevard de Sainte Marguerite, 13274 Marseille Cedex 09, France

[2] INSERM U912 (SESSTIM), 13006 Marseille, France

[3] Fondation Institut Hospitalo-Universitaire Méditerranée Infection, Pôle des Maladies Infectieuses et Tropicales Clinique et Biologique, Fédération de Bactériologie-Hygiène-Virologie, CHU Timone, 264 rue Saint-Pierre, 13385 Marseille Cedex 05, France

[4] Département d'Hématologie, Institut Paoli Calmettes, 232 boulevard de Sainte Marguerite, 13273 Marseille Cedex 09, France

[5] Aix Marseille Université, AP-HM Hôpital de la Timone, Service de Pharmacocinétique et Toxicologie, CRO2 INSERM U911, 13385 Marseille Cedex 05, France

Correspondence should be addressed to I. Poizot-Martin; isabelle.poizot@ap-hm.fr

Academic Editor: Josep M. Ribera

Background. Non-AIDS-defining cancers represent a rising health issue among HIV-infected patients. Nevertheless, HIV testing is not systematic during the initial cancer staging. Here, we report a case of HIV infection diagnosed three years after chemotherapy initiation for multiple myeloma. *Results.* A 57-year-old woman diagnosed with multiple myeloma underwent a first round of chemotherapy by bortezomib/lenalidomide and then with bortezomib/liposomal-doxorubicine/dexamethasone, with partial remission, poor hematological tolerance, and multiple episodes of pneumococcal infection. Allogenic stem cell transplantation was proposed leading to HIV testing, which revealed seropositivity, with an HIV viral load of $5.5 \log_{10}/\text{mL}$ and severe CD4 T cell depletion (24 cells/mm^3). Chemotherapy by bendamustin was initiated. Multidisciplinary staff decided the initiation of antiretroviral therapy with tenofovir/emtricitabin/efavirenz and prophylaxis against opportunistic infections. After 34 months, patient achieved complete remission, sustained HIV suppression, and significant CD4 recovery (450 cells/mm^3), allowing effective pneumococcal immunization without relapse. *Conclusion.* Our case illustrates the drawback that ignored HIV infection is still causing to cancer patients receiving chemotherapy and highlights the importance of early HIV testing in oncology. A multidisciplinary approach including oncologists/hematologists, virologists, and pharmacists is recommended in order to avoid drug interactions between chemotherapy and antiretroviral drugs. Moreover, prophylactic medication is recommended in these patients regardless of CD4+ cell count at the initiation of chemotherapy.

1. Introduction

The incidence of non-AIDS-defining cancers in HIV-infected patients appears to be higher than the general population [1]. However, HIV infection is frequently undiagnosed in cancer patients and HIV testing is not systematic. In Europe, the fraction of HIV-infected people that ignore their HIV status has been estimated to 20 to 40% [2, 3]. Plasma cell neoplasms, of which multiple myeloma (MM) is the most common, represent 20% of all lymphoid malignancies in Europe [4] and stem cell transplantation (SCT) after systemic chemotherapy is currently the standard of care for this malignancy. Although practice is progressively evolving, HIV infection has historically been an exclusion criterion for SCT, while approved chemotherapy for multiple myeloma is frequently associated with hematological toxicity.

Nevertheless, recent observations indicate that well-adapted antiretroviral treatment (cART) may improve the outcome of chemotherapy and even of SCT [5, 6]. Here, we report a case of HIV infection diagnosed three years after the initiation of systemic chemotherapy for MM in a female patient, which illustrates the consequences of ignored HIV infection on patient's outcome.

2. Case Presentation

Patient is a 57-year-old woman that presented with an inflammatory syndrome in February 2008. Clinicians diagnosed her with multiple myeloma on the basis of a positive myelography, a monoclonal IgG-κ gammopathy (M-protein: IgG 40 g/L; Kappa: 373 mg/L; Lambda: 195 mg/L), a β2-microglobulin 2 × ULN, and a diffuse infiltration of the spine detected by MRI. From March 2008 until December 2009, gammopathy was treated with bortezomib followed by lenalidomide, achieving partial remission. In June 2009, spinal MRI was normal and IgG was 30 g/L with no other abnormalities of the blood count and without renal failure. In May and December 2009, this patient received antimicrobial therapy for two episodes of pneumococcal pneumoniae. In November 2010, spinal MRI was normal. In January 2011, a combination of bortezomib, liposomal doxorubicine, and dexamethasone was initiated following worsening of gammopathy (IgG: 53 g/L), with IgA 1.74 g/L, IgM 11.03 g/L, normocytic anemia (107 g/L), platelet count 208 × 10^9/L, creatinine 45 μmol/L, normal calcemia, LDH 2 × ULN with anicteric cholestasis, β2-microglobuline 5 × ULN. Karyotype was normal. After 4 chemotherapy cycles with poor hematological tolerance, IgG was 25 g/L, and allogenic SCT was proposed. Of note, the patient presented with a new episode of pneumococcal pneumonia in March 2011. In August 2011, the patient underwent HIV testing before SCT; she tested positive for HIV with severe immune depression (CD4+ cell count: 24 cells/mm^3; normal value: 600–1200) and HIV viral load 316228 copies/mL (5.5 $\log_{10}$/mL). SCT was cancelled, and chemotherapy with bendamustin was proposed. An antiretroviral regimen combining tenofovir/emtricitabin/efavirenz and opportunistic prophylaxis (against *pneumocystis jiroveci, toxoplasma gondii*, and cytomegalovirus) was proposed by multidisciplinary staff, including a pharmacologist and virologist, to limit the risk of drug-drug interactions. After 34 months of followup, complete and sustained remission of gammopathy (IgG: 15 g/L; Kappa: 21 mg/L; Lambda: 21 mg/L; ratio 1.22) was achieved, associated with sustained HIV suppression and significant immune restoration (CD4+ T cell count: 450/mm^3; 15%; Figure 1), which allowed for effective pneumococcal immunization without relapse.

3. Discussion

Here, we present a case of ignored HIV infection that severely affected the management and outcome of MM. The most likely HIV transmission route for this patient was a blood transfusion that occurred in 1978, which is 30 years prior to the diagnosis of MM and 33 years before diagnosis of

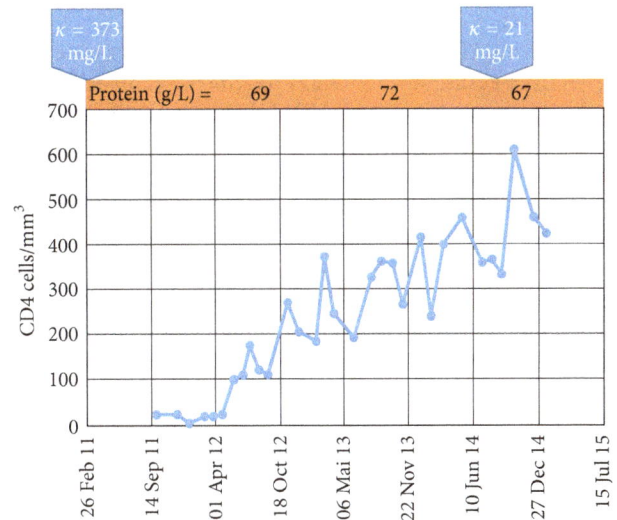

FIGURE 1: Evolution of CD4+ T cell count during and after bendamustine chemotherapy. Graph shows longitudinal evolution of CD4+ cell counts during and after bendamustine chemotherapy (from September 19, 2011, to February 29, 2012). y-axis = CD4 cells/mm^3; x-axis = date. (Top) orange box show plasma protein quantitation (g/L).

HIV. Although monoclonal gammopathies of undetermined significance (MGUS) are frequent in HIV-infected patients [7, 8], our patient presented with plasma M-protein >30 g/L at diagnosis, which classifies for MM according to the International Myeloma Working Group [9]. Nevertheless, a long-term followup of MGUS patients at the Mayo Clinic revealed that around 16% of MGUS cases evolved towards a MM, with a median time of progression of 10.6 years [10]. Thus, we cannot exclude that our patient might have developed an HIV-related MGUS prior to MM.

Several studies in industrialized countries have shown that HIV-infected patients have 2 to 5 times increased risk of developing multiple myeloma compared to the general population [11–17]. Moreover, male HIV-infected patients die three times more frequently of MM compared to uninfected age-matched individuals [18]. Recently, a case-control study including 10 HIV-infected and 28 uninfected patients treated for MM showed that HIV-infected patients receiving highly active antiretroviral therapy (HAART) had longer overall and disease-free survival than uninfected controls [19]. Hence, the awareness of HIV infection and antiretroviral treatment have a proven benefit for MM patients in terms of survival.

Because invasive pneumococcal disease is a frequent complication of HIV infection, the recurrent episodes observed in this patient should have alerted physicians to the need for HIV testing. Unfortunately, missed opportunities for HIV testing are not rare [20], stressing the need to improve HIV-related recognition in all healthcare facilities and this is particularly relevant for oncologists. Indeed, systematic HIV-testing at the initial diagnosis of cancer would allow for cautious initiation of treatment with an immunosuppressive regimen for a potentially immune-compromised patient, as in this case study. Strikingly, more than 30 years after the beginning of the AIDS epidemic, patients with AIDS-defining cancers are not always tested for HIV [21]. Because antiretroviral treatment seems to have a positive impact on survival, HIV-infected patients who also have cancer should keep or initiate a cART while undergoing treatment for malignant disease [6]. However, many chemotherapeutic and antiretroviral drugs are metabolized through the cytochrome P450 (CYP) enzyme system of the liver, increasing the chemotherapy-associated toxicity or decreasing the treatment efficacy. Hence, a multidisciplinary approach to HIV-cancer care that includes physicians, hematologist/oncologists, virologists, and pharmacists is recommended to prevent the risk of drug-drug interactions and optimize clinical management [22]. In our case, the association of the antiretroviral ritonavir, a CYP450-1A2 inducer, with bendamustin, a substrate/inhibitor of CYP450-1A2, could potentially reduce the efficacy of chemotherapy. Therefore, a ritonavir-boosted protease inhibitor-based regimen was contraindicated. Interactions with other medications that are used to treat or to prevent opportunistic infections or chemotherapy side effects should also be evaluated. Indeed, prophylactic medications are recommended in these patients regardless of their CD4+ cell count at the start of chemotherapy.

Currently, scarce data are available on the prevalence of undiagnosed HIV infection among patients who present with non-AIDS-defining cancer [23]. Nevertheless, our case highlights the importance of HIV testing during the initial cancer staging. A multidisciplinary approach to HIV-cancer care that includes physicians, hematologist/oncologists, virologists, and pharmacists is particularly relevant considering the high risk of drug-drug interactions between systemic chemotherapy and antiretroviral drugs. Furthermore, prophylactic medications are recommended in these patients regardless of their CD4+ cell count at the start of chemotherapy.

Abbreviations

SCT: Stem cell transplantation
AIDS: Acquired immune deficiency
cART: Combined antiretroviral therapy.

Consent

Written informed consent was obtained from the patient for publication of this case report.

Acknowledgments

The authors would like to thank the patient for giving consent to publish her case.

References

[1] M. S. Shiels, S. R. Cole, G. D. Kirk, and C. Poole, "A meta-analysis of the incidence of non-AIDS cancers in HIV-infected individuals," *Journal of Acquired Immune Deficiency Syndromes*, vol. 52, no. 5, pp. 611–622, 2009.

[2] F. F. Hamers and A. N. Phillips, "Diagnosed and undiagnosed HIV-infected populations in Europe," *HIV Medicine*, vol. 9, supplement 2, pp. 6–12, 2008.

[3] M. G. Van Veen, A. M. Presanis, S. Conti et al., "National estimate of HIV prevalence in the Netherlands: comparison and applicability of different estimation tools," *AIDS*, vol. 25, no. 2, pp. 229–237, 2011.

[4] R. De Angelis, P. Minicozzi, M. Sant et al., "Survival variations by country and age for lymphoid and myeloid malignancies in Europe 2000–2007: results of EUROCARE-5 population-based study," *European Journal of Cancer*, vol. 51, no. 15, pp. 2254–2268, 2015.

[5] J. L. Díez-Martín, P. Balsalobre, A. Re et al., "Comparable survival between HIV+ and HIV- non-Hodgkin and Hodgkin lymphoma patients undergoing autologous peripheral blood stem cell transplantation," *Blood*, vol. 113, no. 23, pp. 6011–6014, 2009.

[6] A. Makinson, J.-C. Tenon, S. Eymard-Duvernay et al., "Human immunodeficiency virus infection and non-small cell lung cancer: survival and toxicity of antineoplastic chemotherapy in a cohort study," *Journal of Thoracic Oncology*, vol. 6, no. 6, pp. 1022–1029, 2011.

[7] A. S. Fiorino and B. Atac, "Paraproteinemia, plasmacytoma, myeloma and HIV infection," *Leukemia*, vol. 11, no. 12, pp. 2150–2156, 1997.

[8] P. Genet, L. Sutton, D. Chaoui et al., "Prevalence of monoclonal gammopathy in HIV patients in 2014," *Journal of the International AIDS Society*, vol. 17, no. 4, supplement 3, Article ID 19649, 2014.

[9] R. A. Kyle and S. V. Rajkumar, "Criteria for diagnosis, staging, risk stratification and response assessment of multiple myeloma," *Leukemia*, vol. 23, no. 1, pp. 3–9, 2009.

[10] R. A. Kyle and S. V. Rajkumar, "Monoclonal gammopathy of undetermined significance," *British Journal of Haematology*, vol. 134, no. 6, pp. 573–589, 2006.

[11] G. M. Clifford, J. Polesel, M. Rickenbach et al., "Cancer risk in the Swiss HIV cohort study: associations with immunodeficiency, smoking, and highly active antiretroviral therapy," *Journal of the National Cancer Institute*, vol. 97, no. 6, pp. 425–432, 2005.

[12] L. Dal Maso, S. Franceschi, J. Polesel et al., "Risk of cancer in persons with AIDS in Italy, 1985–1998," *British Journal of Cancer*, vol. 89, no. 1, pp. 94–100, 2003.

[13] E. A. Engels, R. M. Pfeiffer, J. J. Goedert et al., "Trends in cancer risk among people with AIDS in the United States 1980–2002," *AIDS*, vol. 20, no. 12, pp. 1645–1654, 2006.

[14] A. E. Grulich, Y. Li, A. McDonald, P. K. L. Correll, M. G. Law, and J. M. Kaldor, "Rates of non-AIDS-defining cancers in people with HIV infection before and after AIDS diagnosis," *AIDS*, vol. 16, no. 8, pp. 1155–1161, 2002.

[15] A. E. Grulich, M. T. van Leeuwen, M. O. Falster, and C. M. Vajdic, "Incidence of cancers in people with HIV/AIDS compared with immunosuppressed transplant recipients: a meta-analysis," *The Lancet*, vol. 370, no. 9581, pp. 59–67, 2007.

[16] A. Newnham, J. Harris, H. S. Evans, B. G. Evans, and H. Møller, "The risk of cancer in HIV-infected people in southeast

England: A Cohort Study," *British Journal of Cancer*, vol. 92, no. 1, pp. 194–200, 2005.

[17] M. Frisch, R. J. Biggar, E. A. Engels, and J. J. Goedert, "Association of cancer with AIDS-related immunosuppression in adults," *The Journal of the American Medical Association*, vol. 285, no. 13, pp. 1736–1745, 2001.

[18] R. M. Selik and C. S. Rabkin, "Cancer death rates associated with human immunodeficiency virus infection in the United States," *Journal of the National Cancer Institute*, vol. 90, no. 17, pp. 1300–1302, 1998.

[19] G. Li, R. D. Lewis, N. Mishra, and C. A. Axiotis, "A retrospective analysis of ten symptomatic multiple myeloma patients with HIV infection: a potential therapeutic effect of HAART in multiple myeloma," *Leukemia Research*, vol. 38, no. 9, pp. 1079–1084, 2014.

[20] K. Champenois, A. Cousien, L. Cuzin et al., "Missed opportunities for HIV testing in newly-HIV-diagnosed patients, a cross sectional study," *BMC Infectious Diseases*, vol. 13, no. 1, article 200, 2013.

[21] V. Mosimann, M. Cavassini, O. Hugli et al., "Patients with AIDS-defining cancers are not universally screened for HIV: a 10-year retrospective analysis of HIV-testing practices in a Swiss university hospital," *HIV Medicine*, vol. 15, no. 10, pp. 631–634, 2014.

[22] P. G. Rubinstein, D. M. Aboulafia, and A. Zloza, "Malignancies in HIV/AIDS: from epidemiology to therapeutic challenges," *AIDS*, vol. 28, no. 4, pp. 453–465, 2014.

[23] S. Shrestha, D. C. Johnson, D. C. Porter et al., "Short communication: lack of occult HIV infection among non-AIDS-defining cancer patients in three academic oncology clinics in the United States," *AIDS Research and Human Retroviruses*, vol. 29, no. 6, pp. 887–891, 2013.

49

West Nile Virus Encephalitis in a Patient with Neuroendocrine Carcinoma

Romina Deldar, Derek Thomas, and Anna Maria Storniolo

Division of Hematology & Oncology, Indiana University School of Medicine, Indianapolis, IN 46202, USA

Correspondence should be addressed to Anna Maria Storniolo; astornio@iu.edu

Academic Editor: Constantine Gennatas

Importance. Oftentimes, when patients with metastatic cancer present with acute encephalopathy, it is suspected to be secondary to their underlying malignancy. However, there are multiple causes of delirium such as central nervous system (CNS) infections, electrolyte abnormalities, and drug adverse reactions. Because West Nile Virus (WNV) neuroinvasive disease has a high mortality rate in immunosuppressed patients, a high index of suspicion is required in patients who present with fever, altered mental status, and other neurological symptoms. *Observations.* Our case report details a single patient with brain metastases who presented with unexplained fever, encephalopathy, and new-onset tremors. Initially, it was assumed that his symptoms were due to his underlying malignancy or seizures. However, because his unexplained fevers persisted, lumbar puncture was pursued. Cerebrospinal fluid analysis included WNV polymerase chain reaction and serologies were ordered which eventually led to diagnosis of WNV encephalitis. *Conclusions and Relevance.* Patients with metastatic cancer who present with encephalopathy are often evaluated with assumption that malignancy is the underlying etiology. This can lead to delays in diagnosis and possible mistreatment. Our case highlights the importance of maintaining a broad differential diagnosis and an important diagnostic consideration of WNV encephalitis in patients with cancer.

1. Case Report

A 58-year-old male presented in the summertime with fever, generalized weakness, and encephalopathy after being found unconscious. Upon arrival to the hospital, he was disoriented to place and time, dysarthric, and amnestic to details of the event. Review of systems was positive for one week of progressive gait instability but negative for any other preceding or ongoing infectious or neurologic symptoms. He had no recent travel or exposure to sick contacts.

Seven months prior to his presentation, the patient had been diagnosed with a poorly differentiated neuroendocrine carcinoma, which presented primarily in his parotid gland. He had completed seven cycles of chemotherapy, with the last cycle given two weeks previously. Two months earlier, he had developed numerous asymptomatic brain metastases. A whole-brain radiation therapy was recommended for him; however, he declined. Other chronic medical problems included a history of prostate cancer in remission, dyslipidemia, and hypertension. He also had a history of

"visual seizures" for which he was taking daily antiepileptic medication.

On presentation, the patient was somnolent but arousable. His vital signs revealed that he was febrile (temperature of 102.4 F) and tachycardic (heart rate of 126), blood pressure was 150/105 mmHg, respiratory rate was 14, and oxygen saturation was 95% on 2 liters per minute nasal cannula. Cardiopulmonary and gastrointestinal examinations were otherwise unremarkable. On neurological examination, the patient exhibited a resting tremor in both upper extremities, which his family reported was new within the past few days. There was no evidence of tongue biting, urinary incontinence, photophobia, or nuchal rigidity. Muscle strength, tone, and deep tendon reflexes were normal and symmetric. Babinski signs were absent. Sensory examination was normal.

Laboratory evaluation was significant only for mild hyponatremia (132 mmol/L) and elevated creatinine kinase (236 mmol/L). Tests for liver function, complete blood count, and urinalysis were unremarkable. Blood cultures and urine cultures were sent upon presentation and eventually revealed no growth. Urine drug screen was positive for cannabinoids only. Chest radiograph revealed no acute abnormalities. A noncontrasted head computed tomography was unremarkable with poor visualization of his known intracranial metastases. Initially, there was suspicion for an infectious etiology or progression of previously known brain metastases; therefore, the patient was started on empiric broad-spectrum antibiotics and systemic glucocorticoids for potential vasogenic edema until further diagnostic evaluation could be performed. His antiseizure medication was also continued.

One day after presentation, the patient's mental status was remarkably improved, although not completely to baseline. The transient nature of his encephalopathy raised suspicion of a generalized seizure as the inciting event with resultant temporary postictal state. Given this, an electroencephalogram (EEG) was obtained, revealing mild-to-moderate generalized background slowing, indicating diffuse encephalopathy, without any epileptogenic foci identified.

Two days after presentation, the patient remained febrile and tremulous; however, his cognition continued to improve. Because no definitive diagnosis had been reached and he continued to have unexplained fevers, a lumbar puncture was performed for further evaluation. Cerebrospinal fluid (CSF) studies revealed lymphocytic inflammation with an elevated glucose (84 mg/dL), elevated protein (89 mg/dL), and elevated total nucleated cell count (95/cumm), with a differential of neutrophils 8%, lymphocytes 53%, plasma cells 25%, and monocytes 14%. CSF Gram stain was negative, and cytology was negative for malignant cells. Herpes Simplex Virus-1 (HSV-1) and HSV-2 reverse transcription-polymerase chain reaction (RT-PCR) tests were negative, as was *Cryptococcus neoformans* antigen. CSF and serologic testing for West Nile Virus (WNV) IgM, IgG, and PCR was also ordered.

Approximately one week after presentation, a final diagnosis of acute WNV encephalitis was made. Although CSF IgG and PCR for WNV were negative, the patient's serum and CSF WNV IgM were qualitatively positive, establishing the diagnosis of WNV neuroinvasive disease [5, 8]. Empiric antibiotics and steroids were discontinued. Brain magnetic resonance imaging was obtained, which revealed stable intracranial metastases compared to one month earlier. Over a period of several days, his mental status improved completely to baseline and his fever and tremors subsided. He did, however, continue to have significant diffuse weakness, presumably secondary to prolonged hospital stay and systemic glucocorticoids. The patient was eventually discharged to a subacute rehabilitation facility.

2. Discussion

Oftentimes, when patients with metastatic cancer present with acute encephalopathy, it is suspected to be secondary to their underlying malignancy. Supporting this rationale is the fact that brain metastases affect 20 to 40 percent of cancer patients who are hospitalized, and neurologic complications are one of the most common reasons for their hospitalization [9]. Nevertheless, other causes of delirium, specifically central nervous system (CNS) infections, electrolyte abnormalities, vitamin deficiencies, seizures, and drug

Table 1: Infectious and noninfectious causes of encephalitis.

Infectious causes	Diagnostic tests (CSF, unless indicated)	Noninfectious causes
Viruses		
Enteroviruses	PCR	Opiates
HSV-1, HSV-2	PCR	Adverse drug reactions
VZV	PCR, virus-specific antibody	ADEM
EBV	PCR	CNS vasculitis
HIV	Western Blot, ELISA (blood)	
WNV	Virus-specific IgM	
TBEV	PCR	
JEV	Virus-specific IgM	
Parasites		
Toxoplasma gondii	PCR, culture	
Trypanosoma cruzi	PCR, culture	
Fungi		
Cryptococcus neoformans	India ink, cryptococcal antigen	
Histoplasma capsulatum	Serum: CSF antibody	
Candida albicans	Culture	
Bacteria		
MRSA	Culture	
Streptococcus	Culture	

HSV, Herpes Simplex Virus; VZV, Varicella Zoster Virus; EBV, Epstein-Barr Virus; HIV, Human Immunodeficiency Virus; WNV, West Nile Virus; TBEV, tick-borne encephalitis virus; JEV, Japanese encephalitis virus; MRSA, methicillin-resistant *Staphylococcus pneumonia*; CSF, cerebrospinal fluid; PCR, polymerase chain reaction; ELISA, enzyme-linked immunosorbent assay; ADEM, Acute Disseminated Encephalomyelitis; CNS, central nervous system.
References: [1–4].

adverse effects, should be considered on initial evaluation. In a retrospective review by De la Cruz et al., opioid-related delirium accounted for 47.31% of missed delirium cases in cancer patients [10]. Primary CNS infection warrants specific consideration in the workup of delirium in cancer patients noting that 16% of patients with CNS infections have primary CNS tumors [11]. Table 1 lists infectious and noninfectious causes of meningoencephalitis worldwide that may affect immunocompromised patients, including cancer patients [11].

Although uncommon in the healthy population, WNV has an increased incidence in immunocompromised patients [12]. WNV can be a difficult diagnosis to make. It requires a high index of suspicion as presenting symptoms are nonspecific and initial brain imaging may reveal no abnormalities [12]. The presentation of WNV infection can vary from asymptomatic to a mild, febrile flu-like syndrome to more severe neurological symptoms. Less than 1% of individuals develop neuroinvasive disease, which manifests as meningitis, encephalitis, or polio-like flaccid paralysis [13].

TABLE 2: Diagnostic tests for acute West Nile Virus infection.

Test	Sensitivity	Specificity
PCR (serum)	10%	100%
PCR (CSF)	55%	100%
WNV-specific IgM (serum)	95%	90%
WNV-specific IgM (CSF)	95%	92%

PCR, polymerase chain reaction; CSF, cerebrospinal fluid; WNV, West Nile Virus.
References: [1, 5–7].

Symptoms such as tremors, myoclonus, or extrapyramidal symptoms may be seen. Immunosuppressed patients, such as those receiving chemotherapy, are at higher risk for neuroinvasive disease [12]. Mortality rate can reach as high as 20% in these populations [14]. Treatments with interferon, intravenous immunoglobulin, and ribavirin have been used but lack high efficacy. Therefore, only supportive measures are recommended in most cases.

In our patient, workups of systemic infection, including blood cultures, urine cultures, and chest imaging, were all negative. CSF evaluation was pursued only after the patient's mental status and fevers did not improve with broad-spectrum antibiotics. Although CSF IgG and PCR for WNV were negative, this is common in acute WNV infection, given their low sensitivity [5]. Both serum and CSF IgM were positive, which is the gold standard for diagnosis of acute WNV encephalitis [15]. WNV-specific IgM antibodies are detectable 3 to 8 days after onset of illness and typically persist up to 90 days, whereas WNV-specific IgG is detectable after 7 days of illness onset and persists indefinitely [8, 16]. A positive IgM result combined with a negative IgG result suggests acute infection [16]. Table 2 illustrates the sensitivities and specificities of various diagnostic tests for WNV infection.

As described above, patients with metastatic cancer who present with encephalopathy are often evaluated with the assumption that malignancy is the underlying etiology. This can lead to delays in diagnosis and possible mistreatment. To date, there have been few case reports detailing the course of WNV infection in patients with malignancy. Our case highlights the importance of maintaining a broad differential diagnosis as well as a relatively rare but important diagnostic consideration of WNV encephalitis in this patient population. Because of its high mortality rate in immunosuppressed patients, timely diagnosis of WNV neuroinvasive disease should be made to ensure proper monitoring and supportive measures. It is therefore critical that multiple etiologies be considered in the workup of acute delirium in the patient with malignancy as determining the underlying diagnosis may obviate unnecessary diagnostic interventions and empiric treatments that could have adverse effects.

References

[1] West Nile Virus (WNV), Molecular Detection, PCR, Plasma. Mayo Clinic Medical Laboratories, http://www.mayomedical-laboratories.com/test-catalog/Clinical+and+Interpretive/87802.

[2] Toxoplasma gondii Encephalitis: Guidelines for the prevention and treatment of opportunistic infections in HIV-infected adults and adolescents, AIDSinfo, 2016, https://aidsinfo.nih.gov/guidelines/html/4/adult-and-adolescent-oi-prevention-and-treatment-guidelines/322/toxo.

[3] E. Lages-Silva, L. E. Ramirez, M. L. Silva-Vergara, and E. Chiari, "Chagasic meningoencephalitis in a patient with acquired immunodeficiency syndrome: diagnosis, follow-up, and genetic characterization of Trypanosoma cruzi," Clinical Infectious Diseases, vol. 34, no. 1, pp. 118–123, 2002.

[4] Centers for Disease Control and Prevention, "Vector-Born Diseases: Diagnostic Testing," http://www.cdc.gov/ncezid/dvbd/index.html.

[5] Mayo Clinic: Mayo Medical Laboratories, "West Nile virus, molecular detection, PCR," http://www.mayomedicallaboratories.com/test-catalog/Clinical+and+Interpretive/86197.

[6] L. Jeha and C. A. Sila, Neurologic Complications of West Nile Virus, The Cleveland Clinic Foundation, Cleveland, Ohio, USA, 2009, http://www.clevelandclinicmeded.com/medicalpubs/diseasemanagement/neurology/neurologic-complications-west-nile-virus/.

[7] A. K. Malan, T. B. Martins, H. R. Hill, and C. M. Litwin, "Evaluations of commercial West Nile virus immunoglobulin G (IgG) and IgM enzyme immunoassays show the value of continuous validation," Journal of Clinical Microbiology, vol. 42, no. 2, pp. 727–733, 2004.

[8] Diagnostic Testing: WNV Antibody Testing. Centers for Disease Control and Prevention, 2016, http://www.cdc.gov/westnile/healthcareproviders/healthcareproviders-diagnostic.html.

[9] H. B. Newton, "Neurological complications of systemic cancer," American Family Physician, vol. 59, no. 4, pp. 878–886, 1999.

[10] M. De la Cruz, J. Fan, S. Yennu et al., "The frequency of missed delirium in patients referred to palliative care in a comprehensive cancer center," Supportive Care in Cancer, vol. 23, no. 8, pp. 2427–2433, 2015.

[11] A. A. Pruitt, "Central nervous system infections in cancer patients," Seminars in Neurology, vol. 30, no. 3, pp. 296–310, 2010.

[12] K. V. Ravindra, A. G. Freifeld, A. C. Kalil et al., "West nile virus-associated encephalitis in recipients of renal and pancreas transplants: case series and literature review," Clinical Infectious Diseases, vol. 38, no. 9, pp. 1257–1260, 2004.

[13] T. Ajayi, A. Bhatia, B. Lambl, and S. Altamimi, "Altered mental status and fever," BMJ Case Reports, Article ID 009238, 2013.

[14] S. Ulbert, "West Nile virus: the complex biology of an emerging pathogen," *Intervirology*, vol. 54, no. 4, pp. 171–184, 2011.

[15] J. J. Mandel, S. Tummala, K. H. Woodman, and I. Tremont-Lukats, "Delayed imaging abnormalities of neuro-invasive West Nile virus in cancer patients," *Journal of the Neurological Sciences*, vol. 350, no. 1-2, pp. 115–117, 2015.

[16] West Nile Virus: Detection with serologic and Real-time PCR assays. Quest Diagnostics, 2016, http://www.questdiagnostics .com/testcenter/testguide.action%3Fdc%3DCF_WestNileVirus.

50

Smooth Muscle Tumor Originating in the Pleura: A Case Report and Updated Literature Review

Santiago Fabián Moscoso Martínez,[1] Vadim Zarubin,[1] Geethapriya Rajasekaran Rathnakumar,[2] and Alireza Zarineh[3]

[1]Department of Hematology and Oncology, The Brooklyn Hospital Center, 121 Dekalb Ave, New York, NY 11201, USA
[2]Department of Internal Medicine, The Brooklyn Hospital Center, 121 Dekalb Ave, New York, NY 11201, USA
[3]Department of Pathology, The Brooklyn Hospital Center, 121 Dekalb Ave, New York, NY 11201, USA

Correspondence should be addressed to Santiago Fabián Moscoso Martínez; sanmoscoso@gmail.com

Academic Editor: Francesco A. Mauri

Smooth muscle tumors (SMTs) of the pleura are exceptionally rare. At present and to the best of these authors' knowledge, there are only 17 cases reported in the literature. We describe a case of a 51-year-old woman who complained of left sided pleuritic chest pain. Further, computed tomography (CT) revealed a left sided localized pleural-based mass involving the 9th rib. She underwent an interventional radiology guided percutaneous core biopsy of the lesion, which disclosed a "Smooth Muscle Tumor of Undetermined Malignant Potential (SMT-UMP)." A video-assisted thoracoscopic surgery (VATS) was performed for diagnosis and treatment purposes. Resections of the pleural-based mass and 9th rib were performed. SMT-UMP was the definitive diagnosis.

1. Introduction

Intrathoracic smooth muscle tumors are uncommon in the respiratory tract (upper and lower respiratory tract). They are seen occasionally in the gastrointestinal tract and commonly seen in the urogenital system [1–3]. However, the existence and diagnostic criteria of smooth muscle tumors originating in the pleura have been controversial and only rare and sporadic case reports have been mentioned in the literature [4]. Table 1 describes all cases that have been reported in the literature. We present a case of SMT-UMP with CT evidence of involvement of the 9th rib.

2. Case Report

A 51-year-old woman presented to the emergency department with persistent posterior left sided chest discomfort. Patient had nonspecific symptoms for over one year. Upon admission patient was noted to have a normal EKG findings; X-Ray of the chest was unremarkable. She underwent a CT which revealed a pleural-based mass 3.3 cm × 2.0 cm of the left lower lobe involving the 9th rib posteriorly, in Figure 1. A CT-guided transthoracic core biopsy of the tumor revealed a smooth muscle tumor of the pleura of undetermined malignant potential (SMT-UMP). The specimen showed a bland proliferation of spindle cells with abundant eosinophilic cytoplasm arranged in fascicles. No necrosis and rare mitotic activity were identified. Due to the pattern of spread that has been shown of these tumors (local growth without metastasis) and the lack of high risk features (no necrosis and rare mitotic activity) CT scan of the chest including the upper abdomen was performed for staging purposes and it did not show metastasis.

She was further treated with complete resection of the pleural-based mass and the 9th rib by video-assisted thoracoscopic surgery (VATS). The final pathology examination revealed a well-capsulated SMT-UMP of pleural origin measuring 3.5 × 3.0 × 2.4 cm with no evidence of rib involvement by the tumor, in Figure 2. Patient tolerated the procedure well without any surgical or medical complications. Unfortunately patient was lost to follow-up. Table 2 shows patient's immunohistochemical staining.

TABLE 1: Clinical and histopathological features of previous case reports and current case report of SMT of the pleura.

Case	Sex	Age	Clinical features	Size[a] (cm)	Histology	Origin of the tumor	Procedure	Follow-up (months)	Clinical course
1[b]	F	21	Asymptomatic	U	SMT of UMP	Vascular smooth muscle (pleura)	Too large for complete resection	4	Alive at 4 M without enlargement or metastasis
2	M	49	Asymptomatic	18	LMS/IG	No detail	Complete resection	8	Alive at 8 M without recurrence
3	F	23	Asymptomatic	10	SMT of UMP	Vascular smooth muscle (pleura)	Too large for complete resection	6	Alive at 6 M without enlargement or metastasis
4	F	44	Empyema	U	LMS/IG	No detail	Complete resection	2	Alive at 2 M without recurrence
5	F	69	Chest pain	11	LMS/HG	No detail	Complete resection	12	Alive at 12 M without recurrence
6	M	32	Asymptomatic	7 (intrathoracic) + 6 (extrathoracic) = 13	SMT of UMP	No detail (pleura)	Complete resection	12	Alive at 12 M without recurrence
7	M	73	Asymptomatic	At least 21	SMT of UMP→LMS	No detail (pleura)	Possible incomplete resection at the apex and received radiation to reduce the risk of local recurrence	14	Alive at 14 M without recurrence
8	F	55	Asymptomatic	1.5	Leiomyoma	Microvascular wall (pleura)	Complete resection	26	Alive at 26 M without recurrence
9	F	40	Asymptomatic	3.5	SMT of UMP	Microvascular wall (pleura)	Complete resection	17	Alive at 17 M without recurrence
10	M	45	Chest pain	9	Leiomyoma	No detail (pleura)	Complete resection	15	Alive at 15 M without recurrence
11	M	33	Asymptomatic	3	Leiomyoma	No detail	Complete resection	Unknown	Unknown
12	F	50	Chest pain	4	SMT of UMP	Vascular smooth muscle (pleura)	Complete resection	53	Alive at 53 M without recurrence
13	F	48	Chest pain	18	Leiomyoma	No detail (pleura)	Complete resection	18	Alive at 18 M without recurrence
14	F	32	Chest pain	2 tumors, unknown size	Leiomyoma	No detail	Complete resection	57	Recurrence after 1 year during follow-up Underwent to chest wall resection. Alive at 57 M without further recurrence

TABLE 1: Continued.

Case	Sex	Age	Clinical features	Size[a] (cm)	Histology	Origin of the tumor	Procedure	Follow-up (months)	Clinical course
15	M	43	Chest pain	2	Leiomyoma	No detail	Complete resection	40	Alive at 40 M without recurrence
16	F	28	Chest pain	4.2	Leiomyoma	No detail (intercostal space)	Complete resection	2	Alive at 2 M without recurrence
17	F	33	Chest pain	5.3	Leiomyoma	Vascular smooth muscle (pleura)	Complete resection	14	Alive at 14 M without recurrence
Present case	F	51	Chest pain	3.5	SMT of UMP	No detail	Complete resection	0	—

[a]Maximum diameter of the tumor in cm.
[b]Cases 1–5 from Moran et al. [5]; case 6 from Proca et al. [6]; case 7 from Al-Daraji et al. [7]; case 8 from Nose et al. [8]; case 9 from Tanaka et al. [9]; case 10 from Qiu et al. [10]; case 11 from Mochizuki et al. [11]; case 12 from Turhan et al. [12]; case 13 from Rodríguez et al. [13]; cases 14 and 15 from Kuman et al. [14]; case 16 from Nakada et al. [15]; case 17 from Ziyade et al. [16].
Note: U, unresectable tumors that were only debulked at surgery; SMT, smooth muscle tumor; UMP, undetermined malignant potential; LMS, leiomyosarcoma; IG, intermediate grade; HG, high grade.

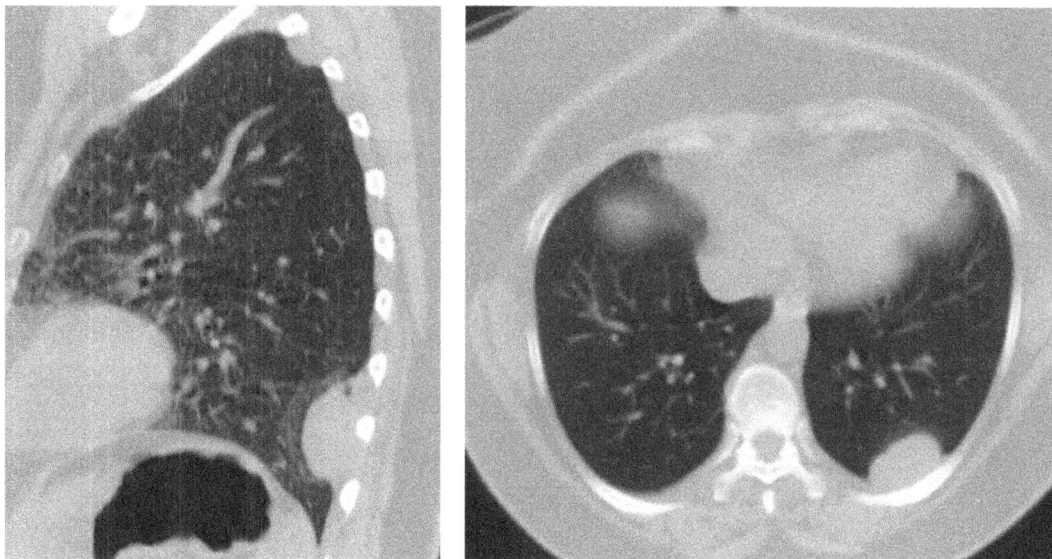

FIGURE 1: Left sided posterior pleural-based mass.

3. Discussion

SMT-UMP originating in the pleura are rare. They tend to have a female predominance (12 out of 18 patients) as per current literature review. Patient's age ranges from 21 to 73 years old (mean 42.7). Leiomyosarcomas (LMS) were found mainly in older patients and SMT of UMP on the other hand tend to happen in younger patients. Our case illustrates that SMT-UMP can present in a relatively older age.

SMTs can be found incidentally on imaging studies done for unrelated issues or they can cause symptoms usually related to tumor size (the largest one has been reported as at least 21 cm) and location. In our case a middle aged women presented with nonspecific pleuritic chest pain where fatal conditions need to be ruled out. These patients should undergo a thorough history and physical examination. Radiological studies should be performed with chest X-ray (CXR), computed tomography, and magnetic resonance imaging that helps identify location, size, and radiological structure of the tumor [6].

Pleural tumors tend to grow locally toward the intrathoracic cavity [15]. There is not a single case reported in the literature showing that these tumors did metastasize. Proca et al. [6] reported a case that was followed up without any surgical intervention for four years and it showed that the tumor did grow locally inside and out of the thoracic cavity but no metastasis was reported. However, due to the rarity of these tumors and short follow-ups reported there is not enough data at the moment to determine if these tumors have the ability to metastasize.

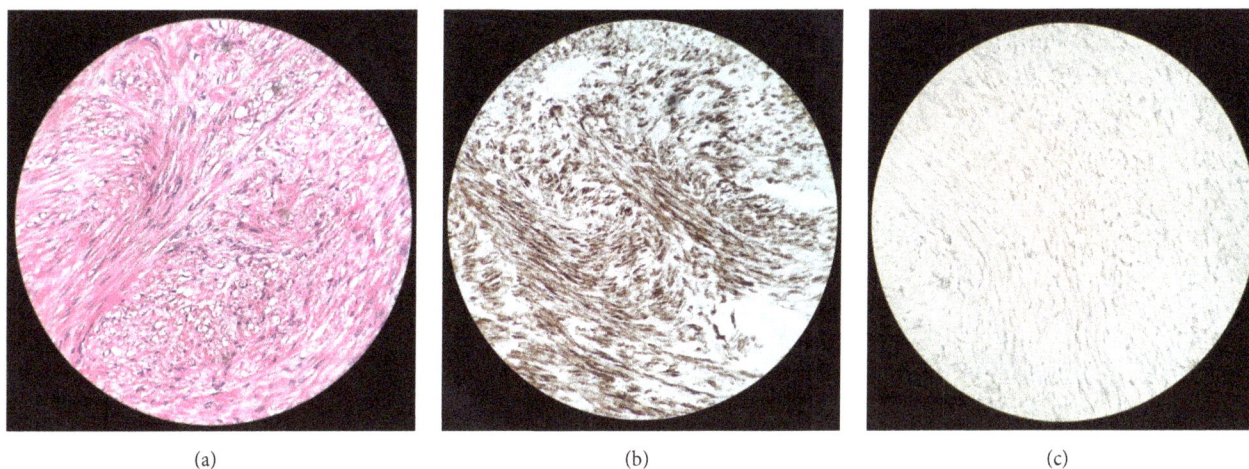

FIGURE 2: (a) Proliferation of bland spindle cells with elongated nuclei and eosinophilic cytoplasm (hematoxylin and eosin, 400x magnification). (b) Desmin immunohistochemical stain is positive (400x magnification). (c) Beta-catenin is negative (400x magnification).

TABLE 2: Immunohistochemical staining.

Immunohistochemical staining	Result
CD34 (focal)	Positive
Smooth muscle actin	Positive
SMMHC	Positive
Desmin	Positive
Vimentin	Positive
CD99	Negative
Beta-catenin	Negative
S-100	Negative
BCL-2	Negative
Ki-67	Less than 2% cells showing nuclear staining
Cytokeratin AE1/AE3	Negative

Confirmation of diagnosis is always made with tissue sample and histological examination. A CT-guided biopsy can be performed, but it has the potential to seed the tissues directly in its path [6]. If surgical excision of the lesion can be done safely with minimal complications it should be done with diagnostic and treatment purposes instead of diagnostic needle biopsy in order to avoid potential seeding and spread of tumor with malignant potential.

Primary pleural tumors are rare since 75% of pleural tumors represent metastatic disease [13]. The differential diagnosis of spindle cell neoplasms from pleural origin includes smooth muscle tumor, solitary fibrous tumor, metastatic spindle cell carcinoma, synovial sarcoma, fibrosarcoma, malignant peripheral nerve sheath tumor, sarcomatous mesothelioma, and spindle cell thymoma [2]. Table 3 describes the main differences between these entities.

Immunohistochemical staining for smooth muscle actin and desmin provides a definitive diagnosis of smooth muscle origin.

In our patient, microscopic examination showed proliferation of bland spindle cells with elongated nuclei, eosinophilic cytoplasm, and rare mitotic figures. Focal areas of increased cellularity and atypia were present, but no necrosis was identified, in Figure 2. The tumor cells reacted with immunohistochemical stains for desmin, smooth muscle actin, SMMHC, CD34 (focal), and vimentin. Additional immunostains were performed, including S-100, BCL-2, CD99, and beta-catenin. All of these were negative. Less than 2% of the cells showed reactivity with proliferation index Ki-67; see Table 2. The pathological findings were diagnostic of a smooth muscle neoplasm. The absence of pleomorphism, increased mitotic figures, necrosis, and poor differentiation distinguished SMT of UMP from LMS [7].

Even when smooth muscle tumors of the pleura appear benign, well-encapsulated, smooth, and without evidence of necrosis and show rare mitotic activity they can possess malignant potential and present as or transform in LMS; see Table 1 [7].

Primary and preferred treatment is surgical resection if feasible which can be performed using minimally invasive surgery such as VATS, if after surgical resection there are positive margins to consider reresection (preferable option) versus observation (watch and wait approach) of the remaining disease with serial imaging studies during follow-up [6]. Smooth muscle tumors may increase in size with local invasion to the mediastinum and other structures, which can jeopardize complete resection with curative intent. If further surgery is contraindicated and disease was left behind perhaps the role of radiation could be explored [17–20]. Al-Daraji et al. [7] reported a case where there was a concern for possible incomplete resection at the apex and this patient received radiation with the intention to reduce the risk of local recurrence. This patient was reported to be alive at 14 months of follow-up and without recurrence. At present, there is no role for adjuvant chemotherapy.

The prognosis appears to be good if the tumor is excised completely with negative margins, but routine follow-up should not be neglected. Due to the rarity of this entity and

TABLE 3: Immunohistochemical pattern in pleural spindle cell neoplasms [6].

Tumor	Vimentin	SMA	HHF-35	SMMHC	Desmin	CD34	S100	BCL-2	CD99	Cytokeratin
Smooth muscle tumor	+	+	+	+	+	+/−	−	−	−	−
Solitary fibrous tumor	+	−/+	−/+	−/+	−	+	−	+	+	−
Metastatic spindle cell carcinoma	+/−	−	−	−	−	−	−	−	−	+
Synovial sarcoma	+	−	−	−	−	−	−	+	+/−	+/−
Fibrosarcoma	+	−	−	−	−	−	−	−/+	−	−
Malignant peripheral nerve sheath tumor	+	−	−	−	−	−	−/+	−/+	−	−
Sarcomatous mesothelioma	+	−	−	−	−/+	−	−/+	−/+	−/+	+
Spindle cell thymoma	−	−	−	−	−	−	−	−/+	−	+

SMA: smooth muscle actin; HHF-35: actin muscle specific; SMMHC, smooth muscle myosin-heavy chain; +, positive staining; +/−, usually positive; −/+, rarely positive; and −, negative.

relative short follow-ups the behavior of this tumor cannot be properly evaluated.

4. Conclusion

Primary SMTs of the pleura are infrequent tumors and should be considered as a differential diagnosis when approaching a pleural mass. It seems to develop from the vascular smooth muscle cells. SMT-UMP tends to affect younger patients and LMS to tends to affect older patients. However, SMT-UMP can present in older patients as in our case. They appear to grow locally and invade nearby structures but there is not yet a single case reporting distant metastasis (the present case was not the exception). Tissue diagnosis and accurate histopathological evaluation are required. Although these tumors seem to possess low malignant potential they can be life threatening (they can grow very large causing serious symptomatology and/or degenerate into malignant tumors) and should be treated as such with appropriate surgical management and close follow-up.

Competing Interests

The authors declare that there is no conflict of interests regarding the publication of this paper.

References

[1] C. A. Moran, S. Suster, G. Perino, M. Kaneko, and M. N. Koss, "Malignant smooth muscle tumors presenting as mediastinal soft tissue masses: a clinicopathologic study of 10 cases," *Cancer*, vol. 74, pp. 2251–2260, 1994.

[2] P. L. Newman and C. D. M. Fletcher, "Smooth muscle tumours of the external genitalia: clinicopathological analysis of a series," *Histopathology*, vol. 18, no. 6, pp. 523–529, 1991.

[3] T. Diamond, M. H. D. Danton, and T. G. Parks, "Smooth muscle tumours of the alimentary tract," *Annals of the Royal College of Surgeons of England*, vol. 72, no. 5, pp. 316–320, 1990.

[4] A. R. Gibbs, "Smooth muscle tumours of the pleura," *Histopathology*, vol. 27, no. 3, pp. 295–296, 1995.

[5] C. A. Moran, S. Suster, and M. N. Koss, "Smooth muscle tumours presenting as pleural neoplasms," *Histopathology*, vol. 27, no. 3, pp. 227–234, 1995.

[6] D. M. Proca, P. J. Ross, J. Pratt, and W. L. Frankel, "Smooth muscle tumor of the pleura: a case report and review of the literature," *Archives of Pathology and Laboratory Medicine*, vol. 124, no. 11, pp. 1688–1692, 2000.

[7] W. I. Al-Daraji, W. D. Salman, Y. Nakhuda, F. Zaman, and B. Eyden, "Primary smooth muscle tumor of the pleura: a clinico-pathological case report with ultrastructural observations and a review of the literature," *Ultrastructural Pathology*, vol. 29, no. 5, pp. 389–398, 2005.

[8] N. Nose, M. Inoue, M. Kodate, M. Kawaguchi, and K. Yasumoto, "Leiomyoma originating from the extrapleural tissue of the chest wall," *Japanese Journal of Thoracic and Cardiovascular Surgery*, vol. 54, no. 6, pp. 242–245, 2006.

[9] T. Tanaka, A. Adachi, S. Iwata, Y. Nishimura, Y. Tanaka, and T. Kakegawa, "A case of leiomyoma of the chest wall," *Nippon Kyōbu Geka Gakkai Zasshi*, vol. 40, no. 9, pp. 1721–1724, 1992.

[10] X. Qiu, D. Zhu, S. Wei, G. Chen, J. Chen, and Q. Zhou, "Primary Leiomyoma of the pleura," *World Journal of Surgical Oncology*, vol. 9, article 76, 2011.

[11] H. Mochizuki, T. Okada, H. Yoshikawa, E. Suzuki, and F. Gejyo, "A case of primary pleural leiomyoma," *Nihon Kokyuki Gakkai Zasshi*, vol. 42, pp. 625–628, 2004.

[12] K. Turhan, A. Cakan, and U. Cagirici, "Leiomyoma: an unusual pleural tumor," *Report of a Case Turkish Respiratory Journal*, vol. 9, pp. 53–55, 2008.

[13] P. M. Rodríguez, J. L. Freixinet, M. L. Plaza, and R. Camacho, "Unusual primary pleural leiomyoma," *Interactive Cardiovascular and Thoracic Surgery*, vol. 10, no. 3, pp. 441–442, 2010.

[14] N. K. Kuman, E. Pabuşçu, and I. Meteoğlu, "Leiomyomas requiring chest wall resection and reconstruction," *General Thoracic and Cardiovascular Surgery*, vol. 62, no. 3, pp. 186–190, 2014.

[15] T. Nakada, T. Akiba, T. Inagaki, T. Morikawa, and T. Ohki, "A rare case of primary intercostal leiomyoma: complete resection followed by reconstruction using a Gore-Tex(®) dual mesh," *Annals of Thoracic and Cardiovascular Surgery*, vol. 20, supplement, pp. 617–621, 2014.

[16] S. Ziyade, M. Ugurlucan, O. Soysal, and O. C. Akdemir, "Leiomyoma of the extrapleural chest wall: an atypical location," *Archives of Medical Science*, vol. 7, no. 2, pp. 356–360, 2011.

[17] Y. Zhang, L. H. Clark, X. Sheng, and C. Zhou, "Successful en bloc venous resection with reconstruction and subsequent radiotherapy for 2 consecutive recurrences of intravenous leiomyoma—a case report," *BMC Cancer*, vol. 16, article 6, 2016.

[18] S. Ma, W. Bu, L. Wang et al., "Radiotherapy treatment of large esophageal leiomyosarcoma: a case report," *Oncology Letters*, vol. 9, no. 5, pp. 2422–2424, 2015.

[19] J. A. Blansfield, H. Chung, T. R. Sullivan Jr., and C. M. Pezzi, "Leiomyosarcoma of the major peripheral arteries: case report and review of the literature," *Annals of Vascular Surgery*, vol. 17, no. 5, Article ID 565e70, pp. 565–570, 2003.

[20] K. M. Alektiar, K. Hu, L. Anderson, M. F. Brennan, and L. B. Harrison, "High-dose-rate intraoperative radiation therapy (HDR-IORT) for retroperitoneal sarcomas," *International Journal of Radiation Oncology Biology Physics*, vol. 47, no. 1, pp. 157–163, 2000.

51

Pancreatic GIST in a Patient with Limited Stage Small Cell Lung Cancer: A Case Report and Review of Published Cases

Minh Phan,[1] Shari Jones,[2] Justin Jenkins,[3] Shubham Pant,[1] and Mohamad Khawandanah[1]

[1]Hematology-Oncology Section, Department of Medicine, The University of Oklahoma Health Sciences Center, Oklahoma City, OK 73104, USA
[2]Department of Internal Medicine, The University of Oklahoma Health Sciences Center, Oklahoma City, OK 73104, USA
[3]Department of Pathology, The University of Oklahoma Health Sciences Center, Oklahoma City, OK 73104, USA

Correspondence should be addressed to Mohamad Khawandanah; mohamad-khawandanah@ouhsc.edu

Academic Editor: Raffaele Palmirotta

Gastrointestinal stromal tumors (GISTs) are the most common mesenchymal tumors of the gastrointestinal tract and usually occur in the stomach and the small intestine. The pancreas is an extremely rare primary site for GISTs and there are 25 reported cases of pancreatic GIST with most being treated with surgical resection. We describe a 52-year-old African-American female who was diagnosed with limited stage small cell carcinoma in November 2009 and treated with concurrent cisplatin/etoposide chemotherapy and radiation. She subsequently achieved complete remission. Two years later she was diagnosed with localized pancreatic GIST by endoscopic ultrasonography guided fine needle aspiration. We treated her with a tyrosine kinase inhibitor (TKI) imatinib 400 mg oral dose daily as she declined surgery. Her disease is stable based on computed tomography imaging scans 40 months after diagnosis without any metastasis. To the best of our knowledge, our case is the second case of localized pancreatic GIST treated with TKI monotherapy.

1. Introduction

Gastrointestinal stromal tumors (GISTs) are the most common mesenchymal tumors of the gastrointestinal tract and usually occur in the stomach and the small intestine. The pancreas is an extremely rare primary site for GISTs. The annual incidence of GIST in the United States is 5000–6000/year and they are more common in the males, blacks, and the elderly [1, 2]. Workup of these lesions includes morphologic study and immunohistochemical and molecular diagnostic analysis. Historically, these neoplasms had been included under a number of diagnostic categories including leiomyoma, leiomyosarcoma, schwannoma, and leiomyoblastoma. Surgery was the only available treatment and this changed in 2001 after discovery of mutational activation of the KIT or PDGFRA genes [3] and the use of targeted therapies.

2. Methods

Abstracts, case reports, and case series of pancreatic GIST in the English literature were identified with no date limits until November 2015, by searching the keywords "pancreatic gastrointestinal tumors", "pancreatic GIST", and "extra gastrointestinal stromal tumors" in the National Library of Medicine, PubMed, OVID, and EMBASE search engines. Bibliographies of publications were also reviewed for additional relevant studies.

3. Case Presentation

A 52-year-old African-American female was diagnosed with limited stage small cell carcinoma in November 2009 and treated with concurrent cisplatin/etoposide chemotherapy and radiation. She achieved complete remission and underwent prophylactic whole brain radiation in March 2010. Two years later she started to complain of vague abdominal pain and this was investigated with computed tomography (CT) scans which revealed a 3.5 cm enhancing lesion in the pancreas in addition to multiple uterine fibroids (Figure 1).

She underwent endoscopic ultrasonography guided fine needle aspiration (EUS-FNA) of the pancreatic lesion

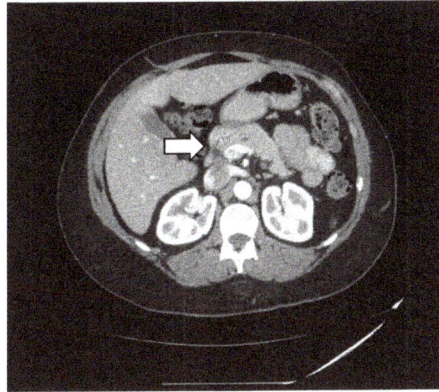

FIGURE 1: CT scan of the abdomen demonstrate a mass, arising from the uncinate process of the pancreas.

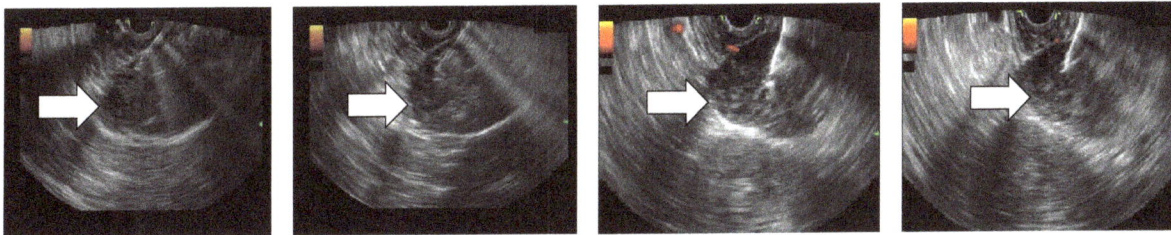

FIGURE 2: EUS showing hypoechoic mass in the pancreatic uncinate process during FNA procedure.

TABLE 1: Immunohistochemical stains performed on our pancreatic GIST case.

Stain	Result
CD117 (c-KIT)	Strongly and diffusely positive in spindle cells
DOG-1	Strongly and diffusely positive in spindle cells
Smooth muscle actin (SMA)	Negative in spindle cells
S-100 protein	Negative in spindle cells
ALK-1	Negative in spindle cells

(Figure 2). Cytopathology revealed atypical cells with spindle cell features. Another EUS-FNA along with core biopsy sampling was performed, yielding the pathological diagnosis of gastrointestinal stromal tumor. Immunohistochemical staining of stromal cells was positive for CD117 (c-kit) and DOG-1 and negative for smooth muscle actin, S-100 protein, and ALK-1 (Figure 3 and Table 1).

We proceeded with medical therapy as patient declined surgical approach, and she was started on treatment with imatinib 400 mg PO daily. During treatment, she experienced imatinib side effects including nausea, vomiting, and leg cramps; we controlled these with promethazine and carisoprodol. Her disease is stable based on CT scans 40 months after diagnosis without any evidence of metastatic disease.

4. Discussion

GISTs are group of tumors showing differentiation or derived from the interstitial cells of Cajal which works as the GI pacemaker cells and like GISTs, these cells express both KIT and CD34 [4, 5]. Eighty percent of GIST cases have a mutation in the KIT gene exon 8, 9, 11, 13, or 17 [6]. In around 7% of cases there are mutations in PDGFR exon 12, 14, 18 D842V, or 18 [7].

Rarely, wild-type adult GIST tumors are associated with activation of the succinate dehydrogenase (SDH) complex like cases of GIST associated with Carney triad or Neurofibromatosis 1 [8]. On the other hand, wild type is very common in pediatric GIST [9] in around 85% cases while only 10–15% of adult cases do not harbor any mutation in the KIT and PDGFR genes [10].

GISTs commonly involve the stomach (60%), jejunum and ileum (30%), duodenum (4-5%), rectum (4%), colon and appendix (1-2%), and esophagus (<1%) and rarely present as primary tumors outside the gastrointestinal lumen such as the omentum, mesentery, and urinary bladder [11–13] or as in our case the pancreas. Both extragastrointestinal GIST and GIST are thought to originate from the gut smooth muscle cells and interstitial cells of Cajal; the former is thought to contribute to the growth outside of the gastrointestinal tract [14]. Another theory is that extragastrointestinal GISTs are mural GISTs which result in extramural growth [14].

The incidence of GIST is around eleven per million population in an Icelandic study [15]. It is difficult to determine the incidence due to the rarity of extragastrointestinal GIST.

(a)   (b)   (c)   (d)

(e)

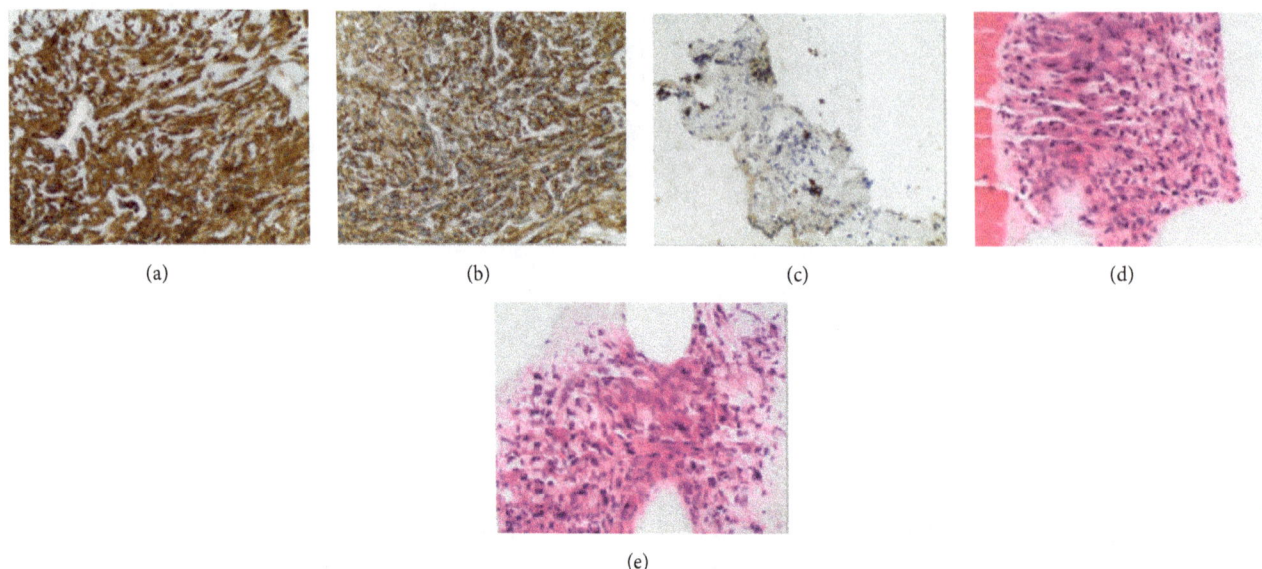

FIGURE 3: Pathology shows spindle cell lesion composed of intersecting fascicles and relatively bland spindle cells. (a) CD117, (b) DOG1, (c) spindled tumor cells which are negative for pancytokeratin, (d) atypical spindle cells on H&E stain, and (e) atypical spindle cells on H&E stain.

The mean age at diagnosis was 63 [1] for GIST compared to 53 for pancreatic GIST from the reviewed case reports. Gender involvement was not different between the pancreatic and extragastrointestinal GIST. A formal statistical analysis was not performed with the available case report data.

GISTs display two morphologic variants represented by the spindle cell and epithelioid subtypes. The spindle cell type is the most frequent, while the histological patterns relate to site of primary origin [16]. The majority of GISTs are strongly positive when stained with antibodies directed against the KIT protein (CD117), and the combination of CD34 and CD117 positivity aids in confirmation of the diagnosis of GIST. There are two targets that have been found to be useful in the diagnosis of GISTs: both C (PKC)-O and DOG1 are expressed in KIT positive and KIT negative GIST [17, 18].

Mutational analysis can aid in determining prognosis or if GIST will be responsive to imatinib therapy, it can also predict which dose level is most appropriate [19, 20]. For example, exon 9 mutant tumors carry the worst prognosis but have superior objective response to tumors with mutations in exon 11, and those patients with documented exon 9 mutations benefit from an 800 mg dose of imatinib rather than the standard 400 mg PO daily dose [21]. Routine mutation analysis is not recommended by the National Comprehensive Cancer Network (NCCN) GIST Task Force due to insufficient data for risk stratification and relapse prognostication [22]. Because of this report, we did not perform the mutation analysis on our patient. This is in contrast to the European Society for Medical Oncology guidelines which support administering an imatinib dose of 800 mg daily for exon 9 mutation [23]. The imatinib 400 mg regimen was chosen due to the Gastrointestinal Stromal Tumor Meta-Analysis Group data [24].

While imatinib can be used in the neoadjuvant or adjuvant setting, sunitinib—which is another tyrosine kinase inhibitor (TKI)—is frequently used as second-line therapy in refractory disease or in case of imatinib intolerance [25]. Sunitinib is administered at 50 mg starting dose in 6-week cycles with 4 weeks on and 2 weeks off treatment and can be also given as 37.5 mg PO daily which appears safe and effective [26]. Regorafenib is a TKI that targets multiple kinases including PDGFR, KIT, and vascular endothelial growth factor receptors; it can be used in advanced GIST after failure of both imatinib and sunitinib [27]. In the third-line setting, other TKIs such as sorafenib and nilotinib have significant clinical activity in imatinib and sunitinib resistant GIST and may represent an alternative for rechallenge treatment with imatinib, which is of limited benefit; nevertheless, it is superior to best supportive care in terms of overall survival [28]. Ganjoo et al. reported the use of pazopanib, another TKI, in a phase 2 clinical trial as a single agent with marginal activity in unselected heavily pretreated patients with advanced GIST [29].

To the best of our knowledge, our case is unique in terms of long survival with single nonsurgical modality and it is the second case of localized pancreatic GIST treated only with TKI. In the English literature there are 25 reported cases of pancreatic GIST (Table 2). Padhi et al. reported nineteen cases of pancreatic GIST gathered from 2000 to 2012 [30]. In 2015, Joseph et al. reported a case of a patient with pancreatic GIST that was started on imatinib but later developed metastatic disease and died 9 months later [31]. If the tumor can be resected, then treatment of choice would be surgery. The stabilization of the lesion in our patient with TKI therapy suggests that this is a reasonable therapeutic course in patients who are not surgical candidates. The lesion should

TABLE 2: List of published cases in English literature of pancreatic GIST.

Number of patients	Age	Gender	Primary treatment	Clinical presentation	Year of report	Author	Reference
1	54	Female	Surgery	Abdominal tumor	2004	Yamaura et al.	[32]
1	48	Female	Surgery	Asymptomatic abdominal mass	2004	Neto et al.	[33]
1	38	Female	Surgery	Not described	2005	Krska et al.	[34]
1	70	Female	Surgery	Asymptomatic abdominal mass	2005	Daum et al.	[35]
1	47	Male	n/a	Nausea/vomiting	2008	Yan et al.	[36]
1	55	Male	Surgery	Poor appetite, abdominal discomfort	2008	Yang et al.	[37]
1	63	Female	Surgery	Flank pain	2009	Harindhanavudhi et al.	[38]
1	58	Male	Surgery	Weight loss, dysuria	2009	Goh et al.	[39]
1	52	Female	Surgery	Epigastric pain	2009	Trabelsi et al.	[40]
1	42	Male	Surgery	Asymptomatic abdominal mass	2011	Meng et al.	[41]
1	42	Female	Surgery	Abdominal pain, loss of appetite, weight	2010	Padhi et al.	[42]
1	31	Male	Surgery	Abdominal pain, fatigue, weight loss	2010	Saif et al.	[43]
1	61	Male	Surgery	Fever, sweating, weight loss	2010	Crisan et al.	[44]
1	84	Male	Supportive	Abdominal distension, confusion, agitation	2010	Joshi and Rustagi	[45]
1	n/a	n/a	Surgery	n/a	2011	Barros et al.	[46]
1	74	Female	Surgery	Abdominal mass	2011	Čečka et al.	[47]
1	40	Male	Surgery	Athenia, abdominal pain, low grade fever, severe anemia, loss of appetite, weight loss	2011	Rao et al.	[48]
1	55	Male	Surgery	Postprandial abdominal discomfort	2012	Kim et al.	[49]
1	55	Female	Surgery	Abdominal pain	2012	Babu et al.	[50]
1	39	Male	Surgery	Weight loss, epigastric pain, constipation, anorexia	2013	Soufi et al.	[51]
1	30	Male	Surgery	Abdominal distension	2013	Serin et al.	[52]
1	74	Female	Surgery	Gastrointestinal bleeding	2014	Hansen et al.	[53]
1	56	Male	Surgery	Gastrointestinal hemorrhage, abdominal pain	2015	Aziret et al.	[54]
1	55	Male	Surgery	Asymptomatic	2015	Stanek et al.	[55]
1	60	Male	Medical	Abdominal pain	2015	Joseph et al.	[31]

be reevaluated for resection within three to four months [56]. Given the limited long term follow-up of patients with the pancreas as the site of origin, it is unclear whether pancreatic GISTs have a different natural history relative to luminal GISTs.

Consent

Written informed consent was obtained from the patient for the publication of this case report.

References

[1] T. Tran, J. A. Davila, and H. B. El-Serag, "The epidemiology of malignant gastrointestinal stromal tumors: an analysis of 1,458 cases from 1992 to 2000," *American Journal of Gastroenterology*, vol. 100, no. 1, pp. 162–168, 2005.

[2] C. D. M. Fletcher, J. J. Berman, C. Corless et al., "Diagnosis of gastrointestinal stromal tumors: a consensus approach," *Human Pathology*, vol. 33, no. 5, pp. 459–465, 2002.

[3] R. P. DeMatteo, J. J. Lewis, D. Leung, S. S. Mudan, J. M. Woodruff, and M. F. Brennan, "Two hundred gastrointestinal stromal tumors: recurrence patterns and prognostic factors for survival," *Annals of Surgery*, vol. 231, no. 1, pp. 51–58, 2000.

[4] C. D. M. Fletcher, J. J. Berman, C. Corless et al., "Diagnosis of gastrointestinal stromal tumors: a consensus approach," *International Journal of Surgical Pathology*, vol. 10, no. 2, pp. 81–89, 2002.

[5] S. Hirota, K. Isozaki, Y. Moriyama et al., "Gain-of-function mutations of c-kit in human gastrointestinal stromal tumors," *Science*, vol. 279, no. 5350, pp. 577–580, 1998.

[6] J. F. Emile, N. Theou, S. Tabone et al., "Clinicopathologic, phenotypic, and genotypic characteristics of gastrointestinal mesenchymal tumors," *Clinical Gastroenterology and Hepatology*, vol. 2, no. 7, pp. 597–605, 2004.

[7] C. L. Corless, A. Schroeder, D. Griffith et al., "PDGFRA mutations in gastrointestinal stromal tumors: frequency, spectrum and in vitro sensitivity to imatinib," *Journal of Clinical Oncology*, vol. 23, no. 23, pp. 5357–5364, 2005.

[8] K. A. Janeway, S. Y. Kim, M. Lodish et al., "Defects in succinate dehydrogenase in gastrointestinal stromal tumors lacking KIT and PDGFRA mutations," *Proceedings of the National Academy of Sciences of the United States of America*, vol. 108, no. 1, pp. 314–318, 2011.

[9] S. Prakash, L. Sarran, N. Socci et al., "Gastrointestinal stromal tumors in children and young adults: a clinicopathologic, molecular, and genomic study of 15 cases and review of the literature," *Journal of Pediatric Hematology/Oncology*, vol. 27, no. 4, pp. 179–187, 2005.

[10] M. Nannini, G. Biasco, A. Astolfi, and M. A. Pantaleo, "An overview on molecular biology of KIT/PDGFRA wild type (WT) gastrointestinal stromal tumours (GIST)," *Journal of Medical Genetics*, vol. 50, no. 10, pp. 653–661, 2013.

[11] M. Miettinen and J. Lasota, "Gastrointestinal stromal tumors: pathology and prognosis at different sites," *Seminars in Diagnostic Pathology*, vol. 23, no. 2, pp. 70–83, 2006.

[12] J. Lasota, J. A. Carlson, and M. Miettinen, "Spindle cell tumor of urinary bladder serosa with phenotypic and genotypic features of gastrointestinal stromal tumor," *Archives of Pathology and Laboratory Medicine*, vol. 124, no. 6, pp. 894–897, 2000.

[13] M. Miettinen, J. M. Monihan, M. Sarlomo-Rikala et al., "Gastrointestinal stromal tumors/smooth muscle tumors (GISTs) primary in the omentum and mesentery: clinicopathologic and immunohistochemical study of 26 cases," *The American Journal of Surgical Pathology*, vol. 23, no. 9, pp. 1109–1118, 1999.

[14] V. Beltrame, M. Gruppo, D. Pastorelli, S. Pizzi, S. Merigliano, and C. Sperti, "Extra-gastrointestinal stromal tumor of the pancreas: case report and review of the literature," *World Journal of Surgical Oncology*, vol. 12, no. 1, article 105, 2014.

[15] G. Tryggvason, H. G. Gíslason, M. K. Magnússon, and J. G. Jónasson, "Gastrointestinal stromal tumors in Iceland, 1990–2003: the Icelandic GIST study, a population-based incidence and pathologic risk stratification study," *International Journal of Cancer*, vol. 117, no. 2, pp. 289–293, 2005.

[16] L. J. Layfield and M. L. Wallander, "Diagnosis of gastrointestinal stromal tumors from minute specimens: cytomorphology, immunohistochemistry, and molecular diagnostic findings," *Diagnostic Cytopathology*, vol. 40, no. 6, pp. 484–490, 2012.

[17] I. Espinosa, C.-H. Lee, M. K. Kim et al., "A novel monoclonal antibody against DOG1 is a sensitive and specific marker for gastrointestinal stromal tumors," *The American Journal of Surgical Pathology*, vol. 32, no. 2, pp. 210–218, 2008.

[18] A. Motegi, S. Sakurai, H. Nakayama, T. Sano, T. Oyama, and T. Nakajima, "PKC theta, a novel immunohistochemical marker for gastrointestinal stromal tumors (GIST), especially useful for identifying KIT-negative tumors," *Pathology International*, vol. 55, no. 3, pp. 106–112, 2005.

[19] K. Kontogianni-Katsarou, E. Dimitriadis, C. Lariou, E. Kairi-Vassilatou, N. Pandis, and A. Kondi-Paphiti, "KIT exon 11 codon 557/558 deletion/insertion mutations define a subset of gastrointestinal stromal tumors with malignant potential," *World Journal of Gastroenterology*, vol. 14, no. 12, pp. 1891–1897, 2008.

[20] C. L. Corless and M. C. Heinrich, "Molecular pathobiology of gastrointestinal stromal sarcomas," *Annual Review of Pathology: Mechanisms of Disease*, vol. 3, pp. 557–586, 2008.

[21] M. Debiec-Rychter, R. Sciot, A. Le Cesne et al., "KIT mutations and dose selection for imatinib in patients with advanced gastrointestinal stromal tumours," *European Journal of Cancer*, vol. 42, no. 8, pp. 1093–1103, 2006.

[22] G. D. Demetri, M. von Mehren, C. R. Antonescu et al., "NCCN Task Force report: update on the management of patients with gastrointestinal stromal tumors," *Journal of the National Comprehensive Cancer Network*, vol. 8, supplement 2, pp. S1–S44, 2010.

[23] European Sarcoma Network Working Group, "Gastrointestinal stromal tumours: ESMO clinical practice guidelines for diagnosis, treatment and follow-up," *Annals of Oncology*, vol. 25, supplement 3, pp. iii21–iii26, 2014.

[24] M. Van Glabbeke, "Comparison of two doses of imatinib for the treatment of unresectable or metastatic gastrointestinal stromal tumors: a meta-analysis of 1,640 patients," *Journal of Clinical Oncology*, vol. 28, no. 7, pp. 1247–1253, 2010.

[25] G. D. Demetri, A. T. van Oosterom, C. R. Garrett et al., "Efficacy and safety of sunitinib in patients with advanced gastrointestinal stromal tumour after failure of imatinib: a randomised controlled trial," *The Lancet*, vol. 368, no. 9544, pp. 1329–1338, 2006.

[26] S. George, J. Y. Blay, P. G. Casali et al., "Clinical evaluation of continuous daily dosing of sunitinib malate in patients with advanced gastrointestinal stromal tumour after imatinib failure," *European Journal of Cancer*, vol. 45, no. 11, pp. 1959–1968, 2009.

[27] S. George, Q. Wang, M. C. Heinrich et al., "Efficacy and safety of regorafenib in patients with metastatic and/or unresectable GI stromal tumor after failure of imatinib and sunitinib: a multicenter phase II trial," *Journal of Clinical Oncology*, vol. 30, no. 19, pp. 2401–2407, 2012.

[28] A. Italiano, A. Cioffi, P. Coco et al., "Patterns of care, prognosis, and survival in patients with metastatic gastrointestinal stromal tumors (GIST) refractory to first-line imatinib and second-line sunitinib," *Annals of Surgical Oncology*, vol. 19, no. 5, pp. 1551–1559, 2012.

[29] K. N. Ganjoo, V. M. Villalobos, A. Kamaya et al., "A multicenter phase II study of pazopanib in patients with advanced gastrointestinal stromal tumors (GIST) following failure of at least imatinib and sunitinib," *Annals of Oncology*, vol. 25, no. 1, pp. 236–240, 2014.

[30] S. Padhi, R. Sarangi, and S. Mallick, "Pancreatic extragastrointestinal stromal tumors, interstitial Cajal like cells, and telocytes," *Journal of the Pancreas*, vol. 14, no. 1, pp. 1–14, 2013.

[31] P. Joseph, R. Goyal, P. Bansal, R. Parmar, and S. Dutt, "Pancreatic extra-gastrointestinal stromal tumour with documentation of C-Kit mutation: a case report," *Journal of Clinical and Diagnostic Research*, vol. 9, no. 4, pp. 17–18, 2015.

[32] K. Yamaura, K. Kato, M. Miyazawa et al., "Stromal tumor of the pancreas with expression of c-kit protein: report of a case," *Journal of Gastroenterology and Hepatology*, vol. 19, no. 4, pp. 467–470, 2004.

[33] M. R. M. Neto, T. N. Machuca, R. V. Pinho, L. D. Yuasa, and L. F. Bleggi-Torres, "Gastrointestinal stromal tumor: report of two unusual cases," *Virchows Archiv*, vol. 444, no. 6, pp. 594–596, 2004.

[34] Z. Krska, M. Peskova, C. Povysil et al., "GIST of pancreas," *Prague Medical Report*, vol. 106, pp. 201–208, 2005.

[35] O. Daum, J. Klecka, J. Ferda et al., "Gastrointestinal stromal tumor of the pancreas: case report with documentation of KIT gene mutation," *Virchows Archiv*, vol. 446, no. 4, pp. 470–472, 2005.

[36] B. M. Yan, R. K. Pai, and J. Van Dam, "Diagnosis of pancreatic gastrointestinal stromal tumor by EUS guided FNA," *Journal of the Pancreas*, vol. 9, no. 2, pp. 192–196, 2008.

[37] F. Yang, J. Long, Y. Di et al., "A giant cystic lesion in the epigastric region," *Gut*, vol. 57, no. 11, pp. 1494–1636, 2008.

[38] T. Harindhanavudhi, T. Tanawuttiwat, J. Pyle, and R. Silva, "Extra-gastrointestinal stromal tumor presenting as hemorrhagic pancreatic cyst diagnosed by EUS-FNA," *Journal of the Pancreas*, vol. 10, no. 2, pp. 189–191, 2009.

[39] B. K. P. Goh, S. M. Kesavan, and W.-K. Wong, "An unusual cause of a pancreatic head tumor," *Gastroenterology*, vol. 137, no. 2, pp. e5–e6, 2009.

[40] A. Trabelsi, L. B. Yacoub-Abid, A. Mtimet et al., "Gastrointestinal stromal tumor of the pancreas: a case report and review of the literature," *North American Journal of Medical Sciences*, vol. 1, no. 6, pp. 324–326, 2009.

[41] L. Meng, S.-H. Fang, and M. Jin, "An unusual case of pancreatic and gastric neoplasms (2010: 12b). Malignant GISTs originating from the pancreas and stomach," *European Radiology*, vol. 21, no. 3, pp. 663–665, 2011.

[42] S. Padhi, R. Kongara, S. G. Uppin et al., "Extragastrointestinal stromal tumor arising in the pancreas: a case report with a review of the literature," *Journal of the Pancreas*, vol. 11, no. 3, pp. 244–248, 2010.

[43] M. W. Saif, S. Hotchkiss, and K. Kaley, "Gastrointestinal stromal tumors of the pancreas," *Journal of the Pancreas*, vol. 11, no. 4, pp. 405–412, 2010.

[44] A. Crisan, E. Nicoara, V. Cucui, G. Cornea, and R. Laza, "Prolonged fever associated with gastrointestinal stromal tumor—case report," *Journal of Experimental Medical & Surgical Research*, vol. 17, pp. 219–224, 2010.

[45] J. Joshi and T. Rustagi, "Pancreatic extra-gastrointestinal stromal tumor: an unusual presentation of a rare diagnosis," *Gastrointestinal Cancer Research*, supplement 1, pp. S29–S30, 2010.

[46] A. Barros, E. Linhares, M. Valadão et al., "Extragastrointestinal stromal tumors (EGIST): a series of case reports," *Hepato-Gastroenterology*, vol. 58, no. 107-108, pp. 865–868, 2011.

[47] F. Čečka, B. Jon, A. Ferko, Z. Šubrt, D. H. Nikolov, and V. Tyčová, "Long-term survival of a patient after resection of a gastrointestinal stromal tumor arising from the pancreas," *Hepatobiliary and Pancreatic Diseases International*, vol. 10, no. 3, pp. 330–332, 2011.

[48] R. N. Rao, M. Vij, N. Singla, and A. Kumar, "Malignant pancreatic extra-gastrointestinal stromal tumor diagnosed by ultrasound guided fine needle aspiration cytology. A case report with a review of the literature," *Journal of the Pancreas*, vol. 12, no. 3, pp. 283–286, 2011.

[49] H.-H. Kim, Y.-S. Koh, E.-K. Park et al., "Primary extragastrointestinal stromal tumor arising in the pancreas: report of a case," *Surgery Today*, vol. 42, no. 4, pp. 386–390, 2012.

[50] S. R. Babu, S. Kumari, Y. Zhang, A. Su, W. Wang, and B. Tian, "Extra gastrointestinal stromal tumor arising in the pancreas: a case report and literature review," *Journal of Gastroenterology and Hepatology Research*, vol. 1, pp. 80–83, 2012.

[51] M. Soufi, M. Bouziane, R. Massrouri, and B. Chad, "Pancreatic GIST with pancreas divisum: a new entity," *International Journal of Surgery Case Reports*, vol. 4, no. 1, pp. 68–71, 2013.

[52] K. R. Serin, M. Keskin, M. Güllüoğlu, and A. Emre, "Atypical localisation of a gastrointestinal stromal tumour: a case report of pancreas gastrointestinal stromal tumour," *Ulusal Cerrahi Dergisi*, vol. 29, no. 1, pp. 42–44, 2013.

[53] C. A. P. Hansen, F. F. José, and N. P. Caluz, "Gastrointestinal stromal tumor (GIST) mistaken for pancreatic pseudocyst—case report and literature review," *Clinical Case Reports*, vol. 2, no. 5, pp. 197–200, 2014.

[54] M. Aziret, S. Çetinkünar, E. Aktaş, O. İrkörücü, İ. Bali, and H. Erdem, "Pancreatic gastrointestinal stromal tumor after upper gastrointestinal hemorrhage and performance of whipple procedure: a case report and literature review," *American Journal of Case Reports*, vol. 16, pp. 509–513, 2015.

[55] M. Stanek, M. Pędziwiatr, M. Matłok, and A. Budzyński, "Laparoscopic removal of gastrointestinal stromal tumors of uncinate process of pancreas," *Wideochirurgia I Inne Techniki Maloinwazyjne*, vol. 10, no. 2, pp. 311–315, 2015.

[56] F. Bormann, W. Wild, H. Aksoy, P. Dörr, S. Schmeck, and M. Schwarzbach, "A pancreatic head tumor arising as a duodenal GIST: a case report and review of the literature," *Case Reports in Medicine*, vol. 2014, Article ID 420295, 4 pages, 2014.

52

Presentation of Two Cases with Early Extracranial Metastases from Glioblastoma and Review of the Literature

Maria Dinche Johansen,[1] Per Rochat,[2] Ian Law,[3] David Scheie,[4] Hans Skovgaard Poulsen,[1,5] and Aida Muhic[5]

[1]Department of Radiation Biology, The Finsen Center, Rigshospitalet, Blegdamsvej 9, 2100 Copenhagen, Denmark
[2]Department of Neurosurgery, The Neurocenter, Rigshospitalet, Blegdamsvej 9, 2100 Copenhagen, Denmark
[3]Department of Clinical Physiology, Nuclear Medicine and PET, Center of Diagnostic Investigation, Rigshospitalet, Blegdamsvej 9, 2100 Copenhagen, Denmark
[4]Department of Pathology, Center of Diagnostic Investigation, Rigshospitalet, Blegdamsvej 9, 2100 Copenhagen, Denmark
[5]Department of Oncology, The Finsen Center, Rigshospitalet, Blegdamsvej 9, 2100 Copenhagen, Denmark

Correspondence should be addressed to Maria Dinche Johansen; mariadinchejohansen@gmail.com

Academic Editor: Didier Frappaz

Extracranial metastases from glioblastoma are rare. We report two patients with extracranial metastases from glioblastoma. Case 1 concerns a 59-year-old woman with multiple metastases that spread early in the course of disease. What makes this case unusual is that the tumor had grown into the falx close to the straight sinus and this might be an explanation to the early and extensive metastases. Case 2 presents a 60-year-old man with liver metastasis found at autopsy, and, in this case, it is more difficult to find an explanation. This patient had two spontaneous intracerebral bleeding incidents and extensive bleeding during acute surgery with tumor removal, which might have induced extracranial seeding. The cases presented might have hematogenous spreading in common as an explanation to extracranial metastases from GBM.

1. Introduction

Glioblastoma (GBM) is the most frequent adult primary tumor of the central nervous system with median survival of 14.6 months in patients with newly diagnosed glioblastoma. The majority of patients experience local progression within the central nervous system [1].

Extracranial metastases (ECMs) are uncommon events seen in these patients, and most patients metastasize to only one or two extracranial foci [2]. Most frequent localization of ECM is regional lymph nodes, mostly cervical, lungs, liver, and bone [2, 3]. The rarity of ECM makes epidemiological analysis challenging, but it has been suggested that the median time from diagnosis to detection of ECM is 8.5 months and the time from ECM to death is 1.5 months [2]. A study has found that 20% of GBM patients have circulating tumor cells in peripheral blood, pointing out the ability to escape the central nervous system [4]. This combined with longer survival time should increase the awareness of ECM.

Here, we report two cases that demonstrate the ability of GBM to metastasize in one case to multiple organs simultaneously.

2. Case Presentations

2.1. Case 1. This case presents a 59-year-old woman with a history of type 2 diabetes, hypertension, and tobacco consumption (20 cigarettes per day for 45 years). The patient visited an ophthalmologist due to three months of blurred vision and two months of headache. This revealed impaired vision (right sided homonymous hemianopsia) and memory and concentration difficulties. Contrast enhanced CT and MRI of the brain showed a $4 \times 5 \times 4$ cm solitaire left sided occipital tumor with midline shift. At this point, helical CT

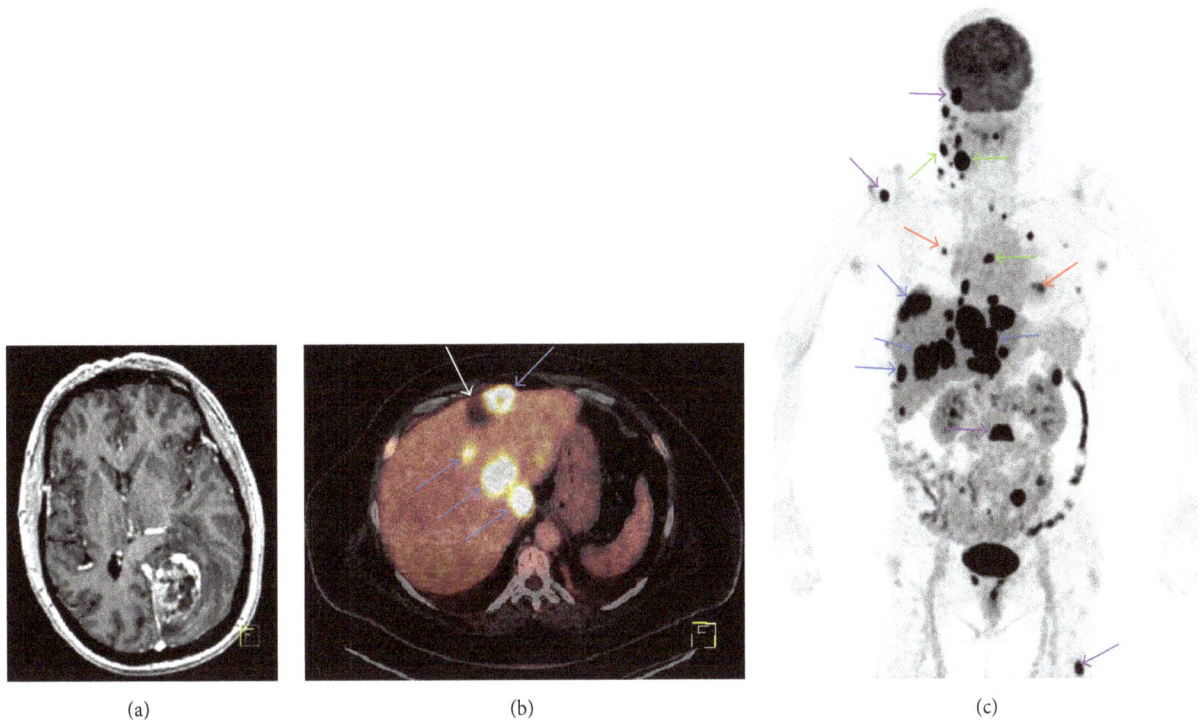

FIGURE 1: Case 1. (a) Preoperative post-contrast enhanced T1 weighted MRI showing the localization of the tumor in close proximity to the falx. (b) Fused FDG PET/CT scanning at liver level 5 months after diagnosis of GBM showing multiple metabolically active metastases (blue) and inactive liver cyst (white). (c) Frontal maximum intensity projection (MIP) image of whole body FDG PET scanning identifying disseminated metastatic spread to lymph nodes (green), lungs (red), bone (purple), and liver (blue). Physiological excretion to intestines, kidneys, and the bladder.

of thorax and abdomen was inconspicuous. The patient was treated with corticosteroids.

Two weeks later macro radical tumor resection was achieved using Gliolan® when the patient underwent left sided occipital craniotomy. During surgery, there was copious venous bleeding. Early postoperative post-contrast T1 weighted MRI showed no measurable tumor. Postoperatively the patient suffered from right sided hemianopsia. Histological examination revealed a cellular astrocytic glioma with pleomorphic nuclei, numerous mitoses, microvascular proliferation, pseudopalisading necrosis, and thrombosed vessels. Upon immunohistochemical examination, the tumor cells stained positive for GFAP, p53 (pronounced and strong in almost all tumor cells), map2, and olig2. Immunohistochemical stainings did not reveal IDH1- or ATRX-mutations. Ki67 was high. These findings were compatible with glioblastoma, WHO grade IV. PCR-analysis revealed an average O^6-methylguanine-DNA methyltransferase (MGMT) promoter methylation of 18%. PET scanning using the radiolabeled amino acid analog O-(2-^{18}F-fluoroethyl)-L-tyrosine (FET) performed at radiation treatment planning revealed a few mL of active tissue close to the cortex. The patient received radiotherapy, 2 Gy/5 days per week, for a total dose of 60 Gy with concomitant chemotherapy (temozolomide 75 mg/m^2 per day) for six weeks. This was followed by adjuvant chemotherapy temozolomide; the first dose was administered at 150 mg/m^2 for five days and second and third cycles were

administered at 200 mg/m^2 for five days. Routine surveillance MRI from the start of the second series of adjuvant chemotherapy found no sign of tumor recurrence. Clinically, however, the patient complained about circumscribed pain on the right abdominal side and on the right side of her neck. This was examined at a local hospital with ultra sound, whole body FDG PET/CT scanning (Figures 1(b) and 1(c)) and three biopsies of the cervical lymph nodes. There were no signs of local recurrence at the resection cavity on brain MRI.

The biopsies were examined by pathologists at the local hospital and reexamined by neuropathologists who specialize in neurooncology. Microscopic examination revealed pronounced tumor necrosis. Tumor cells were large and epithelioid with vesicular nuclei with prominent nucleoli (Figure 2(a)). Spindled cells were also observed. There were numerous mitoses. The tumor cells stained positive for S-100, vimentin, CD56, and GFAP (Figure 2(b)). There was focal staining for olig2 and synaptophysin, while map2 was almost negative. As in the brain tumor, the cells showed strong and pronounced staining for p53. There were negative stainings for pancytokeratin, CK7, CK20, TTF1, melan A, and CD45. The average MGMT promoter methylation was 2%. The diagnosis was lymph node metastasis from malignant tumor, most likely glioblastoma. The conclusion based on scans and histology was multiple glioblastoma metastases to lymph nodes in cervical and mediastinal region, liver, bones, and both lungs.

(a)

(b)

(c)

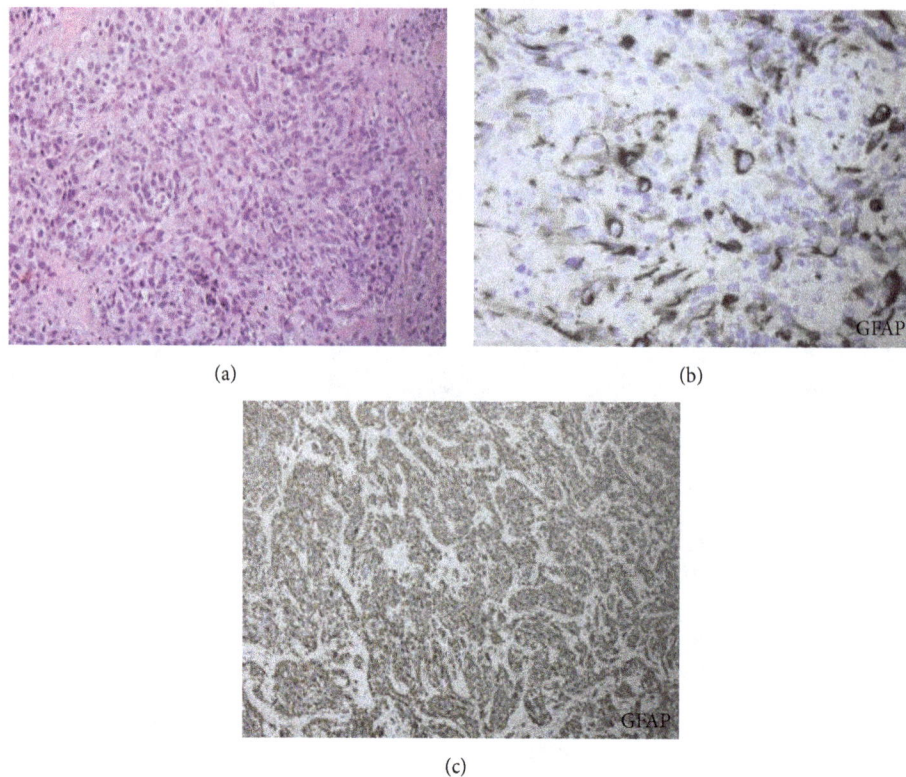

FIGURE 2: Histopathology from both cases. (a) HE staining (×20) of cervical lymph node metastasis from case 1. (b) GFAP staining (×40) of cervical lymph node metastasis from case 1. (c) GFAP staining (×10) of liver metastasis from case 2.

Second line treatment with irinotecan (250 mg) and bevacizumab (1000 mg) was initiated, but this was discontinued after one series due to deterioration of the patient's clinical condition.

During this period—from lymph node biopsy till admission to hospice—blood test showed signs of liver damage with elevated and increasing values of lactate dehydrogenase (LDH; 230–1331 U/L [normal range, <205 U/L]), elevated alkaline phosphatase (134–446 U/L [normal range, <105 U/L]), normal to slightly elevated alanine transferase (ALAT; 22–68 U/L [normal range, <45 U/L]), normal bilirubin (6–12 μmol/L [normal range, 5–25 μmol/L]), and decreased lymphocytes (0.26–1.1 × 10^9 [normal range, 1.0–3.5 × 10^9]). No further diagnostic investigations were performed out of respect for the patient's wish.

The patient was referred to hospice, where she had a rapid decline with confusion, insufficient nutritional intake, nausea, and increased pain. She died eight months after diagnosis with a clinical pattern of liver insufficiency.

2.2. *Case 2.* The second case presents a 60-year-old man with a history of hypertension. He was brought to the emergency room because of several generalized tonic-clonic seizures, and a head CT showed a frontal intracerebral hemorrhage. In the following weeks, two MRI scans had to be cancelled because the patient suffered from claustrophobia and could not cooperate. Contrast CT scan was not performed, even though it would have been relevant. A cerebral angiography

was performed and excluded a vascular cause of the hemorrhage. A frontal tumor was found when the patient had an MRI four months after the initial intracerebral hemorrhage.

The patient suffered from several subsequent seizures. An operation was scheduled for removal of the tumor. The patient was brought to the emergency room a few days before the scheduled surgery with decreasing consciousness, and an acute CT scan revealed a new bleeding from the tumor. He therefore underwent emergency surgery during which there was extensive bleeding during removal of the tumor. The patient had no early postoperative MRI because the hypothesized diagnosis was metastasis from an unknown malignant melanoma. The microscopic examination revealed a malignant astrocytoma with numerous mitoses, microvascular proliferation, and pseudopalisading necrosis. The tumor cells stained positive for GFAP, map2, and olig2. p53 demonstrated weak staining. Immunohistochemical stainings did not reveal IDH1- or ATRX-mutations. Ki67 was high. The findings were compatible with glioblastoma, WHO grade IV. The average MGMT promoter methylation was 42%.

Due to the new intracerebral bleeding, the patient spent one month at an intensive care unit and after this the patient and his family decided not to go through radiation. At this point, the patient was at performance status 4 and was treated at a palliative care unit until his death 10 months after his first hemorrhage. An autopsy was performed, and this revealed well demarcated solid metastasis in the liver. The solid metastasis measured 1 × 1 × 0.5 cm. Microscopic examination revealed a metastasis composed of spindled cells with scattered mitoses. Necrosis or microvascular proliferation was not observed. Immunohistochemical staining revealed strong and uniform staining for GFAP (Figure 2(c)) and S-100 but not IDH1-mutation, and they were negative for map2, olig2, melan A, pancytokeratin, desmin, and actin. P53 staining was weak. These findings were compatible with metastasis from glioblastoma. The MGMT promoter methylation was 37%. There was no suspicion or complaints during the course of the disease that could lead to suspicion of liver metastasis.

3. Discussion

Despite the rarity, ECMs from GBM have been known for many years, with the first documented case in 1928 [5]. In 1955, Weiss established diagnostic criteria for extraneural metastases from primary CNS tumors. These included a clinical history of primary CNS tumor, a complete postmortem examination, and histological correlation between the primary CNS tumor and the presumed extraneural metastases [6]. Today, not all new cases have a complete postmortem examination because of new imaging methods—such as PET/CT scans—making it possible to detect a potential undiscovered primary tumor other than GBM.

In a meta-analysis by Lun et al., 83 published cases of ECM from GBM were found in the period from 1928 to 2009 [2]. Increasing incidence of ECM has been suggested but possible explanations are increased interest among specialists, improved access to health care, improved neuroimaging, and advanced multimodal treatment of gliomas [2, 7]. A meta-analysis by Anghileri et al. supports the idea that prolonged survival of GBM patients is associated with greater risk of ECM and it is emphasized that this finding does not rule out the hypothesis that GBM subclones contribute to tumor cell dissemination [4, 8].

The rarity of GBM may be due to a number of factors: the preference of GBM cells to adhere to neural stroma, the low number of circulating GBM cells compared to the number of circulating monocytes, and the need for a metastatic niche in distant organs in order for GBM cells to establish a metastasis [2].

Most frequent localization of ECM is regional lymph nodes, mostly cervical, lungs, liver, and bone [3]. Although ECMs are mostly seen in patients with preceding intracranial surgery, such as ventriculoperitoneal shunt [9], ECM in the absence of previous surgery has been described [10]. In most previously published cases, the tumor metastasized to either only one or two extracranial organs or the time from diagnosis to detection of ECM was more than 5 months [2]. In their meta-analysis, Lun et al. suggest that it may be more difficult to detect neck and liver metastasis as fast as metastasis in other areas [2].

So far, no standard treatment for ECM exists. This might be because the patients are already in the late stage of the disease when the metastases are discovered, and at that point only palliative care is needed. Ray et al. suggest organ-specific considerations for patients with ECM and that the oncological treatment focuses on systemic chemotherapy [11].

Our case 1 had early multiple metastases to bone, liver, lymph nodes, and lungs. One explanation could be the localization of the tumor (Figure 1(a)). From both the MRI and surgical procedure, it is clear that this tumor had grown into the falx near the straight sinus. It is possible that the tumor spread hematogenously—perhaps even before surgery—due to this intimate contact with the venous structures outside the blood brain barrier. Other interesting observations in case 1 are strong and pronounced staining for p53, in both tumor and metastasis, and change of MGMT status from positive to negative when comparing primary tumor to metastasis (cut-off at 10%). The metastatic potential of the tumor cells increases with a gain-of-function mutation of p53 [12], and the negative MGMT status in the metastasis makes it less vulnerable to treatment with temozolomide [13]. This supports the idea of heterogeneity of the primary tumor and the idea of a subclone of temozolomide resistant cells managing to grow despite chemotherapy. These factors combined could have created an environment suitable for metastases. P53 gene mutations and differential clone selection have been suggested to be related to the metastatic potential of GBM [14]. In distant melanoma metastasis, it has been reported that one-third of the patients had MGMT hypermethylation [15]. It remains unknown if the interaction between MGMT status and temozolomide makes ECM from GBM more likely.

In the second case, the patient had two spontaneous bleeding incidents. These are rare in GBM compared to brain metastasis from malignant melanomas and renal cell carcinoma where bleeding incidents frequently occur. The GBM in this patient might have spread in relation to the intracerebral bleeding incidents but that is only theoretical, and in reality we do not have a plausible reason for spreading of this patient's GBM outside the blood brain barrier.

In conclusion, the cases presented might have hematogenous spreading in common as an explanation to extracranial metastases from GBM. Clinicians should keep in mind the potential of GBM to metastasize in order to diagnose ECM early. Even though this might not prolong the patients' survival, the quality of life and palliative treatment may improve. In the future, it would be relevant to make clinical guidelines to aid the clinicians in handling ECM in GBM patients.

References

[1] R. Stupp, W. P. Mason, M. J. van den Bent et al., "Radiotherapy plus concomitant and adjuvant temozolomide for glioblastoma," *The New England Journal of Medicine*, vol. 352, no. 10, pp. 987–996, 2005.

[2] M. Lun, E. Lok, S. Gautam, E. Wu, and E. T. Wong, "The natural history of extracranial metastasis from glioblastoma multiforme," *Journal of Neuro-Oncology*, vol. 105, no. 2, pp. 261–273, 2011.

[3] M. Piccirilli, G. M. F. Brunetto, G. Rocchi, F. Giangaspero, and M. Salvati, "Extra central nervous system metastases from

cerebral glioblastoma multiforme in elderly patients. Clinico-pathological remarks on our series of seven cases and critical review of the literature," *Tumori*, vol. 94, no. 1, pp. 40–51, 2008.

[4] C. Müller, J. Holtschmidt, M. Auer et al., "Hematogenous dissemination of glioblastoma multiforme," *Science Translational Medicine*, vol. 6, no. 247, Article ID 247ra101, 2014.

[5] L. Davis, "Spongioblastoma multiforme of the brain," *Annals of Surgery*, vol. 87, no. 1, pp. 8–14, 1928.

[6] L. Weiss, "A metastasizing ependymoma of the cauda equina," *Cancer*, vol. 8, no. 1, pp. 161–171, 1955.

[7] J. Undabeitia, M. Castle, M. Arrazola, C. Pendleton, I. Ruiz, and E. Úrculo, "Multiple extraneural metastasis of glioblastoma multiforme," *Anales del Sistema Sanitario de Navarra*, vol. 38, no. 1, pp. 157–161, 2015.

[8] E. Anghileri, M. Castiglione, R. Nunziata et al., "Erratum to: extraneural metastases in glioblastoma patients: two cases with YKL-40-positive glioblastomas and a meta-analysis of the literature," *Neurosurgical Review*, vol. 38, no. 4, article 773, 2015.

[9] A. Narayan, G. Jallo, and T. A. Huisman, "Extracranial, peritoneal seeding of primary malignant brain tumors through ventriculo-peritoneal shunts in children: case report and review of the literature," *The Neuroradiology Journal*, vol. 28, no. 5, pp. 536–539, 2015.

[10] S. Hulbanni and P. A. Goodman, "Glioblastoma multiforme with extraneural metastases in the absence of previous surgery," *Cancer*, vol. 37, no. 3, pp. 1577–1583, 1976.

[11] A. Ray, S. Manjila, A. Hdeib et al., "Extracranial metastasis of gliobastoma: three illustrative cases and current review of the molecular pathology and management strategies," *Molecular and Clinical Oncology*, vol. 3, no. 3, pp. 479–486, 2015.

[12] E. Powell, D. Piwnica-Worms, and H. Piwnica-Worms, "Contribution of p53 to metastasis," *Cancer Discovery*, vol. 4, no. 4, pp. 405–414, 2014.

[13] M. E. Hegi, A.-C. Diserens, T. Gorlia et al., "MGMT gene silencing and benefit from temozolomide in glioblastoma," *The New England Journal of Medicine*, vol. 352, no. 10, pp. 997–1003, 2005.

[14] C. C. Park, C. Hartmann, R. Folkerth et al., "Systemic metastasis in glioblastoma may represent the emergence of neoplastic subclones," *Journal of Neuropathology and Experimental Neurology*, vol. 59, no. 12, pp. 1044–1050, 2000.

[15] M. R. J. Kohonen-Corish, W. A. Cooper, J. Saab, J. F. Thompson, R. J. A. Trent, and M. J. Millward, "Promoter hypermethylation of the O^6-methylguanine DNA methyltransferase gene and microsatellite instability in metastatic melanoma," *Journal of Investigative Dermatology*, vol. 126, no. 1, pp. 167–171, 2006.

53

Metastasis-Induced Acute Pancreatitis Successfully Treated with Chemotherapy and Radiotherapy in a Patient with Small Cell Lung Cancer

Kerem Okutur,[1] Mustafa Bozkurt,[1] Taner Korkmaz,[2] Ercan Karaaslan,[3] Levent Guner,[4] Suha Goksel,[5] and Gokhan Demir[1]

[1]*Department of Medical Oncology, Acibadem University School of Medicine, Buyukdere Caddesi, No. 40, Sariyer, 34453 Istanbul, Turkey*
[2]*Department of Medical Oncology, Acibadem Maslak Hospital, Buyukdere Caddesi, No. 40, Sariyer, 34453 Istanbul, Turkey*
[3]*Department of Radiology, Acibadem University School of Medicine, Buyukdere Caddesi, No. 40, Sariyer, 34453 Istanbul, Turkey*
[4]*Department of Nuclear Medicine, Acibadem University School of Medicine, Buyukdere Caddesi, No. 40, Sariyer, 34453 Istanbul, Turkey*
[5]*Department of Pathology, Acibadem Maslak Hospital, Buyukdere Caddesi, No. 40, Sariyer, 34453 Istanbul, Turkey*

Correspondence should be addressed to Kerem Okutur; keremokutur@gmail.com

Academic Editor: Francesco A. Mauri

Although involvement of pancreas is a common finding in small cell lung cancer (SCLC), metastasis-induced acute pancreatitis (MIAP) is very rare. A 50-year-old female with SCLC who had limited disease and achieved full response after treatment presented with acute pancreatitis during her follow-up. The radiologic studies revealed a small area causing obliteration of the pancreatic duct without mass in the pancreatic neck, and endoscopic ultrasound-guided fine-needle aspiration (EUS-FNA) confirmed the metastasis of SCLC. The patient was treated successfully with systemic chemotherapy and radiotherapy delivered to pancreatic field. In SCLC, cases of MIAP can be encountered with conventional computed tomography with no mass image, and positron emission tomography and EUS-FNA can be useful for diagnosis of such cases. Aggressive systemic and local treatment can prolong survival, especially in patients with good performance status.

1. Introduction

Metastatic involvement of pancreas is rare and accounts for 2–5% of all pancreatic tumors [1]. Its incidence varies from 3% to 12% in autopsy series [2]. Tumors mostly metastatic to pancreas include renal cell carcinoma, melanoma, lung, colon, and gastric cancers. It usually appears as a late manifestation of disease and represents the diffuse spread of primary tumor [2].

Small cell lung cancer (SCLC) is a subtype of lung cancer with aggressive course and poor prognosis. Although it mostly spreads to the lungs, brain, bones, lymph nodes, and adrenal glands, it can involve almost all organs and tissues of the body. Although metastatic pancreatic involvement is a common finding of autopsy series in SCLC, metastasis-induced acute pancreatitis (MIAP) is very rare [2–4]. Here we

reported a 50-year-old woman with SCLC who was admitted for attacks of acute pancreatitis and was diagnosed with MIAP.

2. Case Report

The medical work-up of a 50-year-old female patient who applied for chronic cough revealed a mass in the right lung. She had a 40-year pack smoking history and no history of alcohol abuse. Bronchoscopy showed an occlusive mass in the lateral segment bronchus of the right middle lobe and ^{18}F-fluorodeoxyglucose (FDG) positron emission tomography-computed tomography (PET-CT) demonstrated a primary mass distal to the bronchus of the right middle lobe and hypermetabolic enlarged lymph nodes in the right lower

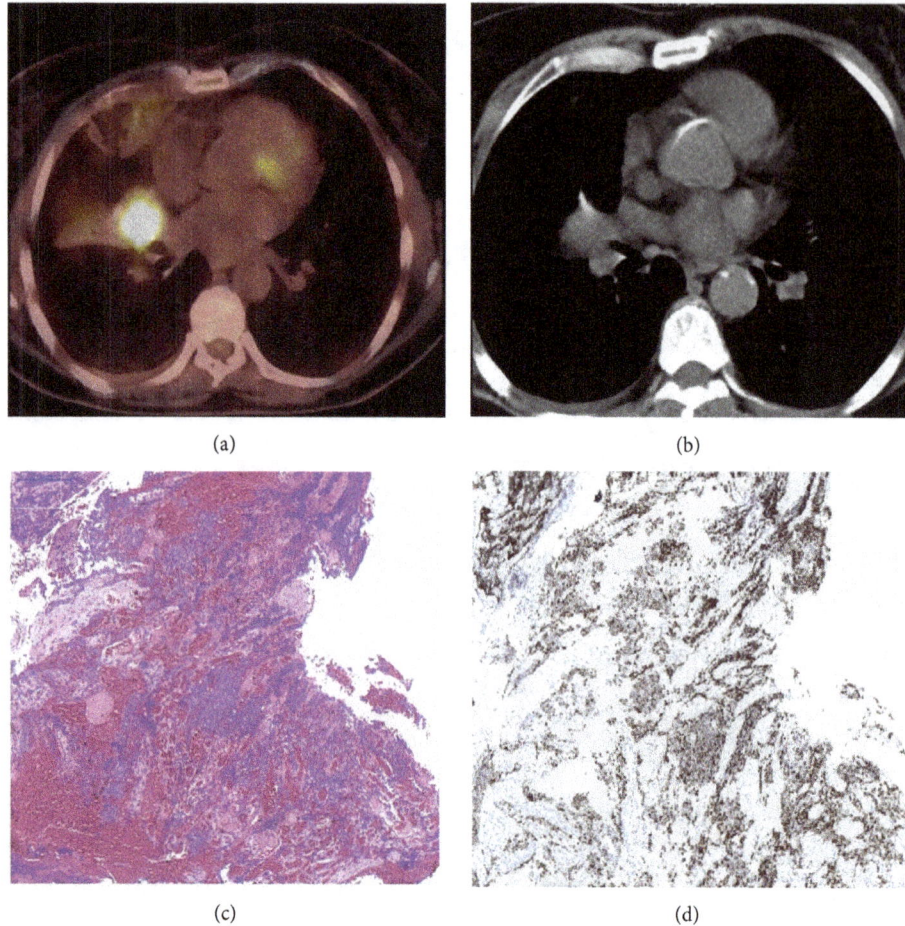

FIGURE 1: ((a) and (b)) A hypermetabolic primary mass distal to the bronchus of the right middle lobe on PET-CT. (c) Infiltration of small cell carcinoma in transbronchial biopsy of the mass (H&E, ×10). (d) Thyroid transcription factor-1 (TTF-1) positive staining of tumor cells (TTF-1, ×10).

and upper paratracheal region and the right supraclavicular region (Figures 1(a) and 1(b)). Bronchoscopic biopsy from the mass confirmed small cell carcinoma (Figures 1(c) and 1(d)). Patient's cranial magnetic resonance imaging (MRI) showed no metastasis, and then she was diagnosed with limited-stage SCLC and started cisplatin-etoposide concurrently with radiotherapy. Treatment was completed without major side effects and a PET-CT was performed after a month, which showed a full metabolic response to the chemoradiotherapy; during follow-up she was provided with prophylactic cranial radiation. The patient was admitted four months after completion of treatment for abdominal pain. The patient reported that she was hospitalized for diagnosis of acute pancreatitis for five days at an outside center two weeks ago; her complaints and amylase level which was initially high were regressed and improved after supportive therapy; however her abdominal pain progressively increased in the last two days. In the physical examination, she had localized pain in the epigastric and periumbilical area; the patient expressed that she felt the pain mostly on the back and lower back. Eastern Cooperative Oncology Group Performance Status (ECOG-PS) was 1 and there was no clinical

finding of acute abdomen. The laboratory tests showed a mild leukocytosis and hyperamylasemia (780 U/L) with moderately high C-reactive protein. The patient's history involved no alcohol intake and cholelithiasis, and abdominal computed tomography (CT) demonstrated three metastatic lesions of 0.5–1 cm in diameter in the liver, nodular metastatic thickening in the right adrenal, and diffuse enlargement of the pancreas, and pancreatic ductus became slightly apparent. In addition to metastatic lesions described on abdominal CT, PET-CT showed abnormal focal FDG uptake in the neck and tail of pancreas with diffusely increased FDG uptake (Figure 2(a)). Magnetic resonance cholangiopancreatography (MRCP) revealed a segmental obliteration in the pancreatic duct and dilatation of its distal part (Figure 2(b)); postcontrast MRI sections demonstrated a poorly marginated hypointense area of around 1 cm at obliteration level in the pancreatic duct on the head-corpus junction of the pancreas (Figure 2(c)). Endoscopic ultrasonography (EUS) indicated a very indistinct area with irregular margins in the neck of pancreas and pancreatic duct interruption at this level. The cytopathological examination of EUS-guided fine-needle aspiration (EUS-FNA) from the lesion showed small cell

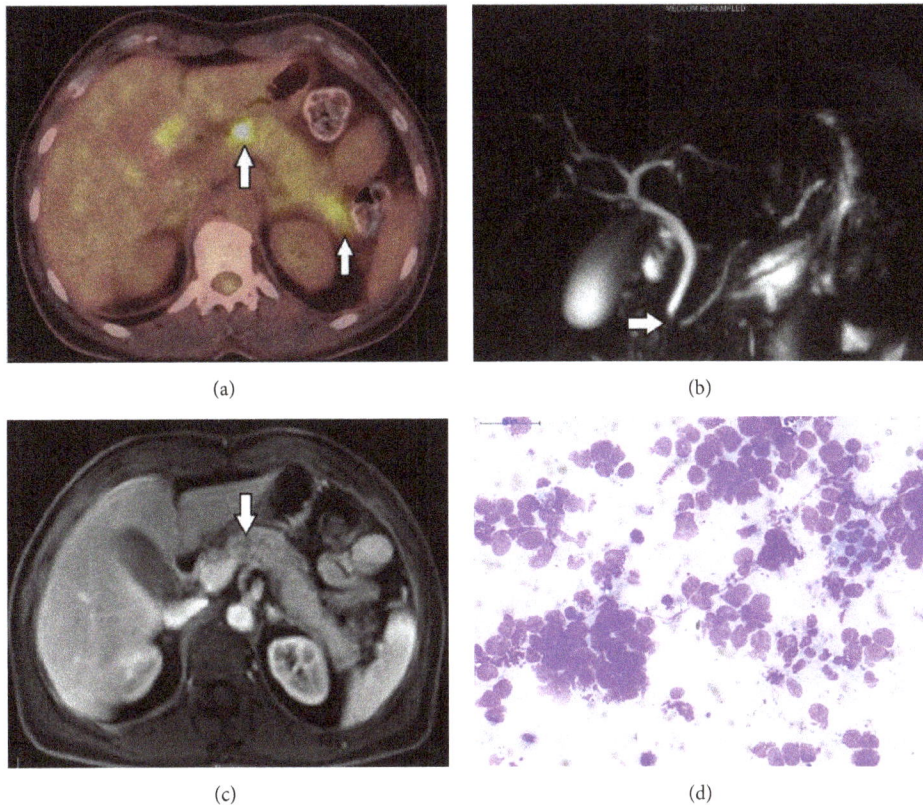

(a)

(b)

(c)

(d)

FIGURE 2: (a) Focal involvement areas of neck and tail of the pancreas on PET-CT (indicated by arrows). (b) Indistinct and nonuniformly circumscribed area of the pancreatic neck on abdominal MRI (arrow). (c) Segmental obliteration of the pancreatic duct on MRCP (arrow) and dilatation to its distal part. (d) Small cell carcinoma as shown by cytopathological examination of EUS-FNA taken from suspected area of the pancreas (MGG, ×40).

carcinoma cells (Figure 2(d)). The patient was discussed at the tumor board, and a second-line chemotherapy with cisplatin and irinotecan (cisplatin 60 mg/m^2 on day 1, irinotecan 60 mg/m^2 on days 1, 8, and 15, every 4 weeks) and intensity-modulated radiotherapy (total dose of 30 Gy administered in daily 3-Gy fractions during 10 days) to pancreatic lesion were started concurrently. The patient's abdominal pain was relieved at the end of the first week of systemic chemotherapy and radiotherapy, and it completely disappeared after 3 weeks. The radiological studies performed after completion of second cycle of chemotherapy showed that metastatic lesions were regressed, and involvement of pancreas and dilatation of pancreatic duct disappeared. No pancreatic attacks were observed during follow-up. The patient is still alive at 14 months after her first diagnosis and 8 months after the first pancreatitis attack.

3. Discussion

The most common subtype of metastatic lung cancer to the pancreas is SCLC, followed by large cell carcinoma, squamous cell carcinoma, and adenocarcinoma [5, 6]. The incidence of metastasis to pancreas was reported to be 24–40% in patients with SCLC as revealed by postmortem studies [3, 4]. More than half of the patients are clinically asymptomatic and

detected on radiological studies during follow-up. The most common symptoms are abdominal pain due to pancreatic invasion and jaundice associated with involvement of biliary tract [7]. In 1973, Levine and Danovitch were first to define acute pancreatitis associated with progression of the disease in a patient with SCLC [8]. Two series of 40 and 60 patients with SCLC reported the incidence of MIAP to be 7.5% and 3.3%, respectively [3, 9]. In a study by Stewart et al. that included the highest number of patients, only one patient was diagnosed with MIAP among 802 patients with lung cancer [10]. Although it is usually a late manifestation and present with extensive metastatic disease, it may rarely manifest as the initial symptom of the disease or as an isolated metastatic involvement [11].

The mechanism that is mostly held responsible for development of MIAP is obstruction/rupture of pancreatic duct due to compression of metastatic mass or enlarged regional lymph nodes. This is followed by vascular compromise/rupture secondary to tumor invasion. Other possible causes associated with development of acute pancreatitis in patients with SCLC include alcohol intake, cholelithiasis, hypercalcemia, and the use of chemotherapy agents such as cisplatin, ifosfamide, and vinorelbine. In cases where no etiological factor exists, paraneoplastic acute pancreatitis may be developed [6, 11].

Most of the cases of MIAP with SCLC in the literature were diagnosed clinically. Tissue diagnosis can be difficult in MIAP due to poor performance status of the patients and false negative rate of biopsy [12]. Therefore, there are no prospective studies on MIAP and most data comes from case reports and retrospective case series including patients with pancreatic metastasis.

The pancreatic metastasis associated with SCLC is commonly localized in the head and corpus of the pancreas. Radiologically, the most common types of pancreatic involvement are solitary metastatic mass (50–73%), diffuse pancreatic enlargement (15–44%), and multiple pancreatic nodules (5–10%), respectively [12, 13]. Ultrasonography's diagnostic value is low as the initial radiologic assessment and it can usually show accompanied biliary calculus and rarely dilatation of pancreatic duct. On a contrast-enhanced CT, a peripheral rim enhancement is typical for pancreatic metastasis and due to hypervascular pattern of tumor with respect to pancreatic parenchyma [6, 12, 13]. This pattern does not only provide detection of the localization of metastatic lesion but also allow differentiating primary pancreas adenocarcinoma that is seen as a mass with no uniformly contrast uptake [12, 13]. On MRI, pancreatic metastases appeared as hypointense and well-circumscribed lesions with peripheral involvement after contrast agent injection similar to CT. However, it was reported that uniform vascular pattern could be observed in lesions smaller than 1.5 cm on CT and MRI, and small lesions could not be demonstrated by imaging methods [12–15]. In our patient, abdominal CT, the initial imaging, showed no mass image in the pancreas except for radiologic findings of acute pancreatitis. However, PET-CT demonstrated two focal hypermetabolic areas with diffuse pancreatic involvement consistent with acute pancreatitis. There is limited data on the use of ^{18}F-FDG PET for pancreatic metastases which is a very useful method for assessment of primary pancreatic tumors. There is only one relevant study by Sato et al. that included 573 patients with lung cancer who underwent PET-CT during initial staging or follow-up, and 11 patients were then diagnosed with pancreatic metastasis [16]. In 3 of these 11 patients, no visible radiologic lesions were observed in the pancreas with standard transaxial CT.

EUS is probably the best method for the evaluation of pancreatic masses. The appearance of primary pancreatic tumors is similar to pancreatic metastases on EUS; however metastatic lesions were reported to usually have more well-defined borders than primary tumors [17]. In our case, MIAP was caused by obstruction of pancreatic duct associated with invasion of a small metastasis localized in the pancreatic neck. In contrast to the literature, the focal involvement area in the pancreatic neck on PET-CT appeared indistinct and nonuniformly circumscribed on both MRI and EUS. Various studies reported diagnostic accuracy of EUS-FNA for pancreatic metastases to be 89–92% [17–19]. EUS-FNA appears to be the most effective method for tissue diagnosis of small pancreatic masses in particular [19]. In our case, the pancreatic lesion was cytopathologically confirmed to be metastasis of SCLC by EUS-FNA.

There is no standard treatment approach for MIAP in patients with SCLC. Endoscopic intrapancreatic stent implantation is a palliative solution, but in some cases it can improve performance status of the patients and consequently make them suitable for receiving chemotherapy [6, 20]. Radiotherapy can be used for palliation of symptoms. Because SCLC is a chemosensitive tumor, a systemic chemotherapy improves outcomes. The survival time varies from 4 months to 6 months after developing MIAP in patients receiving chemotherapy, and the survival of patients who receive no treatment is around 2–4 weeks [9, 10, 21]. A study by Lin et al. found major predictors of survival to be duration of high amylase levels, performance status when MIAP occurred, and the length of chemotherapy after diagnosis of MIAP [22]. The study by Liu et al. reported a better overall survival in patients with a good performance status and receiving systemic chemotherapy. In our case, the longer survival was probably due to a good performance status at diagnosis of MIAP and good tumor response achieved by early initiation of aggressive treatment. The main symptom of the patient was abdominal pain due to pancreatic involvement; however there was also systemic disease with adrenal and liver metastases. Consequently, radiotherapy for the palliation of pain and systemic chemotherapy were started concurrently. The patient experienced no major treatment-related side effect and achieved complete pain relief and systemic disease control.

As a result, MIAP is a rare clinical entity that may occur in the course of disease or as an initial symptom in patients with SCLC. It should be noted that standard imaging methods may not demonstrate a mass image in some cases. In such cases, PET-CT and EUS-FNA can be used to confirm the diagnosis. Rapid and early diagnosis, systemic chemotherapy, and local treatments may have an influence on the palliation of symptoms and survival. An aggressive treatment may prolong survival particularly in patients with good performance status.

References

[1] B. Pan, Y. Lee, T. Rodriguez, J. Lee, and M. W. Saif, "Secondary tumors of the pancreas: a case series," *Anticancer Research*, vol. 32, no. 4, pp. 1449–1452, 2012.

[2] S. L. Showalter, E. Hager, and C. J. Yeo, "Metastatic disease to the pancreas and spleen," *Seminars in Oncology*, vol. 35, no. 2, pp. 160–171, 2008.

[3] K. Y. Yeung, D. J. Haidak, J. A. Brown, and D. Anderson, "Metastasis-induced acute pancreatitis in small cell bronchogenic carcinoma," *Archives of Internal Medicine*, vol. 139, no. 5, pp. 552–554, 1979.

[4] K. Yamanashi, S. Marumo, M. Saitoh, and M. Kato, "A case of metastasis-induced acute pancreatitis in a patient with small cell lung cancer," *Clinical Case Reports*, vol. 3, no. 2, pp. 96–98, 2015.

[5] N. Bouyahia, K. Daoudi, K. Moumna et al., "A case of a metastatic disease to the pancreas from a small-cell lung carcinoma documented by a CT-scan-guided trucut biopsy: the diagnostic role of cytomorphology and immunohistochemistry," *Case*

Reports in Oncological Medicine, vol. 2012, Article ID 520430, 5 pages, 2012.

[6] J.-S. Woo, K. R. Joo, Y. S. Woo et al., "Pancreatitis from metastatic small cell lung cancer: successful treatment with endoscopic intrapancreatic stenting," *Korean Journal of Internal Medicine*, vol. 21, no. 4, pp. 256–261, 2006.

[7] A. D. Sweeney, W. E. Fisher, M.-F. Wu, S. G. Hilsenbeck, and F. C. Brunicardi, "Value of pancreatic resection for cancer metastatic to the pancreas," *Journal of Surgical Research*, vol. 160, no. 2, pp. 268–276, 2010.

[8] M. Levine and S. H. Danovitch, "Metastatic carcinoma to the pancreas. Another cause for acute pancreatitis," *The American Journal of Gastroenterology*, vol. 60, no. 3, pp. 290–294, 1973.

[9] N. M. Chowhan and S. Madajewicz, "Management of metastases-induced acute pancreatitis in small cell carcinoma of the lung," *Cancer*, vol. 65, no. 6, pp. 1445–1448, 1990.

[10] K. C. Stewart, W. J. Dickout, and J. D. Urschel, "Metastasis-induced acute pancreatitis as the initial manifestation of bronchogenic carcinoma," *Chest*, vol. 104, no. 1, pp. 98–100, 1993.

[11] M. A. Khan, F. K. Luni, S. Kamal et al., "Acute pancreatitis first and sole manifestation of small cell carcinoma of lung," *Journal of Medical Cases*, vol. 5, no. 10, pp. 525–528, 2014.

[12] U. Gonlugur, A. Mirici, and M. Karaayvaz, "Pancreatic involvement in small cell lung cancer," *Radiology and Oncology*, vol. 48, no. 1, pp. 11–19, 2014.

[13] I. Tsitouridis, A. Diamantopoulou, M. Michaelides, M. Arvanity, and S. Papaioannou, "Pancreatic metastases: CT and MRI findings," *Diagnostic and Interventional Radiology*, vol. 16, no. 1, pp. 45–51, 2010.

[14] E. M. Merkle, T. Boaz, O. Kolokythas, J. R. Haaga, J. S. Lewin, and H.-J. Brambs, "Metastases to the pancreas," *The British Journal of Radiology*, vol. 71, no. 851, pp. 1208–1214, 1998.

[15] T. Muranaka, K. Teshima, H. Honda, T. Nanjo, K. Hanada, and Y. Oshiumi, "Computed tomography and histologic appearance of pancreatic metastases from distant sources," *Acta Radiologica*, vol. 30, no. 6, pp. 615–619, 1989.

[16] M. Sato, T. Okumura, K. Kaito et al., "Usefulness of FDG-PET/CT in the detection of pancreatic metastases from lung cancer," *Annals of Nuclear Medicine*, vol. 23, no. 1, pp. 49–57, 2009.

[17] J. C. Ardengh, C. V. Lopes, R. Kemp, F. Venco, E. R. de Lima-Filho, and J. S. dos Santos, "Accuracy of endoscopic ultrasound-guided fine-needle aspiration in the suspicion of pancreatic metastases," *BMC Gastroenterology*, vol. 13, no. 1, article 63, 2013.

[18] M. Atiq, M. S. Bhutani, W. A. Ross et al., "Role of endoscopic ultrasonography in evaluation of metastatic lesions to the pancreas: a tertiary cancer center experience," *Pancreas*, vol. 42, no. 3, pp. 516–523, 2013.

[19] I. I. El Hajj, J. K. Leblanc, S. Sherman et al., "Endoscopic ultrasound-guided biopsy of pancreatic metastases: a large single-center experience," *Pancreas*, vol. 42, no. 3, pp. 524–530, 2013.

[20] D. Singh, O. U. Vaidya, E. Sadeddin, and O. Yousef, "Role of endoscopic ultrasound and endoscopic retrograde cholangiopancreatography in isolated pancreatic metastasis from lung cancer," *World Journal of Gastrointestinal Endoscopy*, vol. 4, no. 7, pp. 328–330, 2012.

[21] S.-F. Liu, S. Zhang, Y.-C. Chen et al., "Experience of cancer care for metastasis-induced acute pancreatitis patients with lung cancer," *Journal of Thoracic Oncology*, vol. 4, no. 10, pp. 1231–1235, 2009.

[22] J. Lin, P. Chen, and W. Wang, "Metastasis-induced acute pancreatitis in lung cancer," *Advances in Therapy*, vol. 22, no. 3, pp. 225–233, 2005.

54

Malignant Mesothelioma Mimicking Invasive Mammary Carcinoma in a Male Breast

Mohamed Mokhtar Desouki and Daniel Jerad Long

Department of Pathology Microbiology and Immunology, Vanderbilt University School of Medicine, Nashville, TN 37232, USA

Correspondence should be addressed to Mohamed Mokhtar Desouki; mokhtar.desouki@vanderbilt.edu

Academic Editor: Francesco A. Mauri

Malignant mesothelioma is an uncommon tumor with strong association with asbestos exposure. Few cases of malignant pleural mesothelioma metastatic to the female breast have been reported. Herein, we presented, for the first time, a case of locally infiltrating malignant pleural mesothelioma forming a mass in the breast of a male as the first pathologically confirmed manifestation of the disease. Breast ultrasound revealed an irregular mass in the right breast which involves the pectoralis muscle. Breast core biopsy revealed a proliferation of neoplastic epithelioid cells mimicking an infiltrating pleomorphic lobular carcinoma. IHC studies showed the cells to be positive for calretinin, CK5/6, WT1, and CK7. The cells were negative for MOC-31, BerEp4, ER, and PR. A final diagnosis of malignant mesothelioma, epithelioid type, was rendered. This case demonstrates the importance of considering a broad differential diagnosis in the setting of atypical presentation with application of a panel of IHC markers.

1. Introduction

Malignant mesothelioma is an uncommon tumor with a high mortality rate. The reported incidence of mesothelioma in the United States is approximately 3,300 cases per year [1]. Asbestos exposure, mostly occupational, is a well-known risk factor associated with pleural mesothelioma [2]. Other contributing factors which may be associated with increased incidence of mesothelioma include external radiation at nuclear facilities and exposure to Thorotrast which is a radioactive contrast agent used in diagnostic radiologic procedures among other factors [3, 4]. The incidence of mesothelioma is now declining, which is likely due to significant measures taken to limit asbestos exposure [5].

Metastasis of malignant mesothelioma to distant organs has been reported to the central nervous system, the chest, abdominal and pelvic walls, oral cavity and tongue [6–8]. A case of metastatic malignant pleural mesothelioma to a 51-year-old female breast has been also reported [9]. To the best of our knowledge, there is no reported metastatic or locally extended malignant mesothelioma to a male breast in the English literature. Herein, we presented, for the first time, a case of locally infiltrating malignant pleural mesothelioma forming a 5 cm mass in the right breast of a 77-year-old man as the first pathologically confirmed manifestation of the disease.

2. Case Report

2.1. Clinical Presentation. A 77-year-old male presented with palpable abnormality on the right breast. The past medical history was significant for a recent complicated parapneumonic effusion requiring right thoracotomy and pleural decortication with benign pathologic findings eleven months prior to presenting with the breast mass. The patient also had a history of squamous cell carcinoma and melanoma in situ of the skin. The patient reported an occupational history of asbestos exposure. Family history was significant for breast cancer and BRCA1 mutation positivity in two siblings; the patient's own BRCA status was unknown. On physical examination, there was a fixed, firm mass in the right breast measuring approximately 5 cm in greatest dimension.

2.2. Imaging Studies. Anteroposterior chest X-ray showed pleural thickening along the right lateral chest wall and blunting of the right costophrenic angle (Figure 1(a)). A chest

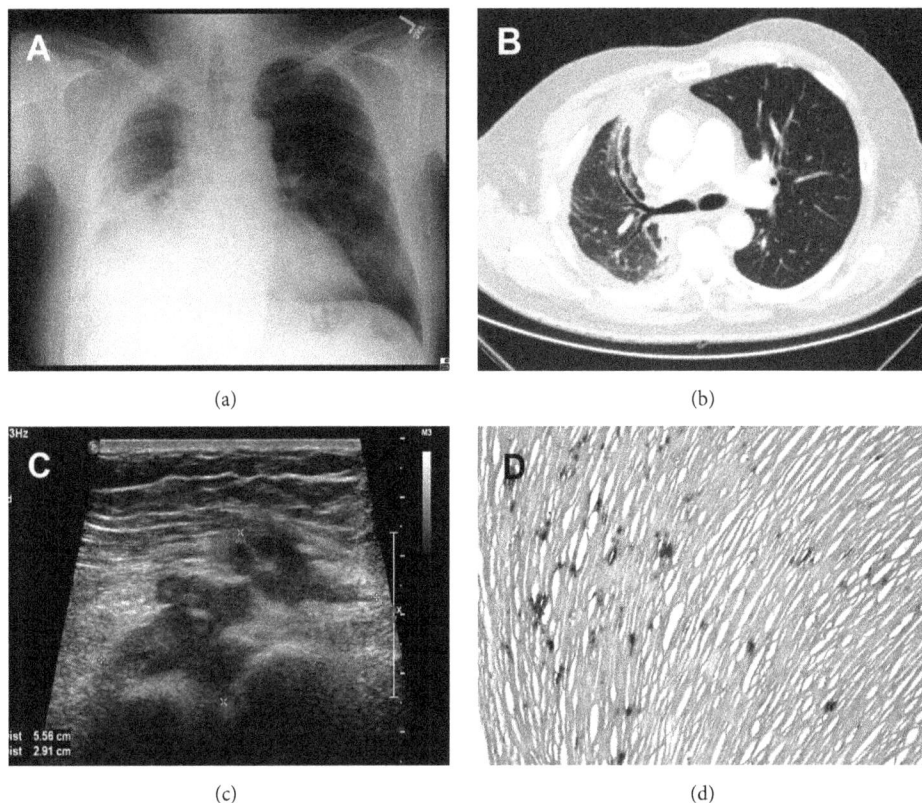

FIGURE 1: (a) Anteroposterior chest X-ray shows pleural thickening along the right lateral chest wall and blunting of the right costophrenic angle. (b) A chest CT scan shows extensive pleural thickening on the right side and calcified pleural plaque on the left side. (c) A breast ultrasound shows an irregular, hypoechoic mass measuring 5.6 × 2.9 × 3.6 cm. A portion of the mass involves pectoralis muscle and extends into the intercostal muscles. (d) Pleural biopsy shows plaque formation with dense fibrosis, minimal inflammation, and dystrophic calcification with no evidence of malignancy.

CT scan with contrast demonstrated a contracted right hemithorax with an irregular pleural-based process that extends through the intercostal muscle and into the subcutaneous adipose tissue indicating direct spread rather than a metastasis in breast tissue. Bronchiectasis of right middle and lower lobes, right middle lobe atelectasis, and prior granulomatous disease have been also reported (Figure 1(b)). A diagnostic breast mammogram revealed predominantly fatty breast parenchyma and no morphologically abnormal lymph nodes in the axilla. A diagnostic breast ultrasound revealed an irregular, hypoechoic mass in the right breast with angular margins measuring 5.6 × 2.9 × 3.6 cm. A portion of the mass appeared to involve the pectoralis muscle and possibly extended into the intercostal muscles (Figure 1(c)). Fine needle biopsy was recommended.

2.3. Histopathology. Biopsy from the right pleural decortication described grossly as a fragment of red-tan tissue measuring 0.9 × 0.7 × 0.2 cm was entirely submitted in one cassette. Microscopic examination was performed at an outside facility and reviewed by expert lung pathologists in consensus at our institution subsequent to the diagnosis of the breast lesion and reported as pleural plaque with dense fibrosis, minimal inflammation, and dystrophic calcification

with no evidence of malignancy (Figure 1(d)). Breast needle core biopsy revealed a proliferation of neoplastic epithelioid cells in cords and nests infiltrating breast parenchyma and skeletal muscles. The neoplastic cells were round to polygonal in shape with moderate cytoplasm, moderate cytologic pleomorphism, and occasional nucleoli mimicking an infiltrating pleomorphic lobular carcinoma (Figures 2(a) and 2(b)). There were focal gland-like and micropapillary structures. Rare mitotic activity was present.

2.4. Immunohistochemistry (IHC). IHC studies showed the tumor cells to be strong and diffusely positive for WT1 (inset in Figure 2(b)), calretinin (Figure 2(c)), CK5/6 (Figure 2(d)), and CK7. The cells were negative for MOC-31, BerEp4, ER, PR, S100 protein, and HMB-45. Based on the morphologic and IHC findings, a final diagnosis of malignant mesothelioma, epithelioid type, was rendered.

3. Discussion

Malignant neoplasms of the male breast, whether primary tumors or metastases from distant sites, are rare. In the United States, the incidence of male breast carcinoma is approximately 1.3 per 100,000 [10], and metastases account for

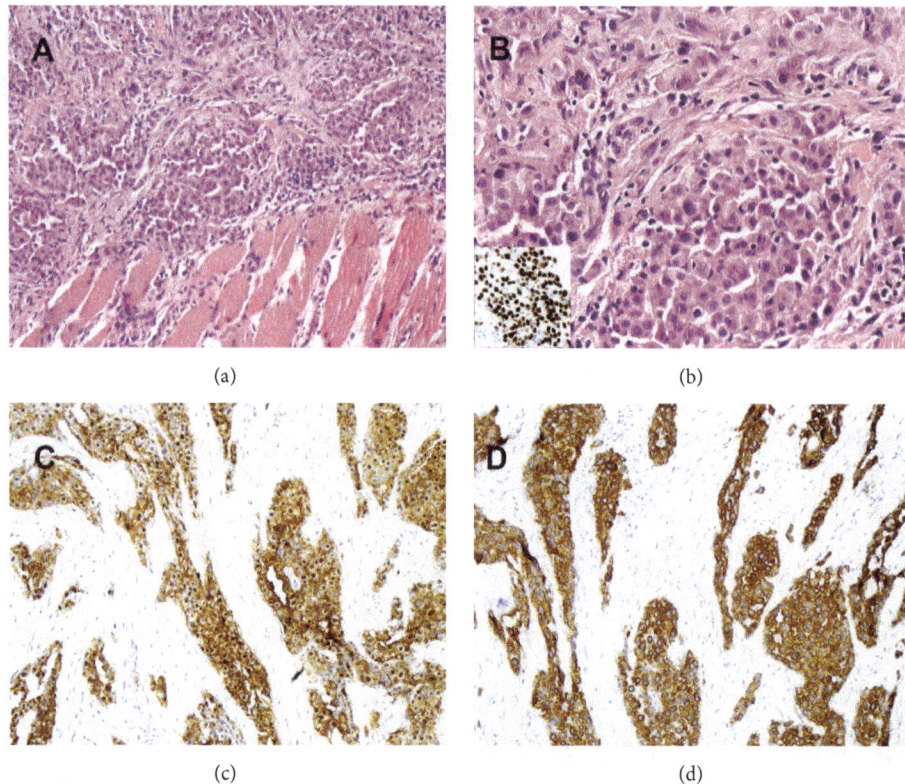

FIGURE 2: Histopathology and immunoprofile of the metastatic malignant mesothelioma to the breast. ((a) and (b)) Representative H&E captions from the metastatic malignant mesothelioma in the breast biopsy which show proliferation of neoplastic epithelioid cells forming cords and nests which infiltrate the breast parenchyma and skeletal muscles. The neoplastic cells are round to polygonal with moderate cytoplasm, moderate cytologic pleomorphism, and occasional nucleoli. The neoplastic cells are positive for WT1 (inset in (b)), calretinin (c), and CK5/6 (d).

approximately 1.3–2.7% of all malignant breast tumors [11]. In this reported case, there were clinical findings concerning both primary mammary carcinoma (clinically palpable breast mass, family history of breast cancer and BRCA1 mutation, and recent benign pleural biopsy) and malignant mesothelioma (history of asbestos exposure and pleural thickening). Given the previous thoracotomy and the predilection of mesothelioma to spread through surgical and drainage sites [12], there is a possibility that this might be causing the chest wall and breast involvement. The morphologic overlap between epithelioid variants of malignant mesothelioma and adenocarcinoma is well described [13]. This overlap is exemplified in this case, with the malignant mesothelioma forming infiltrating nests, cords, and occasional gland-like structures, which impart an overall histologic akin to intermediate grade invasive pleomorphic lobular carcinoma.

Clinical history and morphologic features of a tumor are critically important in the determination of primary versus secondary origin of a breast tumor. However, in cases where the clinical and morphologic data is inconclusive, similar to this reported case, an IHC evaluation may be useful. Approximately 20–25% of mammary cancers are negative for ER, and tumors with a high nuclear grade have the highest proportion of ER-negativity [14]. In the reported case, the morphology and the negativity for ER and PR in the tumor cells raised the

suspicion of an extramammary malignancy, given the tumor's intermediate grade appearance. Although CK7 is positive in greater than 90% of mammary carcinomas [15], many other tumors express CK7, including malignant mesothelioma, as in this case [13]. Another word of caution is the utilization of calretinin which is a known marker for mesothelioma. Approximately 15% of breast carcinomas stain positive for calretinin. These tumors are more likely to be ER- and high-grade tumors of the basal-like phenotype [16]. Therefore, we recommend utilizing a full panel of IHC markers when evaluating the possibility of an extramammary metastasis.

In the reported case, the correct diagnosis of malignant mesothelioma was important, given the significant difference in management between patients with mammary carcinoma and those with malignant mesothelioma. For example, primary surgery is typically considered in patients with nonmetastatic mammary carcinoma, whereas surgical resection is only performed in a subset of patients with malignant pleural mesothelioma. Additionally, there are significant differences between the chemotherapy regimens and radiation therapy protocols utilized for patients with these malignancies [17].

In conclusion, this case of malignant mesothelioma forming a mass lesion, as the first pathologically proven manifestation in a male breast, demonstrates the importance of considering a broad differential diagnosis in the setting of a rare tumor or atypical presentation. When there is concern for an extramammary metastasis/local spread, a panel of IHC markers may be helpful, and malignant mesothelioma should be considered among the potential neoplasms.

Disclosure

The authors of this paper have no relevant financial relationships with commercial interests to disclose.

References

[1] M. J. Teta, P. J. Mink, E. Lau, B. K. Sceurman, and E. D. Foster, "US mesothelioma patterns 1973–2002: indicators of change and insights into background rates," *European Journal of Cancer Prevention*, vol. 17, no. 6, pp. 525–534, 2008.

[2] A. Lacourt, C. Gramond, P. Rolland et al., "Occupational and non-occupational attributable risk of asbestos exposure for malignant pleural mesothelioma," *Thorax*, vol. 69, no. 6, pp. 532–539, 2014.

[3] H. Gibb, K. Fulcher, S. Nagarajan et al., "Analyses of radiation and mesothelioma in the us transuranium and uranium registries," *American Journal of Public Health*, vol. 103, no. 4, pp. 710–716, 2013.

[4] J. T. Peterson Jr., S. D. Greenberg, and P. A. Buffler, "Non-asbestos-related malignant mesothelioma: a review," *Cancer*, vol. 54, no. 5, pp. 951–960, 1984.

[5] B. Price, "Analysis of current trends in United States mesothelioma incidence," *The American Journal of Epidemiology*, vol. 145, no. 3, pp. 211–218, 1997.

[6] C. J. Winfree, W. J. Mack, and M. B. Sisti, "Solitary cerebellar metastasis of malignant pleural mesothelioma: case report," *Surgical Neurology*, vol. 61, no. 2, pp. 174–179, 2004.

[7] Z.-H. Shao, X.-L. Gao, X.-H. Yi, and P.-J. Wang, "Malignant mesothelioma presenting as a giant chest, abdominal and pelvic wall mass," *Korean Journal of Radiology*, vol. 12, no. 6, pp. 750–753, 2011.

[8] D. Kirke, K. Horwood, and B. Wallwork, "Floor of mouth and tongue metastasis from malignant pleural mesothelioma," *ANZ Journal of Surgery*, vol. 80, no. 7-8, pp. 556–558, 2010.

[9] S.-M. Sheen-Chen, Y.-W. Liu, H.-L. Eng, C.-C. Huang, and S.-F. Ko, "Metastatic malignant pleural mesothelioma to the breast," *Southern Medical Journal*, vol. 99, no. 12, pp. 1395–1397, 2006.

[10] American Cancer Society, *Cancer Facts & Figures 2014*, American Cancer Society, Atlanta, Ga, USA, 2014.

[11] I. Alvarado Cabrero, M. Carrera Álvarez, D. Pérez Montiel, and F. A. Tavassoli, "Metastases to the breast," *European Journal of Surgical Oncology*, vol. 29, no. 10, pp. 854–855, 2003.

[12] M. Di Salvo, G. Gambaro, S. Pagella, I. Manfredda, C. Casadio, and M. Krengli, "Prevention of malignant seeding at drain sites after invasive procedures (surgery and/or thoracoscopy) by hypofractionated radiotherapy in patients with pleural mesothelioma," *Acta Oncologica*, vol. 47, no. 6, pp. 1094–1098, 2008.

[13] A. S. Abutaily, B. J. Addis, and W. R. Roche, "Immunohistochemistry in the distinction between malignant mesothelioma and pulmonary adenocarcinoma: a critical evaluation of new antibodies," *Journal of Clinical Pathology*, vol. 55, no. 9, pp. 662–668, 2002.

[14] M. Nadji, C. Gomez-Fernandez, P. Ganjei-Azar, and A. R. Morales, "Immunohistochemistry of estrogen and progesterone receptors reconsidered: experience with 5,993 breast cancers," *The American Journal of Clinical Pathology*, vol. 123, no. 1, pp. 21–27, 2005.

[15] T. Tot, "Cytokeratins 20 and 7 as biomarkers: usefulness in discriminating primary from metastatic adenocarcinoma," *European Journal of Cancer*, vol. 38, no. 6, pp. 758–763, 2002.

[16] G. Powell, H. Roche, and W. R. Roche, "Expression of calretinin by breast carcinoma and the potential for misdiagnosis of mesothelioma," *Histopathology*, vol. 59, no. 5, pp. 950–956, 2011.

[17] J. E. Dowell, F. R. Dunphy, R. N. Taub et al., "A multicenter phase II study of cisplatin, pemetrexed, and bevacizumab in patients with advanced malignant mesothelioma," *Lung Cancer*, vol. 77, no. 3, pp. 567–571, 2012.

55

Primary Intracranial Melanoma with Early Leptomeningeal Spread: A Case Report and Treatment Options Available

Rajesh Balakrishnan,[1] Rokeya Porag,[2] Dewan Shamsul Asif,[2] A. M. Rejaus Satter,[2] Md. Taufiq,[3] and Samson S. K. Gaddam[2]

[1]*Department of Radiotherapy and Oncology, Square HospitalsLimited, Dhaka 1205, Bangladesh*
[2]*Department of Neurosurgery, Square HospitalsLimited, Dhaka 1205, Bangladesh*
[3]*Department of Pathology, Square HospitalsLimited, Dhaka 1205, Bangladesh*

Correspondence should be addressed to Rajesh Balakrishnan; drrajeshb77@gmail.com

Academic Editor: Jose I. Mayordomo

Primary CNS melanomas are rare and they constitute about 1% of all cases of melanomas and 0.07% of all brain tumors. These tumors are aggressive in nature and may metastasise to other organs. Till date less than 25 cases have been reported in the literature. The primary treatment for local intraparenchymal tumours is complete resection and/or radiotherapy and it is associated with good survival. However once there is disease spread to leptomeninges the overall median survival is around 10 weeks. In this case report we describe a primary intracranial melanoma without any dural attachment in 16-year-old boy who had radical excision of the tumor followed by radiotherapy who eventually had rapidly developed leptomeningeal disease and review the literature with a focus on the clinic pathological, radiological, and treatment options.

1. Introduction/Background

Primary CNS melanomas are rare and they constitute about 1% of all cases of melanomas and 0.07% of all brain tumors [1].

Till date less than 25 cases have been reported in the literature [2]. Malignant melanoma arises from either melanocytes or their precursor cells, melanoblasts [3]. As melanocytes are found in normal leptomeningeal tissue, it is not surprising that primary melanomas can grow within the central nervous system. In most instances, melanomas involving the CNS represent metastatic disease. Primary CNS melanomas are aggressive in nature and may metastasise to other organs. The primary treatment for local intraparenchymal tumours is complete resection and/or radiotherapy and it is associated with good survival. Temozolomide is an active drug which crosses the blood brain barrier and is known to be active in brain metastases from melanoma [4]. However once there is disease spread to leptomeninges the overall median survival is around 10 weeks [5]. In this case report we describe an adolescent male who had primary intracranial melanoma with early leptomeningeal disease progression and literature review with a focus on the pathological, radiological, and available treatment options.

2. Case Report

A 16-year-old boy presented with headache, convulsions, blurring of vision, and vertigo. On examination vitals were stable, fully conscious, and oriented, pupils 2 mm both equally reacting, no cranial nerve, motor and sensory deficit. His past medical history was unremarkable. He also had scattered melanocytic naevi over the back since birth without any itching or ulceration. None of the skin lesions were larger than 1 cm. He would fit into Fitzpatrick skin phototype IV. The patient had no family history of melanoma or atypical melanocytic nevus. Contrast enhanced CT brain revealed a heterogeneous high density mass at anterior part of the left temporal lobe with contrast enhancement. MRI brain demonstrated a T1 hyperintense and T2 hypointense mass in the left temporal lobe with perilesional oedema with no

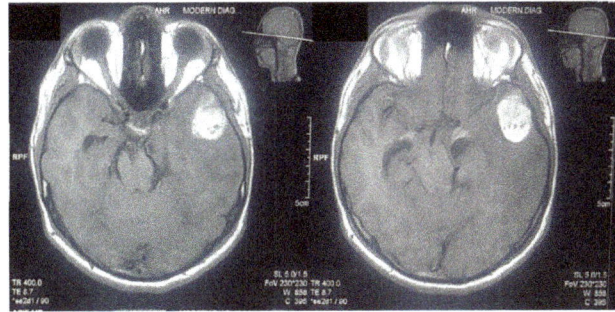

FIGURE 1: Preop MRI showing the lesion in the left temporal lobe with no dural attachment.

dural attachment (Figure 1). There was mild heterogeneous enhancement after administration of gadolinium.

The images prompted consideration of a hemorrhagic brain tumour. He had left temporal craniotomy and gross total excision of the tumor. Histopathological examination (HPE) revealed nervous tissue infiltrated by tumour composed of sheets of moderately large polygonal cells with round to oval pleomorphic nuclei, dispersed chromatin with mitotic activity (8–10/10 HPF). Numerous cells contained coarse, granular intracellular, intracytoplasmic, and extracytoplasmic brownish pigment resembling melanin. Periphery of the tumor showed tumor cells in the Virchow spaces of the brain tissue. On immunohistochemistry the tumor cells showed diffuse positivity for human melanin black-45 (HMB-45) antibody and S100 and weak patchy cytoplasmic positivity for antimelanosomal antibody MART-1 (Melan A) which were all suggestive of melanocytic origin (Figures 2 and 3). Tumor cells were negative for epithelial membrane antigen (EMA) and glial fibrillary acidic protein (GFAP) which effectively ruled out a meningioma or a glial neoplasm. HPE was reported as melanoma. He then underwent whole body PET-CT and it did not reveal any FDG avid regions except for small foci in rectal lumen. He had a colonoscopy which showed a rectal polyp. Biopsies from largest skin naevi found in the left gluteal region were reported as benign intradermal nevus and biopsy from the rectal polyp was reported as juvenile rectal polyp. His fundoscopy did not reveal any uveal melanoma. This suggested that we were dealing with a primary intracranial cerebral melanoma. Postoperative MRI brain showed no residual brain tumor.

He then received adjuvant radiation (Involved Field 3DCRT) along with concurrent Temozolomide to a total dose of 5600 cGy in 28 fractions, 200 cGy per fraction, and five days in week to the postoperative tumor bed using 6 MV linear accelerator (Figure 4). Concurrent Temozolomide was given at a dose of 75 mg/sq·m to a dose of 100 mg for six and half weeks. His MRI brain done four weeks after completion of chemoRT showed no disease recurrence and hence he was started on adjuvant chemotherapy with Temozolomide (Figure 5). He presented one week after starting adjuvant chemotherapy with complaints of severe back pain which was not controlled with analgesics. He also progressed to have constipation and retention of urine. MRI whole spine screening showed multiple tiny T1 hyperintense and T2 hypointense intradural nodular lesions (Figure 6) along the

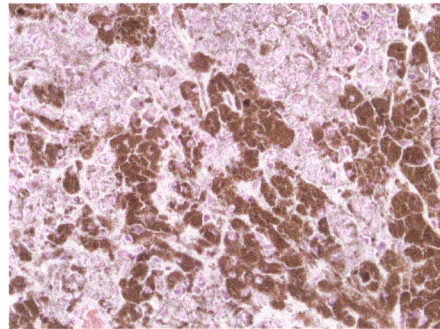

FIGURE 2: H&E stain, ×400, sheets of moderately large polygonal cells with round to oval pleomorphic nuclei, dispersed chromatin with mitotic activity (8–10/10 high power field).

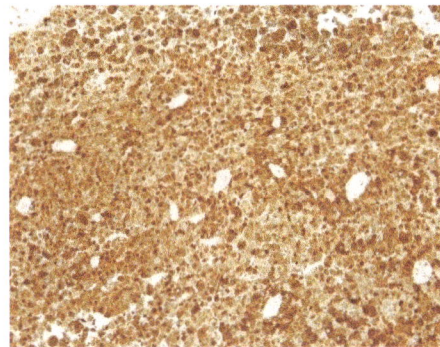

FIGURE 3: S100 staining, ×200, cells diffusely positive for S100.

intrathecal nerve roots along with diffuse enhancement of the lower dorsal cord and along the pons. His repeat metastatic workup did not show any lesions in the liver or lungs. His cerebrospinal fluid (CSF) cytospin done now showed melanoma cells (Figure 7) and he was started on Palliative RT to the lumbosacral region (3000 cGy in 10 fractions). He had marginal symptom relief and he had progression of the leptomeningeal disease. He developed cranial nerve deficits and the patient was not willing for any further treatment. He opted for best supportive care and he died from leptomeningeal disease progression at 7 months after diagnosis. The patient's family has consented for publication of his case and the signed form is available with the author.

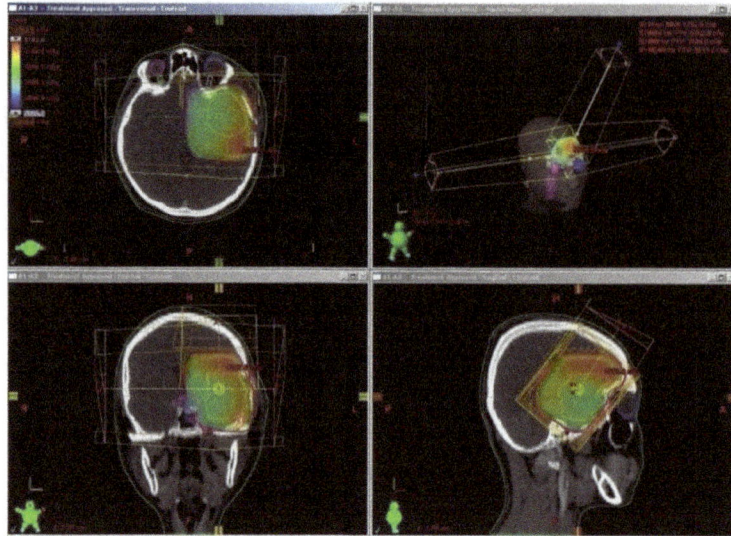

FIGURE 4: Radiotherapy was administered by 3D conformal technique and the dose wash shown in the figure.

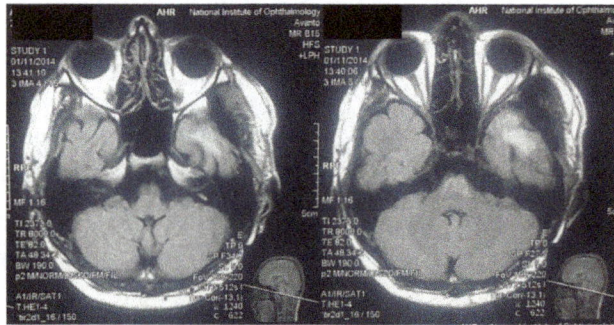

FIGURE 5: Post-ChemoRT images showing no recurrent/residual tumor.

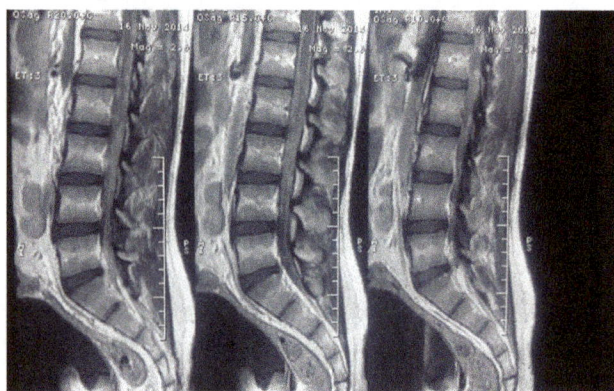

FIGURE 6: Spine MRI showing drop metastases in the lumbosacral spine.

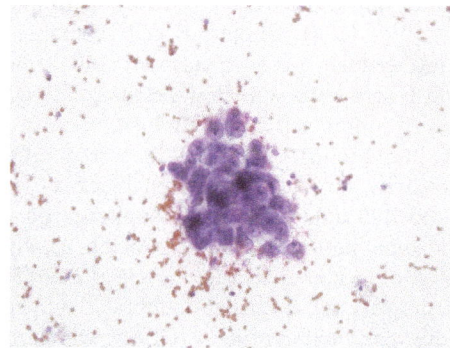

FIGURE 7: CSF cytospin smear showing atypical cells in small clusters with intracytoplasmic melanin pigment.

3. Discussion

Melanocytes are of neural crest in origin and they migrate during development to the skin, eyes, oral cavity, and the leptomeninges. Primary melanoma of the CNS originates from the melanocytes of the leptomeninges. In children it occurs primarily in patients with neurocutaneous melanosis. In children the primary melanoma of the CNS is of poor prognosis unlike in adults and is associated with an overall survival of 8 months from the initial presentation [6].

3.1. Origin of Primary CNS Melanoma. Several histogenetic theories (mesodermal origin, ectodermal origin, and neurogenic origin) have been proposed regarding the origin of melanin cells [7]. The most recent theory is the implication of overexpression of oncogenic NRAS in melanocytes during embryonic development [8]. It is also interesting to note that NRAS mutations are the second most common mutations to occur in melanomas (20%) next to BRAF mutations (50%) [9].

3.2. Diagnosing Primary CNS Melanoma. It is difficult to diagnose a primary CNS melanoma upfront. Majority of patients with intracranial melanomas present with features of raised intracranial tension (43%), neurological deficits (35%), features of subarachnoid haemorrhage (14%), or convulsions

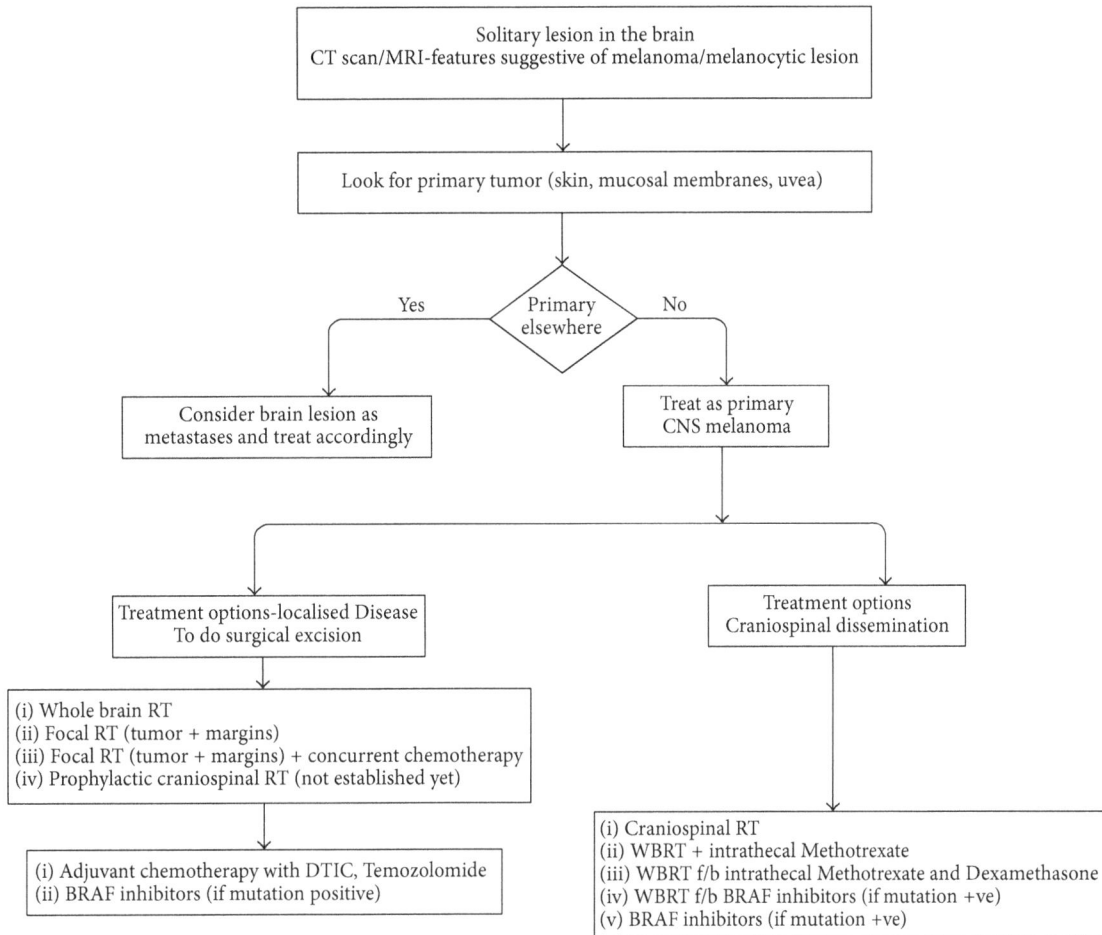

FIGURE 8: Proposed diagnostic/treatment algorithm for primary CNS melanoma.

(12%) [10]. There is a documented male predominance in primary CNS melanomas (same as our patient). It is usually a diagnosis of exclusion of metastatic disease from a skin or oral or uveal melanoma by proper evaluation as brain is the most common site for metastases from breast, lung, or melanoma. Hayward in his landmark publication had set down criteria to classify tumors into primary melanomas, secondaries, and melanin containing variants of other intracranial tumors. According to Hayward, A solitary cerebral lesion, intramedullary or leptomeningeal involvement, hydrocephalus, and pineal/pituitary tumors could be primary melanomas provided that no melanomatous lesions are found outside the CNS [11].

3.3. Neuroradiology. The preoperative diagnosis of primary CNS melanoma is difficult, except in cases associated with neurocutaneous melanosis [12] or when melanin or melanin-containing cells are detected in the cerebrospinal fluid [7]. The CT findings of intracranial melanomas, including high-density mass on precontrast scans, homogeneous enhancement, and marked peritumoral oedema, are not specific [13–15]. MRI brain with gadolinium is the imaging of choice for a patient with suspected CNS melanoma. The MRI findings of a CNS melanoma are so typical that they are hyperintense on T1 weighted images and hypointense on T2 weighted images due to presence of melanin [16]. The radiological differentials are haemorrhage, primary or metastatic malignant intracranial melanomas [17]. These lesions are hyperperfused on perfusion imaging and have an elevated choline and reduced NAA peak on MR spectroscopy. Melanocytomas and meningiomas usually appear isointense on T1WI and display homogenous enhancement. Both display dural attachment and occasionally brain invasion [18]. The differential diagnosis is more difficult in some cases of meningioma with cells containing melanin pigment, ectopic meningioma, or hemorrhagic meningioma [19]. As MRI of our patient shows T1WI hyperintensity and T2WI isointense to hyperintensity with peritumoral edema, our initial impression was a tumor haemorrhage either primary or secondary. In our patient, there was no dural attachment but there was extensive peritumoral edema which could be due to brain invasion. Peritumoral edema seen as T2 hyperintensity reflects the rapid growth rate of the tumor.

The role of FDG PET is also important as it would be of immense help to rule out the presence of disease anywhere else outside the CNS. The whole body FDG PET has specificity of about 91% in diagnosing locoregional disease and for staging of melanomas [20].

3.4. Immunohistochemistry. Primary melanocytic neoplasms of the central nervous system (CNS) consist of a broad spectrum ranging from well differentiated melanocytoma to its overtly malignant counterpart, melanoma [21]. HMB-45, MART-1 (Melan A), S-100, and tyrosinase are almost always diffusely positive in primary melanocytic neoplasms of the CNS. Melanomas do not stain for EMA and this is used to differentiate from meningiomas [22] Occasionally, in cases of neurilemmoma and pigmented malignant schwannoma, more rarely in ependymoma, gliosarcoma, and cerebral primitive neuroectodermal tumors there could be some focal positivity of HMB 45.

Immunohistochemistry results in our patient showed diffuse positivity for HMB-45 and S-100 protein and weak patchy cytoplasmic positivity for Melan A. Also tumor cells were negative for EMA and GFAP. Histopathology and immunohistochemistry of the patient's tumor led us to diagnosis of a malignant melanoma. We reached a diagnosis of primary CNS melanoma after excluding extracranial disease in the skin, uvea, or the mucosa along with the HPE and IHC from the specimen. He fulfilled the Hayward criteria for diagnosing a primary CNS melanoma. BRAF mutations analysis could not be done in this patient as our lab was not equipped with the facilities for doing it. Moreover BRAF inhibitors are not available in our country for patient use.

3.5. Treatment Options. There are no specific guidelines to our knowledge for the management of the primary CNS melanomas as they are a rare tumor. There are no published randomised trials which would help us in the management of these tumours.

Complete excision of the tumor is the mainstay of the management and it helps to reduce the raised ICT. Primary CNS melanocytic tumours have better outcome by surgical intervention, with or without additional adjuvant treatment [23, 24]. Radiotherapy and chemotherapy play an important role after surgery even though it has been considered that melanomas are one of the radioresistant or chemoresistant tumours.

Radiation can be either given whole brain RT or involved field RT with margins with or without concurrent chemotherapy with Temozolomide. The agents that have been tried with RT include BRAF inhibitors, intraventricular chemotherapy, intrathecal Methotrexate+ steroids, and intrathecal recombinant Interleukin-2.

There are reports where RT up to 5400 Gy has been tried to the postoperative tumor bed in conventional fractionation successfully in the adjuvant setting [25].

Involved field radiotherapy at the symptomatic regions or for the bulky disease is component of treatment for patients with leptomeningeal spread. When a patient presents with cranial nerve involvement, RT helps to reestablish the normal CSF flow and these patients have hydrocephalus [26].

IntraCSF chemotherapy has been tried for these tumours with leptomeningeal disease by a few researchers. The primary intent was that since most chemotherapy agents do not cross the BBB they attempted to directly instil the chemotherapy in the CSF to kill the cells directly. Le Rhun et al. had used Methotrexate (15 mg) and Dexamethasone (5 mg) once or twice weekly [27].

Lee et al. had treated patients with advanced melanoma with whole brain RT (30 Gy in 10 fractions) followed by BRAF inhibitors like Vemurafenib [28] and had reported long-term stabilisation of the Leptomeningeal disease for 18 months.

WBRT (40 Gy in 20 fractions) along with concurrent intrathecal Methotrexate (15 mg once weekly for 8 weeks) has been tried and it had resulted in a progression free interval of 8 months [26].

In a retrospective study in advanced malignant melanomas done by Paul et al., he demonstrated significant reduction in CNS relapse in the Temozolomide group compared to DTIC at 19-month follow-up. In view of these results and as the lineage of primary CNS melanomas is similar to melanomas, TMZ could play an important role in the concurrent and adjuvant treatment schema and this needs to be evaluated further [4].

The role of craniospinal irradiation is not yet defined in treating patients with intracranial CNS melanoma as they frequently metastasize to the leptomeninges (LM) in the due course of disease. The benefits and the risks of subjecting the patient to the prophylactic craniospinal axis irradiation need to be weighed before such a treatment is being offered to the patient in patients who do not have leptomeningeal dissemination at presentation. However in case of patient presenting with LM dissemination they could be considered for craniospinal RT [29]. A diagnostic and treatment pathway for these rare tumors is depicted in Figure 8.

4. Conclusion

It is difficult to diagnose primary CNS melanoma in the absence of any cutaneous melanosis. A high index of clinical suspicion along with good pathology reporting is the key in diagnosing these extremely rare tumours. PET CT whole body helps to rule out the presence of occult primary anywhere else. It is necessary to differentiate the benign melanocytomas from the malignant melanomas. The preferred treatment option is total surgical excision if feasible followed by postoperative adjuvant therapy with radiation and chemotherapy. The role of BRAF inhibitors, immunomodulating therapies, prophylactic craniospinal irradiation, and intrathecal chemotherapy needs to be evaluated in future.

Abbreviations

3DCRT: 3-dimensional conformal radiotherapy
BBB: Blood brain barrier
CECT: Contrast enhanced computerised
        tomography
CSF: Cerebrospinal fluid
CNS: Central nervous system
LM: Leptomeningeal
PET-CT: Positron emission
        tomography-computerised tomography
RT: Radiotherapy
WBRT: Whole brain radiotherapy.

Consent

Consent has been obtained from the patient's family for publication of this case report and a copy is available for the editor on request.

Authors' Contribution

Rajesh Balakrishnan was responsible for patient management, writing, and literature review, Rokeya Porag was responsible for writing and literature review, Dewan Shamsul Asif was responsible for patient's management and literature review, A. M. Rejaus Satter was responsible for patient's management and literature review, Md. Taufiq was responsible for patient's management and literature review, and Samson S. K. Gaddam was responsible for patient's management, writing, and literature review.

Acknowledgment

The authors acknowledge the reviewers for their healthy comments that improve the paper.

References

[1] S. G. Crasto, R. Soffietti, G. B. Bradac, and R. Boldorini, "Primitive cerebral melanoma: case report and review of the literature," *Surgical Neurology*, vol. 55, no. 3, pp. 163–168, 2001.

[2] V. V. Suranagi, P. Maste, and P. R. Malur, "Primary intracranial malignant melanoma: a rare casewith review of literature," *Asian Journal of Neurosurgery*, vol. 10, no. 1, pp. 39–41, 2015.

[3] A. W. Kopf and J. C. Maize, "Cutaneous malignant melanoma," *Journal of the American Academy of Dermatology*, vol. 16, no. 3, part 1, pp. 610–613, 1987.

[4] M. J. Paul, Y. Summers, A. H. Calvert et al., "Effect of temozolomide on central nervous system relapse in patients with advanced melanoma," *Melanoma Research*, vol. 12, no. 2, pp. 175–178, 2002.

[5] L. Harstad, K. R. Hess, and M. D. Groves, "Prognostic factors and outcomes in patients with leptomeningeal melanomatosis," *Neuro-Oncology*, vol. 10, no. 6, pp. 1010–1018, 2008.

[6] G. W. J. Makin, O. B. Eden, L. S. Lashford et al., "Leptomeningeal melanoma in childhood," *Cancer*, vol. 86, no. 5, pp. 878–886, 1999.

[7] E. Pappenheim and S. K. Bhattacharji, "Primary melanoma of the central nervous system. Clinical-pathological report of a case, with survey and discussion of the literature," *Archives of Neurology*, vol. 7, pp. 101–113, 1962.

[8] M. Pedersen, H. V. N. Küsters-Vandevelde, A. Viros et al., "Primary melanoma of the CNS in children is driven by congenital expression of oncogenic NRAS in melanocytes," *Cancer Discovery*, vol. 3, no. 4, pp. 458–469, 2013.

[9] J.-H. Lee, J.-W. Choi, and Y.-S. Kim, "Frequencies of BRAF and NRAS mutations are different in histological types and sites of origin of cutaneous melanoma: a meta-analysis," *British Journal of Dermatology*, vol. 164, no. 4, pp. 776–784, 2011.

[10] R. R. Baena, P. Gaetani, M. Danova, F. Bosi, and F. Zappoli, "Primary solitary intracranial melanoma: case report and review of the literature," *Surgical Neurology*, vol. 38, no. 1, pp. 26–37, 1992.

[11] R. D. Hayward, "Malignant melanoma and the central nervous system. A guide for classification based on the clinical findings," *Journal of Neurology, Neurosurgery & Psychiatry*, vol. 39, no. 6, pp. 526–530, 1976.

[12] K. Takakura and A. Teramoto, "Neurocutaneous syndromes and tumors of the central nervous system," *Nō To Shinkei*, vol. 36, no. 1, pp. 36–48, 1984.

[13] S. Ginaldi, S. Wallace, P. Shalen, M. Luna, and S. Handel, "Cranial computed tomography of malignant melanoma," *The American Journal of Roentgenology*, vol. 136, no. 1, pp. 145–149, 1981.

[14] H. Hondo, Y. Sugiyama, S. Kawasaki et al., "An autopsy case of primary intracranial melanoma associated with dermoid cyst (author's transl)," *No Shinkei Geka*, vol. 10, no. 3, pp. 305–310, 1982.

[15] G. M. McGann and A. Platts, "Computed tomography of cranial metastatic malignant melanoma: features, early detection and unusual cases," *British Journal of Radiology*, vol. 64, no. 760, pp. 310–313, 1991.

[16] S.-S. Chio, J. S. Hyde, and R. C. Sealy, "Paramagnetism in melanins: pH dependence," *Archives of Biochemistry and Biophysics*, vol. 215, no. 1, pp. 100–106, 1982.

[17] H. Iizuka, T. Nakamura, and M. Kurauchi, "Primary intracranial melanoma—case report," *Neurologia Medico-Chirurgica*, vol. 30, no. 9, pp. 698–702, 1990.

[18] F. Roser, M. Nakamura, A. Brandis, V. Hans, P. Vorkapic, and M. Samii, "Transition from meningeal melanocytoma to primary cerebral melanoma: case report," *Journal of Neurosurgery*, vol. 101, no. 3, pp. 528–531, 2004.

[19] G. Bradac, R. Ferszt, and B. E. Kendall, *Cranial Meningiomas: Diagnosis, Biology, Therapy*, Springer, Berlin, Germany, 1990.

[20] D. Fuster, S. Chiang, G. Johnson, L. M. Schuchter, H. Zhuang, and A. Alavi, "Is ^{18}F-FDG PET more accurate than standard diagnostic procedures in the detection of suspected recurrent melanoma?" *Journal of Nuclear Medicine*, vol. 45, no. 8, pp. 1323–1327, 2004.

[21] D. J. Brat, C. Giannini, B. W. Scheithauer, and P. C. Burger, "Primary melanocytic neoplasms of the central nervous system," *The American Journal of Surgical Pathology*, vol. 23, no. 7, pp. 745–754, 1999.

[22] T. F. O'Brien, M. Moran, J. H. Miller, and S. D. Hensley, "Meningeal melanocytoma. An uncommon diagnostic pitfall in surgical neuropathology," *Archives of Pathology and Laboratory Medicine*, vol. 119, no. 6, pp. 542–546, 1995.

[23] Y. Kumagai, H. Sugiyama, H. N. Sugiura, K. Kito, and N. Shitara, "A case of intracranial melanoma who has been survived more than 12 years after initial craniotomy was reported (author's transl)," *No To Shinkei*, vol. 31, no. 4, pp. 397–402, 1979.

[24] T. C. Larson III, O. W. Houser, B. M. Onofrio, and D. G. Piepgras, "Primary spinal melanoma," *Journal of Neurosurgery*, vol. 66, no. 1, pp. 47–49, 1987.

[25] T. Wadasadawala, S. Trivedi, T. Gupta, S. Epari, and R. Jalali, "The diagnostic dilemma of primary central nervous system melanoma," *Journal of Clinical Neuroscience*, vol. 17, no. 8, pp. 1014–1017, 2010.

[26] Z. Pan, G. Yang, Y. Wang, T. Yuan, Y. Gao, and L. Dong, "Leptomeningeal metastases from a primary central nervous system melanoma: a case report and literature review," *World Journal of Surgical Oncology*, vol. 12, no. 1, article 265, 2014.

[27] E. Le Rhun, S. Taillibert, and M. Chamberlain, "Carcinomatous meningitis: Leptomeningeal metastases in solid tumors," *Surgical Neurology International*, vol. 4, no. 4, pp. S265–S288, 2013.

[28] J. M. Lee, U. N. Mehta, L. H. Dsouza, B. A. Guadagnolo, D. L. Sanders, and K. B. Kim, "Long-term stabilization of leptomeningeal disease with whole-brain radiation therapy in a patient with metastatic melanoma treated with vemurafenib: a case report," *Melanoma Research*, vol. 23, no. 2, pp. 175–178, 2013.

[29] D. Allcutt, S. Michowiz, S. Weitzman et al., "Primary leptomeningeal melanoma: an unusually aggressive tumor in childhood," *Neurosurgery*, vol. 32, no. 5, pp. 721–729, 1993.

56

High-Grade Leiomyosarcoma Arising in a Previously Replanted Limb

Tiffany J. Pan,[1] Liron Pantanowitz,[2] and Kurt R. Weiss[1]

[1]Department of Orthopaedic Surgery, University of Pittsburgh Medical Center, 3471 Fifth Avenue, Pittsburgh, PA 15213, USA
[2]Division of Anatomic Pathology, University of Pittsburgh Medical Center, 5230 Centre Avenue, Pittsburgh, PA 15232, USA

Correspondence should be addressed to Kurt R. Weiss; weiskr@upmc.edu

Academic Editor: Yoshihito Yokoyama

Sarcoma development has been associated with genetics, irradiation, viral infections, and immunodeficiency. Reports of sarcomas arising in the setting of prior trauma, as in burn scars or fracture sites, are rare. We report a case of a leiomyosarcoma arising in an arm that had previously been replanted at the level of the elbow joint following traumatic amputation when the patient was eight years old. He presented twenty-four years later with a 10.8 cm mass in the replanted arm located on the volar forearm. The tumor was completely resected and pathology examination showed a high-grade, subfascial spindle cell sarcoma diagnosed as a grade 3 leiomyosarcoma with stage pT2bNxMx. The patient underwent treatment with brachytherapy, reconstruction with a free flap, and subsequently chemotherapy. To the best of our knowledge, this is the first case report of leiomyosarcoma developing in a replanted extremity. Development of leiomyosarcoma in this case could be related to revascularization, scar formation, or chronic injury after replantation. The patient remains healthy without signs of recurrence at three-year follow-up.

1. Introduction

Soft tissue leiomyosarcoma is a relatively rare tumor, arising from smooth muscle and comprising approximately 5–10% of all soft tissue sarcomas [1]. Although they typically occur in the uterus, retroperitoneum, intra-abdominal viscera, and blood vessel walls, they can also be found in the bone and soft tissues of the extremities [2].

Few reports exist in the literature of sarcoma occurring in the setting of prior musculoskeletal trauma. Case reports exist in the non-English literature that describe posttraumatic osteosarcoma [3], osteosarcoma arising from posttraumatic myositis ossificans [4], rhabdomyosarcoma after a gunshot wound [5], and sarcoma developing at a fracture site after open reduction and internal fixation [6]. One case report in the English literature regarding rhabdomyosarcoma of the hand following severe trauma was written over half a century ago [7].

We present the case of a patient who sustained a traumatic amputation around the level of the elbow joint as a child and subsequently developed leiomyosarcoma in the replanted limb 24 years later.

2. Case Presentation

At the age of 8, the patient was involved in a tractor accident, and his right arm was severed just distal to the elbow joint. He underwent multiple surgical procedures, resulting in successful replantation of the limb. Of note, immunosuppression was not required given that he had undergone a replantation and not a transplant. Despite suboptimal function, he was working full time in construction at the time of presentation.

24 years subsequent to the accident, the patient returned to the hand surgeon who had performed his replantation as a child when he noticed a mass approximately the size of an orange in his right volar medial forearm. MRI was obtained that demonstrated $10 \times 10 \times 10$ cm heterogenous, subfascial mass, ostensibly originating from the area of the interosseous membrane (Figure 1(a)). His surgeon performed an incomplete excision. Pathology showed a high-grade leiomyosarcoma with 20% necrosis and no angiolymphatic invasion.

He was subsequently referred to our tertiary sarcoma center for evaluation by a musculoskeletal oncologist. At that time, he had essentially normal neurologic hand function

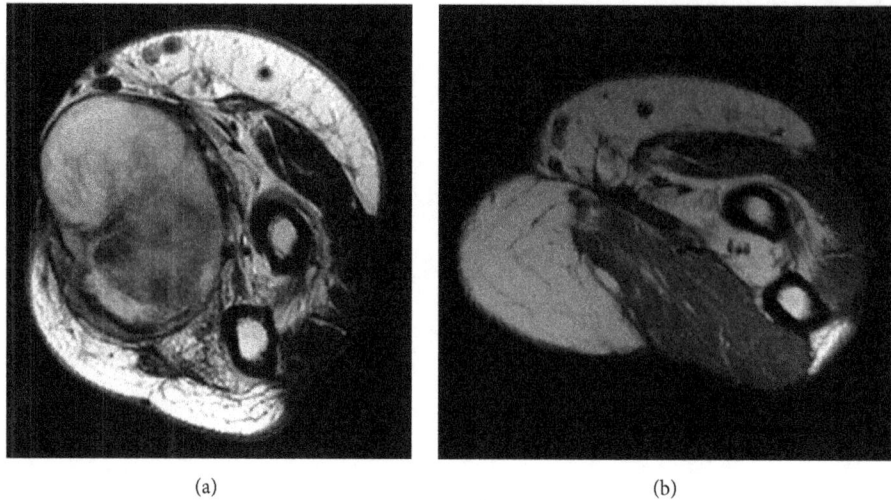

(a)   (b)

FIGURE 1: Preoperative T2 axial MRI image showing a heterogenous, subfascial mass (a) compared with postoperative T1 axial MRI image showing no evidence of residual mass (b).

with a composite grasp and an elbow ankylosed at approximately 30° of flexion. The arm had enumerable scars with evidence of multiple prior soft tissue transfers, but no draining sinuses or evidence of infection. The most recent incision had been made along a previous incision line and extended proximally through the antecubital fossa. A large mass was palpable in this region. Repeat imaging studies 6 weeks after the incomplete excision revealed that the lesion had essentially completely regrown to its preoperative size and shape.

A lengthy discussion was held with the patient, whose primary concern was to salvage the limb if at all possible. Due largely to his extreme physical and emotional investments to save the arm as a child, he was unwilling to accept the possibility of an amputation. An angiogram was performed, identifying the ulnar artery as the only major vessel feeding the distal arm, though there was an extensive collateral tree. It was determined at this time that excision with negative margins would be technically challenging but feasible.

The patient was taken for surgical resection with a limb-sparing procedure and brachytherapy. The median nerve was adhered to the tumor, but the musculoskeletal oncologist was able to salvage it by sacrificing some of the branches. The ulnar artery, however, was encased by tumor. Vascular surgery evaluated the patient intraoperatively and was able to identify a Doppler signal from the brachial artery proximally but could not find a good vessel for a bypass. Therefore, the decision was made to ligate the ulnar artery despite it being the predominant vascular supply to the distal limb. Surprisingly, the radial pulse was dopplerable and the hand remained warm and soft. The tumor was removed en bloc and brachytherapy catheters were placed under a vacuum-assisted-closure (VAC) dressing as described [8].

Postoperatively, the radial pulse remained dopplerable, and the hand remained well perfused. Pathology revealed a 10.8 cm residual high-grade leiomyosarcoma with 5–10% necrosis and 28 mitoses per 10 high-powered fields (Figure 2). Margins were microscopically negative. He underwent brachytherapy and the catheters were removed on postoperative day 8 along with replacement of new VAC dressing. Three days later, he underwent free flap reconstruction of the forearm with split thickness skin grafting and delayed primary closure of the remainder of the wound. The ulnar nerve was transferred to motor branches enervating segmental portions of the flap.

After recovering from these operations, the patient had 4 cycles of ifosfamide and doxorubicin adjuvant chemotherapy. At his most recent follow-up, three years postoperatively, the patient had no evidence of local or systemic recurrence. He was back to work full time as a laborer and his wounds were completely healed (Figures 1(b) and 3).

3. Discussion

Significant trauma has been reported to be a rare risk factor for development of neoplasia, particularly in the case of burns. A review of 80 years of burn literature found 412 case reports of neoplasm arising in burn scars. While squamous cell carcinoma was by far the most common at 71%, 5% of the cases were sarcoma, including one report of leiomyosarcoma [9]. The mean latency interval between time of burn injury and time of tumor diagnosis was 31 years. Healing by secondary intention, nonhealing wounds, and fragile scars were identified as significant risk factors in the development of burn scar neoplasms "Marjolin's ulcer". One review of 11 burn scars over a period of 20 years found a predilection for burn scar carcinomas to arise in the flexion crease of limbs, thought to be a result of repetitive microtrauma from otherwise low impact everyday activities [10].

The pathogenesis of burn scar malignancies is not precisely understood. Initially, it was hypothesized that the

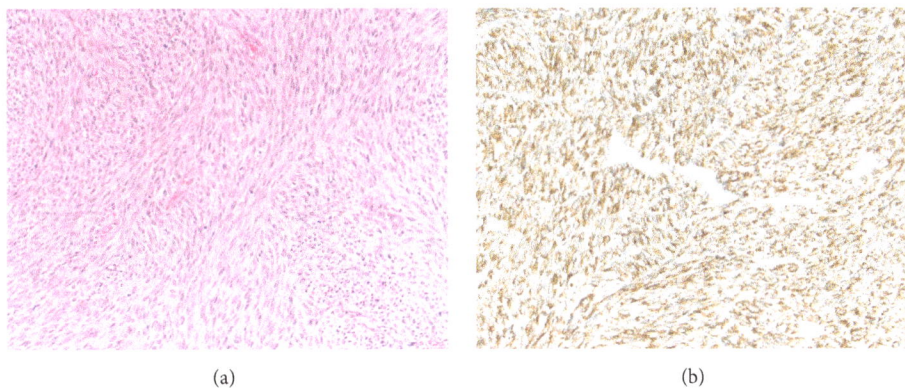

FIGURE 2: Pathology from the time of definitive surgery revealed a high-grade spindle cell sarcoma growing in fascicles that invaded subfascial tissue ((a), H&E). Immunohistochemical stains demonstrated strong, diffuse positivity for desmin ((b), immunostain). A grade 3 leiomyosarcoma was diagnosed with stage pT2bNxMx.

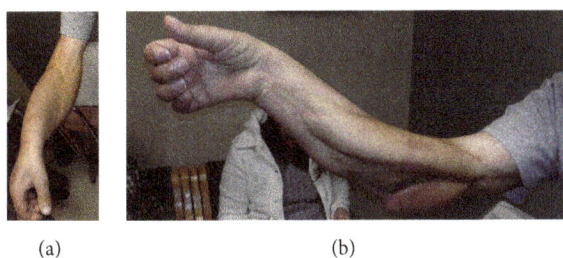

FIGURE 3: At most recent follow-up, the patient is sensate in the median and radial nerve distributions with weak wrist and finger flexion and extension.

damaged tissue released toxins that induced cellular mutations [11]. Another theory regarding the development of skin cancer after trauma is displacement of live epithelial cells into the deep tissue with a concurrent inability of the damaged tissue to regulate against the invading cells [12]. The current prevailing theory is that scar tissue forms an immunologically privileged site due to damage to lymphatic systems that hinders natural immunosurveillance, allowing neoplastic changes to occur [9, 13]. However, there is little scientific data available in the literature to support these postulates. In small series of patients, p53 has been found to be absent or dysfunctional in scar neoplasms, but no large scale scientific studies have been conducted that demonstrate a common pathophysiology for development of burn scar carcinomas [14, 15].

Leiomyosarcoma is typically an intra-abdominal or retroperitoneal tumor, though, in a study that spanned 7 years, 12% were located in the extremities and all but one was subfascial. While a vascular origin was suggested by the relationship of the tumor to the vessels in the majority of cases, definitive diagnosis could only be established in 5 of the cases. Tumor size >10 cm at presentation, mitotic rate >19 per 10 HPF, marginal or intralesional excision, and lack of adjuvant radiotherapy were found to be significant risk factors for progression of leiomyosarcomas located in the extremities. In their series, 2-year and 5-year

disease-free survival rates were 42.3% and 32.6%, respectively [1].

Another series of 66 patients over 22 years with leiomyosarcoma arising from the soft tissues of the extremities found that only 16% were located in the upper extremities. Mortality in this series was similar with 50% survival at a mean of 3 years after diagnosis. Identified risk factors for mortality included tumor size >5 cm^3, MTS stage III, presence of metastases, and axial anatomic location. Radiation and chemotherapy did not appear to directly affect outcome, but patients who underwent surgery with adjuvant therapy trended towards longer survival compared with those treated with surgery alone [2].

To our knowledge, this is the first case reported in the literature of sarcoma development in a replanted limb and joins a very small number of cases of posttraumatic sarcoma in the extremities. The development of leiomyosarcoma in the upper extremity is unusual and even more unique in the setting of a previously replanted arm. While the precise etiology of posttraumatic sarcoma development has not been well established, analogous progression of burn scars into malignancies is proposed to result from development of an immune privileged site that hinders the body's ability to recognize and eliminate cancerous cells. This explanation is also plausible in the setting of severe trauma such as an amputation with multiple procedures required for successful replantation due to disruption of local lymphatic systems in both situations, which prevent tumor specific antigens from being carried to regional lymph nodes and allow for relatively unrestricted tumor growth [13, 16].

In this case, similar to the average latency period seen in burn scar neoplasms, the patient developed a mass 24 years after his initial trauma. Although he presented with several poor prognostic indicators including a tumor size of >10 cm and a high number of mitoses per HPF, he was aggressively treated with wide resection and brachytherapy followed by chemotherapy in accordance with his determination to salvage the limb, minimize the chance of local recurrence, and eradicate micrometastatic disease. He has maintained baseline function of his replanted arm and remains free of local recurrence and evidence of metastases at three-year follow-up.

References

[1] D. Massi, G. Beltrami, M. M. Mela, M. Pertici, R. Capanna, and A. Franchi, "Prognostic factors in soft tissue leiomyosarcoma of the extremities: a retrospective analysis of 42 cases," *European Journal of Surgical Oncology*, vol. 30, no. 5, pp. 565–572, 2004.

[2] H. J. Mankin, J. Casas-Ganem, J.-I. Kim, M. C. Gebhardt, F. J. Hornicek, and E. N. Zeegen, "Leiomyosarcoma of somatic soft tissues," *Clinical Orthopaedics and Related Research*, no. 421, pp. 225–231, 2004.

[3] C.-Y. Wang, C. Yang, S.-Q. Li, and X. Qi, "Posttraumatic osteosarcoma: a case report and review of relative literatures," *Zhongguo Gu Shang*, vol. 27, no. 1, pp. 69–70, 2014.

[4] A. Thyss, S. F. Michiels, C. Caldani, and M. Schneider, "Osteogenic sarcoma of soft tissue after post-traumatic myositis ossificans," *Presse Medicale*, vol. 13, no. 21, pp. 1333–1334, 1984.

[5] G. V. Bykovchenko, "Rhabdomyosarcoma of the knee developing 22 years after a gunshot wound," *Voprosy Onkologii*, vol. 13, no. 8, pp. 118–119, 1967.

[6] T. Witwicki, A. Daniluk, and W. Dulowski, "2 cases of sarcoma developing at the site of fracture and metallic osteosynthesis," *Wiadomosci Lekarskie*, vol. 29, no. 4, pp. 339–343, 1976.

[7] R. J. Cureton and J. D. Griffiths, "Rhabdomyosarcoma of hand following trauma," *British Journal of Surgery*, vol. 44, no. 187, pp. 509–513, 1957.

[8] R. L. McGough, "The BrachyVAC: a new method for managing sarcomas requiring soft tissue reconstruction," *Operative Techniques in Orthopaedics*, vol. 24, no. 2, pp. 68–73, 2014.

[9] A. Kowal-Vern and B. K. Criswell, "Burn scar neoplasms: a literature review and statistical analysis," *Burns*, vol. 31, no. 4, pp. 403–413, 2005.

[10] C.-Y. Huang, C.-H. Feng, Y.-C. Hsiao, S. S. Chuang, and J.-Y. Yang, "Burn scar carcinoma," *Journal of Dermatological Treatment*, vol. 21, no. 6, pp. 350–356, 2010.

[11] A. R. Kadir, "Burn scar neoplasm," *Annals of Burns and Fire Disasters*, vol. 20, no. 4, pp. 185–188, 2007.

[12] Z. Neuman, N. Ben-Hur, and J. Shulman, "Trauma and skin cancer. Implantation of epidermal elements and possible cause," *Plastic and Reconstructive Surgery*, vol. 32, pp. 649–656, 1963.

[13] J. W. Futrell and G. H. Myers Jr., "The burn scar as an 'immunologically privileged site'," *Surgical Forum*, vol. 23, pp. 129–131, 1972.

[14] D. L. Harland, W. A. Robinson, and W. A. Franklin, "Deletion of the p53 gene in a patient with aggressive burn scar carcinoma," *Journal of Trauma*, vol. 42, no. 1, pp. 104–107, 1997.

[15] S. Sakatani, H. Kusakabe, K. Kiyokane, and K. Suzuki, "p53 gene mutations in squamous cell carcinoma occurring in scars: comparison with p53 protein immunoreactivity," *The American Journal of Dermatopathology*, vol. 20, no. 5, pp. 463–467, 1998.

[16] J. Bostwick III, W. J. Pendergrast Jr., and L. O. Vasconez, "Marjolin's ulcer: an immunologically privileged tumor?" *Plastic and Reconstructive Surgery*, vol. 57, no. 1, pp. 66–69, 1976.

57

Multidisciplinary Approach to Hepatic Metastases of Intracranial Hemangiopericytoma: A Case Report and Review of the Literature

Dimitrios K. Manatakis,[1] Spiridon G. Delis,[1] Nikolaos Ptohis,[2] Penelope Korkolopoulou,[3] and Christos Dervenis[1]

[1]Surgical Department, "Konstantopouleio" General Hospital, Nea Ionia, 14233 Athens, Greece
[2]Interventional Radiology Department, "G. Gennimatas" General Hospital, 11527 Athens, Greece
[3]1st Department of Pathology, Medical School, National and Kapodistrian University of Athens, 11527 Athens, Greece

Correspondence should be addressed to Dimitrios K. Manatakis; dmanatak@yahoo.gr

Academic Editor: Francesca Micci

Hemangiopericytoma is a rare primary tumor originating from Zimmerman's pericytes, with significant metastatic potential. Hepatic metastatic disease requires an aggressive approach by a multidisciplinary team of dedicated oncology specialists, to prolong survival in selected patients. We report on a patient with recurrent hepatic metastases of grade II intracranial hemangiopericytoma 5 years after initial treatment, managed by a stepwise combination of liver resection, radiofrequency ablation, and transarterial embolization. Although metastatic disease implies hematogenous dissemination, long-term survival after liver resection has been reported and major hepatectomies are justified in patients with adequate local control. Liver resections combined with transarterial embolization are highly recommended, due to hypervascularity of the tumor.

1. Introduction

Noncolorectal, nonneuroendocrine hepatic metastases are a diverse group of secondary liver neoplasias, exhibiting variable clinical behavior and characteristics. Particularly in cases of rare primary tumors, where limited datasets are available and no official guidelines are published, a multidisciplinary team (MDT) approach is mandated, to provide comprehensive assessment, consultation, and treatment.

We present our experience with a case of recurrent hepatic metastases from an intracranial hemangiopericytoma (HPC), managed by an MDT of oncologic surgeons, medical oncologists, interventional radiologists, and dedicated pathologists.

2. Case Presentation

A 23-year-old Caucasian male underwent a right temporal lobe glomus tumor excision. Seven years later he was diagnosed with local recurrence and underwent two craniotomies to achieve radical resection (Figure 1). Histopathology revealed an HPC grade II. No adjuvant chemoradiotherapy was instituted.

Five years after the last intervention, he was admitted to hospital due to diverticulitis and an incidental finding of a small lesion in the body of T10 vertebra was demonstrated on CT scans, as well as multiple, atypical, hypervascular lesions in both liver lobes, the larger being 8 cm in diameter, initially considered hemangiomas (Figures 2 and 3). Magnetic resonance imaging, however, was consistent with metastatic HPC lesions rather than benign hemangiomas. Although positron emission tomography (PET) revealed strong uptake of the contrast medium in the T10 lesion, no uptake in the liver was documented. Tumor markers (CEA, αFP, and Ca19-9) were within normal limits.

A right hepatectomy plus radiofrequency ablation of one lesion in the left lobe was decided and the patient had an uneventful postoperative course. Histopathology revealed two tumors (8.7 cm and 3.8 cm) consisting of relatively bland

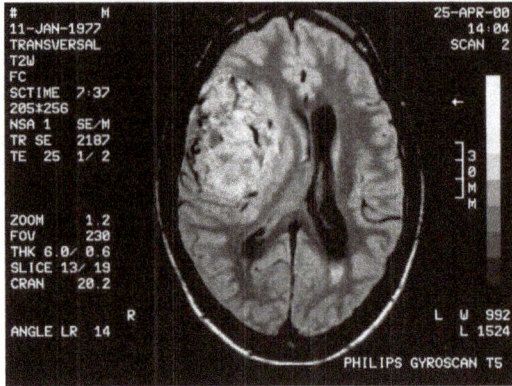

FIGURE 1: Brain primary tumor.

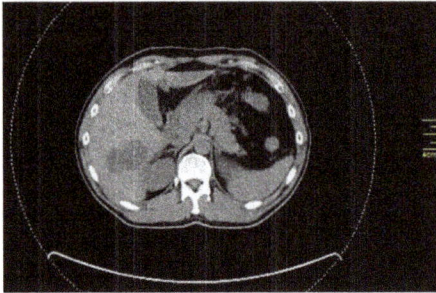

FIGURE 2: Liver metastases, segment VI.

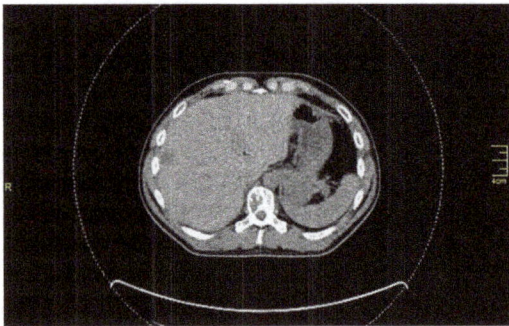

FIGURE 3: Liver metastasis, segment VIII.

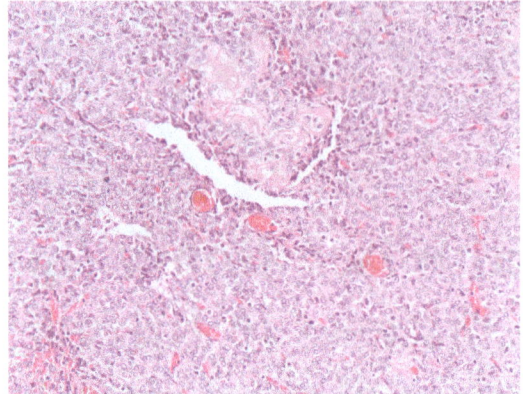

FIGURE 4: H&E stain, 200x.

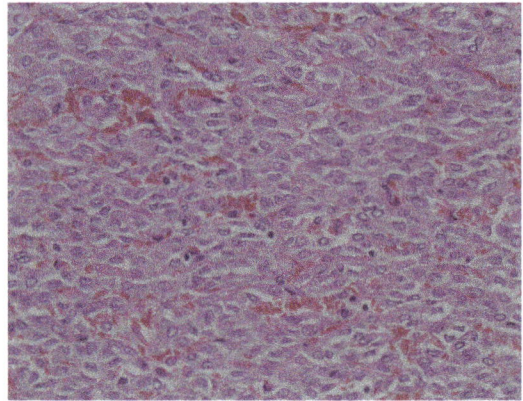

FIGURE 5: H&E stain, 400x.

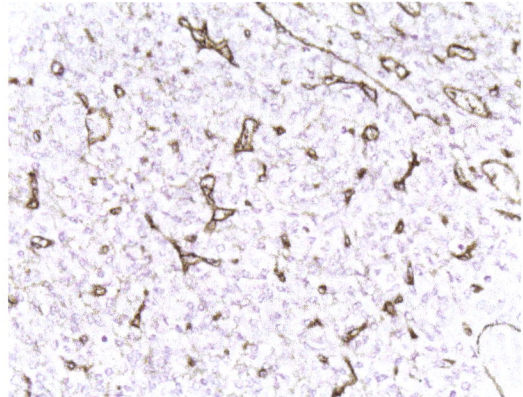

FIGURE 6: CD34 stain, 40x.

mesenchymal cells, with no unique characteristics, packed around an elaborate network of vessels (Figures 4 and 5), confirming the hypervascularity and nonepithelial origin of the neoplasms, which exhibited mild nuclear pleomorphism, low mitotic rate (<5 mitoses/10 HPF), and few areas of necrosis. Immunohistochemistry was positive for CD34 (Figure 6) and vimentin and negative for S100. Stain for EMA was focally positive. The immunoreactivity profile was identical to the previous report of the primary brain tumor.

One year after liver resection, follow-up CT scan revealed no local recurrence in the brain cavity, but three metastatic lesions in the liver parenchyma (segments II and IV) and slow progression of the T10 lesion. The MDT proposed stereotactic radiosurgery for the bone metastasis and elective transarterial embolization (TAE) of the liver lesions, as bridging therapy to a second hepatectomy. Two of the liver lesions were hypervascular, although the caudate lobe metastasis was only slightly vascular with a capillary network. Transarterial embolization was successful, due to hyperselective arterial catheterization (Figures 7 and 8).

3. Discussion

Hemangiopericytoma is a rare mesenchymal tumor, originating from Zimmerman's pericytes, which are contractile spindle cells, surrounding capillaries and postcapillary

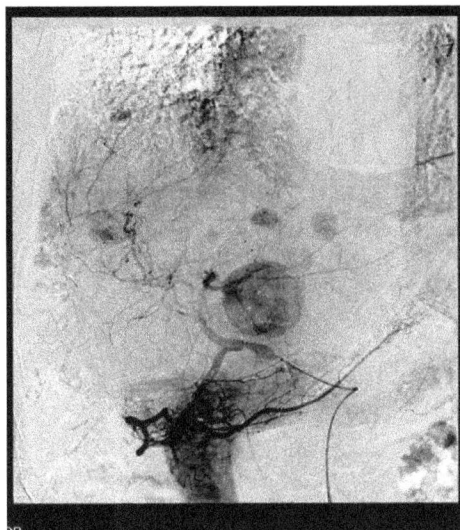

FIGURE 7: Multiple hypervascular hepatic lesions.

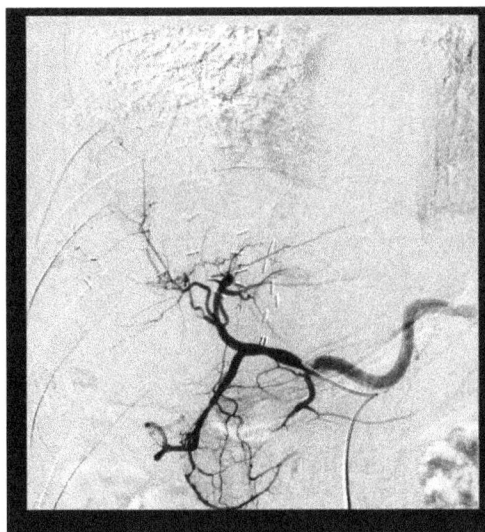

FIGURE 8: Disappearance of hepatic lesions after transarterial embolization.

venules, and regulate capillary flow and permeability [1]. Most common anatomic locations involved are lower extremities, retroperitoneum, and meninges, with both genders equally affected [1, 2]. Intracranial HPCs constitute less than 1% of all intracranial tumors [3].

Generally HPCs are aggressive tumors, with 5-year local recurrence rate of 65% and 5-year distant metastasis rate of 33%, with lung, liver, and bones being the most frequent metastatic locations [3].

Clinical symptoms are vague and nonspecific, depending on tumor location and size [4]. Pain is usually a late presentation, while hypoglycemia represents a unique endocrine paraneoplastic syndrome, caused by oversecretion of insulin-like growth factor II [5].

Hypervascularity is the prominent imaging characteristic and preoperative differential diagnosis from other vascular

lesions is necessary, due to differences in treatment and prognosis. Unenhanced liver ultrasound reveals hypoechoic lesions, which become markedly hyperechoic during the arterial phase of contrast medium administration [6]. On CT scans, HPCs exhibit arterial phase enhancement and usually have well-defined borders [6].

Magnetic resonance imaging reveals well-defined, lobular lesions, with an isointense signal in T1WI and slightly long signal in T2WI unenhanced scans. Following gadolinium administration, a heterogeneous enhancement is observed, due to cystic degeneration, focal tumor necrosis, or flow voids [4, 6].

Unlike meningioma, which has a hyperplastic effect on adjacent bone, HPCs are shown to exert an osteolytic effect. Moreover, no dural tail sign is observed [4, 6].

Fluorodeoxyglucose (FDG) PET may be helpful in revealing multiple distant metastases. As in our case, HPCs show avid enhancement on CT, but low FDG uptake on PET, indicative of low glucose metabolism [7].

Accurate preoperative diagnosis may still be challenging, despite high-tech imaging modalities, and histopathology and immunohistochemistry confirm the diagnosis. Hemangiopericytomas are highly cellular and vascularized tumors, consisting of tightly packed, round to fusiform cells, around a well-developed, elaborate branching "staghorn" vasculature [1, 8].

According to the World Health Organization classification, HPCs are graded as being differentiated (grade II) and anaplastic (grade III) [3]. Signs of anaplasia include high mitotic rate (>5 mitoses per HPF) and/or necrosis, plus at least two of the following features: hemorrhage, moderate to high nuclear atypia, and cellularity [8].

Immunohistochemically tumor cells usually express CD34 and vimentin but not EMA and S100 [1, 3]. Immunoreactivity patterns generally vary among HPCs and no antibody is 100% sensitive or specific [3]. However immunoprofiles are helpful, to exclude meningiomas and solid fibrous tumors [3, 4].

Despite advances in diagnostic and therapeutic modalities, management of HPCs remains challenging and problematic. Due to the tumor's rarity, most published studies are retrospective cohorts with small numbers of patients. Consequently, there are no concrete treatment recommendations based on level I evidence.

Surgery is the mainstay of treatment. Indeed, all authors agree that gross total resection increases overall survival (OS) and recurrence-free interval [3, 9–12]. However, hypervascularity of the tumor and close relation to delicate intracranial structures make complete resection of brain primaries possible in only 50–60% of patients [3, 11]. As for hepatic metastatic disease, there are no guidelines on resection margins and intraoperative ultrasonography may be helpful to achieve R0 resections. Liver transplantation has been reported in a case of refractory hypoglycemia [13].

The role of adjuvant radiotherapy is controversial. Safe conclusions cannot be drawn, due to small sample sizes and retrospective character of available studies. Zweckberger et al. propose radiotherapy to grade II patients with subtotal resections and to all grade III patients [3]. Schiariti et al. found that radiation reduces risk of local recurrence but does not prolong recurrence interval [9]. On the other hand, Rutkowski et al. found no benefit from gross total resection plus radiotherapy when compared to gross total resection alone, and total doses of >50 Gy were associated with increased mortality rates. Similarly, in cases of subtotal resection, addition of radiation offered no survival benefit [10].

Stereotactic radiosurgery (gamma-knife, cyber-knife) has been used in cases of recurrent or residual disease, with promising results [3]. Ecker et al. reported a 93% response rate, with 42 out of 45 tumors obliterated, decreased, or controlled [11]. Veeravagu et al. reported that stereotactic radiosurgery increases time to recurrence and OS [14]. However it does not decrease the risk for distant metastases, which are a cause of significant morbidity and mortality.

Systemic chemotherapy has shown only disappointing results and its role is purely palliative [11, 12]. On the other hand, there is a growing body of evidence on the value of antiangiogenic drugs (sunitinib, sorafenib, pazopanib, bevacizumab/temozolomide, and endostatin/ginsenoside Rg3). The rationale behind their use is the expression of platelet-derived growth factor receptor (PDGFR) and vascular endothelial growth factor receptor (VEGFR) by the HPC tumor cells. Small experimental trials or case reports have been published to date, reporting partial response or stable disease course for several months; however, these results need validation in larger controlled studies [2, 5, 15–17].

Although HPC has been described as borderline malignant, its clinical behavior is difficult to predict and long-term follow-up is indicated, since recurrence and metastasis have been reported even after prolonged disease-free intervals [1, 9, 18]. Factors affecting prognosis are mainly tumor grade and completeness of resection; however, in multivariate analysis, they do not reach statistical significance in most papers due to small sample sizes [9].

Comparison between low- and high-grade tumors has shown that even grade II tumors have significant metastatic potential and often relapse [3]. High-grade tumors recur earlier than low-grade tumors and decrease OS rates [9, 11].

The survival benefit of gross total resection applies to both CNS and extra-CNS HPCs, although extra-CNS tumors tend to be larger and more advanced and with shorter OS [12].

In their study, Damodaran et al. reported OS at 5, 10, 15, and 20 years at 79%, 56%, 44%, and 22%, respectively [19]. For grade II tumors, OS was 216 months, while for grade III tumors OS was 142 months. Local recurrence rates at 5, 10, and 15 years were 20%, 54%, and 77%, while distant metastasis rates at 5, 10, and 15 years were 10%, 31%, and 77%.

Although liver metastatic disease is a surrogate marker of tumor hematogenous dissemination, long-term survival after hepatectomy is reported. Extrahepatic disease is not a contraindication to liver resection in case of local control, as reported in our case. In essence, if the time interval between the primary lesion and the liver metastatic disease is prolonged, major hepatectomy is justified in young individuals. In case of liver recurrence, re-resection combined with TAE is highly recommended, due to the hypervascular nature of the tumor [20].

Consent

This paper is published with the written consent of the patient.

References

[1] M. Koch, G. P. Nielsen, and S. S. Yoon, "Malignant tumors of blood vessels: angiosarcomas, hemangioendotheliomas, and hemangiopericytyomas," *Journal of Surgical Oncology*, vol. 97, no. 4, pp. 321–329, 2008.

[2] X.-D. Li, J.-T. Jiang, and C.-P. Wu, "Combined therapy against recurrent hemangiopericytoma: a case report," *Cancer Biology and Medicine*, vol. 9, no. 2, pp. 141–143, 2012.

[3] K. Zweckberger, C. S. Jung, W. Mueller, A. W. Unterberg, and U. Schick, "Hemangiopericytomas grade II are not benign tumors," *Acta Neurochirurgica*, vol. 153, no. 2, pp. 385–394, 2011.

[4] C. Ma, F. Xu, Y.-D. Xiao, R. Paudel, Y. Sun, and E.-H. Xiao, "Magnetic resonance imaging of intracranial hemangiopericytoma and correlation with pathological findings," *Oncology Letters*, vol. 8, pp. 2140–2144, 2014.

[5] S. W. Lee, E. K. Lee, T. Yun et al., "Recurrent hypoglycemia triggered by sorafenib therapy in a patient with hemangiopericytoma," *Endocrinology and Metabolism*, vol. 29, no. 2, pp. 202–205, 2014.

[6] C. Aliberti, G. Benea, B. Kopf, and U. De Giorgi, "Hepatic metastases of hemangiopericytoma: contrast-enhanced MRI, contrast-enhanced ultrasonography and angiography findings," *Cancer Imaging*, vol. 6, no. 1, pp. 56–59, 2006.

[7] W. S. W. Chan, J. Zhang, and P. L. Khong, "[18]F-FDG-PET-CT imaging findings of recurrent intracranial haemangiopericytoma with distant metastases," *British Journal of Radiology*, vol. 83, no. 992, pp. e172–e174, 2010.

[8] H. Mena, J. L. Ribas, G. H. Pezeshkpour, D. N. Cowan, and J. E. Parisi, "Hemangiopericytoma of the central nervous system: a review of 94 cases," *Human Pathology*, vol. 22, no. 1, pp. 84–91, 1991.

[9] M. Schiariti, P. Goetz, H. El-Maghraby, J. Tailor, and N. Kitchen, "Hemangiopericytoma: long-term outcome revisited," *Journal of Neurosurgery*, vol. 114, no. 3, pp. 747–755, 2011.

[10] M. J. Rutkowski, M. E. Sughrue, A. J. Kane et al., "Predictors of mortality following treatment of intracranial hemangiopericytoma," *Journal of Neurosurgery*, vol. 113, no. 2, pp. 333–339, 2010.

[11] R. D. Ecker, W. R. Marsh, B. E. Pollock et al., "Hemangiopericytoma in the central nervous system: treatment, pathological features, and long-term follow up in 38 patients," *Journal of Neurosurgery*, vol. 98, no. 6, pp. 1182–1187, 2003.

[12] W. A. Hall, A. N. Ali, N. Gullett et al., "Comparing central nervous system (CNS) and extra-CNS hemangiopericytomas in the surveillance, epidemiology, and end results program: analysis of 655 patients and review of current literature," *Cancer*, vol. 118, no. 21, pp. 5331–5338, 2012.

[13] J. Adams, J. P. A. Lodge, and D. Parker, "Liver transplantation for metastatic hemangiopericytoma associated with hypoglycemia," *Transplantation*, vol. 67, no. 3, pp. 488–489, 1999.

[14] A. Veeravagu, B. Jiang, C. G. Patil et al., "CyberKnife stereotactic radiosurgery for recurrent, metastatic, and residual hemangiopericytomas," *Journal of Hematology and Oncology*, vol. 4, article 26, 2011.

[15] M. Delgado, E. Pérez-Ruiz, J. Alcalde, D. Pérez, R. Villatoro, and A. Rueda, "Anti-angiogenic treatment (sunitinib) for disseminated malignant haemangiopericytoma: a case study and review of the literature," *Case Reports in Oncology*, vol. 4, no. 1, pp. 55–59, 2011.

[16] S. J. Lee, S. T. Kim, S. H. Park, Y. L. Choi, J. B. Park, and J. Lee, "Successful use of pazopanib for treatment of refractory metastatic hemangiopericytoma," *Clinical Sarcoma Research*, vol. 4, no. 1, article 13, 2014.

[17] M. S. Park, S. R. Patel, J. A. Ludwig et al., "Activity of temozolomide and bevacizumab in the treatment of locally advanced, recurrent, and metastatic hemangiopericytoma and malignant solitary fibrous tumor," *Cancer*, vol. 117, no. 21, pp. 4939–4947, 2011.

[18] B.-W. Kim, H.-J. Wang, I.-H. Jeong, S.-I. Ahn, and M.-W. Kim, "Metastatic liver cancer: a rare case," *World Journal of Gastroenterology*, vol. 11, no. 27, pp. 4281–4284, 2005.

[19] O. Damodaran, P. Robbins, N. Knuckey, M. Bynevelt, G. Wong, and G. Lee, "Primary intracranial haemangiopericytoma: comparison of survival outcomes and metastatic potential in WHO grade II and III variants," *Journal of Clinical Neuroscience*, vol. 21, no. 8, pp. 1310–1314, 2014.

[20] T. Torigoe, A. Higure, K. Hirata, N. Nagata, and H. Itoh, "Malignant hemangiopericytoma in the pelvic cavity successfully treated by combined-modality therapy: report of a case," *Surgery Today*, vol. 33, no. 6, pp. 479–482, 2003.

Permissions

All chapters in this book were first published in CROM, by Hindawi Publishing Corporation; hereby published with permission under the Creative Commons Attribution License or equivalent. Every chapter published in this book has been scrutinized by our experts. Their significance has been extensively debated. The topics covered herein carry significant findings which will fuel the growth of the discipline. They may even be implemented as practical applications or may be referred to as a beginning point for another development.

The contributors of this book come from diverse backgrounds, making this book a truly international effort. This book will bring forth new frontiers with its revolutionizing research information and detailed analysis of the nascent developments around the world.

We would like to thank all the contributing authors for lending their expertise to make the book truly unique. They have played a crucial role in the development of this book. Without their invaluable contributions this book wouldn't have been possible. They have made vital efforts to compile up to date information on the varied aspects of this subject to make this book a valuable addition to the collection of many professionals and students.

This book was conceptualized with the vision of imparting up-to-date information and advanced data in this field. To ensure the same, a matchless editorial board was set up. Every individual on the board went through rigorous rounds of assessment to prove their worth. After which they invested a large part of their time researching and compiling the most relevant data for our readers.

The editorial board has been involved in producing this book since its inception. They have spent rigorous hours researching and exploring the diverse topics which have resulted in the successful publishing of this book. They have passed on their knowledge of decades through this book. To expedite this challenging task, the publisher supported the team at every step. A small team of assistant editors was also appointed to further simplify the editing procedure and attain best results for the readers.

Apart from the editorial board, the designing team has also invested a significant amount of their time in understanding the subject and creating the most relevant covers. They scrutinized every image to scout for the most suitable representation of the subject and create an appropriate cover for the book.

The publishing team has been an ardent support to the editorial, designing and production team. Their endless efforts to recruit the best for this project, has resulted in the accomplishment of this book. They are a veteran in the field of academics and their pool of knowledge is as vast as their experience in printing. Their expertise and guidance has proved useful at every step. Their uncompromising quality standards have made this book an exceptional effort. Their encouragement from time to time has been an inspiration for everyone.

The publisher and the editorial board hope that this book will prove to be a valuable piece of knowledge for researchers, students, practitioners and scholars across the globe.

List of Contributors

Kerem Okutur and Gokhan Demir
Department of Medical Oncology, Acibadem University School of Medicine, Buyukdere Cad, No. 40, Sariyer, 34453 Istanbul, Turkey

Orhan Onder Eren
Department of Medical Oncology, Yeditepe University School of Medicine, Devlet Yolu, Ankara Caddesi, No. 102-104, Kozyatagi, 34652 Istanbul, Turkey

Mor Moskovitz, Mira Wollner and Nissim Haim
Division of Oncology, Rambam Health Care Campus, 3109601 Haifa, Israel

Kobe Van Bael and Georges Delvaux
Department of Surgery, Laarbeeklaan 101, 1090 Brussels, Belgium

Yanina Jansen, Teofila Seremet and Bart Neyns
Department of Medical Oncology, Laarbeeklaan 101, 1090 Brussels, Belgium

Benedikt Engels
Department of Radiotherapy, Laarbeeklaan 101, 1090 Brussels, Belgium

E. Moussaly and J. P. Atallah
Staten Island University Hospital, 475 Seaview Avenue, Staten Island, NY 10305, USA

Robert Diaz-Beveridge, Marcos Melian, Edwin Navarro, Dilara Akhoundova and Jorge Aparicio
Medical Oncology Department, University Hospital La Fe, Avinguda de Fernando Abril Martorell, No. 106, 46026 Valencia, Spain

Carlos Zac and Melitina Chrivella
Pathology Department, University Hospital La Fe, Avinguda de Fernando Abril Martorell, No. 106, 46026 Valencia, Spain

Zishuo Ian Hu
Department of Medicine, Mount Sinai St. Luke's Roosevelt Hospital Center, New York, NY 10019, USA

Lev Bangiyev
Department of Radiology, Stony Brook University Medical Center, Stony Brook, NY 11794, USA

Roberta J. Seidman
Department of Pathology, Stony Brook University Medical Center, Stony Brook, NY 11794, USA

Jules A. Cohen
Division of Hematology/Oncology, Department of Medicine, Stony Brook University Medical Center, Stony Brook, NY 11794, USA

Ali Ozan Oner
Nuclear Medicine Department, School of Medicine, Afyon Kocatepe University, 03200 Afyon, Turkey

Adil Boz
Nuclear Medicine Department, School of Medicine, Akdeniz University, 07070 Antalya, Turkey

Evrim Surer Budak
Nuclear Medicine Department, Antalya Training and Research Hospital, Antalya, Turkey

Gulnihal Hale Kaplan Kurt
Nuclear Medicine Department, Isparta State Hospital, Isparta, Turkey

Alexander Augustyn
Hamon Center for Therapeutic Oncology Research, University of Texas Southwestern Medical Center, Dallas, TX 75390, USA
Simmons Comprehensive Cancer Center, University of Texas Southwestern Medical Center, Dallas, TX 75390, USA

Mona Lisa Alattar and Harris Naina
Simmons Comprehensive Cancer Center, University of Texas Southwestern Medical Center, Dallas, TX 75390, USA
Department of Hematology and Oncology, University of Texas Southwestern Medical Center, Dallas, TX 75390, USA

Sharang Tenjarla, Theresa M. Kwiatkowski and Sheema Chawla
Department of Radiation Oncology, Rochester General Hospital, 1425 Portland Avenue, Rochester, NY 14621, USA

Lucy Ashley Sheils
Department of Pathology, Rochester General Hospital, 1425 Portland Avenue, Rochester, NY 14621, USA

Alexandra Millet, Sanmeet Singh, Genelle Gittens-Backus and Kim Ann Dang
Howard University College of Medicine, Washington, DC 20059, USA

Babak Shokrani
Department of Pathology, Howard University Hospital, Washington, DC 20060, USA

Bo Zhao, Laura S. Wood and Brian I. Rini
Department of Hematology and Oncology, Cleveland Clinic, 9500 Euclid Avenue R35, Cleveland, OH 44195, USA

Karen James
Department of Cardiovascular Medicine, Cleveland Clinic, 9500 Euclid Avenue J3-4, Cleveland, OH 44195, USA

Alec M. Block, Fiori Alite and Mehee Choi
Department of Radiation Oncology, Stritch School of Medicine, Loyola University Medical Center, 2160 S. First Avenue, Maywood, IL 60153, USA

Aidnag Z. Diaz
Department of Radiation Oncology, Rush University Medical Center, 500 S. Paulina Street, Ground Floor, Chicago, IL 60612, USA

Richard W. Borrowdale
Department of Otolaryngology Head and Neck Surgery, Stritch School of Medicine, Loyola University Medical Center, 2160 S. First Avenue, Maywood, IL 60153, USA

Joseph I. Clark
Department of Medicine, Division of Hematology/Oncology, Stritch School of Medicine, Loyola University Medical Center, 2160 S. First Avenue, Maywood, IL 60153, USA

Monika Pazgan-Simon and Justyna Janocha-Litwin
Infectious Disease Department, Wroclaw Medical University, Wroclaw, Poland

Sylwia Serafinska and Krzysztof Simon
Infectious Disease Department, Division of Infectious Disease and Hepatology, Wroclaw Medical University, Wroclaw, Poland

Jolanta Zuwala-Jagiello
Department of Pharmaceutical Biochemistry, Wroclaw Medical University, Wroclaw, Poland

Meghan E. Kapp, Giovanna A. Giannico and Mohamed Mokhtar Desouki
Department of Pathology, Microbiology and Immunology, Vanderbilt University Medical Center, Nashville, TN 37232, USA

Aleksey Novikov, Horatio Holzer, Ghaith Abu-Zeinah, Tomer M. Mark and Raymond D. Pastore
Department of Internal Medicine, New York Presbyterian Hospital, Weill Cornell Medical College, New York, NY 10065-4897, USA

Robert A. DeSimone and David J. Pisapia
Department of Pathology and Laboratory Medicine, New York Presbyterian Hospital, Weill Cornell Medical College, New York, NY 10065-4897, USA

Shahzaib Nabi
Department of Internal Medicine, Henry Ford Health System, 2799 W. Grand Boulevard, Detroit, MI 48202, USA

Abhijit Saste
Department of Hematology-Oncology, Henry Ford Health System, 2799W. Grand Boulevard, Detroit, MI 48202, USA

Rohit Gulati
Department of Pathology, Henry Ford Health System, 2799W. Grand Boulevard, Detroit, MI 48202, USA

Samer Alsidawi
Department of Internal Medicine, University of Cincinnati, Cincinnati, OH 45267, USA

Abhimanyu Ghose and Neetu Radhakrishnan
Division of Hematology-Oncology, Department of Medicine, University of Cincinnati, Cincinnati, OH 45267, USA

Julianne Qualtieri
Department of Pathology, University of Cincinnati, Cincinnati, OH 45267, USA

Yu Yu Thar and Elizabeth Guevara
Department of Medicine, Division of Hematology and Oncology, The Brooklyn Hospital Center, Brooklyn, NY 11201, USA

Poras Patel
Department of Medicine, The Brooklyn Hospital Center, Brooklyn, NY 11201, USA

Tiangui Huang
Department of Pathology, The Brooklyn Hospital Center, Brooklyn, NY 11201, USA

Mario Metry, Mohamad Shaaban, Magdi Youssef and Michael Carr
Breast Surgery Unit, Northumbria Healthcare NHS Foundation Trust, Woodhorn Lane, Ashington NE63 9JJ, UK

Michael L. Adashek
Department of Internal Medicine, Sinai Hospital, Baltimore, MD, USA

Kenneth Miller
University of Maryland Marlene and Stewart Greenebaum Comprehensive Cancer Center, Baltimore, MD, USA

Arit A. Silpasuvan
Department of Endocrinology, Sinai Hospital, Baltimore, MD, USA

Rubens Barros Costa, Ricardo Costa, Jason Kaplan, Marcelo Rocha Cruz, Hiral Shah, Maria Matsangou and Benedito Carneiro
Developmental Therapeutics Program, Feinberg School of Medicine and Robert H. Lurie Comprehensive Cancer Center of Northwestern University, 233 East Superior Street, Chicago, IL 60611, USA

Sandeep Batra and Stephen C. Martin
Department of Pediatrics, Section of Pediatric Hematology and Oncology, Riley Hospital for Children at Indiana University Health, Indiana University School of Medicine, Indianapolis, IN 46202, USA

Mehdi Nassiri and Amna Qureshi
Department of Pathology and Laboratory Medicine, Indiana University School of Medicine, Indianapolis, IN 46202, USA

Troy A. Markel
Department of Surgery, Section of Pediatric Surgery, Riley Hospital for Children at Indiana University Health, Indiana University School of Medicine, Indianapolis, IN 46202, USA

Renate U. Wahl and Albert Rübben
Department of Dermatology, Euregional Skin Cancer Center, University Hospital of the RWTH-Aachen, Aachen, Germany

Claudio Cacchi
Department of Pathology, University Hospital of the RWTH-Aachen, Aachen, Germany

Yoji Shido and Yukihiro Matsuyama
Department of Orthopaedic Surgery, Hamamatsu University School of Medicine, 1-20-1 Handayama, Higashi-ku, Hamamatsu, Shizuoka 431-3192, Japan

Krishna Adit Agarwal and Myat Han Soe
Department of Medicine, Baystate Medical Center, University of Massachusetts Medical School, Springfield, MA, USA

Nagla Abdel Karim, Ihab Eldessouki, Ahmad Taftaf, Deeb Ayham and Ola Gaber
Department of Hematology-Oncology, University of Cincinnati, Cincinnati, OH, USA

Abouelmagd Makramalla
Department of Interventional Radiology, University of Cincinnati, Cincinnati, OH, USA

Zelia M. Correa
Department of Ophthalmology, University of Cincinnati, Cincinnati, OH, USA

Alina Basnet and Abirami Sivapiragasam
Department of Hematology Oncology, SUNY Upstate Medical University, Syracuse, NY 13205, USA

Aakriti Pandita
Department of Medicine, SUNY Upstate Medical University, Syracuse, NY 13205, USA

Joseph Fullmer
Department of Pathology, SUNY Upstate Medical University, Syracuse, NY 13205, USA

D. Myoteri and E. Carvounis
Pathology Department, Aretaieion University Hospital, Medical School of Athens, Athens, Greece

D. Dellaportas, C. Nastos, I. Gioti, G. Gkiokas and T. Theodosopoulos
2nd Department of Surgery, Aretaieion University Hospital, Medical School of Athens, Athens, Greece

Ravi Maharaj, Sangeeta Parbhu, Wesley Ramcharan, Shanta Baijoo, Wesley Greaves and Dave Harnanan
Department of Clinical Surgical Sciences, University of the West Indies, Eric Williams Medical Sciences Complex, Champ Fleurs, Trinidad and Tobago

Wayne A. Warner
Division of Oncology, Siteman Cancer Center, Washington University School of Medicine, St. Louis, MO 63110, USA
Department of Cell Biology and Physiology, Washington University School of Medicine, St. Louis, MO 63110, USA

Giovanni Faggioni
Medical Oncology Unit 2, Istituto Oncologico Veneto, IRCCS, Padova, Italy

Mara Mantiero, Alice Menichetti, Valentina Guarneri and Pierfranco Conte
Medical Oncology Unit 2, Istituto Oncologico Veneto, IRCCS, Padova, Italy

Department of Surgical, Oncological and Gastroenterological Sciences, University of Padova, Padova, Italy

Matteo Fassan
Department of Medicine, Surgical Pathology and Cytopathology Unit, University of Padova, Padova, Italy

Naomi Fei and Nilay Shah
Department of Internal Medicine, West Virginia University Hospital, 1 Medical Center Dr, Morgantown, WV 26505, USA

Lilit Karapetyan, Manoj Rai and Om Dawani
Michigan State University Department of Medicine and EW Sparrow Hospital, 804 Service Rd, Room B301, East Lansing, MI 48824, USA

Heather S. Laird-Fick
Michigan State University Department of Medicine, 804 Service Rd, Room B316, East Lansing, MI 48824, USA

Mark B. Ulanja, Mohamed E. Taha, Arshad A. Al-Mashhadani, Christie Elliot and Santhosh Ambika
Department of Internal Medicine, University of Nevada Reno, School of Medicine, 1155 Mill Street, Reno, NV 89502, USA

Marwah Muaad Al-Tekreeti
American Public University System, 111 West Congress Street, Charles Town, WV 25414, USA

Nedal Bukhari
Department of Medical Oncology, King Fahad Specialist Hospital, Dammam, Saudi Arabia

Marwah Abdulkader
Department of Pathology, King Fahad Specialist Hospital, Dammam, Saudi Arabia

Reiko Yamada, Hiroyuki Inoue, Takashi Sakuno, Tetsuro Harada, Naohiko Yoshizawa, Hiroshi Miura, Toshihumi Takeuchi, Misaki Nakamura and Yoshiyuki Takei
Department of Gastroenterology and Hepatology, Mie University Graduate School of Medicine, Tsu, Japan

Kyosuke Tanaka, Masaki Katsurahara, Yasuhiko Hamada and Noriyuki Horiki
Department of Endoscopy, Mie University School of Medicine, Tsu, Japan

Kathryn Bower
Section of Hematology/Oncology, West Virginia University, Morgantown, WV, USA

Nilay Shah
Alexander B. Osborn Hematopoietic Malignancy and Transplantation Program, West Virginia University, Morgantown, WV, USA

Tubin Slavisa and Raunik Wolfgang
Institut für Strahlentherapie/Radioonkologie, Feschnigstraβe 11, 9020 Klagenfurt am Wörthersee, Austria

Uroosa Ibrahim, Gwenalyn Garcia and Qun Dai
Department of Hematology/Oncology, Staten Island University Hospital, 475 Seaview Avenue, Staten Island, NY 10305, USA

Amina Saqib
Department of Pulmonary/Critical Care, Staten Island University Hospital, 475 Seaview Avenue, Staten Island, NY 10305, USA

Shafinaz Hussein
Department of Pathology, Staten Island University Hospital, 475 Seaview Avenue, Staten Island, NY 10305, USA

Karan Seegobin, Satish Maharaj, Grant Nelson, Jeremy Carlson, Cherisse Baldeo and Rafik Jacob
Department of Internal Medicine, University of Florida College of Medicine, Jacksonville, FL 32209, USA

Anil Rahul, Fernandes Robin and Hiremath Adarsh
Internal Medicine, MD Anderson Cancer Center, 1400 Pressler Street, Houston, TX 77030, USA

Aristomenes Kollas, George Zarkavelis, Aikaterini Kafantari and Nicholas Pavlidis
Department of Medical Oncology, University Hospital of Ioannina, 45500 Ioannina, Greece

Anna Goussia, Anna Batistatou and Zoi Evangelou
Department of Pathology, University Hospital of Ioannina, 45500 Ioannina, Greece

Eva Sintou
Department of Cytology, University Hospital of Ioannina, 45500 Ioannina, Greece

Jomjit Chantharasamee
Division of Medical Oncology, Department of Medicine, Faculty of Medicine, Siriraj Hospital, Mahidol University, Bangkok, Thailand

Jitsupa Treetipsatit
Department of Pathology, Faculty of Medicine, Siriraj Hospital, Mahidol University, Bangkok, Thailand

Marino Antonio Capurso-García
Departamento de Oncología Mamaria Quirúrgica, Instituto de Enfermedades de la Mama (IEM), La Fundación del Cáncer de Mama (FUCAM), 40980 Mexico City, Mexico
Facultad de Ciencias de la Salud, Universidad Anáhuac México Norte, 52786 Huixquilucan, MEX, Mexico

Alan Pomerantz, Javier Andrés Galnares-Olalde, Ruben Blachman-Braun, Sergio Rodríguez-Rodríguez and Monica Goldberg-Murow
Facultad de Ciencias de la Salud, Universidad Anáhuac México Norte, 52786 Huixquilucan, MEX, Mexico

Verónica Bautista-Piña
Departamento de Patología, Instituto de Enfermedades de la Mama (IEM), La Fundación del Cáncer de Mama (FUCAM), 40980 Mexico City, Mexico

Mingxia Shi, Hongzhi Xu and Xin Gu
Department of Pathology and Translational Pathobiology, Louisiana State University Health Science Center-Shreveport, 1501 Kings Highway, Shreveport, LA 71130, USA

Guillermo P. Sangster
Department of Radiology, Louisiana State University Health Science Center-Shreveport, 1501 Kings Highway, Shreveport, LA 71130, USA

Konstantinos N. Stamatiou
Department of Urology, Tzaneio General Hospital, 18536 Piraeus, Greece

Hippocrates Moschouris, Kiriaki Marmaridou, Michail Kiltenis and Konstantinos Kladis-Kalentzis
Department of Diagnostic and Interventional Radiology, Tzaneio General Hospital, 18536 Piraeus, Greece

Katerina Malagari
2nd Department of Radiology, University of Athens, Attikon Hospital, Chaidari, 12462 Athens, Greece

Brenen P. Swofford
University of Arizona College of Medicine-Phoenix, Phoenix, AZ, USA

Jade Homsi
University of Texas Southwestern, Dallas, TX, USA

Rebecca M. Plato, William F. Morano, Nicholas DeLeo and Wilbur B. Bowne
Department of Surgery, Drexel University College of Medicine, Philadelphia, PA, USA

Luiz Marconcini and Michael Styler
Department of Medicine, Division of Hematology/Oncology, Drexel University College of Medicine, Philadelphia, PA, USA

Beth L. Mapow
Department of Pathology and Laboratory Medicine, Drexel University College of Medicine, Philadelphia, PA, USA

S. Brégigeon, O. Zaegel-Faucher, V. Obry-Roguet, A. Ivanova and C.E. Cano
Aix Marseille Université, APHM Hôpital Sainte-Marguerite, Service d'Immuno-Hématologie Clinique, 270 boulevard de Sainte Marguerite, 13274 Marseille Cedex 09, France

I. Poizot-Martin
Aix Marseille Université, APHM Hôpital Sainte-Marguerite, Service d'Immuno-Hématologie Clinique, 70 boulevard de Sainte Marguerite, 13274 Marseille Cedex 09, France
INSERM U912 (SESSTIM), 13006 Marseille, France

C. Tamalet
Fondation InstitutHospitalo-Universitaire Méditerranée Infection, Pôle desMaladies Infectieuses et Tropicales Clinique et Biologique, Fédération de Bactériologie-Hygiène-Virologie, CHU Timone, 264 rue Saint-Pierre, 13385 Marseille Cedex 05, France

R. Bouabdallah
D´epartement d'Hématologie, Institut Paoli Calmettes, 232 boulevard de Sainte Marguerite, 13273 Marseille Cedex 09, France

C. Solas
Aix Marseille Université, AP-HM Hôpital de la Timone, Service de Pharmacocinétique et Toxicologie, CRO2 INSERM U911, 13385 Marseille Cedex 05, France

Romina Deldar, Derek Thomas and Anna Maria Storniolo
Division of Hematology and Oncology, Indiana University School of Medicine, Indianapolis, IN 46202, USA

Santiago Fabián Moscoso Martínez and Vadim Zarubin
Department of Hematology and Oncology, The Brooklyn Hospital Center, 121 Dekalb Ave, New York, NY 11201, USA

Geethapriya Rajasekaran Rathnakumar
Department of Internal Medicine, The Brooklyn Hospital Center, 121 Dekalb Ave, New York, NY 11201, USA

Alireza Zarineh
Department of Pathology, The Brooklyn Hospital Center, 121 Dekalb Ave, New York, NY 11201, USA

Minh Phan, Shubham Pant and Mohamad Khawandanah
Hematology-Oncology Section, Department of Medicine, The University of Oklahoma Health Sciences Center, Oklahoma City, OK 73104, USA

Shari Jones
Department of Internal Medicine, The University of Oklahoma Health Sciences Center, Oklahoma City, OK 73104, USA

Justin Jenkins
Department of Pathology, The University of Oklahoma Health Sciences Center, Oklahoma City, OK 73104, USA

Maria Dinche Johansen
Department of Radiation Biology, The Finsen Center, Rigshospitalet, Blegdamsvej 9, 2100 Copenhagen, Denmark

Per Rochat
Department of Neurosurgery, The Neurocenter, Rigshospitalet, Blegdamsvej 9, 2100 Copenhagen, Denmark

Ian Law
Department of Clinical Physiology, Nuclear Medicine and PET, Center of Diagnostic Investigation, Rigshospitalet, Blegdamsvej 9, 2100 Copenhagen, Denmark

David Scheie
Department of Pathology, Center of Diagnostic Investigation, Rigshospitalet, Blegdamsvej 9, 2100 Copenhagen, Denmark

Hans Skovgaard Poulsen
Department of Radiation Biology, The Finsen Center, Rigshospitalet, Blegdamsvej 9, 2100 Copenhagen, Denmark
Department of Oncology, The Finsen Center, Rigshospitalet, Blegdamsvej 9, 2100 Copenhagen, Denmark

Aida Muhic
Department of Oncology, The Finsen Center, Rigshospitalet, Blegdamsvej 9, 2100 Copenhagen, Denmark

Kerem Okutur, Mustafa Bozkurt and Gokhan Demir
Department of Medical Oncology, Acibadem University School of Medicine, Buyukdere Caddesi, No. 40, Sariyer, 34453 Istanbul, Turkey

Taner Korkmaz
Department of Medical Oncology, Acibadem Maslak Hospital, Buyukdere Caddesi, No. 40, Sariyer, 34453 Istanbul, Turkey

Ercan Karaaslan
Department of Radiology, Acibadem University School of Medicine, Buyukdere Caddesi, No. 40, Sariyer, 34453 Istanbul, Turkey

Levent Guner
Department of Nuclear Medicine, Acibadem University School of Medicine, Buyukdere Caddesi, No. 40, Sariyer, 34453 Istanbul, Turkey

Suha Goksel
Department of Pathology, Acibadem Maslak Hospital, Buyukdere Caddesi, No. 40, Sariyer, 34453 Istanbul, Turkey

Mohamed Mokhtar Desouki and Daniel Jerad Long
Department of Pathology Microbiology and Immunology, Vanderbilt University School of Medicine, Nashville, TN 37232, USA

Rajesh Balakrishnan
Department of Radiotherapy and Oncology, Square Hospitals Limited, Dhaka 1205, Bangladesh

Rokeya Porag, Dewan Shamsul Asif, A. M. Rejaus Satter and Samson S. K. Gaddam
Department of Neurosurgery, Square Hospitals Limited, Dhaka 1205, Bangladesh

Md. Taufiq
Department of Pathology, Square Hospitals Limited, Dhaka 1205, Bangladesh

Tiffany J. Pan and Kurt R. Weiss
Department of Orthopaedic Surgery, University of Pittsburgh Medical Center, 3471 Fifth Avenue, Pittsburgh, PA 15213, USA

Liron Pantanowitz
Division of Anatomic Pathology, University of Pittsburgh Medical Center, 5230 Centre Avenue, Pittsburgh, PA 15232, USA

Dimitrios K.Manatakis, Spiridon G. Delis and Christos Dervenis
Surgical Department, "Konstantopouleio" General Hospital, Nea Ionia, 14233 Athens, Greece

Nikolaos Ptohis
Interventional Radiology Department, "G. Gennimatas" General Hospital, 11527 Athens, Greece

Penelope Korkolopoulou
Department of Pathology, Medical School, National and Kapodistrian University of Athens, 11527 Athens, Greece

Index

www.ingramcontent.com/pod-product-compliance
Lightning Source LLC
Chambersburg PA
CBHW061329190326
41458CB00011B/3946